ALLE · ZEIT · WACH
SJ
1842

Urolithiasis: Etiology · Diagnosis

Edited by

Hans-Joachim Schneider

Contributions by

M. Peacock
W. G. Robertson
H.-J. Schneider
W. Vahlensieck

With 168 Figures

Springer-Verlag
Berlin Heidelberg New York Tokyo

Handbook of Urology · Volume 17/I

Continuation of Handbuch der Urologie · Encyclopedia of Urology

ISBN-13:978-3-642-70581-6 e-ISBN-13:978-3-642-70579-3
DOI: 10.1007/978-3-642-70579-3

Library of Congress Cataloging in Publication Data. Main entry under title: Urolithiasis: etiology, diagnosis. (Handbook of urology; vol. 17/I. Includes bibliographies and index. 1. Calculi, Urinary. I. Peacock, M. II. Schneider, Hans-Joachim, 1931– III. Series. RC916.U76 1985 616.6'22 85-14751. ISBN-13:978-3-642-70581-6 (U.S.)

Softcover reprint of the hardcover 1st edition 1985

2122/3130-543210

List of Contributors

SCHNEIDER, H.-J., Professor Dr.
Ludwigsplatz 11, D-6300 Giessen

PEACOCK, M., Dr.
MRC Mineral Metabolism Unit, The General Infirmary,
Great George Street, Leeds LS1 3EX, Great Britain

ROBERTSON, W. G., Professor Dr.
MRC Mineral Metabolism Unit, The General Infirmary,
Great George Street, Leeds LS1 3EX, Great Britain

VAHLENSIECK, W., Professor Dr.
Direktor der Urologischen Universitätsklinik Bonn,
Sigmund-Freud-Str. 25, D-5300 Bonn 1

Preface

The handbook on lithiasis edited by Kurt Boshamer and originally brought out in 1961 was for more than two decades the standard work in this field for researchers and clinicians alike. However, our knowledge of urolithiasis has been increased so enormously – by worldwide interdisciplinary research into the genesis of urinary calculi, by the new treatment possibilities opened up principally by advances in technology, and by the success achieved in prevention of recurrence – that it is almost impossible to take in all the relevant journal articles, books chapters, monographs, and proceedings.

It was therefore our aim in this, the first of two independent volumes, to provide a concise but comprehensive summary of current knowledge concerning the morphology and composition of calculi, epidemiology, pathogenesis, and diagnostic techniques. The most recent developments are described, and nothing in the world literature is ignored. A second volume will cover medical therapy, operative, instrumental and noninvasive treatment, and prophylaxis.

To have any chance of success, treatment and prophylaxis must be based on knowledge of calculus formation. Study of the composition of calculi has yielded important information regarding the conditions for formation, and this underlines once again the great value of analysis of urinary concretions. Evaluation of epidemiological data has important consequences for the individual patient.

The authors of the central chapter on pathogenesis are probably the leading experts in this field, whose many research programs have made vital contributions to solving the problems encountered. The chapter on diagnosis of urolithiasis as a precondition for therapy comes from an experienced clinician whose symposia on urinary calculi have been invaluable in promoting cooperation between researchers and practicing urologists. My most heartfelt gratitude goes to these authors for the work they have put into this book.

If the book spurs young colleagues to research into urinary calculi and is used as a work of reference, and if the dissemination of our knowledge concerning urolithiasis leads to reductions in the recurrence rate and in the numbers of new cases, we will have achieved our goal.

I would like to take this opportunity to thank the many colleagues who offered constructive criticism and ideas, and to extend my gratitude to Mr. W. Bergstedt of Springer-Verlag for his creative and patient efforts in the preparation of the book.

Giessen Hans-Joachim Schneider

Contents

Epidemiology of Urolithiasis. H.-J. SCHNEIDER.
With 17 Figures

Pathogenesis of Urolithiasis. W. G. ROBERTSON and M. PEACOCK. With 48 Figures

Diagnosis of Urinary Calculi. W. VAHLENSIECK.
With 1 Figure

Morphology of Urinary Tract Concretions

H.-J. SCHNEIDER

With Contributions by W. BERG

I. Definitions

Calculous disease of the urinary tract is probably as old as mankind itself. Attempts at cure and prevention of this painful affliction may be traced back to the very beginning of the healing art. In the meantime there has been no alteration in the composition of calculi but a very considerable shift in their relative distribution within the urinary tract: bladder and other calculi related to infection are nowadays overshadowed by calcium oxalate calculi of the kidney and ureter. Despite our understanding of the tendency for such calculi to occur in showers and in the face of all the recent successes in prophylaxis and treatment, most countries have seen a trend toward an increasing incidence of urinary calculi. The consequences represent a medical, social and an economic problem. The worldwide extent of the usually interdisciplinary research effort directed at urinary calculi is reflected both in the extensive literature, reviewed for the period to 1960 in the Handbook of Urology, Volume X (BOSHAMER et al. 1961) and in the number of symposia on the topic in recent years. Such international meetings have been held in Leeds (HODGKINSON and NORDIN 1969), Madrid (CIFUENTES DELATTE et al. 1973c), Davos (FLEISCH et al. 1976), Williamsburg (SMITH et al. 1981), Garmisch-Partenkirchen (SCHWILLE et al. 1984) and indeed since 1970 symposia have been held on a regular basis in Jena and in Bonn or Vienna.

Yet the urinary calculus is only the final product and chief symptom of a many-facetted disease picture of multifactorial etiology. From the mineralogist's point of view it is merely a solid aggregate of complex composition, precipitated from a supersaturated solution.

The following definition of a urinary calculus has been arrived at by adding to that given by SCHULTHEIS (BOSHAMER 1961):

"Uroliths are solid structures which arise from disturbances of the physicochemical balance and/or of the hydrodynamic system of the urine and the urinary tract from the collecting system down to the urethra. These structures have a minimal size of 1000 microns, and consist mainly of crystalline and (to a lesser degree) of amorphous organic and/or inorganic components, which may be mixed with a non-crystalline high molecular substance (matrix)." (SCHNEIDER 1982).

The term "secondary calculus" is frequently used (usually in relation to calculi arising in infected urine or around foreign bodies), yet is etiologically more confusing than enlightening. The term should therefore be discarded, since any calculus is secondary in resulting from a number of causal factors.

The mean recurrence rate lies in the region of 50%, and it is these recurrent calculi which are the measure of our successes in the treatment and prevention of urolithiasis.

Nevertheless a generally valid definition of calculus recurrence presents some difficulties, since there are no uniformly accepted terms of reference. One might consider the same organ, the same side, the same type of calculus or a limited period of time. Some authors completely reject such a concept and prefer to distinguish between active and sporadic calculus formers (FINLAYSON and REID 1978).

With due respect to all these restrictions the following comprehensive definition has been suggested as a basis on which to compare the results of therapy:

"Any occurrence of a second or any further urolith is referred to as recurrent stone disease, irrespective of its composition, localisation, or the time interval after the first stone episode. This term does not include continuous crystalluria without clinically manifest concrements" (SCHNEIDER 1982).

If recurrence rates are to be discussed in terms of some other definition (same type of calculus, same location, limited time span), this should be expressly stated.

II. External Appearance of Urinary Calculi in Relation to Site of Recurrence and Type of Stone

For the purpose of clinical communication, it is important to refer to stones not only by their chemical or mineralogical name but also in terms of their current or permanent location (Table 1). Depending where they first occurred or subsequently enlarged, calculi may be of highly variable shape (SCHNEIDER 1973a, 1983). As early as 1663 ROLFINK (Jena) had classified uroliths by size, shape, color and surface. He postulated that these characteristics depended on the site of occurrence and the type of stone.

According to HODGKINSON et al. (1969) 50% of all calculi weigh less than 0.1 g and 76% less than 0.5 g. MAURER (1969) presented similar results with 50% of all calculi lighter than 25 mg.

A variety of metabolic diseases, intoxications and intestinal bypass procedures may lead to the occurrence of intracellular, intrabular or interstitial crystals, *crystal aggregates* or *microliths*. Where these consist of oxalates of calcium they are particularly clearly visualised by polarized light (Figs. 1, 2) (BOTHOR and BERG 1980; DAS et al. 1979; ERNEST et al. 1980; HIENZSCH et al. 1979; LILIEN et al. 1981; SCHNEIDER et al. 1976, 1977b). In advanced cases the clinical presentation is that of nephrocalcinosis.

ARNOLD and SEEMANN (1968) found among 60 stone-containing kidneys 40 cases of oxalate crystals throughout the renal parenchyma. One frequently comes across *papillary calcification*, of typical swallowtail configuration when removed (Figs. 3, 32) (CIFUENTES DELATTE et al. 1984). If such calculi are un-

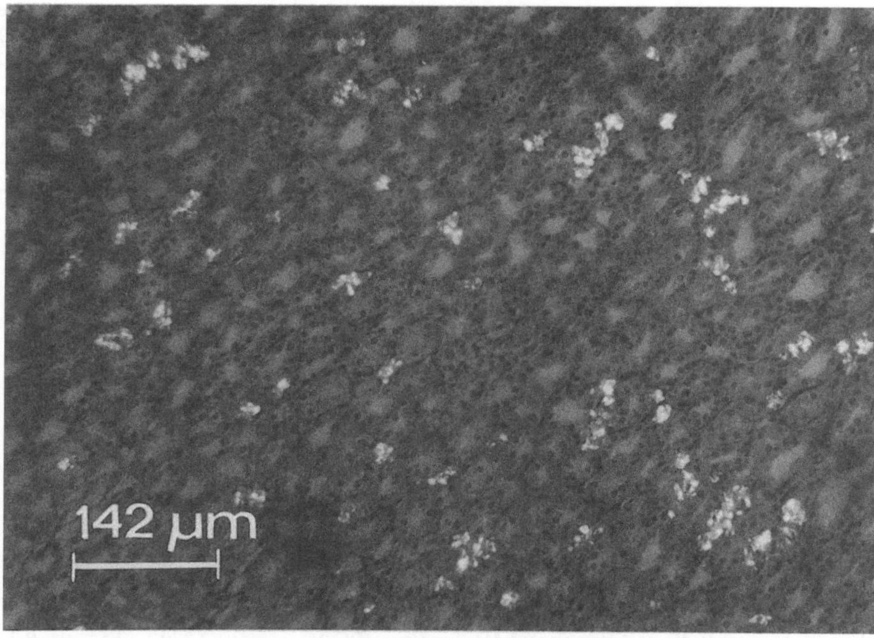

Fig. 1. Microlithic whewellite within the kidney of a glyoxylate poisoned rabbit (crossed polarizing filters)

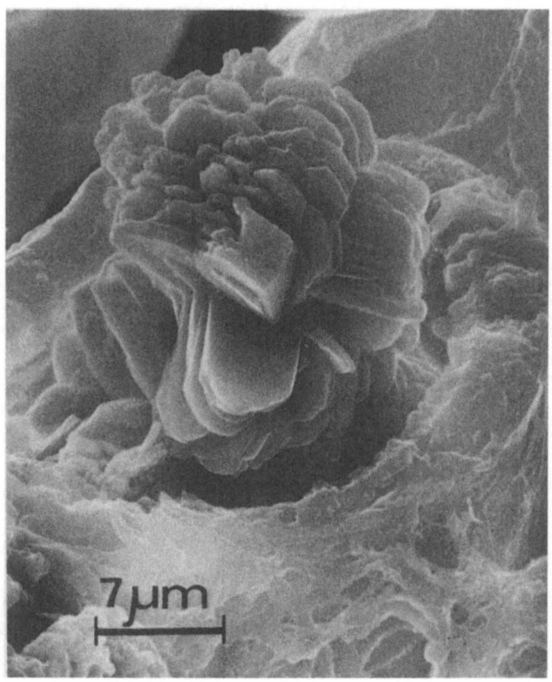

Fig. 2. Whewellite microlith in fan configuration within a tubule (SEM)

Table 1. Types of urolith and their frequency in terms of principle components and the sex ratio of patients in which they occur (X-ray diffraction and infra-red spectroscopy, n = 95,780)

Mineral	Chemical Name		Absolute frequency	%		Sex ratio
	Uric acid	$C_5H_4N_4O_3$	10,916	11.4	14	2.6
	Uric acid dihydrate	$C_5H_4N_4O_3 \cdot 2\,H_2O$	2,534	2.6		1.7
	Ammonium dihydrogenurate	$C_5H_7N_5O_3$	369	0.4		1.6
	Sodium hydrogenurate monohydrate	$NaC_5H_3N_4O_3 \cdot H_2O$	24	0.02		1.4
	Cystine	$C_6H_{12}N_2O_4S_2$	180	0.2		1.0
	Xanthine	$C_5H_4N_4O_2$	2	–		–
	Protein		476	0.5		0.8
Whewellite	Calcium oxalate monohydrate	$CaC_2O_4 \cdot H_2O$	56,056	58.6	72.4	2.1
Weddellite	Calcium oxalate dihydrate	$CaC_2O_4 \cdot 2\,H_2O$	13,255	13.8		2.4
Whitlockite	Tricalcium phosphate	$Ca_3(PO_4)_2$	65	0.07		0.6
Hydroxyapatite	Pentacalcium hydroxyphosphate	$Ca_5(PO_4)_3OH$	1,494	1.6		0.7
Carbonate apatite (Dahllite)	Basic calcium phosphate with carbonate	$Ca_{4.75}(PO_4)_{2.65}(OH)_{0.85}(CO_3)_{0.35}$	3,320	3.5		0.7
	Octacalcium phosphate	$Ca_8H_2(PO_4)_6 \cdot 5\,H_2O$	2	–		–
Newberyite	Magnesium hydrogen-phosphate trihydrate	$MgHPO_4 \cdot 3\,H_2O$	4	–		–
Struvite	Magnesium ammonium phosphate hexahydrate	$MgNH_4PO_4 \cdot 6\,H_2O$	4,875	5.1		1.2
	Magnesium ammonium phosphate monohydrate	$MgNH_4PO_4 \cdot H_2O$	14	0.01		2.5
Brushite	Calcium hydrogen-phosphate dihydrate	$CaHPO_4 \cdot 2\,H_2O$	242	0.2		1.9
Calcite, Vaterite, Aragonite	Calcium carbonate	$CaCO_3$	94	0.1		0.7
Opal, Trydimite	Silicon dioxide	SiO_2	1,836	1.9		0.6
Gypsum, etc.	Calcium sulfate dihydrate	$CaSO_4 \cdot 2\,H_2O$				
Bobierite [a]	Trimagnesiumphosphate octahydrate	$Mg_3(PO_4)_2 \cdot 8\,H_2O$				
Hopeite [a]	Zinc phosphate hexahydrate	$Zn_3(PO_4)_2 \cdot 4\,H_2O$				
Monetite [a]	Calcium hydrogen phosphate	$CaHPO_4$	(BECK et al. 1974)			
	Trimagnesium ortho-phosphate pentahydrate	$Mg_3(PO_4) \cdot 5\,H_2O$	(CARMONA et al. 1980)			
	Trimagnesium phosphate 22-hydrate [a]	$Mg_3(PO_4)_2 \cdot 22\,H_2O$	(ARMBRUSTER 1978)			
Hannayite [a]	Trimagnesium ammonium phoshate octahydrate	$Mg_3(NH_4)_2H_4(PO_4)_4 \cdot 8\,H_2O$	(GIBSON 1974)			

Table 1. (continued)

Mineral	Chemical Name		Absolute frequency	%	Sex ratio
Monohydroxycalcite [a]	Calcium carbonate monohydrate	$CaCO_3 \cdot H_2O$	(DOSCH 1981)		
Humboldtine [a]	Iron oxalate dihydrate	$FeC_2O_4 \cdot 2\,H_2O$	(GEBHARDT 1974)		
Collophane [a]		$(Ca_3(PO_4)_2)_3$ $CO_3(OH)_2F_2 \cdot NH_2O$	(KOSLOWSKI et al. 1977)		
	2,8-dihydroxyadenine [a]	$C_5H_5N_2O_2$	(ASPER et al. 1982, JOOST et al. 1981)		
	Potassium dihydrogenurate [a]	$KC_5H_3N_4O_3$	(CIFCUENTES DELATTE et al. 1981, DOSCH 1981 a)		
	Calcium hydrogenurate [a]	$CaC_5H_2N_4O_3$	(DOSCH 1981 a)		
	Zinc, Lithium, Magnesium, Strontium (unknown stoichiometric composition)		(DOSCH 1981 a, DOSCH u. MOTZKE 1984)		

[a] These urolith components are mentioned in the literature but did not occur in our analytical material

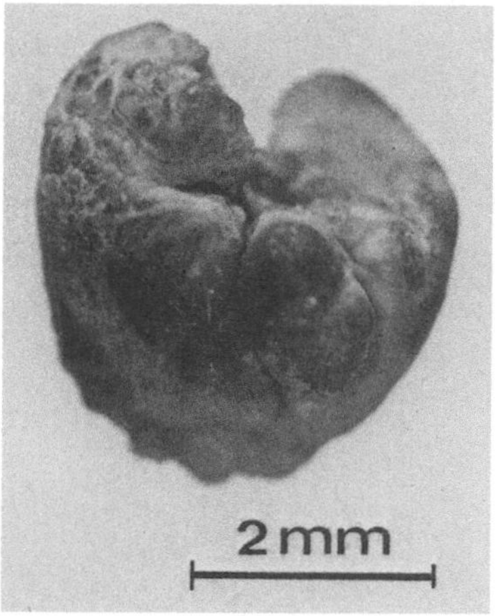

Fig. 3. Whewellite papillary cast

able to pass spontaneously they continue to enlarge within the individual calyx or the renal pelvis. Renal pelvic stones occur in sizes and shapes ranging from a pea-sized round oval or pyramidal concrement right up to casts of monstrous proportions and they may be single or multiple (Figs. 4, 5). Further growth by directional apposition frequently leads to bizarre shapes.

Ureteric calculi are usually small stones which have succeeded in passing the pelviureteric junction, the first physiological narrowing. They frequently dis-

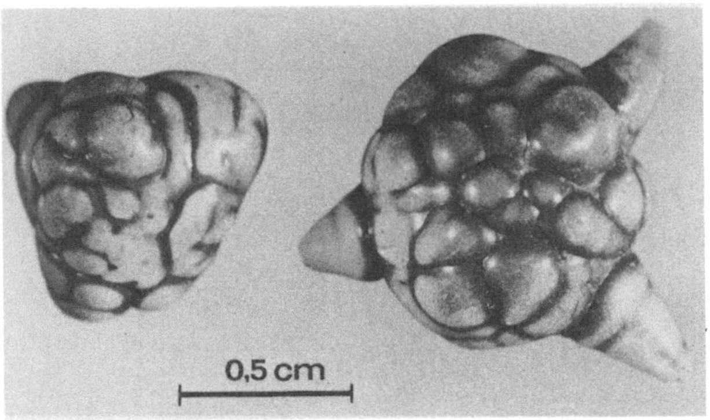

Fig. 4. Whewellite mulberry stone with staghorn processes, formed in the renal pelvis

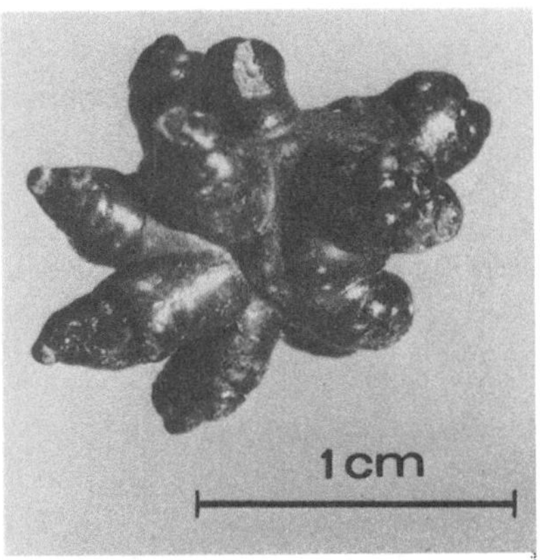

Fig. 5. Stellate renal pelvic calculus of black whewellite

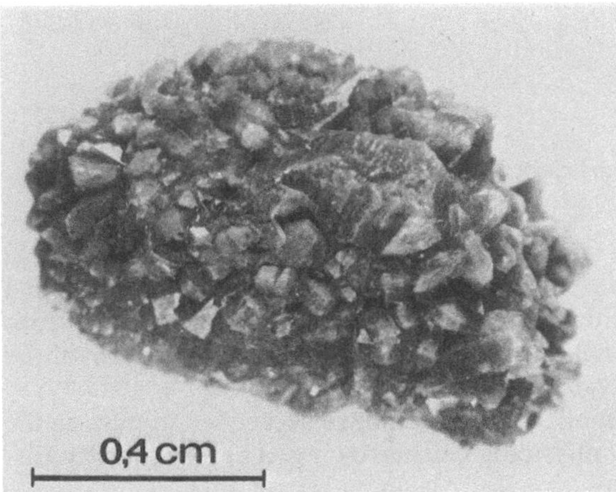

Fig. 6. Rough-surfaced weddellite ureteric calculus

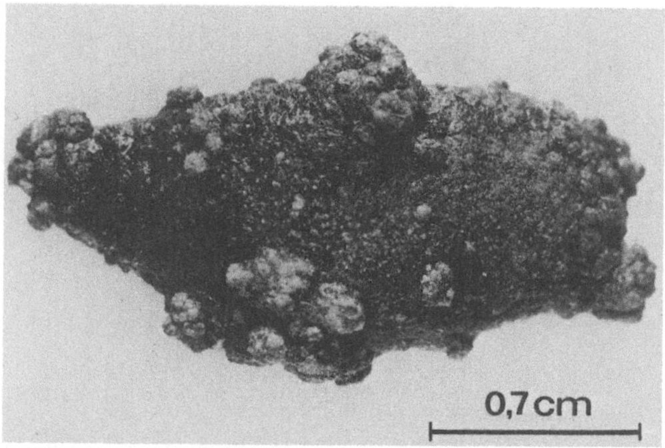

Fig. 7. Whewellite calculus with rough warty excrescences, formed within a ureterocele

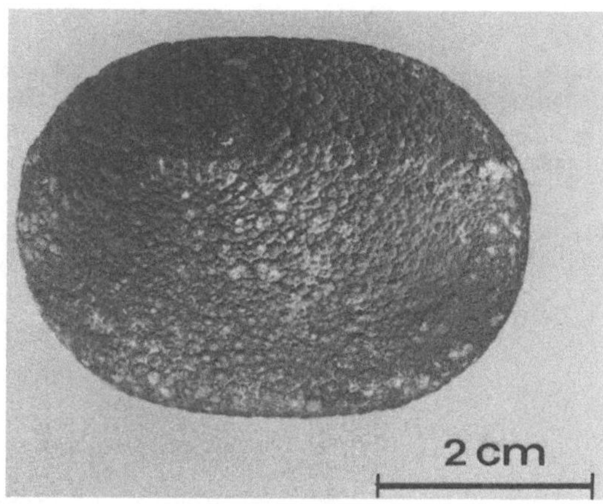

Fig. 8. Large solitary bladder stone of uric acid

integrate within the ureter and pass in numerous small fragments, occasioning the patient severe pain out of all proportion to their size. If they come to rest at a stenosis or stricture these stones may increase in size and reach considerable proportions (Figs. 6, 7).

Bladder calculi show great variability in shape and size. They may be single or multiple and range from poppy seed to fist size, occasionally filling the entire bladder and possessing interlocking facets (Figs. 8–10). Typical hourglass calculi occur after injury or surgery to the bladder neck and are waisted according to the configuration of the sphincter region (Fig. 11).

Urethral stones are usually arrested ureteric calculi which have subsequently enlarged at the site of an obstruction or diverticulum.

Foreign body calculi are found mainly in the urethra and bladder, encasing a wide variety of objects such as catheter tips, needles, wires, etc. as well as suture material and hair (Figs. 12, 13).

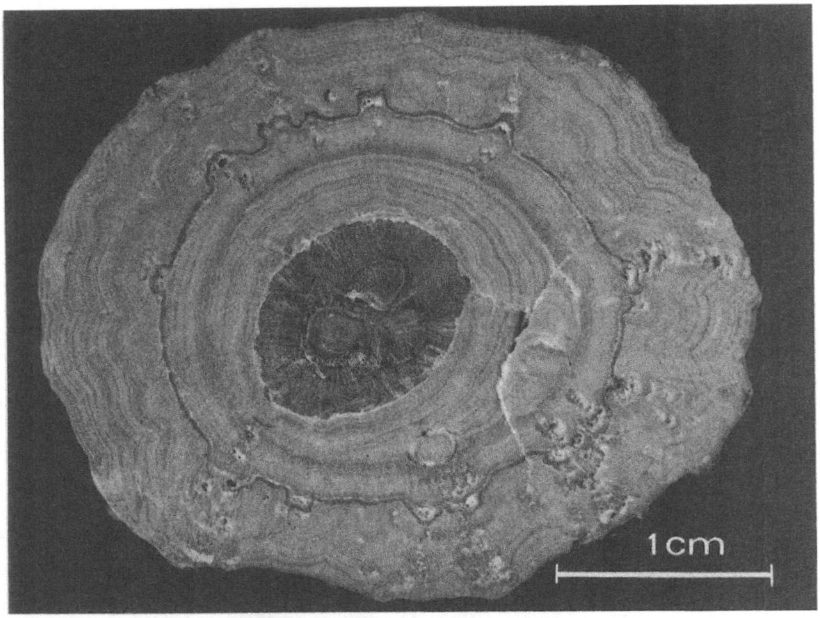

Fig. 9. Polished cross-section of a layered bladder stone of uric acid with a calcium oxalate nucleus

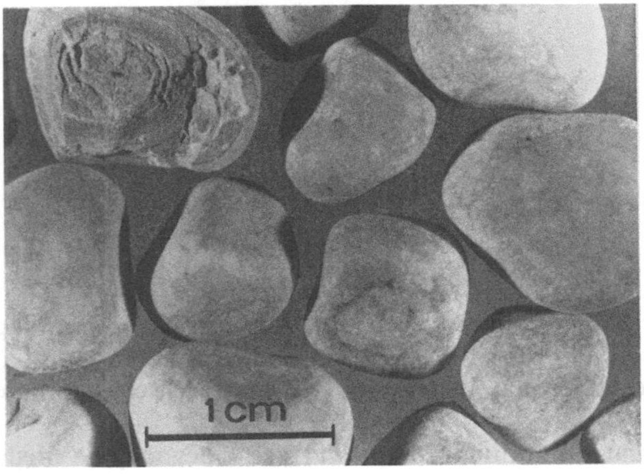

Fig. 10. Multiple struvite and carbonate apatite bladder calculi with articulating facets

Prostatic calculi are not really related to uroliths. They arise as encrustations of prostatic secretion and are frequently composed purely of apatite of hydroxyapatite and a protein fraction (GACA and DOSCH 1981; JOOST et al. 1978; SPECTOR et al. 1981). Only when pathological change allows the entry of urine into the prostatic acini does urate deposition occur. The mineral involved is then chiefly struvite although whewellite, weddellite, ammonium dihydrogenürate, cystine, uric acid and uric acid dihydrate have all been documented

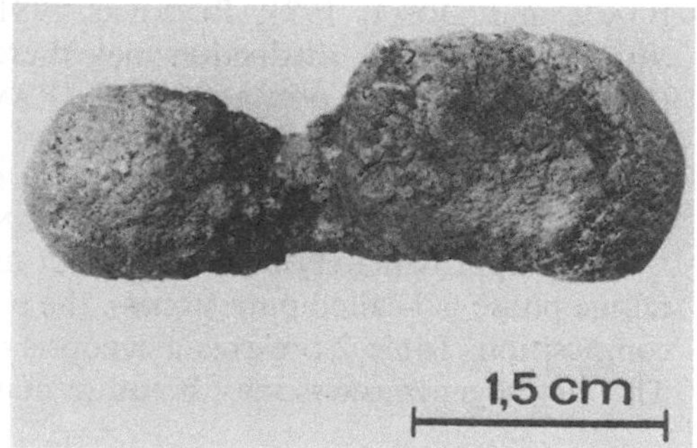

Fig. 11. Struvite urethral stone (hour-glass calculus)

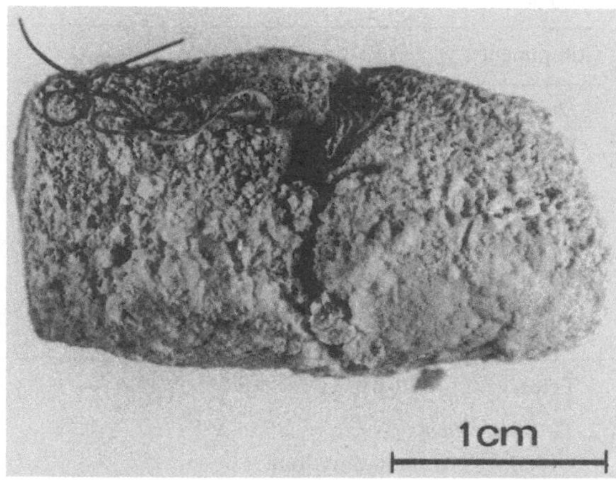

Fig. 12. Struvite foreign-body calculus formed around non-absorbable suture material in an ileal conduit

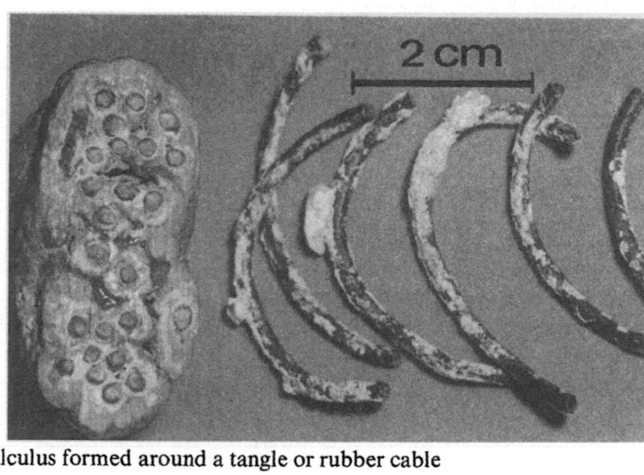

Fig. 13. Struvite bladder calculus formed around a tangle or rubber cable

(GACA and DOSCH 1981; RODGERS 1981a; SANTOS et al. 1976; SUTOR and WOOLEY 1974b). A distinction may therefore be made between endogenous (true) and exogenous prostatic calculi (RAMIREZ et al. 1980a).

A greater effect on the appearance of calculi than that of the organ or organs of formation and their interaction is exerted by the chemical composition and structure of the calculus itself (HINMAN 1979).

Only approximately one-third of all uroliths is composed of a single crystalline phase (so-called pure stones), the majority being of heterogeneous phase composition. Table 2 presents a synopsis of the more important combinations. This heterogeneousness may be quite marked, particularly where one type of

Table 2. The commonest combinations of various components found among 105,303 uroliths analysed

Component	Number	%
1. *One component* (monophasic calculi)		
Uric acid	5,865	5.56
Uric acid dihydrate	827	0.78
Cystine	194	0.18
Whewellite	28,284	26.85
Weddellite	2,926	2.77
Carbonate apatite	956	0.90
Struvite	1,720	1.63
Silica	800	0.75
Total	44,694	42.44
2. *Two components*		
Uric acid/Uric acid dihydrate	5,247	4.98
Uric acid/Ammonium dihydrogenurate	375	0.35
Uric acid/Whewellite	2,662	2.52
Ammonium dihydrogenurate/Struvite	293	0.27
Whewellite/Weddellite	22,250	21.12
Whewellite/Carbonate apatite	2,681	2.54
Whewellite/Apatite	5,351	5.08
Weddellite/Apatite	1,132	1.07
Weddellite/Carbonate apatite	979	0.92
Struvite/Carbonate apatite	3,310	3.14
Total	47,192	44.81
3. *Three components*		
Uric acid/Uric acid dihydrate/Ammonium dihydrogenurate	87	0.08
Uric acid/Whewellite/Weddellite	1,132	1.07
Whewellite/Weddellite/Apatite	6,132	5.82
Whewellite/Weddellite/Carbonate apatite	3,719	3.53
Total	13,253	12.58
4. *Four components*		
Total	164	0.15

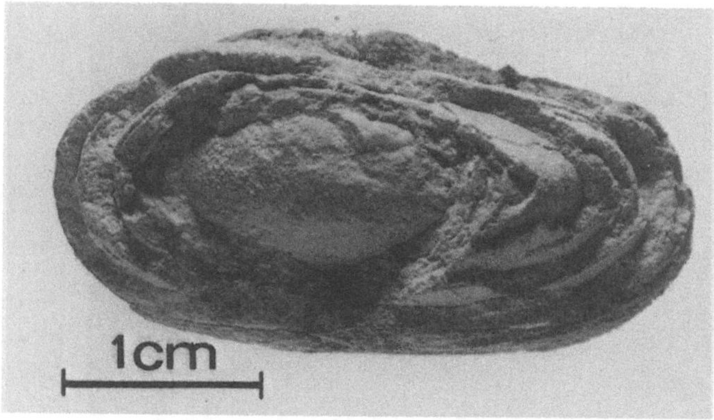

Fig. 14. Fracture plane of a layered calculus with a carbonate apatite nucleus and struvite shell

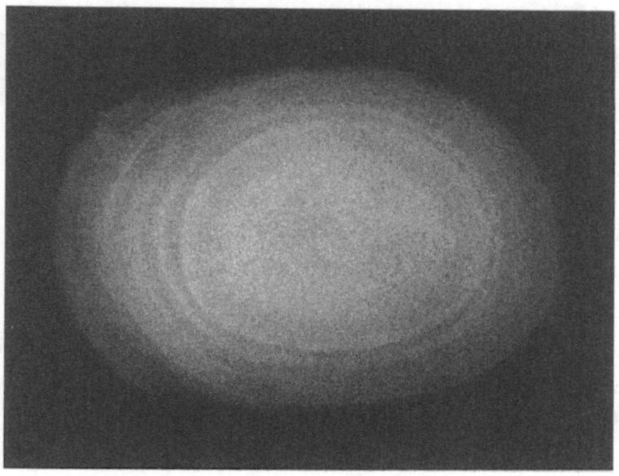

Fig. 15. Radiograph of a layered struvite calculus (same calculus as Fig. 19)

crystal is capable of transmutation into another, e.g. weddellite to whewellite (see Section V, 4a). In other calculi the individual layers may be discerned by the naked eye (Fig. 14). Thus a calculus originating in the kidney, but arrested in the bladder by an outflow obstruction, may possess a mantle of uric acid and subsequently become encased in a layer of struvite in the wake of a urinary infection that lead to alkalinization of the urine. In order to reach valid conclusions as to the mode of formation of these uroliths and thus to take effective therapeutic and preventive measures, it is therefore of some importance to analyse visibly different layers separately (see Section VI).

At the same time, discoloration, variations in packing density and changes in aggregation behaviour may suggest a difference in composition where the basic crystal is unchanged (Figs. 15, 16).

In any consideration of the primary site of calculus formation, particular importance attaches to the central portion, the so-called nucleus of the stone. One may safely assume that the phase composition and the type of aggregation

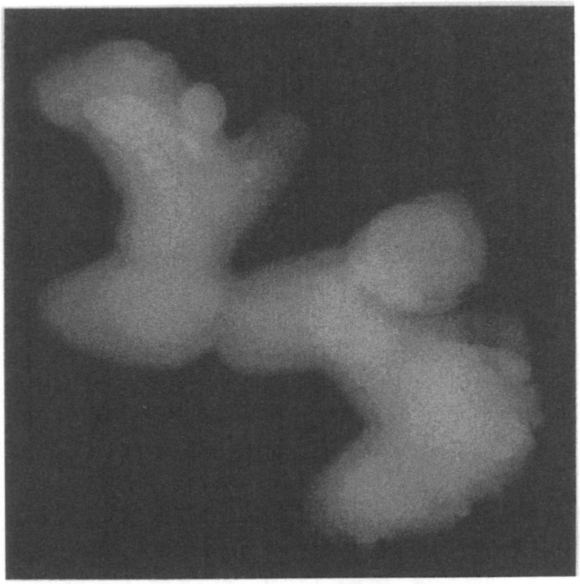

Fig. 16. X-ray contrast variations within a monomineral cystine calculus

found within the nucleus most accurately represent the physico-chemical conditions under which stone formation was initiated (KOLPAKOW and GLIKI 1965a, b; SCHNEIDER and SEYFARTH 1980).

By the nucleus is meant a defined, usually centrally placed section of the calculus. The term is thus a morphologic-topographic one and thin section studies in particular have revealed that a number of calculi possess multiple growth centers (Figs. 38, 39) (see Section V/2). Wherever there is recognizable layering, nucleus and shell(s) should therefore be analysed separately. The best method for differentiating nucleus and shell is thin section microscopy (BICK and BRIEN 1976; BRIEN et al. 1982; CIFUENTES DELATTE et al. 1973b; KOLPAKOW 1971; SCHUBERT et al. 1983). No definite relationship can be established between the phase composition of nucleus and shell (BASTIAN and GEBHARDT 1974). Any combination of nucleus and shell is possible (GEBHARDT and BASTIAN 1976a, b), and an obvious nucleus is frequently of the same phase as the remainder of the stone ("pseudonucleus"). Approximately half of all nuclei are composed of a single mineral and 46% consist of whewellite (BICK et al. 1977; BRIEN 1982; BRIEN et al. 1978; HODGKINSON and MARSHALL 1975). Polyphasic nuclei consist of mixtures of oxalate and phosphate in the majority of cases, whilst the combination of uric acid and phosphate has never been documented (RAMIREZ et al. 1980b, c).

On analysing the nucleus of 101 bladder and urethral stones HAZARIKA et al. (1974) found whewellite tobe the most common and ammonium dihydrogen urate to be the rarest substance. In the study of UNNI MOOPPAN et al. (1979) hydroxyapatite was the dominant component of the nucleus, yet 198 calcium oxalate calculi contained not a single uric acid nucleus. Not infrequently the center of a stone is composed of non-crystalline or organic substances, a fact which may be related to the conditions of formation or to dissolution processes (SCHNEIDER and SEYFARTH 1979) (see Section V). On the other hand MEYER et al. (1976) found uric acid nuclei to occur more frequently in whewellite stones and consider this to be an influence of uric acid crystals on the epitaxial growth of calcium oxalate crystals. Our own polarizing microscopic studies confirm these findings (SCHNEIDER et al. 1977a).

Brushite is a common nuclear component of phosphate calculi (HODGKINSON and MARSHALL 1975), and phosphate micronuclei are occasionally apparent as minute spheres (GIESEK et al. 1982; SCHMANDT and BLASCHKE 1978). More rarely bone mineral or typical renal structures with calcified tubuli have been observed within the stone nucleus (CIFUENTES DELATTE et al. 1976; MEDINA and CIFUENTES DELATTE 1983). Differing distributions of major and trace elements were found by SCOTT et al. (1980) within the nucleus and shell of phosphate and oxalate stones. Magnesium was commoner in the nucleus than in the shell of either type and the reverse was true of calcium. There was a notably higher iron and yttrium content in oxalate than in phosphate stones.

BRIEN (1978, 1981) has studied nucleus and shell of 10,000 calculi extensively (Table 3). Whilst uric acid was fairly equally distributed between nucleus and shell, weddellite and uric acid dihydrate were noticeably commoner in peripheral zones (BERENYI et al. 1972; ELLIOT 1968; REVEILLAUD et al. 1976; SCHNEIDER et al. 1977a; SZABO et al. 1976a). Whilst the thermogravimetric analysis of calcium oxalate stones by ROSE and WOODFINE (1976) was alone in showing more weddellite in the center than in the periphery, LEUSMANN and TOELLE (1984) have demonstrated that the bulk of uric acid dihydrate is found in the mantle. This distribution may reflect transformation of the dihydrate phase into whewellite or uric acid (BÖRNER et al. 1981; HESSE et al. 1976a, 1975, 1972b). The approximately equal distribution of struvite is all the more noticeable since it might have been suspected to prefer the outer zones.

Table 3. Frequency of urolith phases among 10,000 calculi, tabulated according to complete stone, nucleus and shell (BRIEN 1981)

Urolith phase	Whole calculus	Nucleus	Shell
Whewellite	8,265	7,933	7,645
Weddellite	5,910	2,830	4,882
Apatite	2,781	2,433	2,752
Uric acid	1,227	1,028	1,161
Struvite	901	773	843
Uric acid dihydrate	660	521	645
Ammonium dihydrogenurate	75	75	71
Brushite	49	46	45
Cystine	27	27	27
Whitlockite	21	18	20
Sodium dihydrogenurate monohydrate	8	8	7
Octacalcium phosphate	8	8	8

To the extent of their independence of the environment or of adjacent stones, shape, surface, color and cross-section of individual types of calculus are characteristic and allow an approximate classification although this cannot replace exact analysis (Schneider 1968 b, c). Color is only partly conditioned by the innate composition of uroliths. Urinary pigments, hemoglobin, colored metabolites in the urine and drug-derived pigments exert a considerable influence.

There are numerous reports of truly *pigmented stones*, e.g. after the administration of anthraquinones (Berg et al. 1979c; HESSE et al. 1974a; Lonsdale 1969; Tscharnke et al. 1972), of metylene blue, after certain urinary antiseptics, after ingestion of a variety of analgesics (phenazopyridine hydrochloride) (Mulvaney et al. 1972) and in cases of alkaptonuria (Krizek 1971, 1984; Pirlich and Schwarzer 1966; Sutor et al. 1970).

Uric acid calculi are pale yellow to dark reddish-brown, of round or oval shape and possess a smooth surface, only occasionally covered in warty excrescences. Their size varies from that of a grain of sand to fist-sized casts of the urinary bladder or renal pelvis. Occasionally a quantity of spherical calculi the size of a lentil or cherry stone are clustered together. Cleavage planes and polished surfaces reveal a number of regularly concentric layers, radially banded and of varying color (Figs. 8, 9, 17).

Uric acid dihydrate stones are macroscopically indistinguishable from uric acid concretions. However they seldom exceed the size of a lentil, or maximally that of a bean, and generally present as sand or semolina grains (Berenyi 1975).

Urate stones (ammonium dihydrogenurate and sodium hydrogenurate monohydrate) contributed less than 1% in our series. Cifuentes Delatte et al. (1978a) were able by infra-red spectroscopy and thin section techniques to detect monosodium urate in 50 of 3000 calculi (1.66%). There was usually a combination with whewellite, only 6 calculi being pure. We have never documented calcium urate. In a few cases (probable) potassium dihydrogenurate (Cifuentes Delatte et al. 1981; Dosch 1981 a, b) and calcium hydrogenurate (Dosch 1981 a) have been reported. Their significance as components of uric acid concrements has been suggested by Dosch (1981 a, b) to lie in a structural chemical relationship to the cationic stabilization of otherwise thermodynamically unstable uric acid dihydrate.

Urates occur relatively frequently in endemic areas and either as nuclear substance or in thin layers between other calculus components (Armbruster 1979; Cifuentes Delatte et al. 1973b; Sutor 1972). They are generally softer than uric acid stones, of more coarsely granular structure and of yellowish-grey coloration.

Cystine stones have a pale to honey-yellow color and are waxy with occasionally somewhat greasy or shiny surface, granular only in zones of growth. They may occur in any size up to pelvicalyceal casts and are usually monomineral in composition (Hambraeus and Lagergren 1962; Krizek et al. 1973).

Xanthine stones are rare. They were first described by Marcet in 1818, and to date there are approximately 40 reports in the literature (Castro-Mendoza et al. 1972; Cifuentes Delatte and Castro-Mendoza 1967; Rapado 1973; Seegmiller 1968; Terhorst 1969). Occasionally they occur as a complication

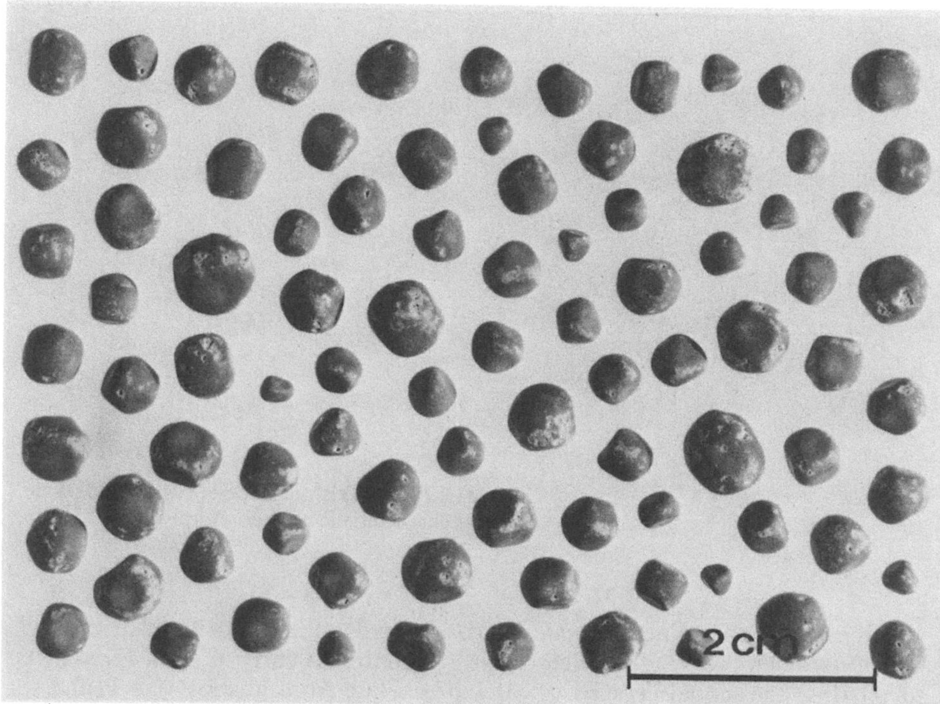

Fig. 17. A quantity of uric acid bladder calculi ranging from lentil to cherry stone size. Growth interactions between individual calculi give rise to the characteristic facets

of allopurinol therapy (GREENE et al. 1968). The concretions are round or oval, yellow to brown, and soft with a laminated interior. A calculus which occurred in our own practice was reddish-brown, smooth, brittle and crumbly in structure (SCHNEIDER et al. 1973b).

Proteinaceous and matrix stones, first described by MARCET in 1818 as fibrin stones, are dirty-white or clay-yellow and of highly variable shape. They range from millet seed-sized firm concrements right up to soft masses filling the entire renal pelvis. They contain urates in varying quantity and these determine the consistency (ASSLAMASOW 1974; BECKER and GASTEYER 1968; HAWOTTE 1972; HORN and HESSE 1972; KOIDE et al. 1977; WILLIAMS 1963).

Calcium oxalate represents an important type of calculus, and in its two chief phases of whewellite and weddellite may give rise to a wide variety of forms.

Whewellite forms hard, grey to blackish-brown concrements, usually with a smooth surface. A mulberry configuration is typical for this type of stone (Fig. 18). Generally the calculi are small, but they may nevertheless achieve considerable size as renal pelvic casts. The somewhat paler planes of cleavage reveal prominent layering and banding. Growth fronts correspond to the often bizarre excrescences and are usually of a paler color.

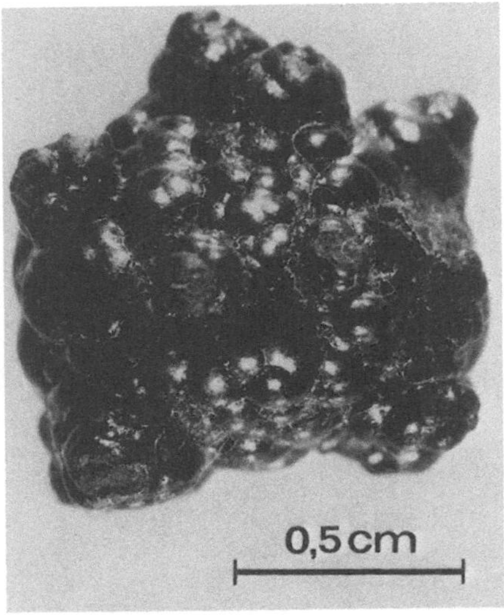

Fig. 18. Blackish renal pelvic whewellite stone of characteristic mulberry form

The name of the mineral *weddellite* corresponds to its first site of discovery by BANNISTER in the Weddell Sea of the Antarctic. As early as 1884 HARTING had purified tetragonal crystals of calcium oxalate from guano (VON PHILIPSBORN 1950). Such renal calculi are usually small, pale yellow to pale brown with an extremely irregular surface. Typically ureteric calculi present as aggregations of coarse, sharp-edged, individual crystals (Fig. 6). Weddellite frequently occurs in a strictly localized fashion on the surface of smooth darker whewellite stones.

Phosphate calculi occur in at least 10 different phases, of which only hydroxyapatite, carbonate-apatite and struvite occur in significant quantities.

Struvite stones may be found throughout the urinary tract, occur in any size and are the typical representatives of foreign body stones (SUTOR 1975). They are usually dirty grey, although in their pure form they may be almost white (Fig. 19). The surface is rough and jagged, the consistency rather soft, and cleavage planes reveal a loose conchoidal arrangement (Fig. 14). Aging and warming may lead to the formation of magnesium-ammonium phosphate monohydrate (HESSE et al. 1973c). The relationship between infected urine and calculus formation was recognized by HIPPOCRATES, and the mineral was given its name in 1845 in honor of the Russian scientist H. C. G. VON STRUVE (GRIFFITH 1978).

TOGGENBURG and BANDHAUER (1980) found urinary tract infection among 84% of patients presenting with struvite calculi and 93% of struvit stones themselves contained bacteria.

Carbonate apatite occurs naturally as dahllite and is usually combined in uroliths with struvite. It is of similar appearance (Fig. 20).

Brushite generally occurs as a contaminant of phosphate and oxalate calculi. We know of one case in which it occurred as a very pure cast. The color was

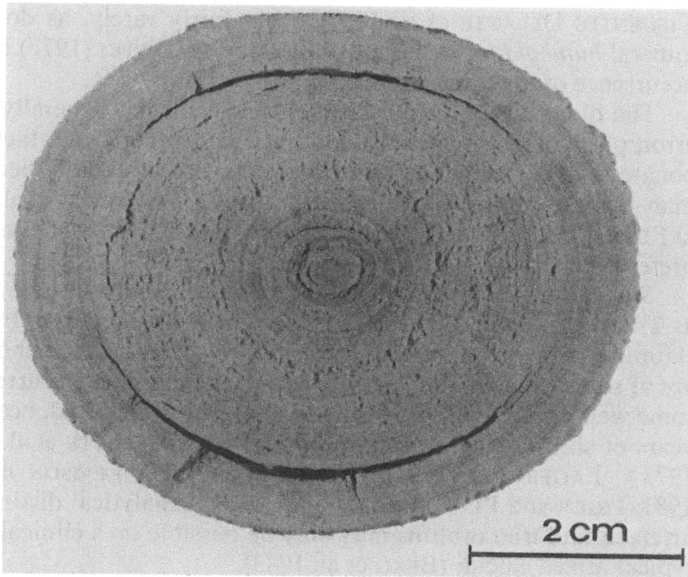

Fig. 19. Polished section across a pure white struvite stone of layered structure

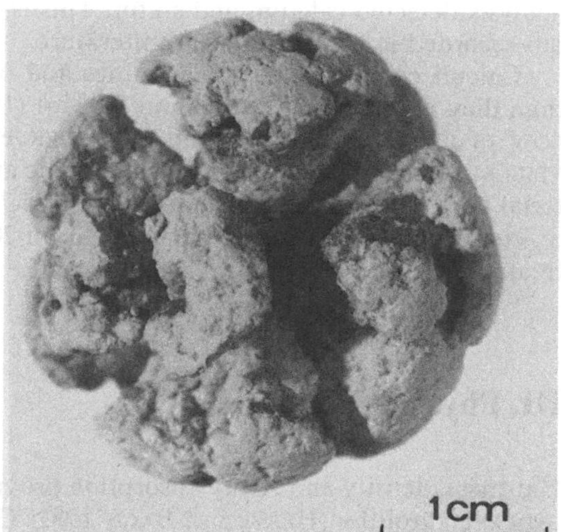

Fig. 20. Bladder calculus resembling pumice and mainly composed of carbonate apatite

greyish-brown and the surface rough. Fracture planes reveal a radiate structure (CIFUENTES DELATTE 1978; JONES and SMITH 1962). The remainder of phosphate calculi strongly resemble each other in external appearance (BECK et al. 1974; MURPHY and PYRAH 1962; NORDIN et al. 1965). The phosphates of magnesium, *newberyite* (MIÑON CIFUENTES and SANTOS 1981; LONSDALE and SUTOR 1966; SUTOR 1968), *hannayite* (GIBSON 1974), *bobierite* (CARMONA et al. 1980;

CIFUENTES DELATTE et al. 1977) occur fairly rarely, as does the iron oxalate mineral *humboldtine* (GEBHARDT 1974). KOSLOWSKI (1977) has documented the occurrence of the mineral *collophane* in uroliths.

The diagnosis of *calcium carbonate* calculi has generally been an analytical error, particularly in chemical analysis. The mineral is in fact nearly always carbonate apatite. *Aragonite* and *vaterite* have occasionally been described in human bladder stones (BECK and BENDER 1969; KOIDE et al. 1982; SUTOR and O'FLYNN 1973), and DOSCH (1981) describes a case of a monohydroxycalcite ureteric stone.

Silicates make up the main bulk of so-called artefacts (in our series as much as 2% of all calculi!). These are calculi which the patient brings his physician, claiming them for a variety of reasons to be uroliths, although they probably are of some other origin. Silicate calculi are a typical occurrence in animals and some well-documented human cases have been reported, occasionally related to years of silicate-rich medication (CIFUENTES DELATTE et al. 1978c; JOKES et al. 1973h; LAGERGREN 1962; MEDINA et al. 1978; LEVISON et al. 1982; MEDINA 1981; PRIEN and PRIEN 1968; PYRAH 1979). Analytical distinction between such artefacts and true uroliths may only be possible on a clinical basis or in cases of typical mixed calculi (BERG et al. 1983).

By infrared spectroscopy and by electron microscopy CIFUENTES et al. (1983) have been able to demonstrate calcium sulfate dihydrate crystals in a series of apatite stones from the same female patient. Electron microprobe analysis detected calcium and sulfur. This is only the sixth case of sulfate crystals recorded in the world urolith literature.

Calculi composed of sulfonamides and other drugs are considerably rarer than they used to be. SCHOLZ and WALCH (1970) described sulfonamide, BÜHLOW et al. (1977) bactrim and ETTINGER et al. (1979, 1980) as well as REVEILLAUD and DAVIDOU (1984) triamterene and its metabolites as a urolith material (181 among 50,000 calculi = 0.4% and 7 among 2200 = 0.3% respectively). SUTTON et al. (1984) report renal calculi in 28 of a series of about 350 patients treated for glaucoma with acetazolamide.

III. Physical Properties

Hardness, density and X-ray absorption provide important data for the identification of uroliths (HESSE and BACH 1982; GEBHARDT et al. 1977; GÖTZ 1973; RODGERS et al. 1981).

1. Hardness

Hardness is measured either on the Mohs hardness scale (talcum = 1, diamond = 10) or in Knoop values (BURNS et al. 1984). Because of the sometimes highly inhomogeneous composition of uroliths and since the individual components often differ only slightly in hardness, the smallest possible grains should be studied.

For this reason WACHTER and MATOUSCHECK (1977) studied the microscopic hardness of ground surfaces by measuring the impression made at 400× magnification under polarized light. Their results are in good agreement with ours of 1973 (SCHNEIDER et al. 1973b) (Table 4). The former authors arrive at the following conclusion:

1. There is no uniformity of hardness among uroliths.
2. For equal chemical composition there remain zones of varying hardness, corresponding to different crystal structures.
3. Different types of crystal have different hardness values.

The hardness of calculi may be of therapeutic significance. Thus urate stones have been noted to be more resistant to electrohydraulic litholapaxy than are by comparison oxalate or phosphate calculi (BRUNDIG and SCHNEIDER 1980).

2. Density

The density of uroliths is most easily determined by the hydrostatic balance method. This involves weighing them in air (a) and in water (b) so as to determine their buoyancy. Density may be calculated according to the following formula:

$$D = \frac{a}{a - b} \; (g/cm^3) .$$

Because of the frequency with which mixed calculi occur, the pyknometric method of ASPER and SCHMUCKI (1980) seems inadequate for determining the density of uroliths.

3. X-Ray Absorption

A plain X-ray film is often used to display some types of calculi in vivo, or at least for a differentiation between calcium-containing "radio-opaque" and organic "non-opaque" calculi. For the following reasons however such a distinction is not truly possible:

1. varying thickness of the calculus in the plane of exposure
2. varying composition of mixed calculi
3. varying porosity of the stone.

There is thus a high margin of error (GEBHARDT et al. 1977). A whewellite crystal will need to be twice as thick and a uric acid crystal even 15 times as thick as an apatite crystal to achieve the same density of shadow (GEBHARDT 1980a). A mixed calcium oxalate–uric acid stone cannot be distinguished radiographically from a pure struvite calculus. The same is true of other mixed stones. The various X-ray absorption values (Table 4) depend not on the

Table 4. Hardness, density and X-ray absorption of various calculi

Type of calculus	Hardness		Density (g/cm^3)	Mass absorption coefficient (after DALICHO 1967)	X-ray absorption (after SCHLECHT)	Absorption capacity (greater than water) (BOSHAMER 1961)
	Moh's scale	Knoop values				
Uric acid	2.5	47.8	1.89	0.019	0.97	1.38
Cystine	2.0	25.7	2.06	0.07	1.18	3.7
Whewellite	2.5–3.0	99.6	2.23	0.15	1.36	10.8
Weddellite	4.0		1.99		1.36	
Apatite	5.0	21.3	3.16–3.22	0.16	1.33	22
Brushite	2.0	90.9	2.32	–	–	–
Struvite	2.0	39.6	1.71	0.09	1.20	4.1

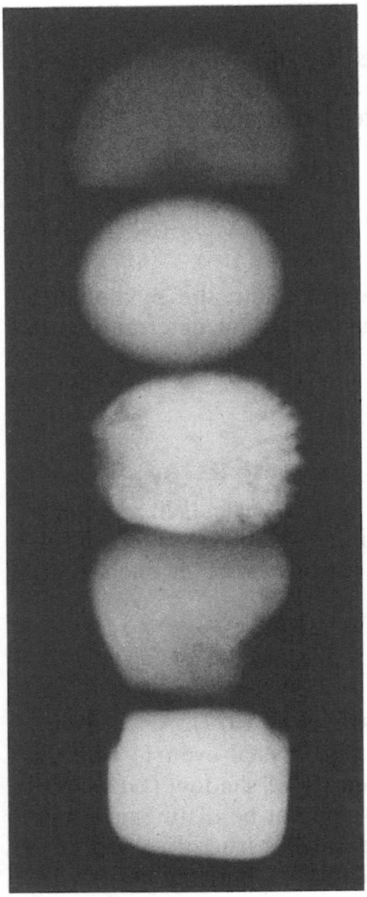

Fig. 21. Radiographic contrast density of varying types of calculus. From above downwards: uric acid, cystine, calcium oxalate, struvite, carbonate apatite

molecular weight of various calculous phases but on density and crystal structure (BOSHAMER 1961) (Figs. 15, 16). Layered strucutre may be visible on radiographs (Fig. 21). Radio-opacity decreases for the series brushite, whitlockite, apatite, struvite, cystine, uric acid (DALICHO 1967). Cystine is only 0.45× as radio-opaque as calcium oxalate, yet 40× as radiodense as uric acid (ROTH and FINLAYSON 1973). Of all inorganic calculi brushite is the most and struvite the least easily demonstrable on X-ray.

IV. Chemical Composition of Uroliths

Following a suggestion by HELLER (1860) uroliths may be classified according to the predominant anion into oxalate, phosphate, uric acid, urate, xanthine, cystine and carbonate calculi. BOSHAMER (1961) suggested a distinction between inorganic stones, of which calcium is the predominant feature, and organic crystalline forms, for which the dominant anion is of principal importance. ELLIOT (1968) thinks the term calcium stone inadvisable and prefers to distinguish between oxalate and phosphate stones.

To date 25 crystalline components of uroliths have been described (DOSCH 1980), and a wide variety of major and trace elements are involved in the composition of calculi (SCHNEIDER 1973b).

Urine is the environment within which stones occur, and thus all components of urine may be expected to occur in uroliths.

1. Compounds

Components of calculi occur chiefly as compounds corresponding to various crystalline phases into which individual elements may be incorporated. The chief groups of compound are uric acid and its salts, cystine, xanthine, the various calcium, magnesium and zinc phosphates, calcium oxalate and the rarer iron oxalate, calcium carbonate, silica, calcium sulfate and also (in animals) citrates. CIFUENTES DELATTE et al. (1978a) detected citrate ions on the surface of human apatite stones. These may substitute either for PO_4^{---} on the surface of the apatite crystal or they may be chemically bound to hydroxyapatite.

In contrast to herbivorous mammals such as horses, cattle, sheep and goats, in which calcium carbonate as calcite or aragonite is the principle type of calculus, calcium carbonate occurs in man chiefly as carbonate apatite. It is not yet entirely clear whether carbonate is incorporated as an integral part of the crystal lattice, mixed in as amorphous $CaCO_3$ or adsorbed onto the surface. Pure calcium carbonate calculi are certainly a great rarity in man. (KOIDE et al. 1982)

Besides inorganic or organic crystalline and amorphous components, most calculi also contain amorphous organic substances, making up 2–3% of the dry weight (matrix). Cystine stones contain as much as 9–11% (BOYCE 1969). Struvite stones may contain even greater proportions and the rare, so-called protein calculi consist almost purely of such substances (KOIDE et al. 1977). This matrix probably has the function of a ground substance (ISMAIL and TAWASHI 1980), binding individual crystals and preventing pH-dependent dissolution (OGBUJI et al. 1984; RESNICK 1984).

According to CARMONA et al. (1973) there is a process of chemical adsorption on the ionic surface involving interactions of apatite hydroxyl groups and carboxylate anions of organic substances.

Variations in the composition and morphology of matrix (7 different morphologic types have been identified, RAO et al. 1978) for individual types of stone suggest that this adsorption is not haphazard but an active process involved in calculus formation (BABA et al. 1983). Analysis of matrix by element leads to values similar to those for protein calculi and largely independent of mineral structure (Table 5). Two-thirds of matrix consists of protein, one-third of carbohydrates (PEREZ CASTRO 1967; SZABO and MODIS 1980).

Electrophoretic studies of the matrix of phosphate and oxalate stones reveal the fractions in Table 6.

Variations in the composition of matrix were also found by KRAMPITZ and GOETZ (1984); SHAKER et al. (1983); SZEDERKENYI and JOZSA (1968); WHITESIDE et al. (1983). Oxalate stones contained on average more protein, glucose, fucose and hexosamine than phosphate calculi, the same quantity of galactose and less hexuronic acid. Calcite and calcite aragonite calculi from horses and cows revealed no species-related variations in the quantities of protein, hexosamine, hexoses and uronic acids (GRÜNBERG 1971). Similar differences occurred in the amino acid patterns of various types of calculus (Table 7).

Glutamic and aspartic acids were predominant in calcium oxalate and struvite calculi whilst the high glutamic acid content of whewellite stones is particularly remarkable (FLACH et al. 1978). The total amino acid content of whewellite calculi was 5.79 μmol/100 mg and of struvite stones 2.89 μmol/100 mg, the corresponding glutamic acid content being 0.85 and 0.43 μmol/100 mg respectively. FLACH et al. (1978) were unable to demonstrate hydroxyproline and hydroxylysine in uroliths and conclude from this that the mucoprotein of urinary calculi is collagen-free.

Following the demonstration in 1971 of Gm(a)-substance in gallstones KERDE et al. (1980) have reported its occurrence in renal calculi. The serum

Table 5. Elementary composition of matrix (HORN and HESSE 1972)

Element	Proportion (in %)
Carbon	48 – 57
Hydrogen	4 – 7.5
Nitrogen	10
Oxygen	24 – 33
Sulfur	0.53 – 0.98

Table 6. The composition of matrix (KIMURA et al. 1976)

Substance	Proportion (in %)
Protein	57.5
Hexose	17.5
Hexosamine	6.6
Uronic acid	4.5
Fucose	3.0
Pentose	1.0
Sialic acid	Trace
Others	9.7

Table 7. Amino acid composition of the ECTA-soluble, nondialyzable proteins of renal calculi (LIAN et al. 1977)

Amino acids	Calcium oxalate		Hydroxy-apatite	Struvite	Apatite struvite	Uric acid	Cystine
	residues/1,000 amino acids						
Hyp	–	–	–	–	–	–	–
Asp	307	212	237	171	165	103	127
Thr	50	50	55	61	54	50	55
Ser	78	76	63	109	78	61	97
Glu	202	179	172	152	150	110	155
Pro	39	26	45	57	32	53	43
Gly	60	82	55	111	107	217	96
Ala	53	66	56	89	71	105	75
Half Cys	4	9	15	3	11	14	–
Val	26	40	49	45	42	40	46
Met	7	7	2	1	7	–	1
Ile	19	19	28	21	29	24	36
Leu	53	56	71	49	69	56	92
Tyr	20	27	20	16	33	35	23
Phe	13	33	33	28	27	25	43
Lys	20	41	50	61	47	47	42
His	22	34	26	9	31	25	27
Arg	25	37	31	16	23	31	38
Gla	25	23	25	0.9	14	0.7	0.6

Gm-factors as well as Inv (1) factor were also present in all the calculi studied, independent of type. Immunoglobulins, or at least their Gm and Inv marker bearing moieties are apparently always detectable in matrix. A quantitative difference between inflammatory and aseptic calculi is suggested but unproven.

2. Ash and Mass Elements

The ash content is an important feature distinguishing uric acid, urate and cystine stones on the one hand and oxalate and phosphate calculi on the other. Oxalate and phosphate stones contain more than 50% ash with calcium at 18.5% and phosphate at 17.6% representing the major components. All other elements are far less frequent than these two.

There is no significant correlation between ash and calcium content of calculi (SCHNEIDER 1968a). This is not surprising, since calcium oxalate (without water of crystallization), carbonate apatite, hydroxyapatite and whitlockite all contain a similar proportion of calcium at 31–39% by formula. Ash content is thus more suitable for the characterization of inorganic stones than is the calcium content.

There is a definite correlation between the ash and phosphate content of stones (Fig. 22). This confirms the dependence of ash content on phosphate.

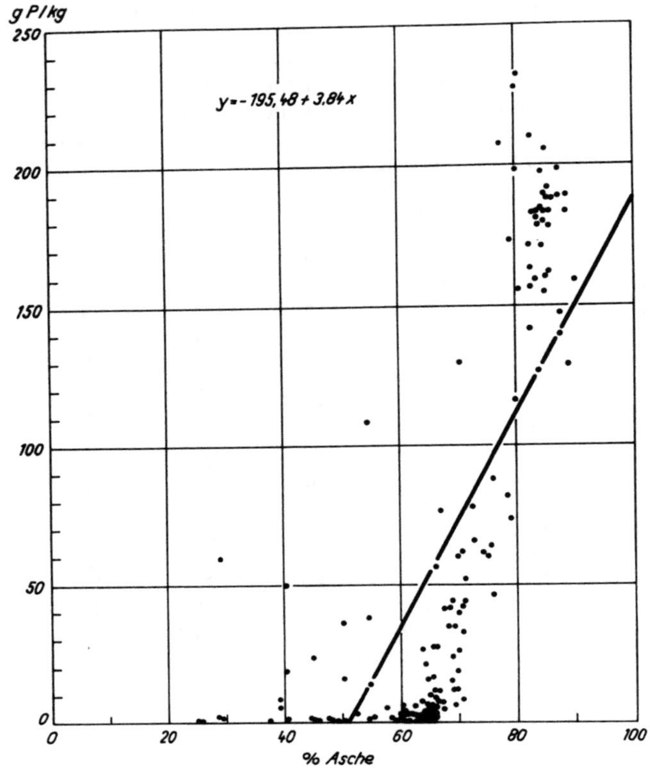

Fig. 22. Relationship between ash and phosphate content of renal calculi

For mixed calcium oxalate-phosphate stones there was a continous frequency distribution from pure oxalate to pure phosphate with a limiting value at 79% ash.

Five groups of calculus may be more closely defined by means of ash and phosphate concentration:

1. Organic crystalline stones with an ash content of 0.1 to maximally 10% and a phosphate content of less than 1 g/kg dry weight.
2. Stones with an ash content of 10–55% are mixed organic-inorganic calculi. The phosphate content distinguishes between admixture of calcium oxalate and phosphate.
3. Calcium oxalate stones contain 55–70% ash.
4. Calculi with more than 70% ash and 50 g phosphorus/kg are mixed stones of calcium oxalate and phosphate.
5. Phosphate calculi contain more than 80% ash and 130 g phosphorus/kg.

Major or principal elements are arbitrarily defined as those present at > 1 g/kg dry weight in inorganic calculi, trace elements generally being limited to mg/kg concentrations. Ash and major element contents are summarized in Table 8.

Table 8. Ash-, calcium-, magnesium-, phosphorus-, potassium- and sodium content of a variety of kidney stones (SCHNEIDER 1968a)

		Organic crystalline calculi	Mixed organic/ inorganic calculi	Oxalate stones		Phosphate calculi
				Oxalates	Pseudo-phosphates	
Ash %	$\bar{x}$	1.61	44	65	74	85
	s	2.06	9	3	3	3
Ca g/kg	$\bar{x}$	5.7	152	200	200	184
	s	13.3	49	41	62	77
Mg g/kg	$\bar{x}$	0.26	7.1	5.0	16	56
	s	0.25	14.3	11.9	19	42
P g/kg	$\bar{x}$	0.24	15.3	12.9	69	176
	s	0.21	25.3	16.6	43	25
K g/kg	$\bar{x}$	1.1	2.6	1.6	2.8	3.2
	s	1.3	2.9	2.2	4.5	1.1
Na g/kg	$\bar{x}$	1.46	4.76	5.12	9.25	9.35
	s	1.82	3.09	1.85	6.34	3.74

The lower calcium content of phosphate stones by comparison to calcium oxalate calculi is explained by the presence of struvite and other magnesium phosphates in which calcium is substituted by magnesium and ammonium. Phosphate stones thus have the highest magnesium content.

Phosphate concentration increases with ash content. There are only small variations in calcium content while sodium concentration rises in proportion to the ash content.

Certain interesting correlations emerge between the various elements involved in calculus formation.

There is an inverse relationship between phosphorus and calcium, calcium content decreasing as that of phosphorus increases (Fig. 23).

HODGKINSON et al. (1969) were able to observe that with increasing total stone weight there was an increase in phosphate content at the expense of oxalate. Hydroxyapatite, carbonate apatite and brushite contain approximately .18% phosphorus by formula. This is exactly the mean value we found for phosphate calculi. The greater the struvite content the less calcium would be expected. A roentgenologically pure struvite stone contained, e.g. only 2% calcium, yet 24% phosphorus. A corresponding proportional relationship may be expected between phosphorus and magnesium content (Fig. 24) and if one disregards rare magnesium-phosphate minerals such as newberyite and bobierite the magnesium concentration in phosphate calculi may be used to estimate their struvite content. The considerably higher magnesium content of weddellite stones compared with that of whewellite may possibly be explained by the stabilizing function of magnesium in this type of crystal (BERG et al. 1976a; HESSE et al. 1977; SCHÄFER and DOSCH 1975; SZABO et al. 1976a). On the other hand in the clinical material of LEWINSON et al. (1978) twice the quantity of magnesium was found in whewellite stones.

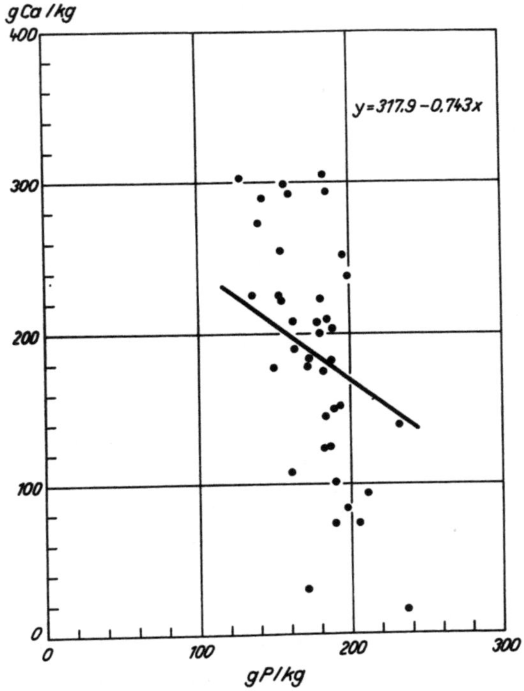

Fig. 23. Relationship between phosphate and calcium content of phosphatic calculi

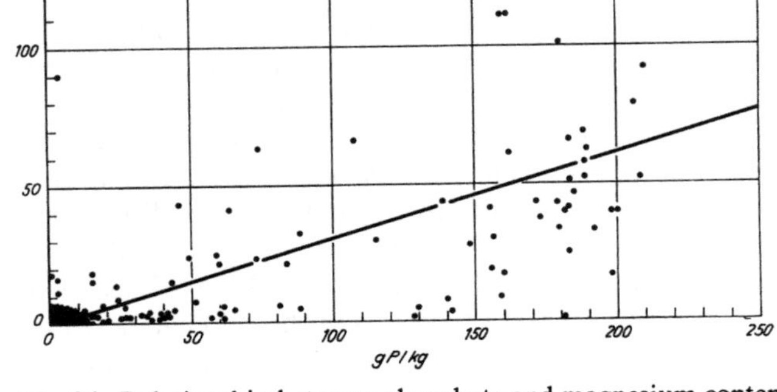

Fig. 24. Relationship between phosphate and magnesium content of uroliths

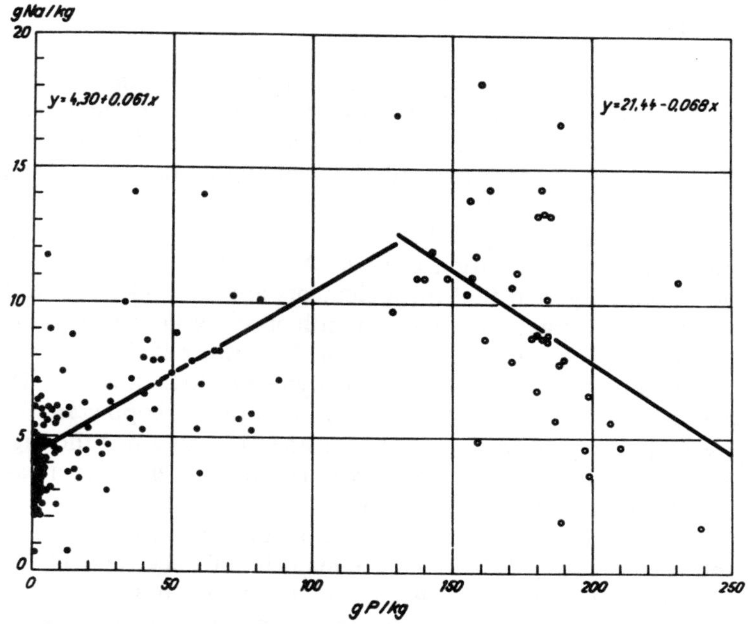

Fig. 25. Relationship between phosphate and sodium content of uroliths

Magnesium also has a decisive influence on the polymorphic modifications of calcium carbonate. In the presence of low urinary magnesium concentrations, calcite precipitates out, with an increasing proportion of aragonite, and finally pure aragonite, as the magnesium content rises (GRÜNBERG 1971). Magnesium carbonate is also said to be regularly incorporated in an isomorphic fashion into the crystal lattice of urolith calcites (GRÜNBERG and PREISINGER 1969). For horses the concentration is 12 mol% magnesium carbonate, for cattle 21 mol%.

The relationship between phosphorus and sodium content only became apparent after separate computation for phosphate and other types of calculi (Fig. 25). Sodium occurs in ionic association with apatite, and its concentration in oxalate stones thus increases with the phosphate content. In phosphate calculi its concentration decreases with the struvite content, struvite being sodium-poor.

HODGKINSON et al. (1969) also found a positive correlation between phosphorus and sodium in mixed stones. The stone nucleus is frequently of a different composition to that of the other layers and often contains more organic substances. MARTI et al. (1969) recorded 14 elements in the nuclear region, in the following order of frequency: Calcium = magnesium > lead > sodium = iron = strontium > copper > aluminium > potassium > chromium > sulfur > lead > magnesium = nickel.

3. Trace Elements

Over the last 20 years the presence of trace elements in uroliths and their influence on stone formation has been studied with increasing intensity corresponding to the advent of improved analytical methods. Nevertheless the data of individual authors varies markedly, depending on the methods employed. There are at present still many gaps in our understanding of the role of trace elements in urolithogenesis. As yet there is no evidence of a direct influence of trace elements on stone formation in man (ANKE and SCHNEIDER 1973). It has, however, been suggested that trace elements are more likely to accumulate in certain types of crystal and that they influence crystallization and stability (BERG et al. 1976a; HESSE et al. 1976a, b, 1978a; HOOFT et al. 1964; SCOTT et al. 1980). On the basis of his spectroscopic analyses FORNITSCHEW (1971) suspects an active role in urolithogenesis for silicon, aluminium, copper and lead, zinc being a passive participant. A finding of considerable note was the high concentration of rubidium in bladder calculi from children in endemic areas, far exceeding that of zinc (POPELIER et al. 1976).

Table 9 gives the mean trace element concentration in relation to ash content. NAGY et al. (1963) found the majority of trace elements in phosphate calculi, silicon, copper, lead, strontium, zinc, manganese, barium, aluminium, silver, cadmium and bismuth occurring in order of decreasing frequency. By means of plasma emission spectrography LEVINSON et al. (1978) were able to demonstrate 20 trace elements in 186 calculi. Only the lead, silicon, strontium and zinc concentrations varied from one type of calculus to another. The same is true for other bivalent cations, e.g. Mg^{++}. By means of wave lenght dispersive electron probe microanalysis, iron, copper, aluminium and silicon have been demonstrated in phosphate stones in concentrations of over 0.1% (HESSE et al. 1979b). Zinc was generally present in even greater concentration, yet never in a self-sufficient zinc phosphate phase. There were significant differences between whewellite and weddellite stones for chlorine, silicon, iron, fluorine, aluminium and bromine (HESSE et al. 1977). SCHÄFER and DOSCH (1975) found the same variation for strontium and were able to demonstrate certain relationships be-

Table 9. Mean trace element content (in ppm)[a] divided up according to ash content of the calculus (n = 512) (ANKE and SCHNEIDER 1973)

Ash %	10	10–55	55–70	70–79	79
Zn	53	210	321	525	568
Fe	65	146	127	83	59
Cu	13	23	27	28	23
Mn	4.0	13	18	13	12
Mo	2.5	1.3	1.1	0.4	0.4
Cd	0.2	3.3	5.1	4.1	4.1
Li[b]	3.3	31.5	17.7	4.9	3.0

[a] ppm = mg/kg dry weight
[b] (SCHNEIDER and HESSE 1971)

Table 10. Mean fluorine content of various types of urolith (in ppm) occurring in regions without (A) and with (B) fluorination of drinking water (HESSE et al. 1978c)

Type of calculus	A	B
Whewellite (n = 40)	801	2,005
Weddellite (n = 40)	959	2,100
Carbonate apatite (n = 20)	405	451
Struvite (n = 20)	358	406
Uric acid (n = 20)	345	529

tween trace element content and stone structure (SCHÄFER and BAUCH 1979). High iron and strontium content generally coexists with stabilized weddellite whilst lower proportions of iron and strontium are found in relation to radiate whewellite crystals.

As a rule the same elements were found in uroliths as were present in drinking water (HAZARIKA and RAO 1974).

SCHULZ et al. (1980a) subjected uric acid and calcium oxalate stones to laser microspectroscopy, measuring 15 individual points on each calculus. At each point calcium, phosphorus, magnesium, sodium, silicon, iron and aluminium could be demonstrated in oxalate calculi, with silver, copper, manganese, nickel, lead and titanium occurring in certain statistically distributed regions.

In uric acid calculi phosphorus, silver, copper and iron could be found at each point. The microprobe also revealed iron, copper, aluminium and silicon in a minimum concentration greater than 0.1% in phosphate calculi (HESSE et al. 1980). Zinc was generally present in greater concentrations but never in an independent zinc phosphate phase.

In view of drinking water fluorination for the prophylaxis of dental caries, fluorine content of uroliths has also been studied (AUERMANN and KÜHN 1969). The fluorine concentration varies from one type of stone to another (HERING et al. 1984). The highest fluorine values, at 2 mg fluorine per g stone were found in calcium oxalate stones from areas with fluorinated drinking water (Table 10).

The data did not, however, allow of any conclusion in relation to the overall frequency of urolithiasis in these regions.

There was, on the other hand, a relationship between the degree of crystallization within the calculi and their fluorine content. The highest crystallinity correlated with a high fluorine content and suggested contraction of coherent lattice regions, i.e. there were decreased angle values in the elementary cell. This may relate to the formation of well-crystallized fluoro-apatite. A similar

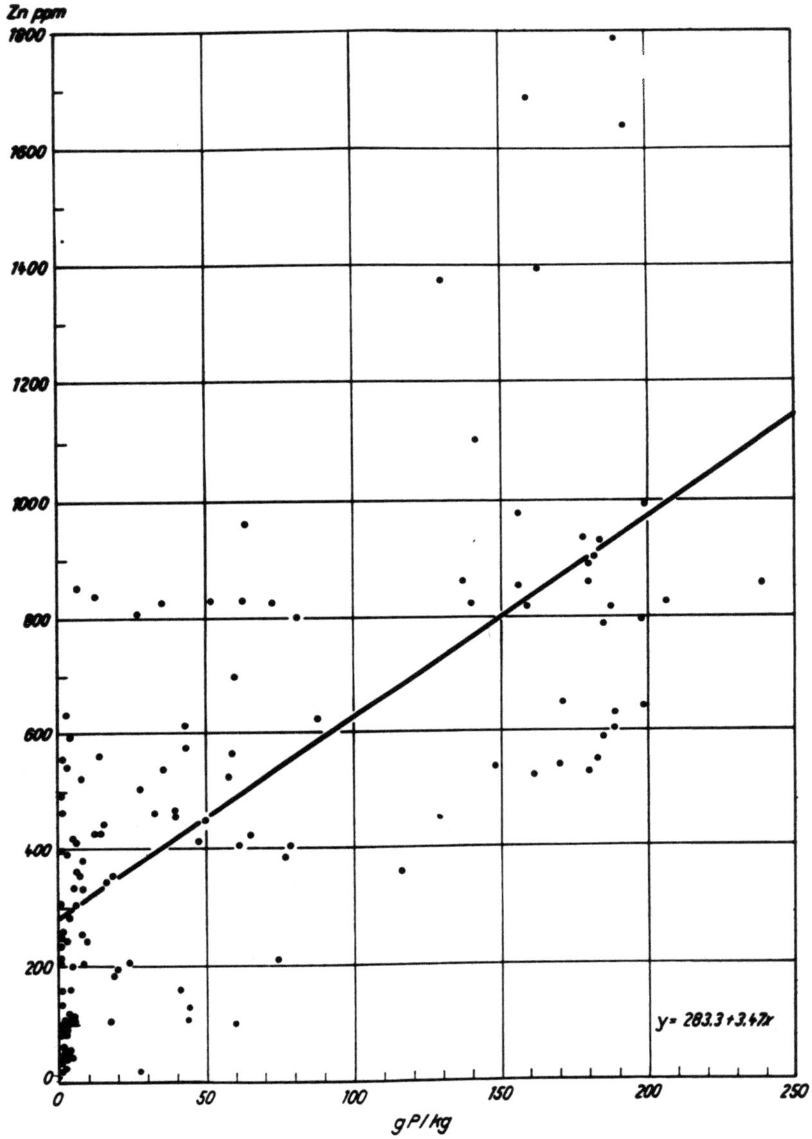

Fig. 26. Relationship between phosphate and zinc content of renal calculi

influence to that of fluoride ions may be exerted by strontium and zinc ions on the crystallization of carbonate apatite (FEATHERSTONE et al. 1981).

An analogous phenomenon to that in regions with fluorinated drinking water may be observed for areas with heavy metal pollution: these elements are all taken up into the structure of uroliths in a similar way, studied in detail for cadmium (SCHNEIDER et al. 1979). The toxic element cadmium is accumulated

Table 11. The cadmium concentration in different types of urinary stones from areas without and with non-ferrous metal smelting industries, in ppm (SCHNEIDER et al. 1979)

Type of stone	Without			With		
	n	s	$\bar{x}$	$\bar{x}$	s	α
Uric acid	26	0.11	0.05	0.58	1.0	<0.05
Weddellite	9	0.20	0.16	0.48	0.34	>
Whewellite	45	0.14	0.19	0.63	0.34	>
Struvite	22	0.13	0.30	1.83	2.4	<0.01

chiefly in the kidney, leading to hypercalciuria and its immediate consequence urolithiasis (KASANTZIS 1979; ADAMS et al. 1969). Pari passu with an increase in urinary calcium concentration there is an increased cadmium content of uroliths in affected areas. Uric acid and struvite calculi are more affected than calcium oxalate stones (Table 11).

Whether or not cadmium has a direct influence on crystallization and stone structure cannot at present be stated with certainty.

An interesting relationship has also been detected between mass and trace elements in uroliths. Phosphorus and zinc are more strongly correlated with calculi of greater than 10% ash content (SCHNEIDER 1969; SCHNEIDER et al. 1970c, Fig. 26). Since the rare zinc phosphate mineral hopeite is of no quantitative significance, zinc is probably taken up into the apatite lattice. The zinc content of phosphate calculi decreases with increasing magnesium content. For this reason it may be assumed that struvite will contain barely any zinc.

The manganese content of renal stones decreases with rising phosphorus concentration.

Although calcium is the chief component of renal calculi by weight, phosphate must nevertheless assume the central role for the formation of inorganic renal stones. It has a highly precise influence on the ash content of calculi, and from it may be derived relationships to the occurrence of magnesium, zinc, sodium and manganese.

V. Structural Composition of Uroliths

The complexities of etiology and pathology in urolithogenesis in situ is mirrored in the structure of a representative cross-section through a stone, just as it is in the multiplicity of various possible phase combinations. The alternating phase sequences which may be observed in urolith structure result from control by qualitative and quantitative variations in the concentration of lithogenic substances. There are variations in the degree of crystallinity, a multiplicity of crystallization and growth centers, numerous phenotypes of phase adsorption and metamorphosis as well as processes of growth stagnation, phase dissolution and transformation, all of which testify to a complexity in urolithogenesis which is characteristic of biomineralization processes and which is impressively demonstrated by polarising microscopic studies of uroliths in thin section (BAUSCH and SORGER 1975; BERG et al. 1978a, b; BRIEN et al. 1980; CAVERO 1972, 1973; CIFUENTES DELATTE et al. 1973b; KOLPAKOW and GLIKI 1965a, b; PINTO 1976; SEYFARTH et al. 1974; SUTOR and WOOLEY 1972b; SZABO 1973). A historical review of thin section studies in the 19th Century has been given by CIFUENTES DELATTE (1981).

Additional high resolution structural detail, morphologic peculiarities and detailed understanding of the processes involved have resulted from scanning electron microscopy of submicroscopic phase samples (ALONSO and SOMACARRERA 1973; BASTIAN 1979; BERG et al. 1979a, b; BLOMEN 1981; DOSCH and KOESTEL 1975; GARCIA-RAMOS et al. 1984; HESSE et al. 1981a; LEUSMANN 1981; PINTO 1976; SCHUBERT et al. 1983). The polymorphic aggregation behaviour of urinary calculi may easily be classified into a few aggregation types having a number of features in common and allowing conclusions as to their formation processes in temporal sequence, as well as a classification of the various changes that occur in their aggregate structure. As early as 1879 ARNO KRÜCHE applied the method of mineralogical thin section to urate stones for their structural classification. He was thus able to derive fundamental rules governing the possible structural forms.

1. Aggregate Structural Description

SEYFARTH et al. (1974) consider the predominant configurational feature to be the clear discontinuity between aggregation in the central nucleus and in the peripheral shells of a urolith, a distinction to which A. KRÜCHE (1879) had already drawn attention. These parts may be distinguished both in calculi of uniform chemical structure and in those of differing phase composition. Whatever their relative sizes they will be more or less sharply separated by a hiatus.

This state of affairs is emphasized by the multitude of studies concerned with separate analytical descriptions of nucleus and shell (BASTIAN and GEBHARDT 1974; BICK et al. 1977; BRIEN et al. 1978; ELLIOT 1973a, b; HINMAN 1979; KOLPAKOW 1971; UNNI MOOPPAN et al. 1979).

Note that any phase involved in the structure of uroliths may represent the starting point of lithogenesis. No urolith component shows a typical preference for any particular region of the calculus, although whewellite is the commonest substance in the nucleus.

The nucleus may be interpreted as the center of growth but is not necessarily the geometric center of the stone. It merely represents a morphologic-topographic function of thin sections, characterized by a more or less concentric arrangement of all subsequently arising calculous phases around it in a shell. Thin section studies by SEYFARTH et al. (1974), as well as scanning electron microscopic studies by LEUSMANN (1981), suggest that uroliths tend to possess but one or two primary centers of growth, frequently coexisting with a number of secondary growth centers of irregular distribution. The latter are then responsible for the frequently irregular form and surface of uroliths (Figs. 38, 39) (KOLPAKOW 1971; DOSCH 1980b).

a) Central Region

According to SEYFARTH et al. (1974), SCHNEIDER and SEYFARTH (1980) and HAHNE and EISMANN (1979) growth centers may be divided into a few basic types.

- The central region is completely isotropic and without recognizable texture (Fig. 27).
- Beside isotropic material crystals are irregularly aggregated in a cobble-stone configuration.
- The crystalline moiety predominates in a nucleus consisting of irregularly arranged fine and coarse-grained crystal aggregates (Fig. 28). Spheroliths occur more rarely, aggregated into a dense conglomerate.
- The center is characterized by cavity formation (Figs. 29).

Studies of the nucleus by SCHNEIDER and SEYFARTH (1980) suggest the conclusion that adsorption of material to individual crystals plays a subordinate role in the formation mechanism of uroliths. Aggregation behaviour in the central region is characterized to a varying degree by intermicellary crystallization or by the presence of matrix proper, the latter partly permeated by colloidal or cryptocrystalline inorganic excretions (SEYFARTH and SCHNEIDER 1978). The

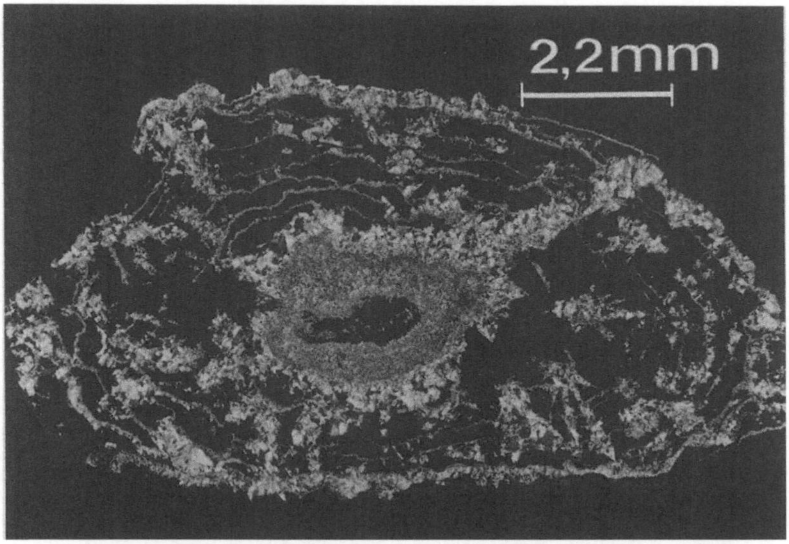

Fig. 27. Optically isotropic central zone and layered concentric texture in peripheral zones, also chiefly of optically isotropic material (apatite). The whole configuration is permeated discordantly by radially arranged, finely crystalline, secondary whewellite formations (crossed polarizing filters)

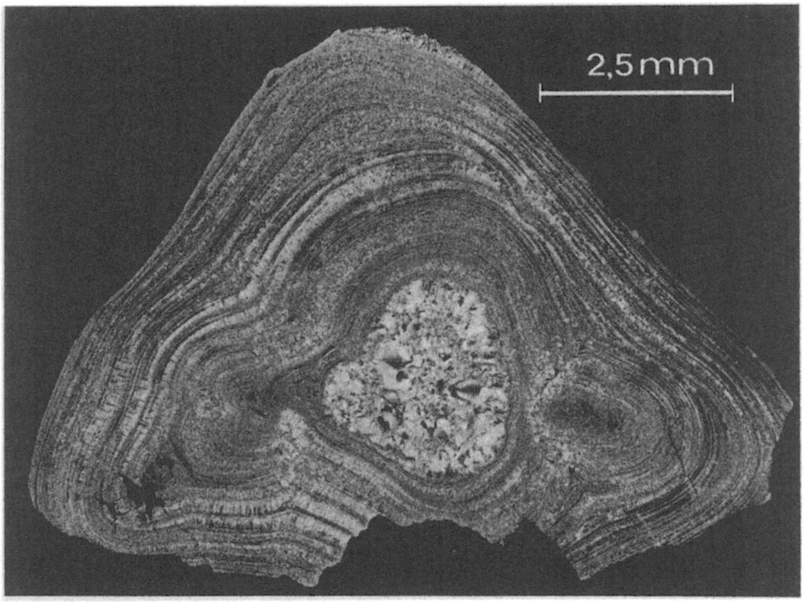

Fig. 28. Growth nucleus of randomly arranged, coarse grained whewellite. The peripheral zones consist of layers of fine grained uric acid (dark) and whewellite in an alternating sequence (crossed polarizing filters)

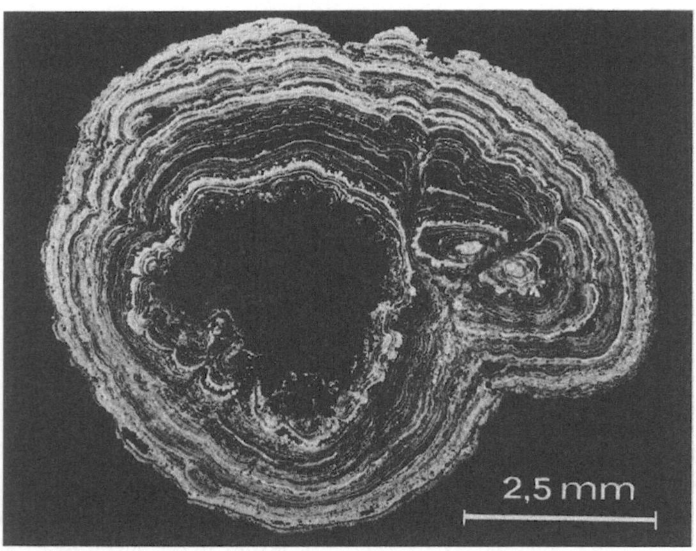

Fig. 29. In the center is a cavity. The periphery consists of alternating concentric layers of whewellite and apatite (extinguished). Two subsidiary whewellite nuclei and obvious features of dissolution aggregation (in discordant section) (crossed polarizers) (see Section V/3)

findings thus suggest subsequent spherolithic crystallization with the formation of thin layers of concentration of inorganic and/or organic substances (new material) within a pre-existing gel matrix (old substance).

There is good agreement between this hypothesis and the observations of BUTHLIASCHWILI (1979), KOLPAKOW (1971), LEUSMANN (1981) and SCHUBERT and BICK (1978). According to SEYFARTH and SCHNEIDER (1980) the precursor of such an isotropic matrix gel could be a "macroflake" arising from a sol–gel transformation. Damaged cellular elements and blood coagula might equally represent the starting point of lithogenesis (BERENYI 1981; KOLPAKOW 1971). On the other hand other authors follow the crystallization theory, considering the formation of crystal seedlings or crystal aggregates to be urolith precursors which then become fixed, mechanically, epitaxially or hydrodynamically within a gel somewhere in the urinary tract. These entities would then subsequently grow to become the starting point of clinical calculus formation (ARMBRUSTER 1978; BLOMEN 1981; BOTHOR and BERG 1980; CAVERO 1972; DOSCH 1975a; GEBHARDT 1974, 1978; HINMAN 1979; MANDEL and MANDEL 1981).

b) Peripheral Region

This region represents a record of the originally adsorbed materials and of subsequent change. According to characteristic internal configurational features the following aggregate types may be discerned (SCHUBERT and BRIEN 1980; HAHNE and EISMANN 1979 and SEYFARTH et al. 1974).

– *Concentric shell structure.* Individual small crystals are arranged in a pallisade perpendicular to the direction of layering and result in a structure of a high degree of organization (whewellite, uric acid, brushite). This type typically contains alternative layers of different phase sequences and varying grain sizes (Figs. 30, 31, 47).

– *Filamentous aggregates* with a strictly radial arrangement of fine submicroscopic filaments (< 0.2 μm) orientated around a nuclear center. Such structures often mimic large crystals and may be marked by a large number of very fine concentric, parallel curved lines around the nucleus. These lines may be explained as growth fronts or as the intermittent incorporation of fine deposits of apatite or organic substances (Figs. 31, 32, cf. also Fig. 47).

Both laminar and radial aggregate configurations are primary participants in stone formation, giving rise to a "year ring" arrangement. They may be interpreted as crystal apposition and/or subsequent crystallization of a primary gel deposit.

One impressive aspect of urolith aggregation behaviour, documented by SUTOR and WOOLEY (1972b), is the property of directional growth. There would appear to be a strict relationship between crystal axis and the radial arrangement of crystallites, the latter showing a marked preference for perpendicular arrangement within an individual layer (year ring structure).

This directional principle may be applied to the structural emergence of virtually all urolith phases, indeed it relates to the epitaxial growth of one

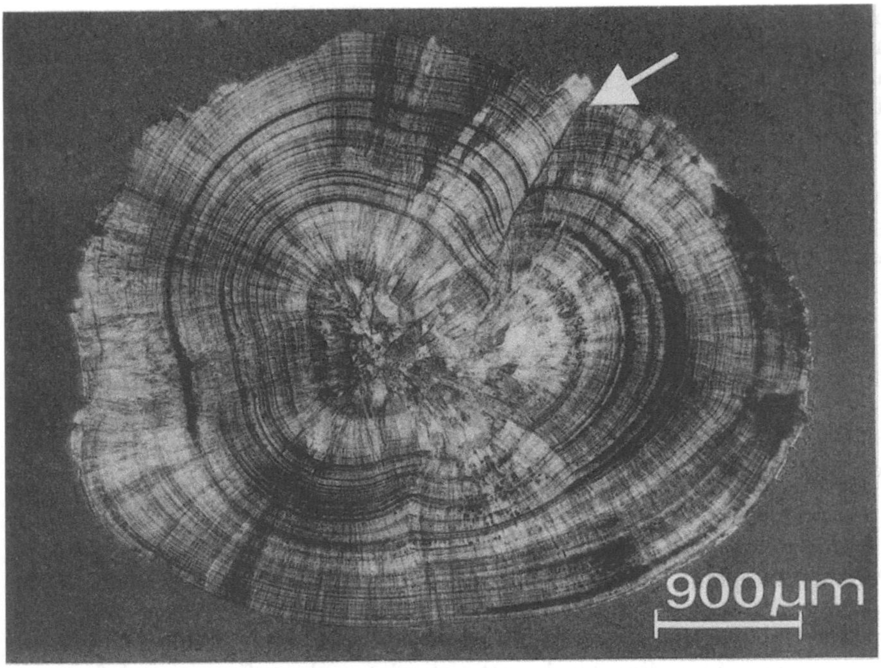

Fig. 30. Whewellite calculus of year-ring configuration. Marked radiate texture and concentrically-layered zonal structure. Pronounced banding with densely pigmented, isotropic material – an appositional and stagnation aggregate. Note also discordant transection of a region displaying dissolution features (arrow). Random arrangement of whewellite crystals in the nucleus (crossed polarizers)

phase upon another. The fact that a stone of uniform material may nevertheless on cross-section reveal a layered series of phases and modulations of grain size suggests some variability in the conditions of deposition. The unfettered radial growth of large crystals (e.g. whewellite) denotes a metastable supersaturation, whilst the deposition of layers of small crystallites is more in favor of higher degrees of supersaturation.

– The grains are generally arranged in an irregular fashion. Regions near the center of a calculus reveal a more or less dense cobble-stone configuration of coarse grain whilst crystal aggregation in outer zones tends to be radiate (characteristic of whewellite) (Fig. 33).

– *Complete irregularity* of idiomorphic crystals (typical of weddellite) embedded in an isotropic or pseudoisotropic substance (apatite). Processes of metamorphosis are still visible as relics of primary crystal structure (cf. transformation of weddellite to whewellite) (Fig. 34).

– Generally large xenomorphous grains are embedded in bands within a gel matrix (apatite) and result in a *string of beads* crystallite arrangement. Such structures tend to be disorderly and of little mechanical strength. They are typical of struvite and apatite.

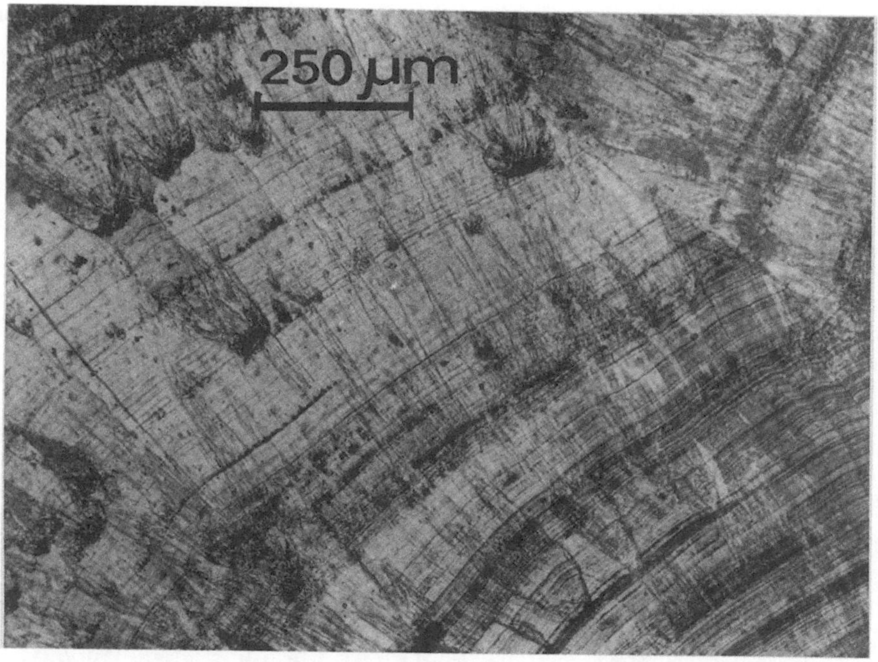

Fig. 31. Whewellite calculus (detail). Year-ring structure, alternating sequential layers of coarse and fine-grained texture

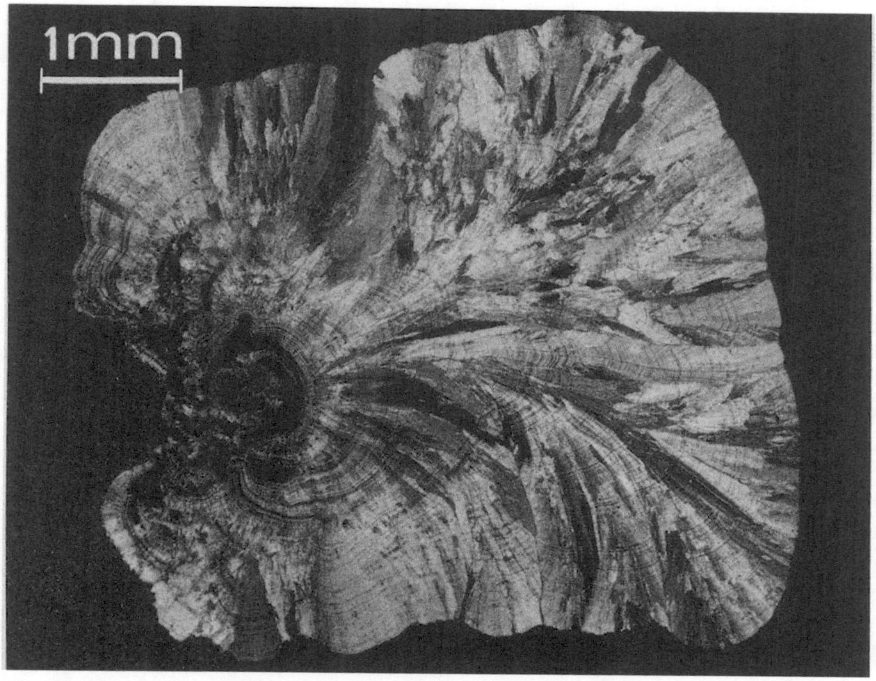

Fig. 32. Papillary cast of whewellite. Nucleus permeated with organic substance. A filamentous aggregate simulating the appearance of large crystals and pervaded with minute concentric lines parallel to the nucleus (crossed polarizers)

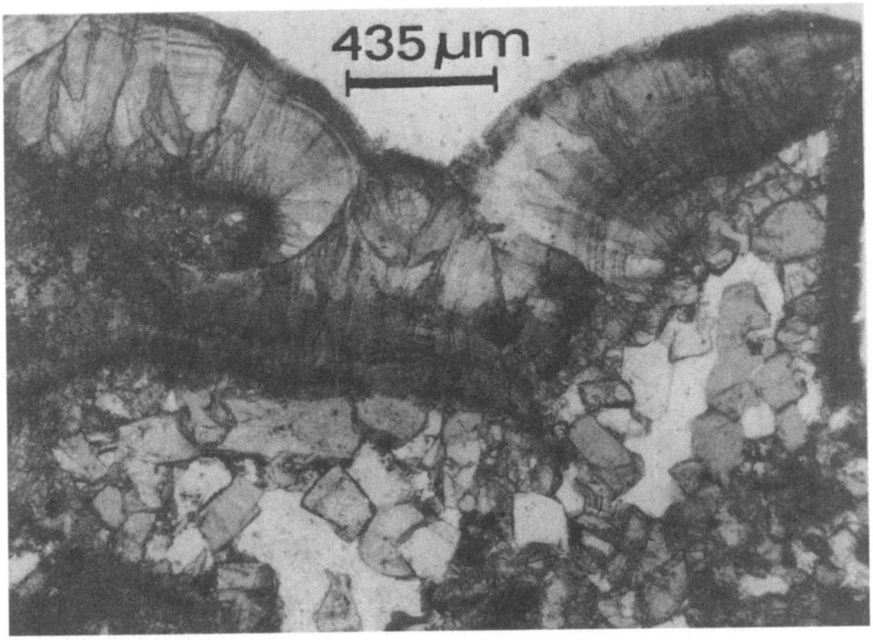

Fig. 33. Periphery of a calculus showing whewellite grains in cobble-stone configuration; adjacent whewellite of radiate texture (polarizers uncrossed)

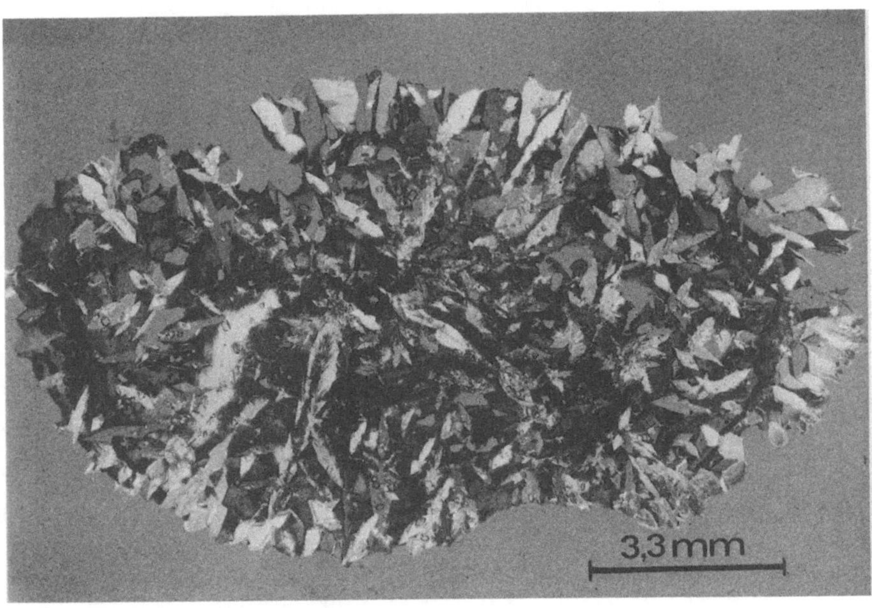

Fig. 34. Random arrangement of idiomorphous, lanceolate whewellite crystals (with some new formations) bedded in apatite and loosely interlocking (polarizers uncrossed)

This description of aggregate configuration may be applied to virtually all urolith phases, although the fundamental arrangement is naturally often blurred by the change and interplay of a large number of variables during urolithogenesis. Any understanding of postgenetic change and its precipitating factors must be in terms of the size, fusion and degree of order of grains.

2. Urolithogenesis as the Basis of Aggregate Configuration

Like its descriptive counterpart a *genetically based nomenclature* of aggregate configuration is subject to observer interpretation. Nevertheless such a nomenclature represents an attempt to categorize descriptively defined calculi in terms of the chief primary and secondary processes of crystallization involved in urolithogenesis (SCHNEIDER and SEYFARTH 1980).

An individual configuration is frequently the result of a number of genetic events and thus represents the aggregation over time of a series of formation stages and processes.

Appositional Aggregation

Crystalline substance from the surrounding solution is laid down on the surface of a pre-existing nucleus by a process involving both the incorporation of film-forming organic substances and the emergence of layered structure under the control of cyclic concentration changes (Figs. 28–31).

Stagnational Aggregation

This aggregation pattern is characterized by clear evidence for periodic interruption of calculous growth. There is a concomitant increase in the incorporation of isotropic inorganic or organic substance, resulting in prominent pigment banding within the aggregate (Fig. 30).

Dissolutional Configuration

Depending on their degree of organization and on concentration variations within the urinary environment, pre-existing calculous zones and layers may dissolve, either concordantly, i.e. corresponding to their pre-existing layered structure) or discordantly (transecting layer boundaries). Subsequent resumption of calculous growth results in aggregate structures with regularities of their own, not apparently related to and frequently abruptly transecting elements of the primary aggregate (Figs. 29, 30).

Metamorphic Configuration

This type of aggregate results from subsequent change within primary appositional aggregates. There may be deposition of aggregates with fine elongated

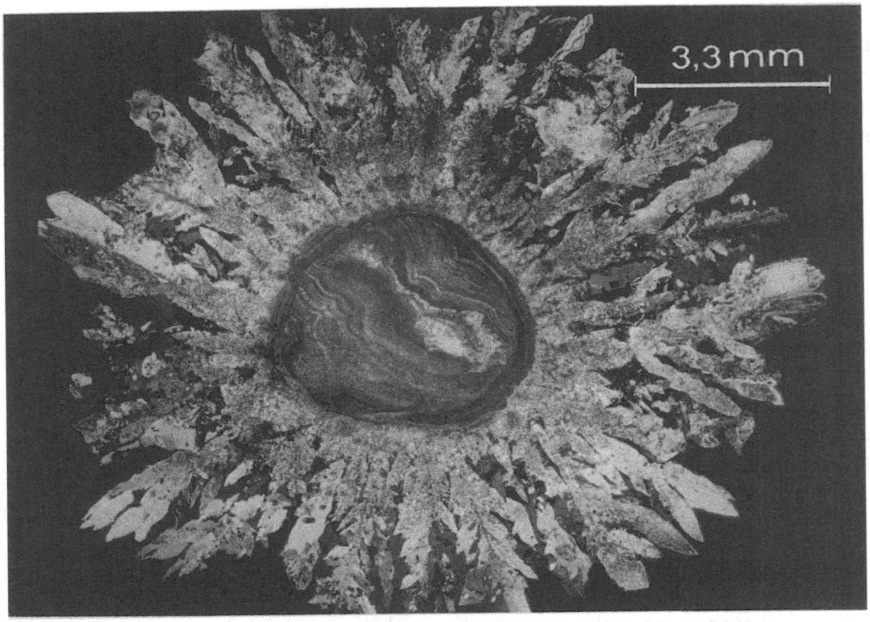

Fig. 35. Calcium oxalate calculus showing the configuration of a displacement aggregate (metamorphic aggregation). Whewellite covered in a growth of coarse weddellite crystals, their bases in a state of advanced metamorphosis to whewellite – crossed polarizers

crystals in definite layers of pronounced radial arrangement. They are thus rendered as discordant to the nucleus as large individual crystals (Fig. 27). Either of these details of aggregation behaviour may demonstrate subsequent infilling of radial clefts and layered secondary crystallization concentric to the growth center. They thus point to phenomena perhaps related to the previously discussed processes of aging and shrinkage in primary gel deposits.

A third metamorphic type is represented by the displacement configuration of calcium oxalate crystals. In this case weddellite is displaced by whewellite (Fig. 35). Such a transformation process may result in the formation of pseudomorphoses.

For a detailed description of the morphology and formation of a large variety of urolith phases along with their optical data the reader should refer to PRIEN and PRIEN (1968).

The existence of such a variety in aggregation behaviour requires that we scrutinize possible relationships between urinary pathology and configurational features within an individual phase (BRIEN et al. 1980; CIFUENTES DELATTE 1978; PRIEN 1949, 1955).

Qualitative and quantitative variations in urine composition might be expected to result in the deposition of differing urolith phases. Nevertheless the grain structure of such individual phases may be closely similar despite variations in urine composition, if only the conditions of deposition and growth remain closely matched. The reverse is true for similar phase composition with variations in urine supersaturation, when a variety of structures will result. This situation will indeed be underlined by the following description of typical urolith phases and their texture. For crystallographic data see Section VI, 8., Table 20.

3. Urolith Phases

a) Calcium Oxalate

Whewellite

As suggested in the preceding Chapters 2 and 3 it is the grain configuration of calcium oxalate monohydrate which may give rise to the widest variety of aggregation types. Virtually all the patterns previously discussed are represented.

Whewellite thus frequently crystallises as fine layers of radial columns and in concentric lamellae, giving rise to the typical dense arrangement of "year ring" structure with a high degree of organization (Figs. 30–32) (BAUSCH and SORGER 1975; BRIEN et al. 1980; CAVERO 1972, 1973, 1981, 1982; CIFUENTES DELATTE et al. 1973b; KOLPAKOW and GLIKI 1965a; MEDINA et al. 1977; SCHÄFER and DOSCH 1978; SEYFARTH et al. 1974, 1975; SUTOR and WOOLEY 1972b; SZABO 1973; 1974).

Thin section studies have also revealed transitions in the regular arrangement of crystallites in individual layers with a tendency to radiate structure. The same may occur within an irregular cobble-stone configuration (Fig. 36) (SEYFARTH et al. 1975).

Scanning electron microscopic studies by DOSCH and KOESTEL (1975) and by HESSE et al. (1979a) have confirmed that the grains represent a dense structure of columns and foliate sequences of minute monocline plates (Figs. 40, 41). The latter frequently fan out from a common growth center.

Studies by KOLPAKOW (1971), SCHUBERT and BICK (1978), and SEYFARTH et al. (1975) suggest this year ring structure may arise by crystallization from the colloid or gel state, which not infrequently also leads to the formation of spheroliths (Fig. 37). The concentric banding visible in Figs. 30 and 31 within the finely laminated radiate zone structure may mean successive variations in oxalate availability and cyclic incorporation of pigments, apatite and organic substances (SCHÄFER and DOSCH 1978; SEYFARTH et al. 1974; WARPEHOSKI et al. 1981).

Crystallographic studies confirm both a primary and a secondary route of formation for whewellite (SCHUBERT et al. 1981).

Whereas the year ring structure of whewellite may be interpreted as a consequence of primary monohydrate crystallization, all other textures are frequently subject to individual observer interpretation. It seems not unreasonable and indeed logical to postulate their secondary formation from weddellite (or calcium oxalate trihydrate) and by subsequent recrystallization processes (see weddellite).

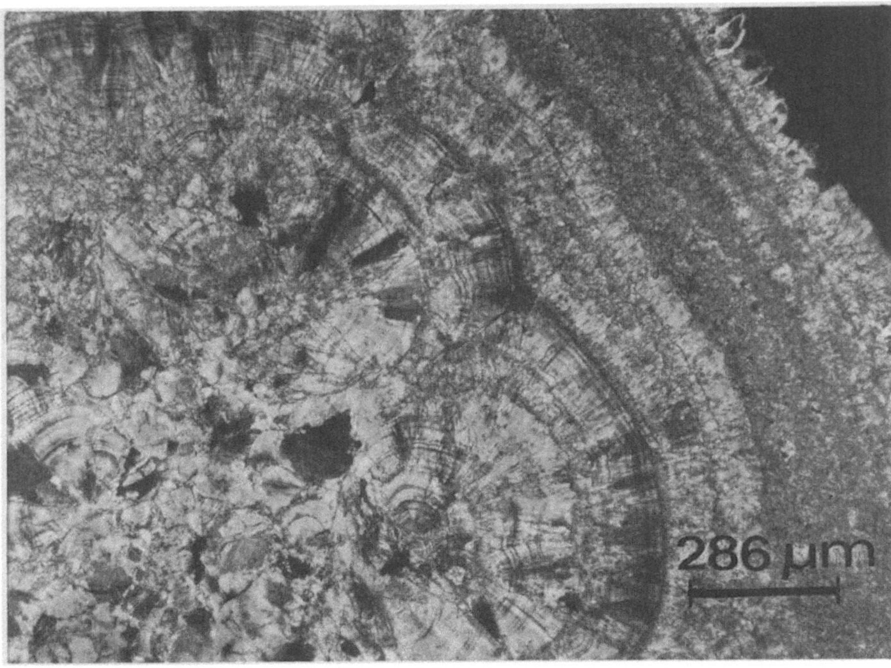

Fig. 36. Whewellite in thin section. Varying degrees of regularity among the crystallites, fine grained layering near the surface, tending towards a radial arrangement (crossed polarizers)

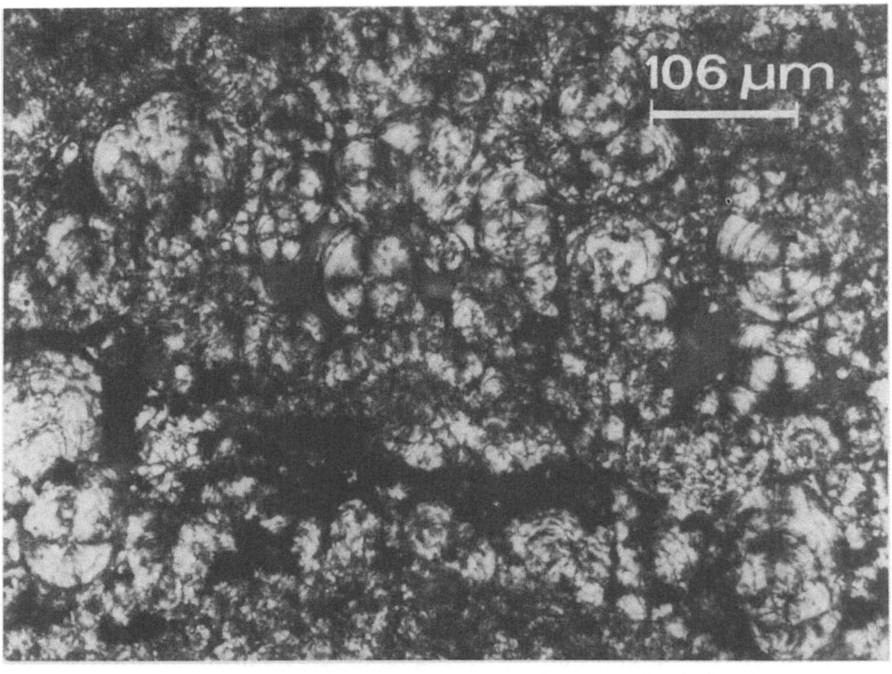

Fig. 37. Whewellite spheroliths in pseudoisotropic apatite (crossed polarizers)

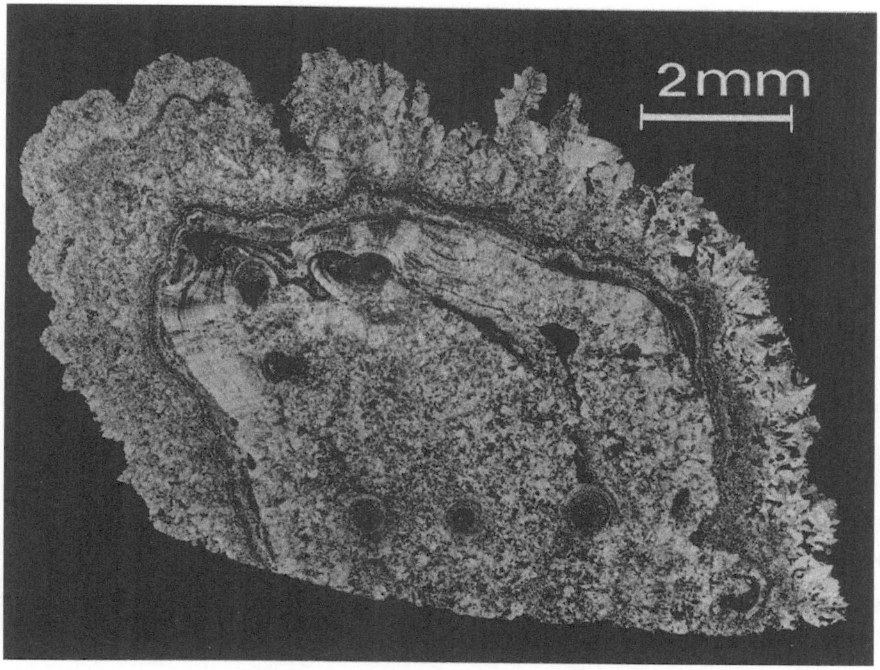

Fig. 38. Whewellite calculus containing multiple secondary growth centers of fine grained uric acid (crossed polarizers)

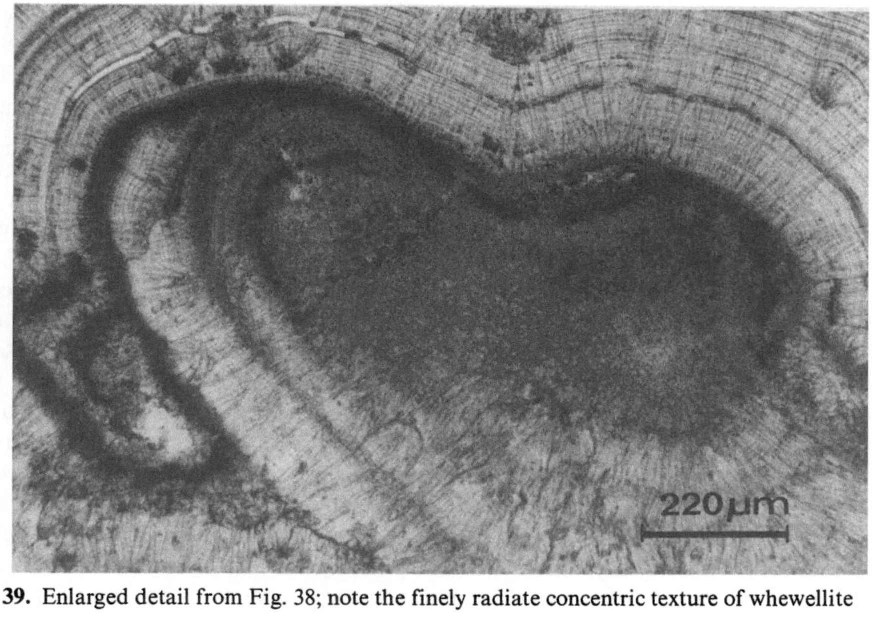

Fig. 39. Enlarged detail from Fig. 38; note the finely radiate concentric texture of whewellite

40 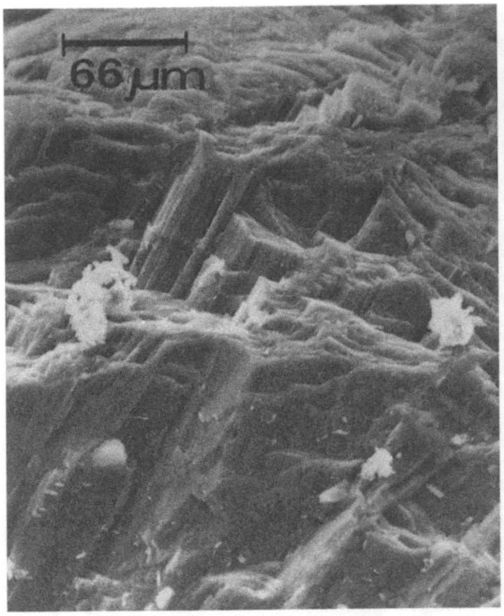

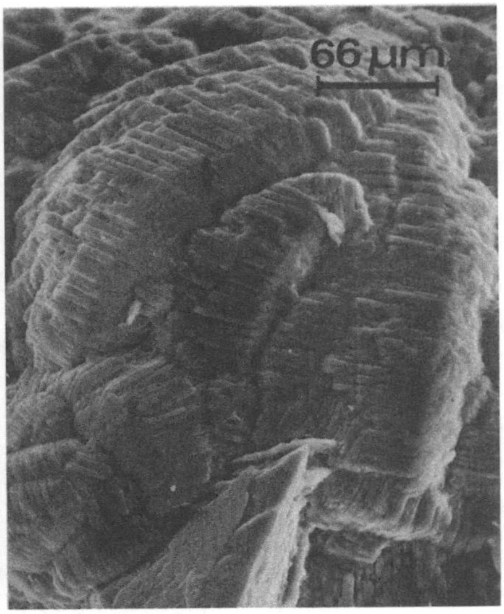

41

Fig. 40. Whewellite showing columnar texture (SEM)

Fig. 41. Micaceous layers of whewellite plates stacked up and fused into radial columns (SEM)

As well as a series of whewellite pervasion twins fused in a rosette configuration and large individual idiomorphous crystals (Fig. 42), fine grain aggregations of polycrystalline whewellite may also be encountered, the latter conjoined throughout a considerable volume (Fig. 43). In the absence of weddellite relics these crystallisates can be regarded as primary precipitates of whewellite, probably from urine of high oxalic acid concentration (BRIEN et al. 1980). Thin sections of whewellite reveal dissolutional and metamorphic configurations as an impressively recurrent structural principle of this urolith phase (Figs. 30, 46). Violation by whewellite of the usual lamellar structure typically seen in thin sections is considered by BAUSCH and SORGER (1975) to represent a secondary recrystallization of fine grain crystals into large idiomorphous whewellite crystals (Fig. 33).

A typical feature of whewellite is its frequent occurrence as a nuclear component (upto 70%) (BASTIAN and GEBHARDT 1974; BICK et al. 1977; ELLIOT 1973a, b) considers this the extent to which it acts as an initiator substance in urolithogenesis. Other urolith phases are frequently associated with calcium oxalate monohydrate, the layered structure consisting of an alternating phase sequence of whewellite and uric acid or urate, whewellite and apatite or variously whewellite, and brushite in concentric laminations (Figs. 28, 29). In this connection there continues to be discussion of the influence of apatite and uric acid crystals as well as high molecular weight organic substances on the crystallization of whewellite, as documented by crystallographic studies of growth centers; see also Section V, 4b, c, and i (BERG

42
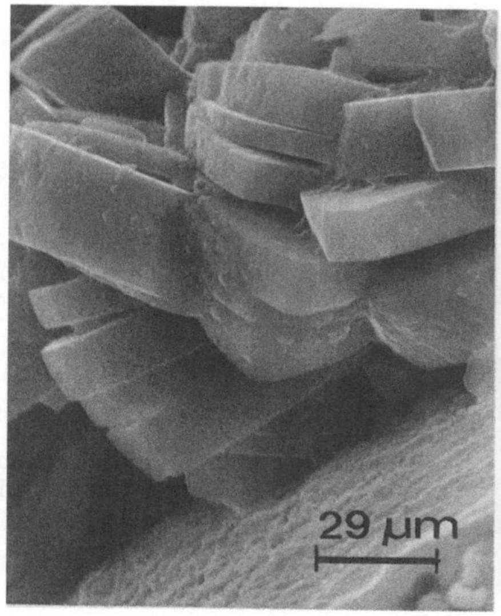

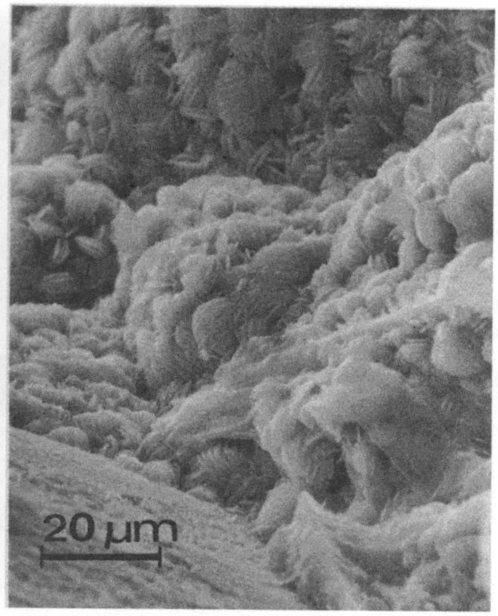

43

Fig. 42. Coarse, idiomorphous whewellite crystals, partially fused by pervasion twins (SEM)

Fig. 43. Fine grain aggregation of polycrystalline whewellite (SEM)

et al. 1978a, b; BLASCHKE and SCHMANDT 1978; ELLIOT 1973b; MEYER et al. 1975, 1976; SMITH et al. 1984; ZAREMSKI and GRIEVE 1976). In such centers whewellite may be seen with its characteristic radial structure spreading out into the phase volume (Figs. 32, 38, 39).

Weddellite

Calcium oxalate dihydrate represents a metastable form of calcium oxalate and generally gives rise to interlocking or ameboid aggregates of irregularly arranged lanceolate individual crystals (Fig. 34), characteristically tetragonal bipyramidal in habit (Fig. 44), frequently already in the process of metamorphosis to whewellite. The extent to which the metastable phase is preserved depends on the varying frequency of incorporation of stabilizing cations – especially magnesium ions – into the weddellite lattice (HEIDE et al. 1978).

As a result of observations made by SZABO (1978) on the uroliths of children, the development of weddellite stones is generally held to result from rapid crystallization.

An impressive bulk of literature testifies to the dominance of dehydration processes acting on primary weddellite crystals as a route of formation for whewellite stones, and this mechanism would thus appear well-established (BAUSCH and SORGER 1975; BERG et al. 1978b, 1979a; HEIDE et al. 1978; HESSE et al. 1976a, b; LEPAGE and TAWASHI 1982; SCHÄFER and BAUSCH 1979; SCHNEIDER

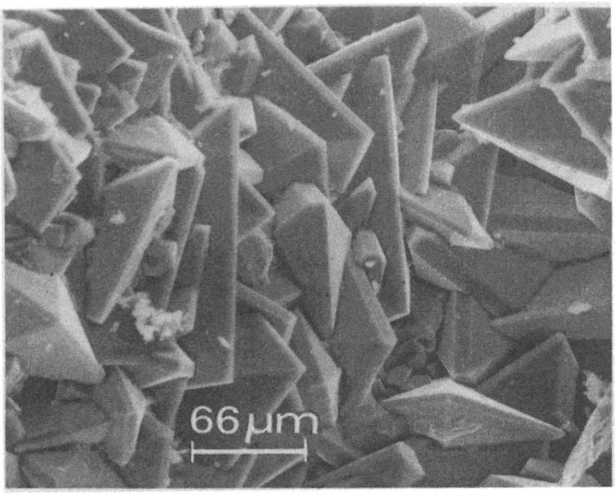

Fig. 44. Typical tetragonal-bipyramidal habit of whewellite crystals (SEM)

et al. 1977a; SCHUBERT and BRIEN 1978; SEYFARTH and HAHNE 1978; SZABO et al. 1976a).

Fundamental features of the weddellite (STERLING 1965) and whewellite (COCCO 1961) crystal structure suggest the formation of whewellite from weddellite by crystal structure transformation (SCHUBERT et al. 1980). Relationships between the crystal structures and comparison of their lattice constants imply partial preservation of weddellite structural elements during dehydration.

Whereas only ROSE and WOODFINE (1976) have described weddellite crystals as a typical nuclear substance in oxalate stones, all other communications report preferential crystallization on the surface of whewellite calculi (BERG et al. 1978b, BRIEN et al. 1978; ELLIOT 1973a, b; HELMAN 1979; SCHNEIDER et al. 1977a; SZABO 1973). The "Jackstone" configuration is a particularly impressive example. Fig. 35 is a thin section through a calcium oxalate calculus demonstrating primary whewellite crystallization in the center. Weddellite crystals are apposed to the exterior of this, their bases revealing a state of advanced erosion into fine grain whewellite. According to observations by BERG et al. (1979a, b), HAHNE and EISMANN (1979), SCHUBERT and BRIEN (1978) and SEYFARTH et al. (1974) the transformation of weddellite (phase B) to whewellite (phase A) may take place both on the surface of idiomorphic weddellite crystals and in the interior of the crystals themselves. Thin section studies allow displacement structures of A to be distinguished within B. Phase metamorphosis from without would appear inevitably associated with a degree of solvation attack, and in this respect there seems to be a thermodynamic preference for the lattice energies occurring along the edges and at the corners of tetragonal bipyramids (BERG et al. 1979b, 1980). Where the transformation is initiated within a weddellite grain, monocrystalline whewellite inclusions may be observed in one or several areas within the crystal. On the other hand metamorphosis involving the entire weddellite crystal leads mainly to the appearance of polycrystalline whewellite without the alternative of provisional re-

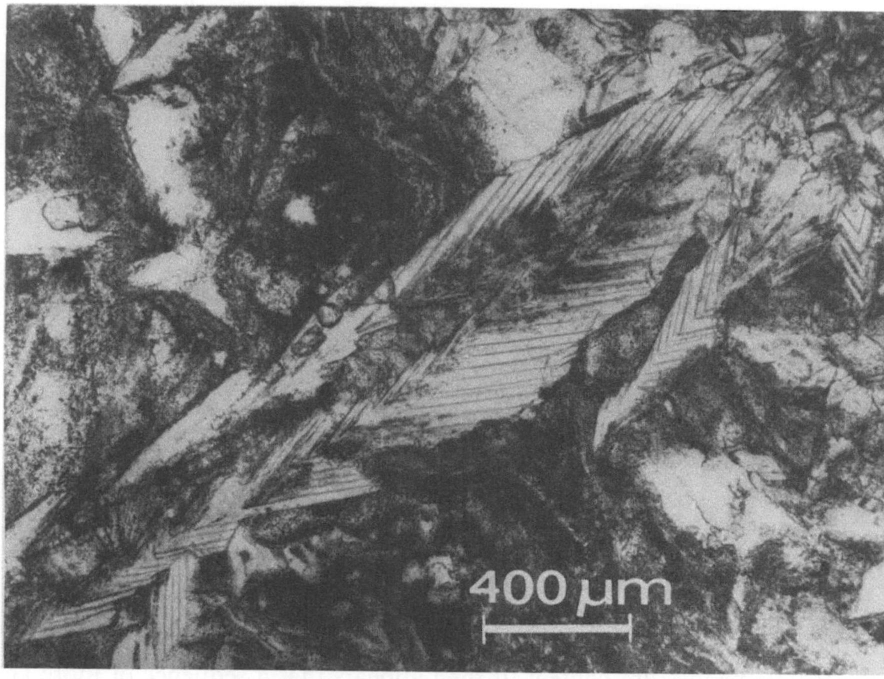

Fig. 45. Growth layers (V-banding) in weddellite crystals (crossed polarizers)

crystallization (SCHUBERT and BRIEN 1978). In special cases this phase metamorphosis occurs with preservation of the original weddellite crystal habit, thus giving an impressive example of pseudomorphosis, as described by BERG et al. (1979a, b), CIFUENTES DELATTE et al. (1973b), SCHÄFER and DOSCH (1978), SCHUBERT et al. (1981) and SZABO (1973) in some detail. The scanning electron microscope reveals this metamorphosis of weddellite to whewellite as involving the more or less pronounced formation of square scars on the pyramid surfaces of weddellite crystals, with strict orientation within the lattice geometry. The first transformation products to appear are gel forms of whewellite crystallisate which then undergo subsequent recrystallization to individual idiomorphous crystals. These coarse crystals frequently fill empty spaces and are thus not the originators of urolithogenesis. Within the overall structure of a stone such transformation processes are generally revealed by the presence of weddellite relics (HAHNE and EISMANN 1979; SCHUBERT and BICK 1978) and by a low packing density of grains (GEBHARDT et al. 1977; SEYFARTH et al. 1975).

Thin section frequently reveal V-shaped growth bands across weddellite crystals giving rise to an obvious stratification (Fig. 45, see also Fig. 55) (CAVERO 1981; CIFUENTES DELATTE et al. 1973b; KOLPAKOW and GLIKI 1965a; SZABO 1967). The scanning electron microscope gives a particularly impressive demonstration of these elements if the crystals were previously incubated with

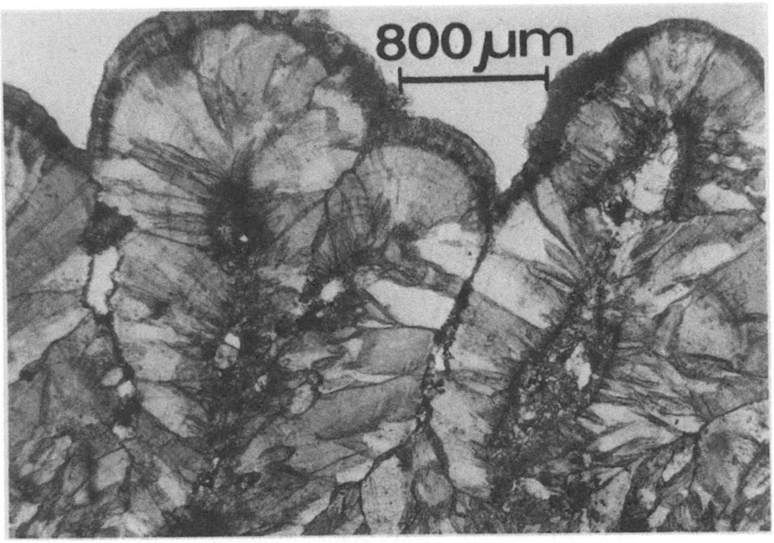

Fig. 46. Pseudomorphosis of whewellite crystals to weddellite, explaining the mulberry surface of whewellite calculi – see Fig. 18 (polarizers uncrossed)

urine of low magnesium content. It then appears that a sequence of more and less solvation-resistant strata constitutes the cyclically recurrent structural principle of weddellite crystals (BERG et al. 1979a, 1980; GEBHARDT 1980b). Such zonal structure is compatible with biorhythmic control of the excretion of lithogenic substances, stabilizing ions and/or of organic substances (BERG et al. 1982a; KOLPAKOW 1965a).

Beside calcium oxalate dihydrate GARDNER (1975), SCHÄFER and BAUSCH (1979) and TOMAZIC and NONCALLAS (1979) ascribe a key role in calcium oxalate calculus formation to the thermodynamically unstable trihydrate, a substance also discussed in connection with the dense shell structure of whewellite concretions (SCHÄFER and DOSCH 1978). Crystallographic data on the lattice structure of the trihydrate may be found in DEGANELLO et al. (1981).

The fact that previously idiomorphic weddellite crystals are able to determine the external habit of whewellite stones, e.g. mulberry stones (Fig. 18) is frequently apparent in the very macroscopic external appearance of the stone. Thin section studies by DOSCH (1980a) and SCHUBERT and BRIEN (1978a) have given a vivid illustration of this interesting aspect of stone architecture, fused radiate spheroliths of whewellite being loosely aggregated with whewellite pseudomorphosed to weddellite. The spherolithic hemispheres shown in Fig. 46 may be interpreted as whewellite growing in a perpendicular direction on the weddellite surface and thus finally giving rise to the mulberry bumps on the surface of the whewellite stone. Many other macroscopic types of calcium oxalate stone owe their existence to the presence of such discontinuities within the aggregate structure (see Figs. 4, 5) (DOSCH 1980a; KRÜCHE 1879; KOLPAKOW 1971).

KIM (1983) has observed mulberry particles around red blood cells incorporated into weddellite stones. The red cells appeared to aid crystal growth by acting as foci for surface nucleation or by forming an encrusting layer on the surface of the native bipyramids. An additional layer of calcium oxalate would then be deposited on this coating.

HINMAN (1979) derives the multiplicity of surface structures occurring in whewellite stones from the pronounced aggregation tendency of whewellite crystallites and particularly from local influences within the urinary tract. In so doing he draws attention to a point of some interest. The degree of mobility or fixation of the growing calculus provides an explanation for the spectrum of surfaces ranging from smoothly rounded through bosselated to bizarre morning star morphology, and also enables a relationship to be established between directional growth of the calculus and fine intermittent secondary deposits of apatite and mucoid materials.

There has been no shortage of attemps to classify the multiplicity of calcium oxalate aggregates by aggregation behaviour or to correlate these with formation in urine of various composition (BRIEN et al. 1980; CIFUENTES DELATTE 1978; HESSE et al. 1984; SCHÄFER and DOSCH 1978; SCHUBERT et al. 1981).

b) Uric Acid – Uric Acid Dihydrate

Two modifications of uric acid have been described – a monocline pseudorhombic (I) and a monocline (II) form (DOSCH 1981b; SHIRLEY and SUTOR 1967). The latter may occur during the dehydration of uric acid dihydrate as a metastable intermediate phase within urinary calculi.

Uric acid stones are characterized by a high degree of mineralization and by a concentrically conchoidal structure of characteristically radial texture, comparable to that of whewellite. Within this structure growth fronts may be prominent and be made even more pronounced by the incorporation of pigments and organic substances (Fig. 47) (BAUSCH and SORGER 1975; BERG et al. 1978b; BRIEN et al. 1980; HAHNE and EISMANN 1979; SZABO 1974).

Within the nucleus of uric acid stones HESSE et al. (1979a) generally found irregularly arranged monocline crystals (Figs. 48, 49), the stratified arrangement of peripheral zones being chiefly characterized by filamentous aggregation sequences of varying coarseness. Scanning electron microscopic studies reveal morphologic compatibility with crystallization of metastable uric acid dihydrate (YONG GO et al. 1980; HESSE et al. 1979a). Cracks and fissures perpendicular to the long axis of uric acid dihydrate columns testify to extensive phase metamorphosis into uric acid, thus illustrating processes of metamorphosis analogous to those pertaining in calcium oxalate (Fig. 50). Apart from the typical form with monocentrically packed fine crystals, multigrain uric acid stones are also described, and not infrequently "seams" within their structure testify to transitory dissolution processes followed by renewed apposition of material (cf. whewellite).

Uric acid calculi are generally rounded structures with a smooth external surface, and oviod growth is therefore likely (BAUSCH and SORGER 1975; DOSCH

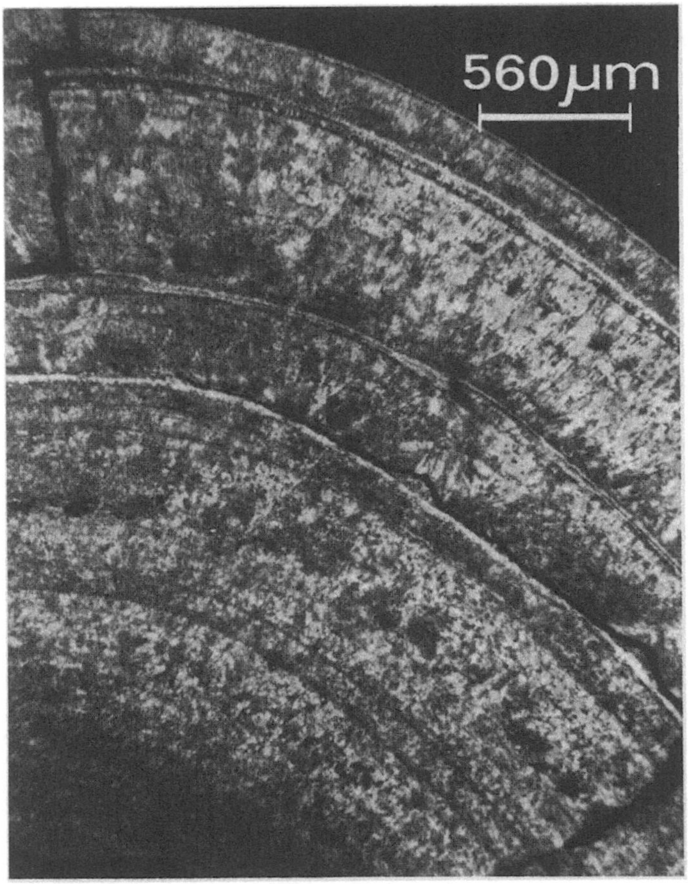

Fig. 47. Detail of a uric acid calculus showing sequential concentric layers of predominantly radiate texture. The nucleus is of fine grain monocline uric acid, the periphery showing a preference for uric acid dihydrate

and KOESTEL 1975). In addition there are warty excrescences on the surface similar to the polymorphic appearance of whewellite, explained by DOSCH (1980a) on the basis of thin section studies as dense radiate overgrowths at points of discontinuity within the stone structure.

In common with whewellite fine grained uric acid often occurs within an alternating sequence of other urolith phases (Fig. 28). Furthermore its occurrence within small finely crystalline growth centers suggests a function as an initiator substance for whewellite deposition (Figs. 38, 39), although it is considerably rarer than whewellite as a nuclear component (7 – 14%) (BICK et al. 1977; BRIEN et al. 1978 and ELLIOT 1973a, b). By the same token sodium dihydrogenurate deposition has been documented in central zones of stratified whewellite concretions by CIFUENTES DELATTE et al. (1978b). It crystallizes as elongated prisms with radial or fan texture, and is deposited in neutral or faint-

48 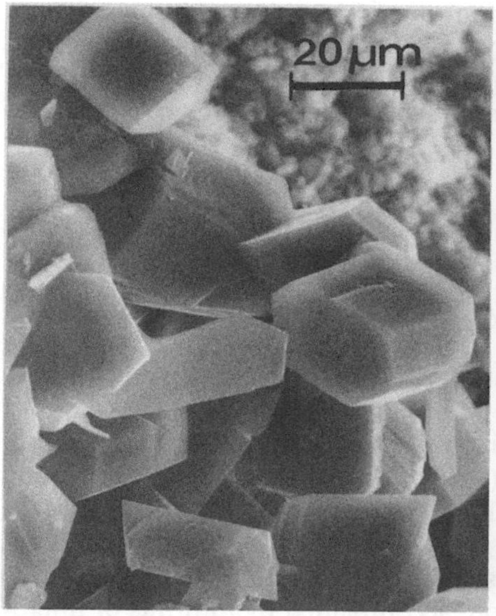

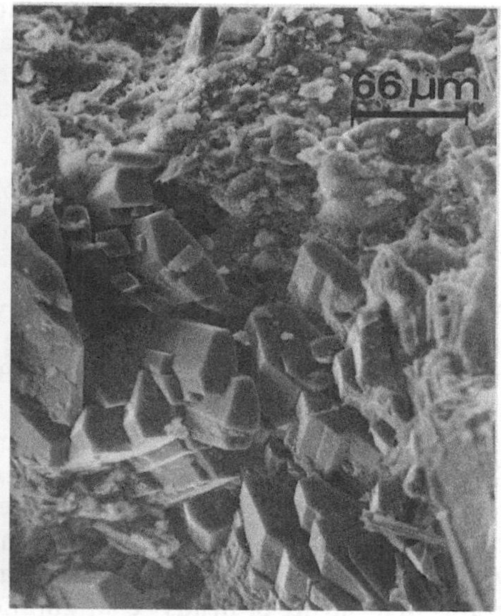 49

Figs. 48 and **49.** Monocline uric acid crystals, some of them columnar (SEM)

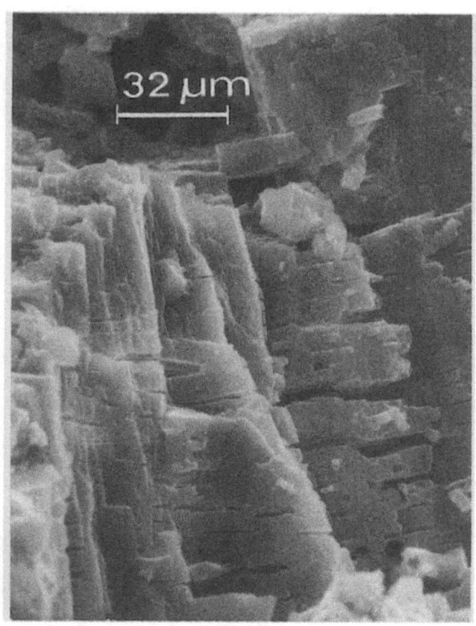

Fig. 50. Tall columnar crystals of uric acid dihydrate, massive cleft formation indicating early transition to anhydrous uric acid (SEM)

ly alkaline urine with a high concentration of uric acid and sodium. Sodium, potassium and potassium urates may play a role in the stabilization of uric acid dihydrate (DOSCH 1981 b).

It may be significant that weddellite and uric acid have hardly been described in immediate sequence.

c) Apatite

Apatite is precipitated from the urinary environment mainly in cryptocrystalline radio-amorphous form, appearing pseudoisotropic under the polarizing microscope (ARMBRUSTER 1978, 1979; BERG et al. 1978b; DOSCH and KOESTEL 1974; GEBHARDT 1975).

Polarizing and scanning electron microscope studies by HESSE et al. (1979a), SORGER and BAUSCH (1971) and SZABO (1967, 1974) have led to the description of flow aggregates of gel-derived lamellar structure occurring within apatite concretions (Fig. 51). This phenomenon is highlighted by the inclusion of struvite, whewellite, weddellite and occasionally ammonium dihydrogenurate grains in a "string of beads" configuration, accompanied by imprints of microorganisms, usually bacteria and colonies of cocci, underlining the causal role of urinary infection (CIFUENTES DELATTE and SANTOS 1977; DOSCH and KOESTEL 1975; HIENZSCH et al. 1975; MINAMI 1961; RODGERS 1981a). HESSE et al. (1978b, 1979b) have used the scanning electron microscope and the electron microprobe to demonstrate a uniform distribution of incorporated magnesium ions within apatite calculi, a phenomenon suggesting the substitution of calcium by magnesium. Furthermore, they were able to document sulfur accumulation within calcium-rich phosphate phases, probably due to the inclusion of proteins.

Observations by ARMBRUSTER (1978), DOSCH and KOESTEL (1975), and SEYFARTH and SCHNEIDER (1980) suggest that the characteristic configuration of

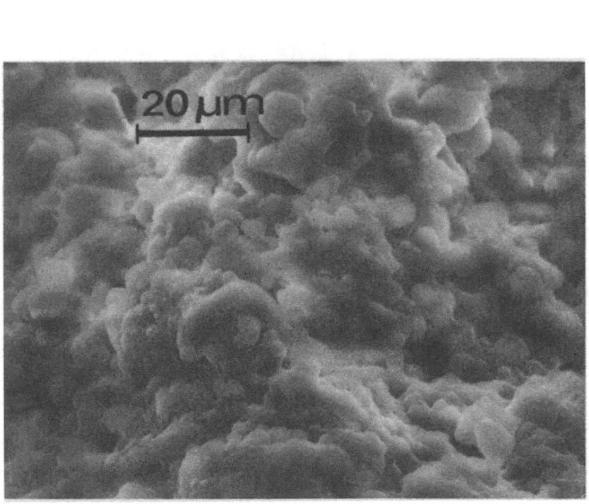

Fig. 51. Typical gel precipitation of apatite (SEM)

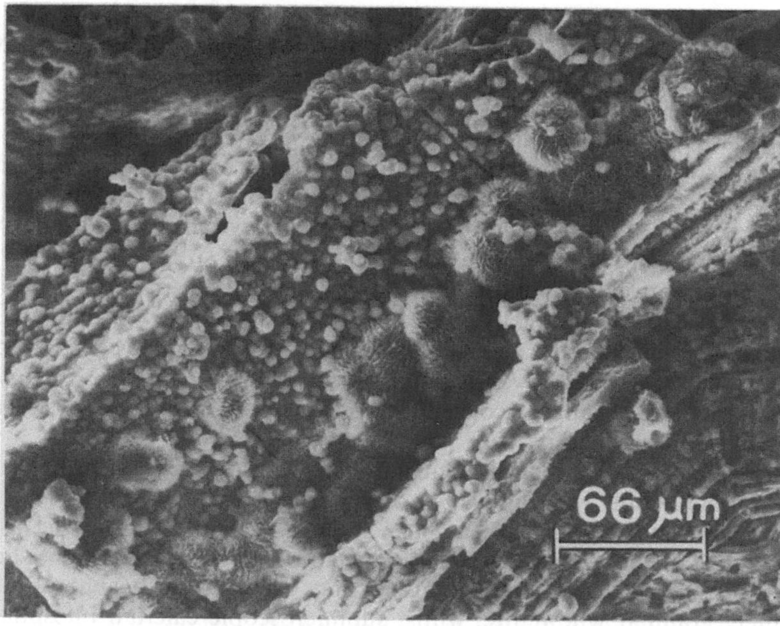

Fig. 52. Spheroliths of minute apatite spicules and surrounded by smaller, smooth surfaced apatide globules (SEM)

apatite concretions arises from the primary precipitation of voluminous flakes of water-rich colloidal material. Aging processes within this "jelly" lead to partial crystallization going hand-in-hand with the appearance of shrinkage fissures and folds, as well as with secondary new formations. Such a mechanism of formation would go some way toward explaining the lack of mechanical strength typical for apatite concretions.

Spherolithic phenotypes of concentrically spiculate or smooth-surfaced structure may also be observed (Fig. 52) (Armbruster 1978; Berg et al. 1979a; Leusmann 1981; Spector et al. 1976, 1978).

It would appear that apatite plays a highly controversial role in any interpretation of urolithogenesis. It occurs as approximately 15% of nuclear substance and in varying propertions as a component of virtually all uroliths (Fig. 29) (Brien et al. 1978; Elliot 1973a, b; Garcia-Ramos et al. 1984; Smith et al. 1984; Unni Mooppan et al. 1979), a fact which has led various workers to propose an initiator role in urolithogenesis for the deposition of an apatite gel matrix (Leskovar and Allgayer 1979; Malek and Boyce 1977; Seyfarth et al. 1974). Thus Blaschke and Schmandt (1978) found a densely matted conglomerate of apatite spheroliths of concentrically conchoidal structure within nuclear zones of calcium oxalate calculi. Like Leusmann (1981), Meyer et al. (1975) and Zaremski and Grieve (1976), these workers considered this phenomenon to have led to secondary calcium oxalate crystallization. At approximately 1 µ the diameters of these spheroliths correspond to that typical of protein precipitates. Similar structures have been detected by GUSEK et al. 1982 and MEYER-JÖRGENS et al. (1981) in biopsied renal tubuli from actively stone-forming patients. In their structure these spheroliths are however said to differ from those found as deposits on the surface of idiomorphous calcium oxalate crystals (Fig. 52) or as alternating strata within mixed stones.

Because of its viscous nature apatite gel could also conceivably form a mantle around crystal aggregates of foreign mineralogic composition, a circumstance which DÖSCH and KOESTEL (1975) believe to favor idiomorphous crystallization.

Observations by GEBHARDT (1975) have tended to confirm the hypothesis that apatite is rhythmically deposited as a gel coating of varying viscosity across growth fronts, where it acts as a diffusion barrier and leads to rhythmic precipitation of crystallites of varying size. Such a process would be a plausible explanation for the coarsely concentric stratification in the year ring structure of many urinary calculi.

Other types of apatite nuclear substance have been described as "calcium phosphate milk" or aggregates of spherolithic ellipsoidal "shot" of oolithic structure and a grain size of 0.5–2 mm (CAVERO 1972; CIFUENTES DELATTE et al. 1979; CIFUENTES DELATTE and MEDINA 1981; SOMACARRERA and ALONSO 1977). The center of such aggregates may contain apatite spheroliths alongside finely granular whewellite, whilst submicroscopic calcium phosphate deposits may occur within the narrow confines of the mantle. According to CIFUENTES DELATTE et al. (1973a, 1976) this material is embedded in organic ground substance in a fashion similar to that occurring in bone and other calcified tissue. The phenomenon of osseous tissue occurring within urolith nuclei may indicate a relationship with the widely debated role of organic matrix in the center of urinary calculi. The hypothesis has variously been advanced that calcium phosphate mineralization of organic macromolecules might generate "host material". The latter would in turn initiate epitaxial crystallization of calcium oxalate (see Section V., 3i).

In a few exceptional cases CIFUENTES et al. (1978) were able to demonstrate the presence of citrate-apatite on the surface of apatite concretions, citrate ions being bound to hydroxyapatite by substitution. By way of contrast WILLIAMS and SALLIS (1981) have described phosphocitrates as native crystallization inhibitors.

Scanning electron microscopy confirms the characteristic ability of carbonate apatite to infill clefts and blank spaces between the individual crystals of an aggregate (see Fig. 57–60) (ARMBRUSTER 1979; DOSCH and KOESTEL 1975; HESSE et al. 1978b, 1979b). This deposition may occur syngenetically during the growth of a concretion or, alternatively, by subsequent postgenetic diffusion of apatite sol into the interstices of the calculus. From a genetic point of view this latter variant may be of special significance. If primary urolith crystallization were followed by a period of selective phase dissolution, the ensuing possibility of apatite sol diffusing into the spaces thus created might offer an explanation for the presence of apatite within urolith nuclei.

BASTIAN and GEBHARDT (1975a, b), BERG et al. (1979a), GEBHARDT et al. (1978) and ZECHNER et al. (1984) have conducted in vitro experiments on uroliths using both synthetic and natural urine in an impressive reconstruction of such processes of growth, dissolution and subsequent apatite deposition.

d) Struvite

In the majority of studies magnesiumammoniumphosphate hexahydrate presents as an aggregate of irregular and variably interdigitated cobble-stone configuration (Fig. 53). More rarely a concentric conchoidal arrangement has been described (BERG et al. 1978b; SCHUBERT and BRIEN 1980; CIFUENTES DELATTE et al. 1973b; GEBHARDT 1975), usually said to be pervaded by discordant radially arranged, coarsely crystalline struvite of later date. By the incorporation of urea-splitting bacteria the grains acquire an obvious dark pigmentation (Fig. 54) (BICK and BRIEN 1975; KOLPAKOW and GLIKI 1965b). The grain appear-

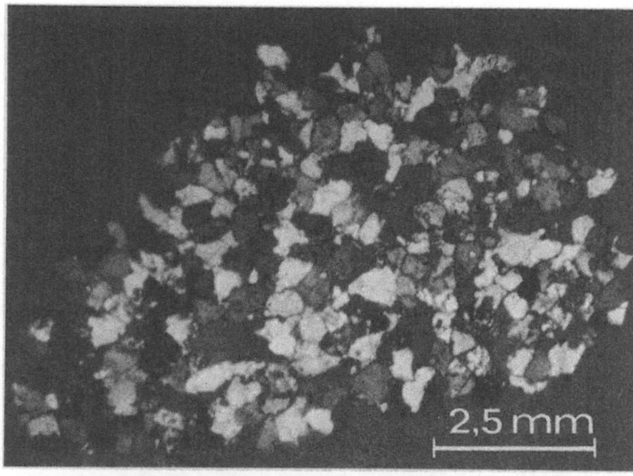

53

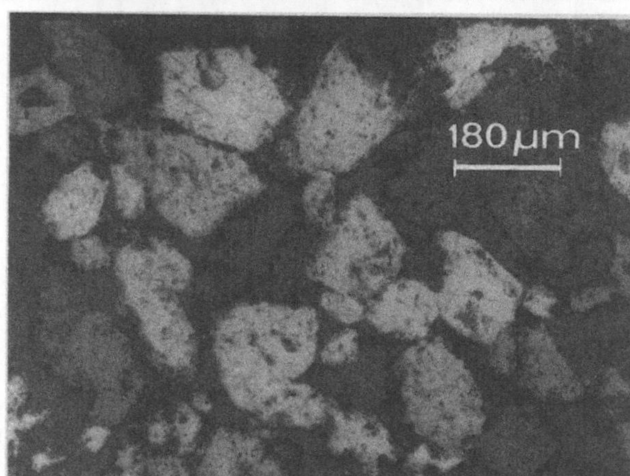

54

Figs. 53 and **54.** Cobbe-stone aggregate of struvite giving a mosaic texture. Incorporation of bacteria is responsible for the dark pigmentation of grains in Fig. 54 (crossed polarizers)

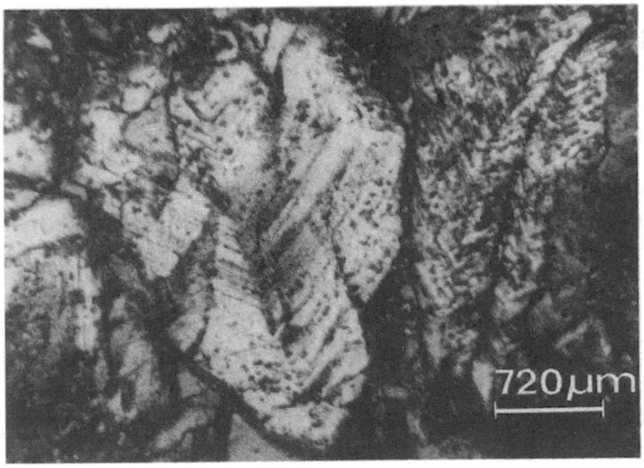

Fig. 55. The growth bands of struvite grains, see Fig. 45 (polarizers uncrossed).

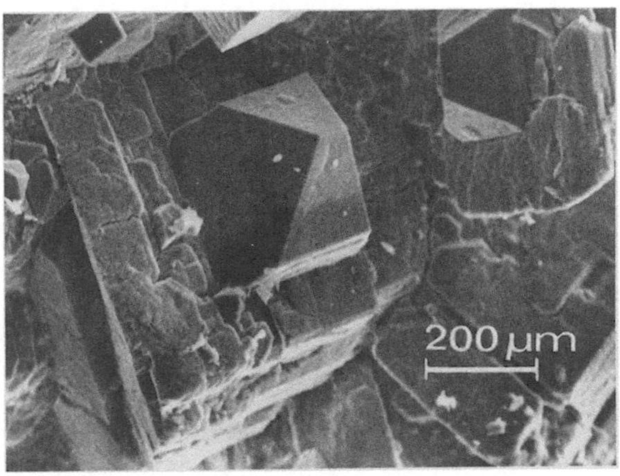

Fig. 56. Coarse struvite pavement surrounding "coffin-lid" crystals of triple phosphate (SEM)

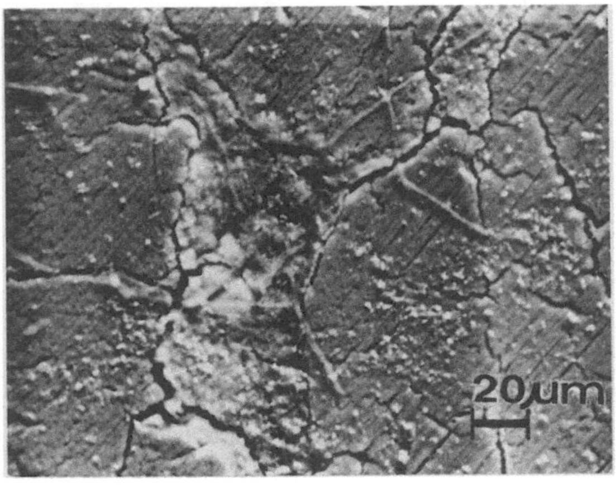

Fig. 57. Ground surface of a struvite calculus showing apatite deposition along grain margins and in fissures; scanning electron micrograph under composition contrast

ance may include a similarity to the chevron banding which gives a form of zonal structure to weddellite crystals. This phenomenon has been traced back to the inclusion of organic substances (Fig. 55, see also Fig. 45). Individual grains may even have such an orderly concentric conchoidal arrangement as to give rise to banded struvite inclusions within an apatite gel matrix. By analogy to the carbonate apatite model this behaviour may be considered to be further evidence for the causal role of infection in the process of precipitation. The degree of organization within an aggregate may be quite variable, usually resulting in calculi of no more than moderate mechanical strength.

Scanning electron microscopy seldom reveals any microcrystalline habit which would be absolutely typical of struvite (Dosch and Koestel 1975; Gebhardt 1974, 1975; He et al. 1984; Hesse et al. 1979a). Nevertheless a coarsely crystalline struvite pavement may occur in broad sheets representing a mosaic configuration, within the framework of which are occasionally fixed the "coffin lid" forms so typical of triplephosphate crystals in urinary sediment (Fig. 56). Besides large crystal aggregates one frequently encounters deposits which may be finely crystalline, take the form of a gel or occasionally present in an ellipsoidal habit, fissured by shrinkage and variably permeated by apatite (Figs. 57–60), bacteria and colonies of cocci (Cifuentes Delatte and Santos 1977; Dosch 1975b; Hesse et al. 1978b, 1979b). Struvite deposits are often found in association with ammonium dihydrogenurate in the peripheral zones of aseptic urolith phases, suggesting subsequent infective events. Szabo and Modis (1980, 1981) demonstrated a high content of organic ground substance by topooptical analysis of reactions within thin sections of struvite (see Section V., 3i).

e) Ammonium Dihydrogenurate

Ammonium dihydrogenurate is frequently found in the presence of carbonate apatite and struvite and so is yet another substance associated with the infective causation of urinary calculi (Armbruster 1979; Cifuentes Delatte 1978; Hienzsch et al. 1975; Garcia de la Peña and Cifuentes Delatte 1981; Rodriguez-Miñon 1976). Cifuentes Delatte et al. (1973b) demonstrated by polarizing microscopy the occurrence of this mineral as deeply stained, yellowish, luminescent spheroliths of fine spicules. Under the scanning electron microscope these may be seen to embody "lawns" of densely matted material (Figs. 61, 62) sometimes occurring intermittently between layers of whewellite (Gebhardt 1975). Such clinging together of spheroliths at the micron level of magnitude has been described both by Dosch and Koestel (1975) and by Hesse et al. (1979a) and may represent mechanisms of stone formation in their own right. Thin section studies of coherent urate deposits usually appear as a deeply stained gel, although interference at fracture margins (see Section VI., 8, Grain preparations) gives rise to intensive yellow luminescence.

In addition ammonium dihydrogenurate has been characterized by Cifuentes Delatte (1978) and Garcia de la Peña and Cifuentes Delatte (1981) as a finely granular material occurring in sterile urine and displaying brilliant interference coloration. This habit of ammonium dihydrogenurate may be demonstrated as an inclusion in a variety of calculous phases.

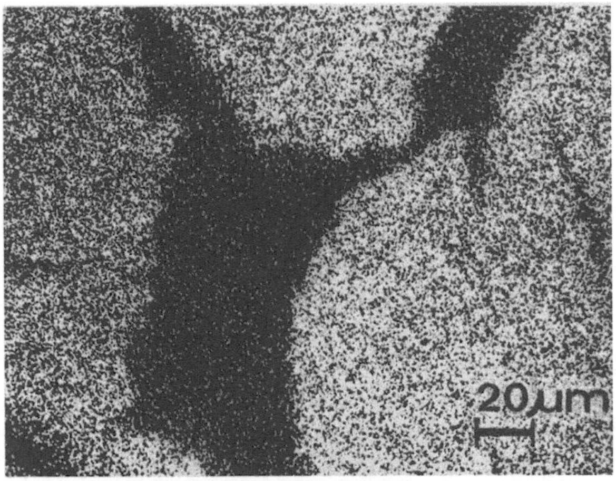

Fig. 58. Magnesium distribution from Fig. 57. Mg-K_α radiation; 100 sec (RAP crystal)

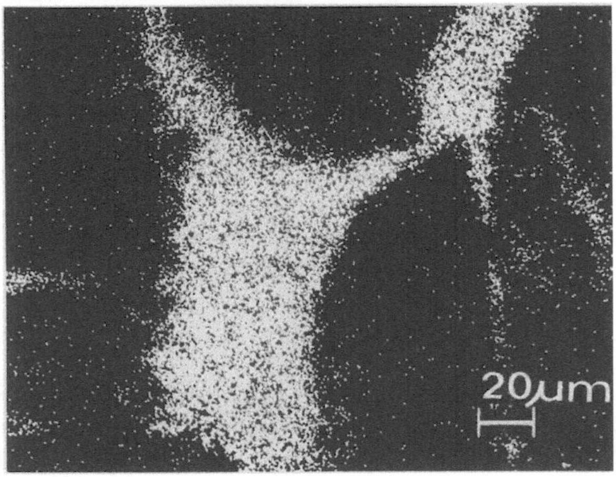

Fig. 59. Calcium distribution from Fig. 57. Ca-K_α radiation, 50 sec (PET crystal)

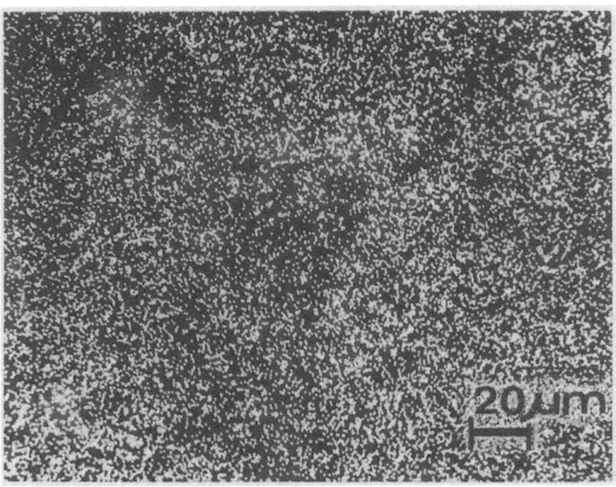

Fig. 60. Phosphorus distribution from Fig. 57. P-K radiation, 100 sec (RAP crystal)

61 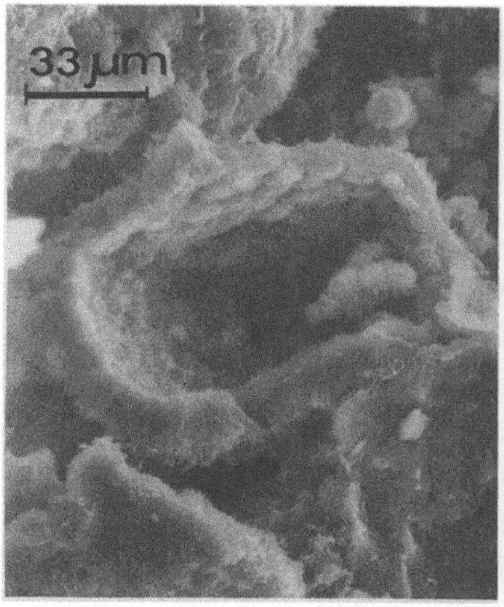

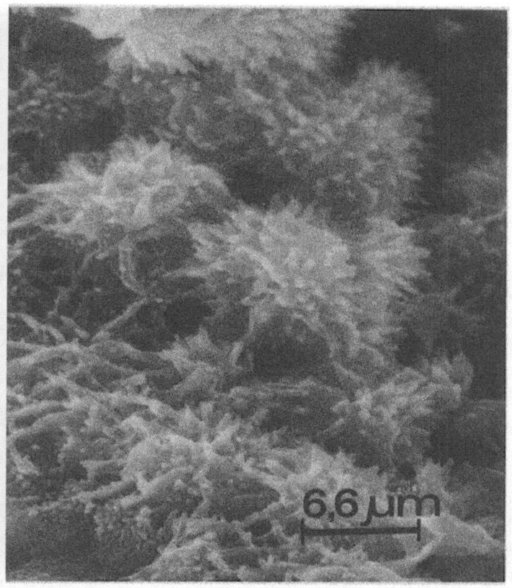 62

Figs. 61 and **62.** Spheroliths of ammonium dihydrogenurate needles matted into dense aggregates (SEM)

f) Brushite

A fan configuration is characteristic of the texture of brushite (Figs. 63, 64) (ARMBRUSTER 1978; BERG et al. 1978b; CIFUENTES DELATTE et al. 1978a; GEBHARDT 1980; SZABO 1974).

The overall crystal configuration may consist of a loose aggregate of fine spicules or plates arranged in spherolithic rosettes.

ARMBRUSTER (1978), BERG et al. (1978b), CIFUENTES DELATTE (1978), DOSCH and KOESTEL (1975), HESSE et al. (1979a) and SZABO (1974) have all given detailed morphologic descriptions.

Columns of fused crystals are sometimes to be found either radiating out from the center of the calculus or in parallel bands with their long axis arranged along the direction of stone growth (Figs. 63, 65). Rhythmic increase coupled with inclusions of whewellite and apatite may impose upon the overall structure a concentric year-ring character. Crystal aggregates fan out from the center and may even reach the outermost limit of a concretion. Communications by ARMBRUSTER (1978), BERG et al. (1976d) and by CIFUENTES DELATTE (1978) all demonstrate that the formation and eventual magnitude of brushite granules crystallizing out of weakly acid hypercalciuric and hyperphosphaturic urine is chiefly determined by the urinary magnesium concentration. According to CIFUENTES DELATTE (1978) layers of octacalcium phosphate sporadically encountered at the base of brushite crystals are to be regarded as transformation products of brushite.

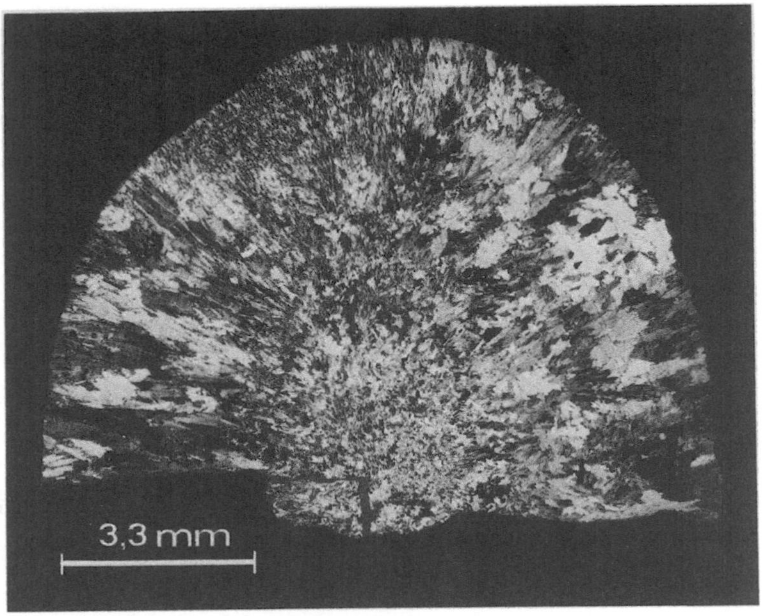

Fig. 63. Coarse fan texture of radiating brushite crystals (crossed polarizers)

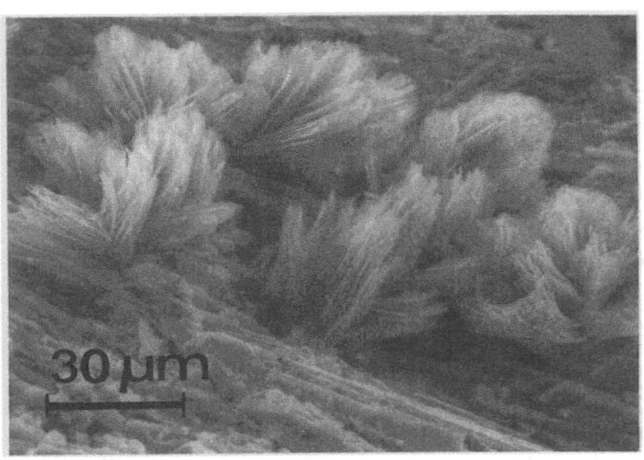

Fig. 64. Brushite spheroliths in fan configuration (SEM)

g) Cystine

Cystine calculi are usually of high purity. However, DOSCH (1975a) has drawn attention to substantial proportions of macromolecular organic substances, HESSE et al. (1979a) have repeatedly observed inclusions of calcium oxalate monohydrate and DIMOPOULUS et al. (1983) sodium urate. Cystine has been characterised by BERG et al. (1978b), by CIFUENTES DELATTE et al. (1973b) and by SZABO (1974) as consisting of fine hexagonal crystal plates which may be seen in thin section to assume either a coarsely radial texture or to lie in a mosaic configuration without any obvious nucleus. The scanning electron microscope reveals a degree of directionally orientated fusion between some crystals as well as a staggered staircase layering of others in all gradations right up to hexagonal columns (Fig. 66a, b).

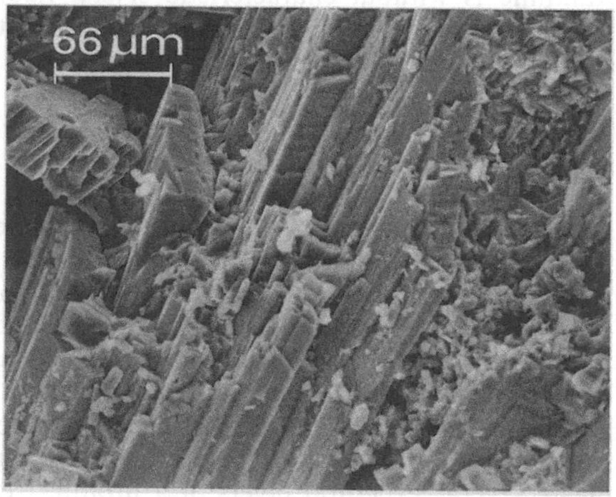

Fig. 65. Brushite columns in parallel arrangement (SEM)

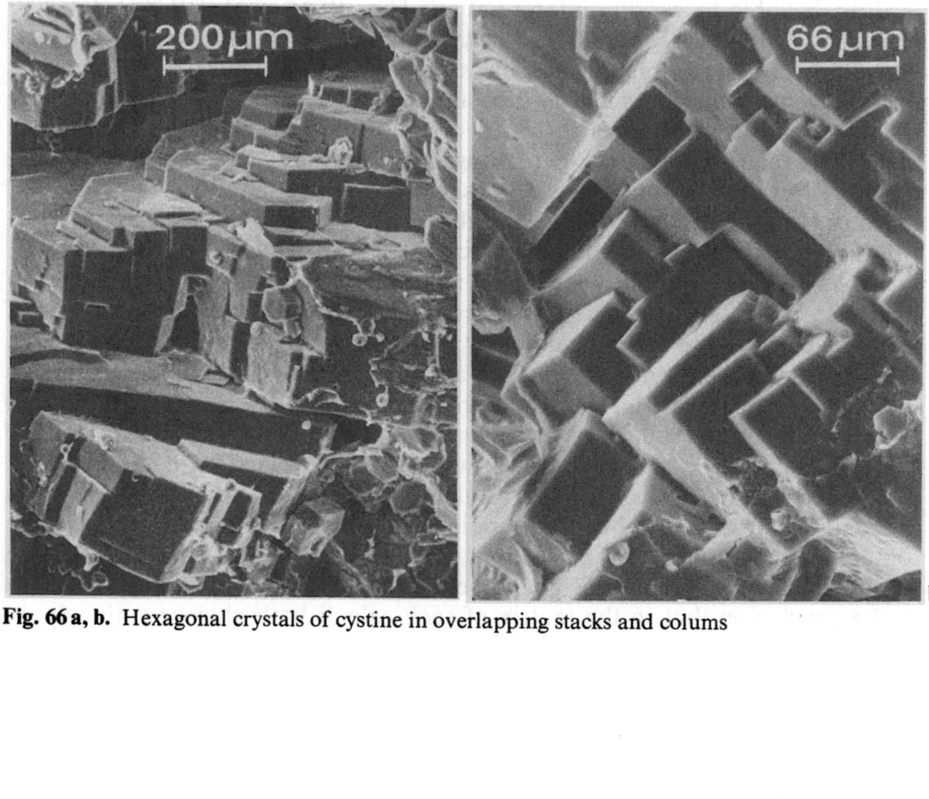

Fig. 66 a, b. Hexagonal crystals of cystine in overlapping stacks and colums

h) Xanthine

Xanthine has rarely been demonstrated to be a urolith phase, and as a consequence there are scanty data for its microscopic characterization. Berg et al. (1978 b) and Szabo (1974) have reported polarizing microscopic studies on thin sections of xanthine. The substance was markedly birefringent with a deep brownish-yellow pigmentation analogous to that of uric acid and the urates. Its aggregation behaviour is characterized by a fine grain densely-packed texture. Xanthine is without characteristic crystal habit under the scanning electron microscope and is strongly reminiscent of apatite gel deposits (Fig. 67) (Hesse et al. 1979 a; Pinto 1976).

i) Organic Matrix

According to Boyce (1973) organic macromolecules make up approximately 2 – 3% w/w of the phase composition of uroliths. Topooptic scrutiny by Szabo-Földvary and Modis (1980, 1981, 1984) of chemical reactions, and scanning electron microscopic studies by Dosch and Koestel (1975), Gebhardt (1975), Krampitz and Goetz (1984), Pinto (1976) and Rao and Argaval (1979) have confirmed these macromolecular organic substances (glycoproteins and glucose aminoglycans) as consisting of a three-dimensional filamentous network or honeycombed structure of variable regularity. This system may permeate several structural layers of a urolith, frequently forming broad fibrous sheets parallel to the mineral layers, or giving rise to amorphous sheaths around crystal aggregates (Fig. 68). The role of this film formation in the production of uroliths is liable to varying interpretation. Thus Berg et al. (1978 a), Cavero (1972), v. Philipsborn (1958) and Warpehoski et al. (1980) speak of coincidental adsorption of organic substances without any recognizable influence on overall events. This statement is substantiated by a variety of work including electron microscopic studies in which organic filaments are found in a completely irregular arrangement, pervading idiomorphous weddellite crystals, and organic films may be found in a gel ensheathing whole sequences of crystal aggregates (Fig. 69). On the other hand these macromolecules possess characteristic functional groups in their chemical structure (Malek and Boyce 1977; Pinto 1980) which render them capable of mineralization. This in turn leads to the assumption that organic substances might represent the starting point of urolithogenesis. Thin section studies by Kolpakow (1971) and Seyfarth et al. (1974) provide some evidence for such an alternative role of organic substances in urolith formation (Fig. 32). Color reaction studies by Hilman (1979) and Szabo and Modis (1980, 1981) are in agreement with this concept, to the extent that organic matrix occurred preferentially in apatite and with marked preponderance in struvite calculi. An originating role of reactive moieties within the matrix may therefore be important in the formation of infective calculi. The topooptically most intensive reactions took place on the surface of struvite stones. Analysis of the optical phenomena in demineralized thin sections leads to the conclusion that in the matrix of such calculi both glucose aminoglycan

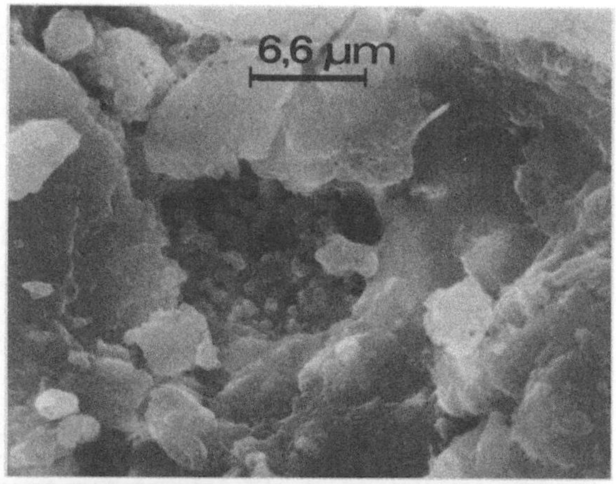

Fig. 67. Xanthine, deposited mainly but uncharacteristically as a gel (SEM)

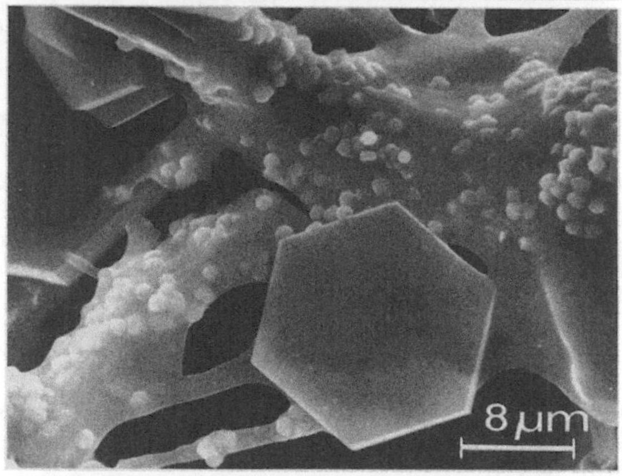

Fig. 68. Three-dimensional network structure of high molecular weight organic matrix clearly demonstrating mineralisation. In the center a hexagonal cystine crystal (SEM)

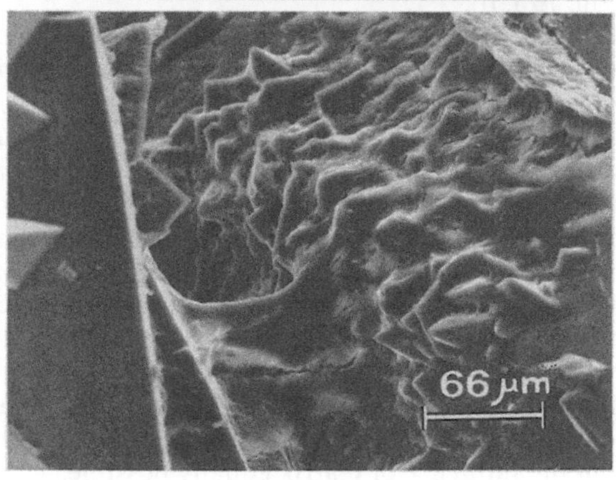

Fig. 69. Weddellite crystals coated in organic tissue (SEM)

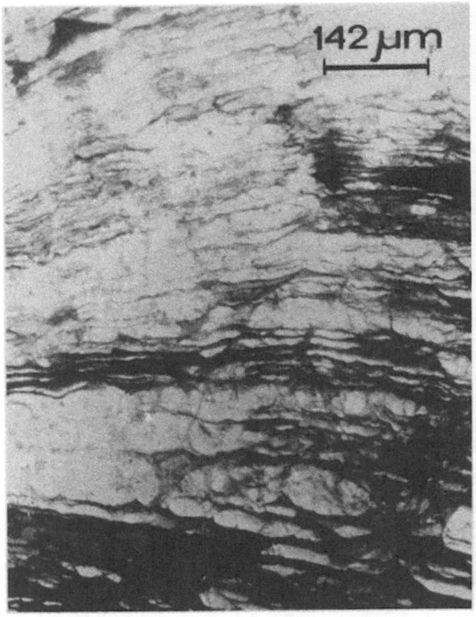

a

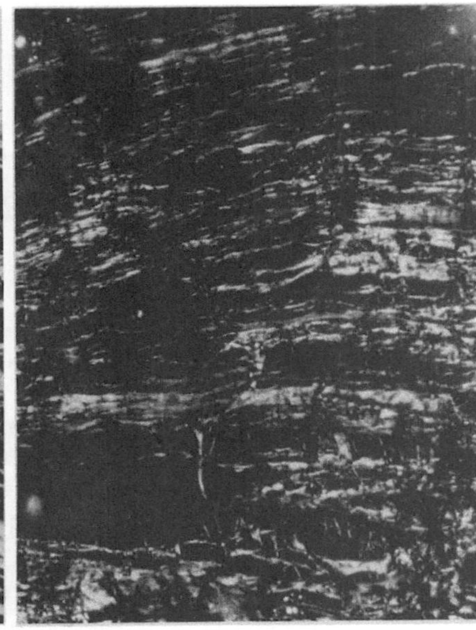
b

Fig. 70 a, b. Topooptic staining of organic matrix with dimethylmethylene blue and pseudoisocyanine in a decalcified thin section of whewellite. **a** Uncrossed polarizers. **b** Crossed polarizers. Birefringence (pale zones) within the matrix corresponds to the orderly extensively lamellar structure of glucose aminoglycans. (Photographs kindly provided by Dr. SZABO-FÖLDVARI, Debrecen)

chains and the oligosaccharide side-chains of glycoproteins are arranged parallel to the filamentous structure of calculi as seen in the optical microscope (see Fig. 70a, b).

The EDTA insoluble fraction may be studied by conventional microscopy to yield information on the nature and precise location of matrix in the interior of stones (KHAN et al. 1983, 1984).

The question raised by BORGNO and PEROLINO (1962) of crystallization in obstructive and non-obstructive urine may be important in any discussion of the role of organic macromolecules. The most important criterion by which this urolithogenic initiator function is postulated remains the capacity for mineralization by calcium phosphate. This property would allow directional growth of urolith phases with an influence on architecture and aggregation behaviour of the emergent stone (BERNSHTAM and PINTO 1976; EL-SAYED and COSSLETT 1977; KOIDE et al. 1977; PINTO 1973, 1976, 1980; SPECTOR et al. 1976). RAO and ARGAVAL (1979) have described such directional crystallization around filamentous matrix moieties, although these authors consider crystallization without the influence of matrix equally possible.

Studies by MALEK and BOYCE (1977) suggest that primary mineralization may occur even at the mitochondrial level within the nephron. Their studies also confirm a relationship between apatite and matrix. In the same connection RESNICK (1984) and RESNICK and BOYCE (1978) have dicussed the role of spheroidal corpuscles of calcium-polysaccharide-protein complexes as primary matrix components in actively stone-forming urines, and they draw a comparison to calcification products of the proximal and distal renal tubule.

The interaction between matrix and nucleation has been ably demonstrated in matrix calculi by KOIDE et al. (1977). A coarsely fibrous reticule beset with submicroscopic deposits of calcium phosphate and struvite appears to form a supporting archwork throughout the calculus. By acting as a crystal "captor" such a network structure could conceivably have a urolithogenic function.

SEM studies of calcium oxalate stones by OGBUIJI and FINLAYSON (1981) suggest that matrix ensures cohesion between individual crystallites. RODGERS (1981 a) also discusses organic substances acting as cements during the formation and aggregation of uroliths.

The finding of osseous tissue within growth nuclei also underlines the initiator role of macromolecular organic substances (CIFUENTES DELATTE et al. 1973a, 1976).

Such a role is however contradicted by the concentric integration of organic substance within the layered structure of a variety of aggregate configurations, as discussed by WARPEHOSKI et al. (1980) and HAHNE and EISMANN (1979). These appearances suggest deposition across growth fronts leading to rhythmic precipitation of crystallites and are strictly similar to the inclusion of apatite within calculi of concentrically conchoidal structure. Such a model also goes some way to explaining external morphological details and contours of calculi (BUSCEMI et al. 1981). According to studies by WARPEHOSKI et al. (1981) certain surface domains of whewellite calculi contain a mean of 5.7% proteins and carbohydrates whereas nuclear zones contain only 2.7%.

It may thus be seen that there may never be a simple positive or negative answer to the question of the role of organic macromolecules in urolithogenesis. Two mechanisms of formation – involving either primary crystallization or a specific role for ground substance (see also Apatite), and a variety of intermediate phenomena – are equally possible. Depending on the pathologic state of the urine and urinary tract these two mechanisms would vary in their relative causal significance (cf. Section V, 2a).

VI. Urolith Analysis

"I cannot forgo this opportunity to stress how undesirable it is for surgeons to seal up calculi in glass phials without investigating their chemical properties." (MARCET 1818).

This demand remains of equal importance today. Happily surgeons and patients alike increasingly appreciate the need to analyse every spontaneously passed or surgically removed stone.

The chemical analysis of uroliths must form the basis for any effective treatment or measures to prevent recurrence (BASTIAN and GEBHARDT 1976; SCHNEIDER and HESSE 1977; SCHNEIDER and HIENZSCH 1970). Amongst a multiplicity of clinical presentations the only factor common to all urolithiasis remains the

Table 12. Etiological classification of renal lithiasis in a series of 1936 patients (RAPADO et al. 1976)

Of known cause	No. of cases	%
Uric acid	250	13.0
Hypercalciuria	213	11.1
Urinary infections	191	9.9
Urologic malformation	87	4.4
Alkali abuse	57	2.9
Hyperparathyroidism	54	2.7
Cystinuria	21	1.1
Metabolic bone disease	19	1.0
Hyperoxaluria	8	0.4
Renal tubular acidosis	6	0.3
Xanthinuria	1	–
Idiopathic lithiasis	1029	53.2

Table 13. Methods of urolith analysis compared (ASPER and SCHMUCKI 1980)

	Method				
	Chemical analysis	Polarizing microscopy	Thermo-analysis	IR-spectro-scopy	X-ray diffrac-tion
Specificity	Ions	Substance structure	Substance	Substance group	Substance structure
Identification of unknown substances	?	?	?	?	+
Point analysis	?	+	?	+	+
Average analysis	+	–	+	+	+
Semiquantitative analysis	–	–	?	+	+
Limiting sensitivity (%)	$\ll 1$	?	10	10	<10
Minimal sample (mg)	10	$\ll 1$	20	5	1
Differentiates between					
– Oxalates	–	+	+	?	+
– Urates	–	–	+	+	+
– Phosphates	–	+	+	?	+
Identification of amorphous apatite	–	–	+	+	–
Semi-skilled personnel	–	–	(+)	+	+
Man hours (min)	15	30	30	15	5
Equipment utilization (min)	(15)	30	200	20	5
Samples/technician/day	30	15	4	20	80
Capital investment (×1,000 Fr.)	1	5	50	40	60
Amortisation time (years)	5	20	10	15	20
Cost (Fr./Stone reported)	4	7	14	7	4

+ = always possible, (+) = conditionally possible, ? = possible with difficulty, – = impossible. Cost comparison based on 1,000 analyses/year.

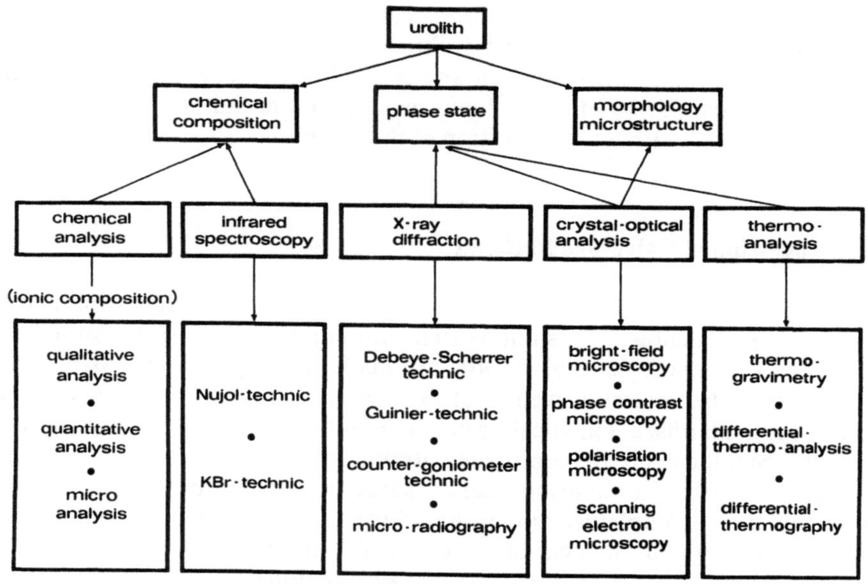

Fig. 71. Analytical methods applicable to uroliths

presence of a urine-derived solid phase somewhere within the urinary tract. The causes of stone formation (Table 12) are only apparent in about 50% of cases. The remainder have to be labelled as idiopathic. Only stone analysis, therefore, will provide any pointers as to the conditions of formation and requirements for prevention of further stones.

In 1973, 8 urologists were asked for their views on urolith analysis (ALKEN et al. 1973). They considered

1. Analysis of very individual stone to be essential.
2. Chemical analysis to be preferable to no analysis at all.
3. X-ray diffraction to be the most suitable technique.

The crystalline components of uroliths are an expression of certain characteristic chemical conditions in the urine from which they were formed. Urolith analysis is capable of mirroring these conditions.

Both DOSCH and ALTROCK (1974) and GEBHARDT (1979b) have given a detailed description of the analytical power and technical requirements of various techniques. Fig. 71 (SCHNEIDER and SEYFARTH 1980) gives a synopsis, and the various methods are also compared in Table 13.

1. Qualitative Chemical Analysis

Chemical analysis of urinary stones is the oldest technique, having been recommended as long ago as 1860 by HELLER in largely the same form as still employed with minor modifications in most countries of the world (BACH et al.

1977; BURRIEL et al. 1969; ESTABAN et al. 1969; KLEEBERG 1968; KOLLWITZ 1968; KREUTZMANN and ECKE 1971; SINGH et al. 1969). The method enjoys the advantage of being practicable in any clinical laboratory, the difficulty being that correct estimation of individual ions does not permit any conclusive statement about actual phase composition of the calculus.

a) Processing of Calculous Material

Analytical accuracy is strongly dependent on preliminary processing and sampling of the calculus. The stone is first thoroughly rinsed with distilled water, dried and weighed. Careful records are made of weight, color, shape, surface and fracture behaviour as well as of the degree of separation into shell and nucleus. A standardised analytical protocol permits automatic data logging (DOSCH 1975b). Small calculi are completely ground up and part of the powder so produced is subjected to analysis. Larger stones are sawn through in the middle, one half being completely ground up whilst the other acts as a source of individual samples from nuclear and recognizable individual shell regions. Part of the material should be held back for re-examination.

b) Analytic Procedure

The standard analytic procedure is given in Fig. 72. A preliminary sample is reduced to ash in order to distinguish between organic and inorganic calculi. If the sample is combusted without residue the stone was organic, and a variety of reactions are employed for the detection of uric acid and urates, xanthine and cystine. Any residue will be of calcium oxalate or phosphate and oxalate, magnesium, calcium, phosphate, ammonium and carbonate are then tested for. In the light of their experience in analysing 1300 calculi KREUTZMANN and ECKE (1971) have opted to omit incineration and the carbonate reaction.

Chemical analysis has been rendered considerably simpler by the appearance on the commercial market of customized sets of reagents and test combinations for urolith analysis (e.g. Temmler urolith analysis reagents, Merckognost, Oxford Reagents, Renal Calculi and others). MAURER (1976) has been extensively involved in the development of these sets of reagents and has also drawn attention to their weaknesses (SCHNEIDER 1976). Their requirement for relatively large quantities of test material is a distinct disadvantage, since at least half of all calculi weigh less than 25 mg, and there is considerable variation in the reliability of individual test reactions. Calculi weighing less than 10 mg cannot be examined by these methods (BRÜCKNER and BERNSTEIN 1979).

The rapid microtechnique of VISKELETY (1965) or LASKOWSKI (1965) may be suitable for very small calculi or minute samples from individual layers within a stone. These techniques involve microscopic observation of reactions taking place on a slide. The microanalyses put forward by MAURER (1969) or REDINGER (1970) also only require a sample of a few milligrams.

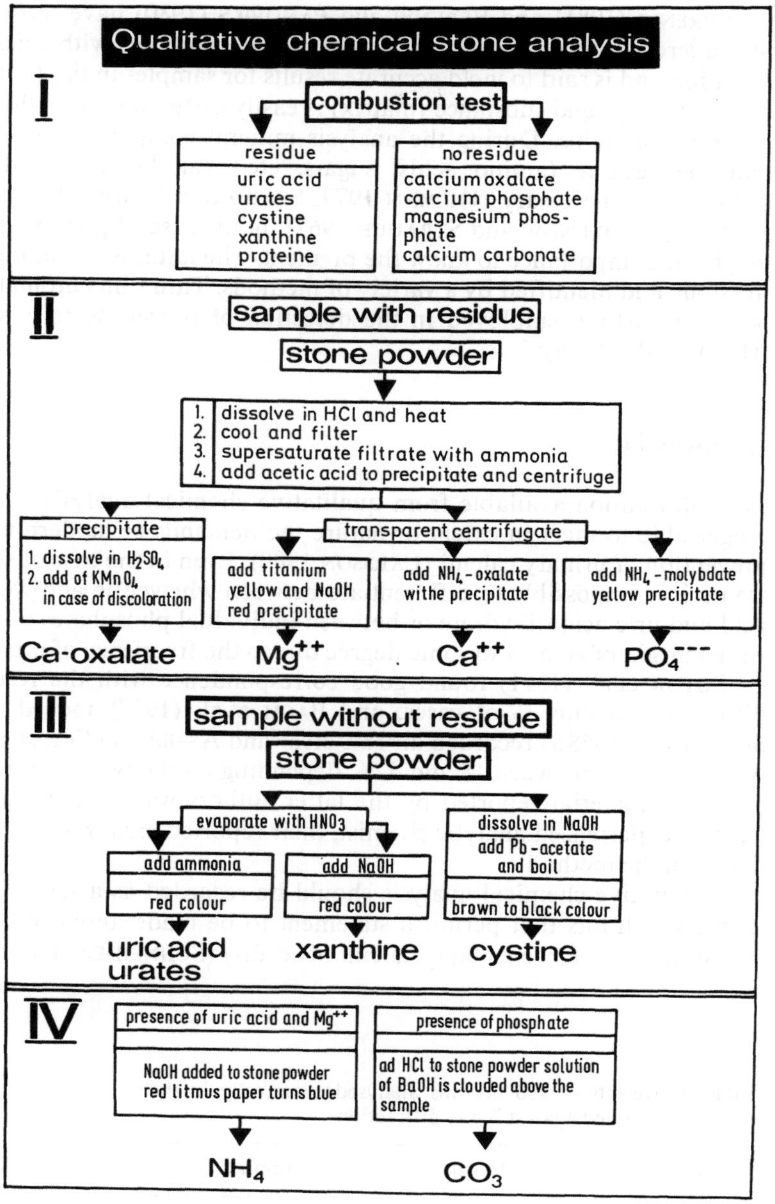

Fig. 72. Protocol for qualitative chemical analysis (SCHNEIDER et al. 1973b)

BERENYI (1981) and BERENYI and PANOVICS (1980) have recommended an ultramicrochemical analysis technique which combines with microscopic observation and is said to yield accurate results for samples in the 1 – 10 µg range.

Organic ground substance (matrix) is easily distinguished in thin sections by a variety of stains. During the analysis mineral components are dissolved so that the residue (amino acids, sugars, etc.) can be estimated, by microtechniques if necessary (HILMAN 1979; SZABO and MODIS 1980, 1981; WATANABE 1972; WILLNOW and STRAUCH 1967). In the case of pigment stones it may be of some importance to know the pigment. The latter is therefore eluted from the stone and identified by a variety of methods. Thin film chromatography has been successfully employed in the detection of purpurine in a reddish stone (HESSE et al. 1974a).

c) Discussion

The information available from qualitative chemical analysis is nowadays no longer able to meet in extent or nature the demands of modern treatment and prevention of urinary calculi (LARSSON 1980). Even in the case of so-called pure stones it is impossible to differentiate between whewellite and weddellite, uric acid and uric acid dihydrate or between individual phosphates of calcium. The wide margin of error is to some degree due to the frequency of mixed calculi.

SUTOR et al. (1971) found good correspondence with the results of X-ray diffraction in only ⅔ of cases, and BACH et al. (1977) indeed in only 57%. SCHNEIDER (1968a) recorded an 18% error and ASPER and SCHMUCKI (1980) reported rates of between 18 and 42%, depending on the type of stone (Table 14). Since the material reported by the latter authors was all examined by an extremely experienced analytic chemist, their reported error rate is likely to be inherent in the method.

Qualitative chemical analysis should be regarded as a screening tool, with theoretical limits that permit a statement to be made about 50% of all stones (i.e. sufficiently large primary calculi of adults) (SCHNEIDER et al. 1985).

Table 14. Results of 150 uroliths analysed chemically in the wet and controlled against X-ray diffraction

Substance	Result	Number	%
Phosphate	False-positive	81	54
	False-negative	1	1
Oxalate	False-positive	5	3
	False-negative	5	7
Uric acid	False-positive	3	2
	False-negative	1	1
Calcium carbonate	False-positive	15	10

2. Quantitative Chemical Analysis

Quantitative chemical analytical methods are employed in the detection of major- and trace elements and of organic compounds. The technique is able to give exact information on certain components involved in the make-up of uroliths (ESTEBAN et al. 1969; HODGKINSON 1971; SCHNEIDER 1969b; THOMAS et al. 1978; WESTBURY 1974).

a) Sample Processing

A mixed sample of approximately 500 mg powdered calculus is dessicated at 105 ° C until the weight is constant and reduced to ash at 550 ° C in a muffle. The ash is weighed and dissolved in hydrochloric acid, in which form it may be stored (Fig. 73).

b) Analytic Procedure

Major and trace elements are estimated in the hydrochloric acid decoction and given in g or mg/kg dry weight. Special techniques suitable for the estimation of trace elements are atomic absorption spectroscopy and mass spectroscopy. In terms of ash, phosphate and magnesium content alone it has been possible to characterize 5 categories of calculus (Fig. 74).

c) Discussion

This quantitative technique is too laborious for routine urolith analysis. It remains of value in comparative studies and for research purposes.

A new method for quantitative chemical analysis in the wet has been described by LARSSON (1984), who also discusses the principles of calculating results and mass recovery by algorithm. Calcium, magnesium, ammonium, phosphate, oxalate, uric acid, cystine and protein are individually determined and the total mass recovery calculated on a microcomputer.

3. X-Ray Diffraction

Since uroliths are chiefly composed of crystalline material, various modifications of the X-ray diffraction technique are suitable for the study of urinary calculi. In recent years X-ray diffraction has indeed become the method of choice.

The London group headed by Dame KATHLEEN LONSDALE has over the past 20 years published a large volume of material (HERRING 1962; LONSDALE 1969; LONSDALE and MASON 1966; LONSDALE and SUTOR 1969; LONSDALE et al. 1968a, b; SUTOR and WOOLEY 1970, 1971, 1972a, 1974a, 1975; SUTOR et al. 1974).

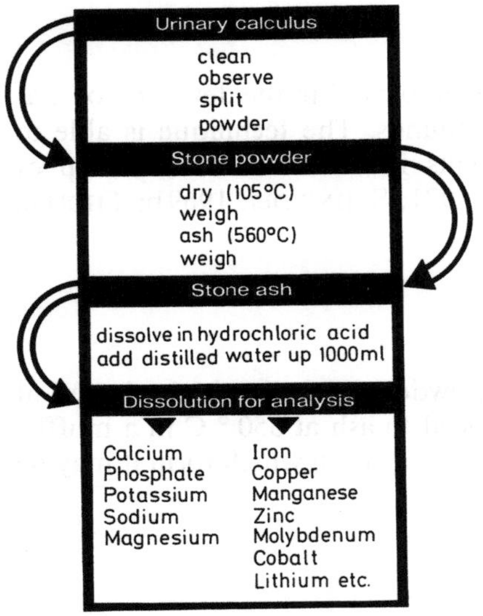

Fig. 73. Protocol for quantitative chemical stone analysis (SCHNEIDER et al. 1973b)

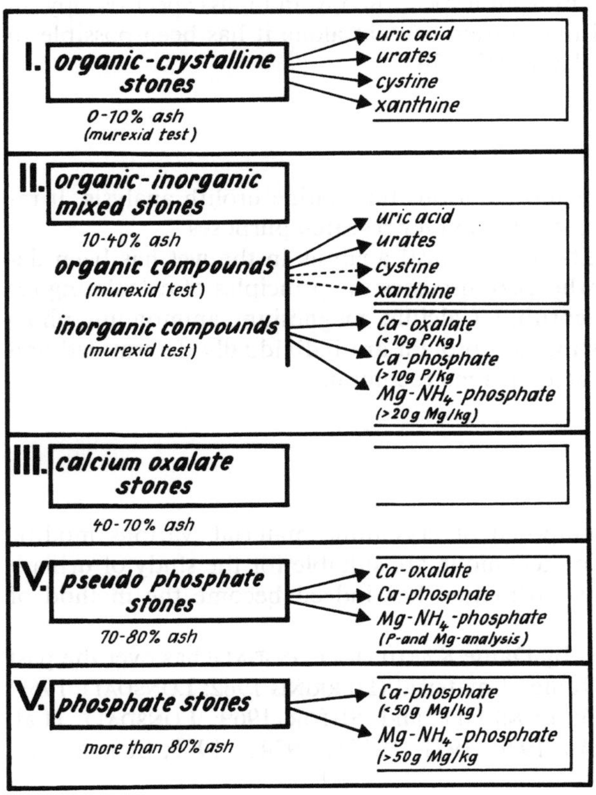

Fig. 74. Classification of calculi according to their composition on quantitative chemical analysis (SCHNEIDER et al. 1973b)

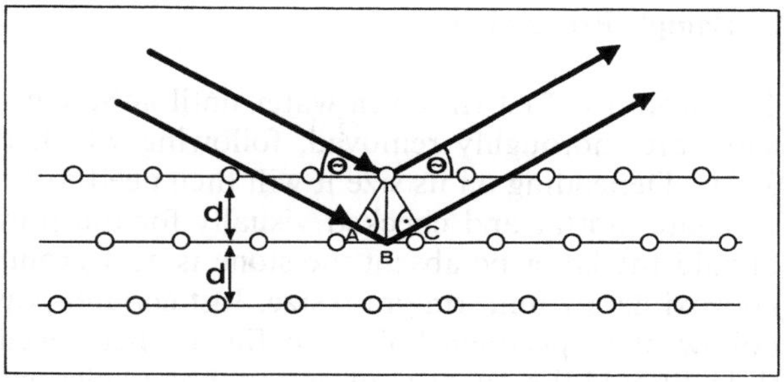

Fig. 75. X-ray diffraction by lattice plane boundaries. Diagram explaining the derivation of the Bragg equation

The techniques employed were those of Debye-Scherrer, Guinier and the goniometer method, all of which yield both qualitative and quantitative results (BAER et al. 1972; BRIEN and BRAUN 1973; CIFUENTES DELATTE et al. 1967; GEBHARDT and BASTIAN 1975; GÖTZ 1974; HESSE and BACH 1982; KAZOHIKO et al. 1983; KOSLOWSKI 1973; LAGERGREN 1961; MATOUSCHEK and HERRIG 1967; MORRIS and BEELER 1967; OTNES 1983; SCHNEIDER and HESSE 1973; SCHNEIDER et al. 1970a, b, 1974a, b).

a) Basic Principle

Whenever monochromatic X-ray impinge on the crystal lattice of a urolith component diffraction will occur at certain defined lattice planes. Suitable monochromatic rays are generated by filtering out the K_β-rays from a copper anode X-ray tube, leaving only K_α-radiation ($Cu_{K\alpha} = 0.1542$ nm). If this radiation passes through crystalline material, electrons of the atomic shell interact with the electromagnetic waves leading to X-ray diffraction and the generation of interference patterns (Fig. 75). The Bragg equation gives a direct relationship between the diffraction angle θ and the "d-value".

$$n \times \lambda = 2\,d \text{ sine } \theta,$$

n = order (1, 2 etc.), λ = wave length (nm), d = lattice plane interval (nm), θ = diffraction angle (°).

Diffraction angle is thus determined by crystal lattice structure and, like the d-values is specific at a constant wave length for substance and crystal type. For known wave length and lattice plane interval the intensity of a given diffraction ray may be compared to that in the diffraction pattern of reference substances (ASTM Index 1971), thus yielding quantitative and qualitative data on urolith samples.

Any given urolith phase is characterised by a multitude of interference effects which are substance specific in position and intensity.

b) Sample Processing

The urolith is first rinsed in water until adherent urine, blood and tissue remnants are thoroughly removed, following which the calculus is desiccated at 38 °C. Depending on its size it will then need to be sawn up or broken down in an agate mortar and checked visually for the presence of a layered structure. Should the latter be absent the stone is next ground to a crystalline powder of approximately uniform grain size. Just enough powder is then deposited in the hollow of a specimen holder to fill it when levelled with a glass microscope slide. Should the quantity of material be inadequate, a carefully roughened flat specimen support may be used and the sample firmly pressed onto it (aliquots of less than 10 mg).

Where a layered structure was noted within the urolith, representative samples will need to be taken from individual layers and treated as above, the layers being labelled from within outwards as nucleus and shell, or shells 1 and 2 respectively. Following individual analysis the test material is returned to the whole and a representative specimen of the entire calculus analysed.

In the Debye-Scherrer technique powdered calculus is inserted into a radiolucent capillary tube which is then fastened to the Debye-Scherrer camera and accurately centered.

c) Exposure Techniques

The exact type of equipment used for X-ray diffraction analysis of uroliths varies from country to country, so that individual apparatus will not be described in great detail. Modern instruments are extensively automated, being provided with mechanical sample transport and with computing equipment.

α) Debye-Scherrer Technique

Once the capillary tube of ground calculus has been carefully centered in the beam (inadequate attention to this leads to broadening of the interference rings on the emulsion) the camera is loaded with film under darkroom conditions and attached to the X-ray tube. The film is then exposed, the time required being specific to the individual apparatus. Figure 76 shows the X-ray beam pathway in the Debye-Scherrer apparatus, whilst Figs. 77a, b demonstrate the diffraction diagrams of major urolith components.

β) Guinier Technique

This method is characterized by extremely high resolving power and excellent sharpness of interference lines (SEIFERT and GEBHARDT 1979).The interference pattern of low intensity peaks is still recognizable even if they lie close together, but this excellent resolution is only achieved by the use of strictly monochromatic radiation and careful focussing of the interference pattern on the film

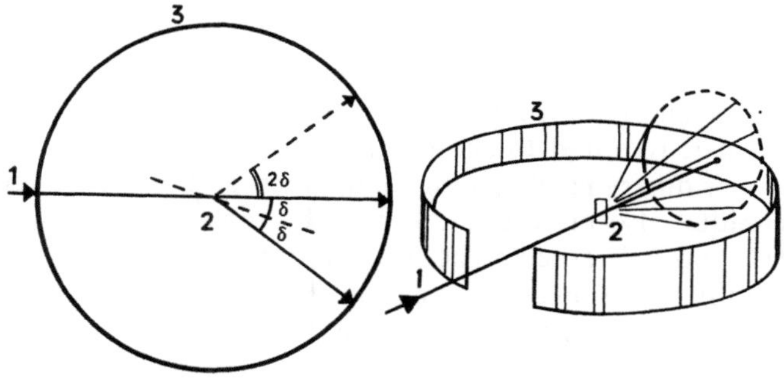

Fig. 76. X-ray beam path for Debye-Scherrer technique (SCHNEIDER et al. 1974b). *1* = X-ray beam, *2* = Specimen, *3* = X-ray film

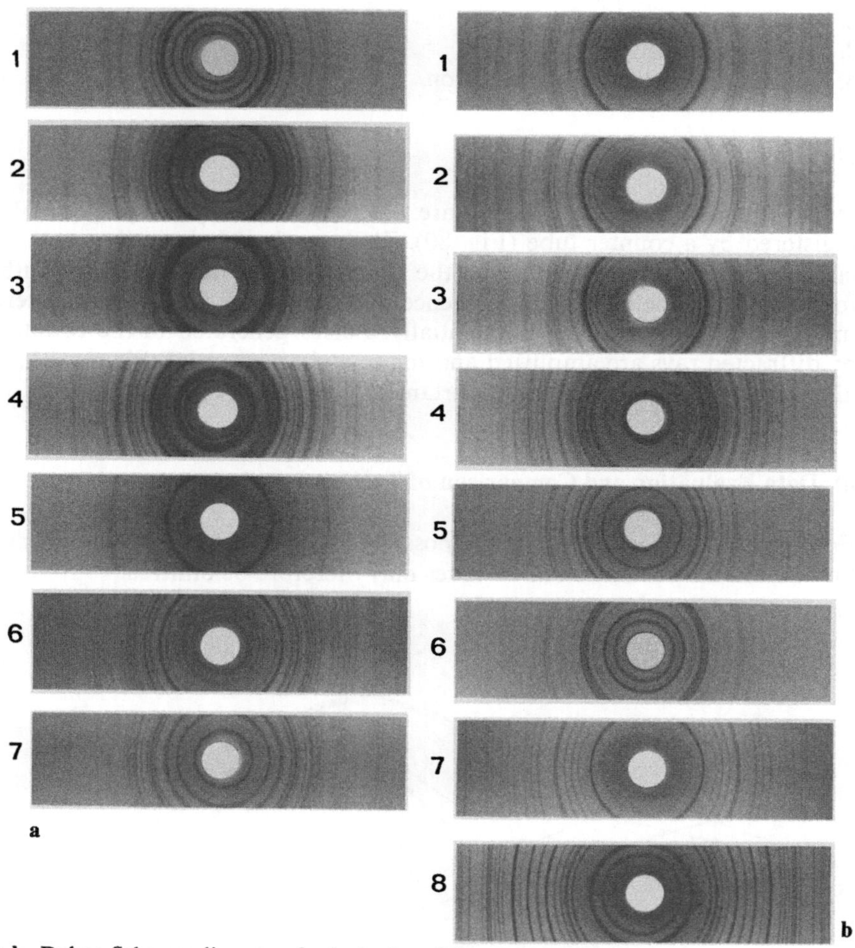

Fig. 77 a, b. Debye-Scherrer diagram of principal urolith components
a *1* = Uric acid, *2* = Uric acid dihydrate, *3* = Ammonium dihydrogenurate, *4* = Cystine, *5* = Xanthine, *6* = Weddellite, *7* = Whewellite
b *1* = Whitlockite, *2* = Hydroxyapatite, *3* = Dhallite, *4* = Newberyite, *5* = Brushite, **6** = Struvite, *7* = Calcium carbonate, *8* = Silicon dioxide

plane. The beam is usually rendered monochrome by the insertion of a thin sheet of quartz in front of the GUINIER chamber (Fig. 78). Careful sample processing is required to achieve a fine grain in the test specimen. Fig. 79 gives Guinier diagrams of urolith components and reference substances. The Guinier technique also permits the film to be replaced by a counter tube (GEBHARDT 1979a), which executes both a rotatory movement around its own axis and a carefully synchronised translation. The specimen is kept at a fixed point for all values of diffraction angle and remains in strict orientation to the primary beam.

This technique has the following advantages over the Debye-Scherrer method:
1. Improved resolving power
2. Smaller sample size
3. Increased intensity of reflection
4. Facilities for measuring absorption.

γ) Diffractometer Technique

In this method diffracted X-rays are not recorded on photographic film but registered by a counter tube (Fig. 80). The sample is held in the center of the circular field of measurement and the counter tube rotates around it with two-fold angular velocity. The interference pattern is now no longer registered simultaneously but recorded sequentially. Pulses generated in the counter tube by diffracted rays are amplified and fed to a chart recorder. Figures 81 a and b give goniometric diagrams of important urolith components.

d) Data Evaluation and Comparison of Techniques

Four routine clinical purposes the possible range of urolith components will be known and the estimation of d-values may therefore be omitted.

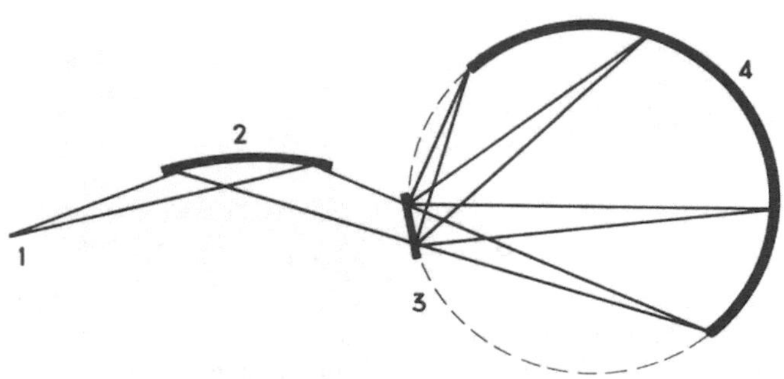

Fig. 78. X-ray beam path in Guinier technique (SCHNEIDER et al. 1974b). *1* = X-ray tube, *2* = Monochromator, *3* = Specimen, *4* = X-ray film

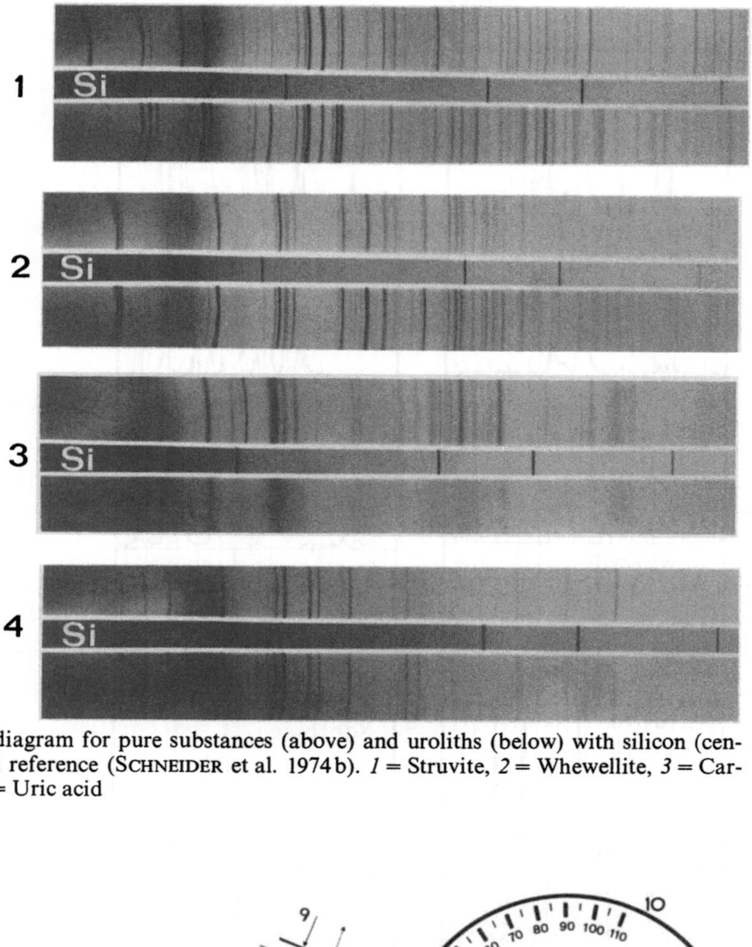

Fig. 79. Guinier diagram for pure substances (above) and uroliths (below) with silicon (center) as an internal reference (SCHNEIDER et al. 1974b). *1* = Struvite, *2* = Whewellite, *3* = Carbonate apatite, *4* = Uric acid

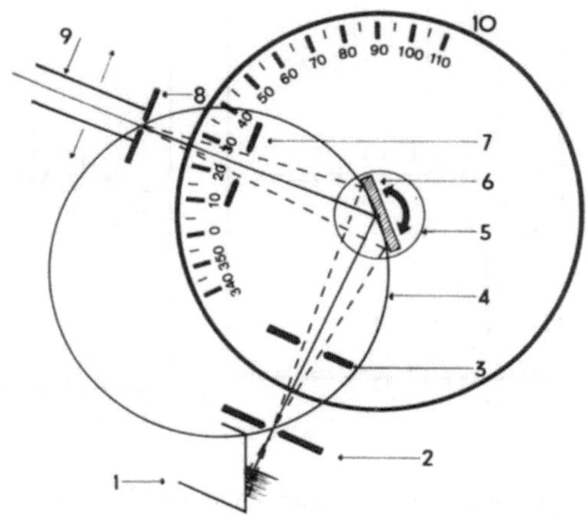

Fig. 80. X-ray beam path in counter goniometer technique (SCHNEIDER et al. 1974b). *1* = X ray tube (pencil beam), *2* = Inlet diaphragm, *3* = Divergence diaphragm, *4* = Focussing arc, *5* = Specimen stage, *6* = Specimen, *7* = Anti-scatter diaphragm, *8* = Counter diaphragm, *9* = Counter tube, *10* = Scale

a

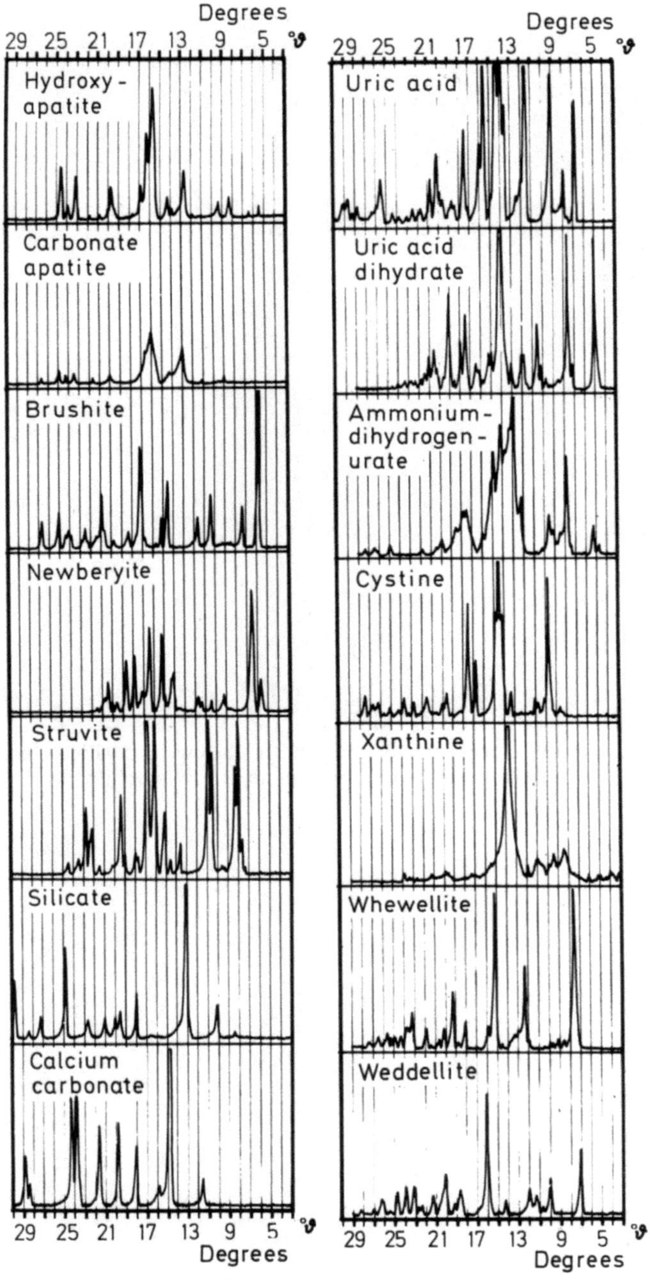

b

Fig. 81 a, b. Goniometer diagrams of principal urolith components

Debye-Scherrer films are interpreted by comparing them with films of chemically pure standards on an illuminated viewing box. The composition of mixed calculi is identified by comparison with serial mixtures of pure substances made up in steps of 10% by weight. Equally a transparent template may be made of pure substance diagrams and compared with the test material by superimposition.

Goniometer diagrams of so-called pure stones can also be identified by templates derived from the pulse density distribution of reference substances. This template method becomes inaccurate for mixed calculi and has to be replaced by analysis after NARAY-SZABO and PETER (1967) (Fig. 82).

$$X_A\,(\text{mole\%}) = \frac{I_A \times f_A}{I_A \times f_A + I_B \times f_B \ldots + I_N \times f_N},$$

X_A = mole% of component A
$I_A \ldots I_N \ldots$ Intensity of the pulse density peaks for components A ... N (height in mm)
$f_A \ldots f_N \ldots$ Reference factors for components A ... N.

The reference factors $f_A \ldots f_N$ are developed from mixtures of urolith reference substances and MgO as an internal standard. Their values are specific to the apparatus employed and characteristic for individual peaks found for each urolith component. They are calculated by the equation

$$f_{A \ldots N} = \frac{X_{A \ldots N} \times I_{MgO}}{X_{MgO} \times I_{A \ldots N}},$$

$X_{A \ldots N}$ mole% reference substance
X_{MgO} mole% MgO
$I_{A \ldots N}$ Amplitude of the pulse density peak characteristic for the reference substance (mm)
$I_{MgO} \ldots$ Amplitude of a pulse density peak for MgO (mm).

$I_A \ldots I_N$ are chosen to correspond to the most intense material – specific pulse density peaks that fail to coincide with other peaks derived from the analytical sample (Table 15).

At a constant angular velocity of 1°/min the whole analytical process including grinding up, processing, evaluating and recording data requires approximately 30 min/stone (REBENTISCH et al. 1981 b). It is convenient to state concentrations in phase mixtures in terms of mole%.

Indeed the eye alone is quite capable of estimating the molar proportions of a mixture from a comparison of the most intense analysis peaks. The main impetus to introducing mole percentages on a broad basic came from the high molar weights of struvite and carbonate apatite, whereas most other urolith phases, possessed of similar molecular weight, did not give rise to wide divergences between the values for mole% and %weight for weight.

The limits of analytical accuracy have been determined for the 7 most common 2- and 3-component mixtures in urinary calculi (REBENTISCH et al. 1981 a,

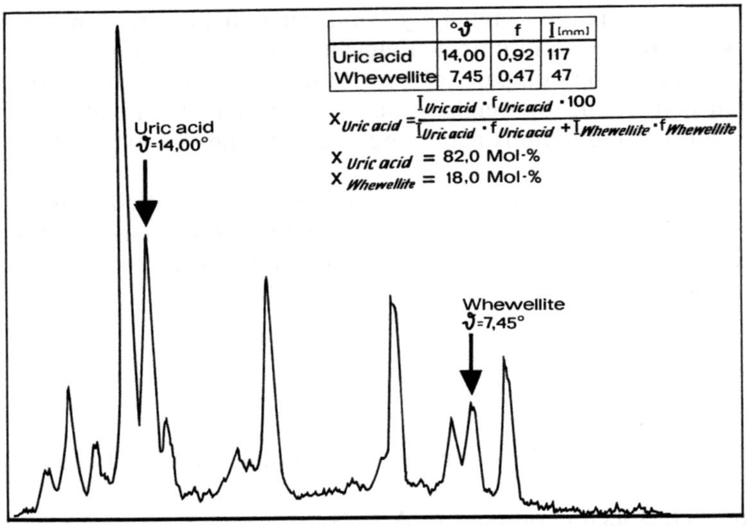

Fig. 82. X-ray diffraction map of a mixed uric acid-whewellite stone with sample Naray computation (SZABO and PETER 1967)

Table 15. Principle analytical peaks for characteristic urolith phases (REBENTISCH et al. 1981 a)

Urolith phase	θ (°)	d-Value (nm)
Whewellite (56.4%[a]) $CaC_2O_4 \cdot 1\ H_2O$	7.45 12.20 15.20	0.694 0.365 0.295
Weddellite (15.1%) $CaC_2O_4 \cdot 2\ H_2O$	7.15 16.15	0.619 0.277
Carbonate apatite (3.62%) $Ca_{4.75}(PO_4)_{2.65}(OH)_{0.85}(OH_3)_{0.35}$	13.00 15.95	0.342 0.280
Struvite (5.87%) $MgNH_4PO_4 \cdot 6\ H_2O$	8.00 10.95 16.85	0.536 0.406 0.266
Brushite (0.28%) $CaHPO_4 \cdot 2\ H_2O$	5.85	0.755
Uric acid (11.9%) $C_5H_4N_4O_3$	5.80 14.00 14.40	0.651 0.318 0.310
Uric acid dihydrate (3.07%) $C_5H_8N_4O_5$	5.05 10.55	0.875 0.421
Monoammonium urate (0.43%) $C_5H_7N_5O_3$	7.90 12.95	0.561 0.344
Monosodium urate $C_5H_7N_4O_5Na$	14.70	0.304
Cystine (0.22%) $C_6H_{12}O_4N_2S_2$	9.50	0.467
Magnesium oxide MgO	21.40	0.212

[a] The values in brackets indicate the relative frequency of each phase in a cohort of 50,000 analyses

c; REBENTISCH and BEYER 1983). These limits lie between 5 and 10 mole%, in the majority of cases ≤ 5 mole%. An analytical limit of 10 mole% for one component of mixed calculi appears adequate in present day diagnostic and therapeutic practice. Problems may nervertheless arise in differentiating phosphate phases. Brushite, struvite and newberyite are unequivocally distinct, whilst hydroxyapatite, carbonate apatite and whitlockite are often difficult to distinguish by X-ray diffraction (SCHUBERT 1981; SUTOR 1968a). Only carbonate apatite may be distinguished from the other members of the group by an additional hydrochloric acid test.

The occasionally poor crystallinity of phosphates also tends to obscure differences in their diffraction pattern. Several hours of tempering at 900° C are required to improve their degree of crystallinity, leading to sharper reflection patterns and more accurate separation of phases (DOSCH and ALTROCK 1974). Figure 83 shows the effect of tempering an apatite calculus. The process is not suitable for carbonate apatite from which carbon dioxide would be liberated, nor for mixed calculi within which reactions might take place between individual components (GEBHARDT 1979a).

DOSCH (1980a), whose knowledge of urolith analysis must be without parallel, considers X-ray diffraction to be the only acceptable method of phase analysis. Calculi of any size greater than 1 mg may be analysed with a minimum of preliminary preparation and an analytical accuracy in the region of 1 – 5% w/w for individual components.

DOSCH and ALTROCK (1974) have made up binary mixtures in the ratio 95:5 w/w employing whewellite, weddellite, hydroxyapatite, struvite, brushite and uric acid. The analytical accuracies obtained (both for X-ray diffraction and infra-red spectroscopy) are set out in Fig. 84. The effect of crystallinity on analytical power is particularly striking.

The effect on analytical accuracy of varying admixtures in the range 5 – 15% has been demonstrated by GEBHARDT and BASTIAN (1976a) in relation to a

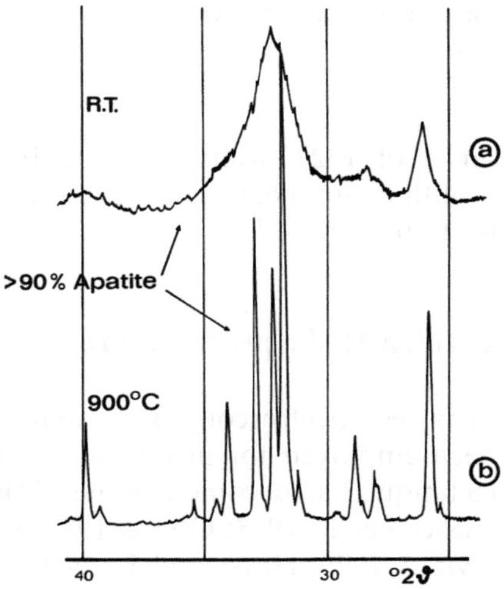

Fig. 83. a, b. Improved X-ray detection of apatite after tempering at 900 °C. Urolith containing > 90% apatite, **a** before and **b** after heating (DOSCH and ALTROCK 1974). R.T. = room temperature

Main components	Whewellite	Weddellite	Uric acid	Struvite	Brushite	Hydroxy-apatite poorly crystallized	Hydroxy-apatite well crystallized
Whew.		**3** 5 / no	**2,5** 7 / 4bd	**3** 3 / 1bd*	**2** 6 / 2bd	**25** / 1bd*	**5** 8
Ur. ac.	**1** 24 / no	**2,5** 26 / no		**2** 14 / no	**1** 27 / no	**25** / no	**5** 35
Struvite	**2,5** 9 / 2bd+*	**5** 10 / 2bd+*	**2,5** 2 / 2bd*		**1** 11 / no	**50_K** / no	**20_K** 15
Brushite	**3** 4 / no	**3** 5 / no	**3** 7 / 7bd	**5** 2 / no		**15** / no	**5** 7
Apatite	**3** 3 / 2bd+*	**5** 3 / 2bd+*	**3** 0,5 / 2bd+*	**5** 2 / no	**5** 4 / no		
μ (cm^2g^{-1})	55,0	50,2	8,4	26,5	60,3	87,4	

+ = IR-bands of Whewellite and Weddellite identical
* = IR-bands of struvite and apatite identical

Fig. 84. Binary mixtures of six principal urolith components. The numbers in heavy print give the minimum quantities of secondary components in % w/w, which are still just detectable in the presence of each principal component. The numbers to the right of the heavy print give the percentage intensity of X-ray interference still recordable in mixtures of which the secondary component constitutes 5%. The box below each heavy printed numeral gives information on infra-red spectrographic detectability, relating to binary mixtures with 5% secondary components (DOSCH and ALTROCK 1974)

Table 16. Percentage frequency of urolith components for varying analytic accuracy (n = 1327 calculi) (GEBHARDT and BASTIAN 1976a)

Type of stone	Patients each impurity level		
	5%	10%	15%
Oxalate stones	40.02	47.63	50.41
Phosphate stones	17.70	18.84	19.52
Uric acid stones	6.64	8.60	9.04
Mixed uric acid-oxalate stones	8.14	2.79	1.43
Mixed oxalate-phosphate stones	16.05	15.07	13.79
Mixed phosphate-oxalate stones	1.89	1.66	0.98

series of 1327 uroliths (Table 16). The distribution of the more important urolith components varies according to frequency of occurrence and mass proportion (Table 17).

4. Infra-Red Spectroscopy

Infra-red spectroscopy is an analytical technique of proven value, having first been employed for urolith analysis by BEISCHER (1955). In the meantime the technique has become routine (ADRIAN 1972; ARNOLD and SEEMAN 1968; BELLANATO et al. 1973; CORNS 1983; FREYE and CHAN 1972; GARCIA-CUERPO and AVILLA 1979; HESSE and KLEE 1974; HESSE and BACH 1982; KISTERS and TER-

Table 17. Frequency of principle components among 1327 calculi (GEBHARDT and BASTIAN 1976a)

Component	Incidence %[a]	Mass %[b]	Bonn reference calculus %[c]
Whewellite	66.69	55.18	30.80
Weddellite	54.56	41.40	22.59
Apatite	32.71	37.87	12.39
Struvite	15.45	67.51	10.43
Uric acid	19.59	43.66	8.55
Uric acid dihydrate	9.04	31.79	2.87
Ammonium dihydrogenurate	16.80	7.28	1.22
Sodium dihydrogenurate monohydrate	15.37	6.94	1.07
Brushite	3.24	59.42	1.93
Octacalcium phosphate	1.28	13.82	0.18
Whitlockite	2.56	21.32	0.55
Newberyite	1.06	14.29	0.15
Bobierite	0.08	10.00	0.01
Cystine	1.28	99.41	1.27

[a] Percentage of calculi containing this component
[b] Mean proportion (%) of a calculus containing any of this material
[c] Mean proportion of this material found in all 1327 stones analysed

HORST 1973; KLEE 1970; OHNMACHT and JOBST 1977; OSCHURKOW et al. 1978; OTTO and IHMANN 1967; RICHTER and SÜCKER 1967; SCHNEIDER et al. 1973a, b; SÜCKER 1963; TAKASAKI 1974; TRY 1981; TSAY 1961).

a) Basic Principle

In the infra-red range of the spectrum between 2.5–50 μ or 4000–200 cm^{-1} the incident energy is capable of exciting oscillation within molecules and crystals. The interaction between infra-red electromagnetic waves and the substance under examination is completely defined by the equation

$$\tilde{\nu} = \frac{1}{\lambda} = \frac{1}{2\pi c} \times \sqrt{\frac{K}{\mu}},$$

$\tilde{\nu} = \frac{1}{\lambda}$ = Quantity of irradiated energy (in cm^{-1}), c = Velocity of light, K = Binding constant, μ = Reduced mass.

Depending on the type of substance specific molecular excitation there will be a discrete attenuation within the irradiated spectrum, giving rise to absolutely characteristic absorption bands on the spectral record. The totality of absorption within a given region of the spectrum is termed the absorption spectrum characteristic of an individual substance. Both the organic and inorganic compounds found in individual urolith components have typical absorption bands. Infra-red spectrophotometers with a wave number range of 100 – 4000 cm^{-1} are suitable for analysing urinary calculi. Just as in X-ray diffraction, fully automated infra-red equipment is available with mechanical sample transport and on-line or off-line data processing equipment (HESSE 1979, 1983).

b) Sample Processing

Material from the calculus must be uniformly distributed through a medium which itself has no or only minimal absorption within the spectral range employed, and in which the sample is suspended or embedded. In the former case powdered calculus is dispersed in a paraffin oil (Nujol) as a film suspended between the two windows of a cuvette. The resulting infra-red spectrum is that due to unaltered test material. However, difficulties in reproducibility make this process unsuitable for quantitative work. For such purposes high pressure embedding is preferable. 1–2 mg of urolith material are ground up with 200 mg potassium bromide in a shot grinder for 2–5 minutes. A hydraulic press with a special die then compresses the powder at 5–7000 kp/cm^2 into a pellet of 12 mm diameter. BELLANATO et al. (1973) were able to take this process down to a sample size of 0.1 mg. One problem lies in the hygroscopic behaviour of potassium bromide, since prolonged grinding of stone material with this substance and their proximity enforced by the pelleting press may lead to chemical change within the sample. Just as in X-ray diffraction methods, sample processing should therefore be designed to avoid any change within the sample material, the hydrates being particularly at risk. Because of its low sample requirement, its reproducibility of sample processing and its overall general ease of application, pressure embedding has become the routine technique for urolith analysis.

c) Measurement Technique and Data Evaluation

The grinding time of the potassium bromide/sample mixture is of great importance for perfect infra-red spectroscopy. Large grains will introduce dispersion and falsify the absorption pattern, leading to difficulties in interpretation. The transparent sample pellet and a control cuvette are equally irradiated with infra-red energy. A rotating mirror directs radiation from each cuvette alternately into a monochromator. Spectrally refracted wave lenghts are then sensed by the receiver, whose amplified output controls both the orifice plate and a pen recorder (HESSE and KLEE 1974, Fig. 85).

By means of a range of reference spectra for all the known components of uroliths, both as pure substances and in serial mixtures in 10% w/w increments, a comparison may be drawn to the spectral pattern of the sample. Thus the nature of even mixed stones may be elucidated with an acceptable error in the 10–15% range (Fig. 86a, b).

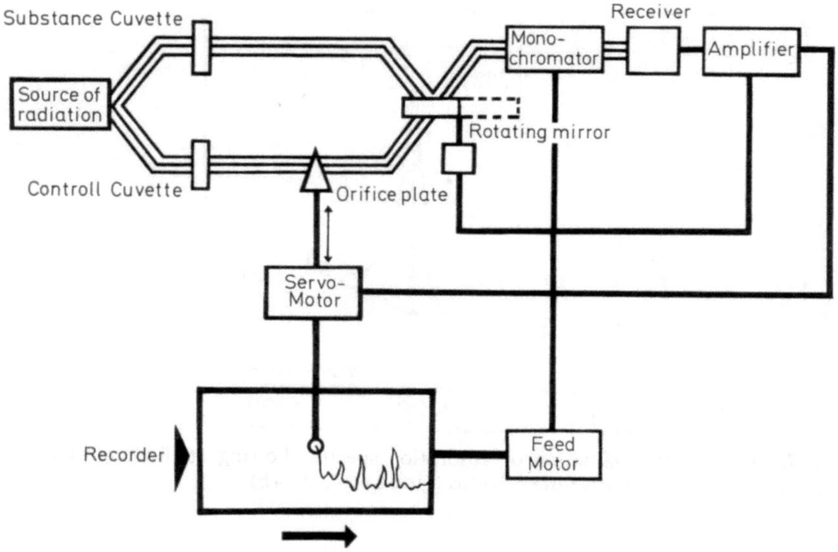

Fig. 85. Basic principle of infra-red spectroscopy (HESSE and KLEE 1974)

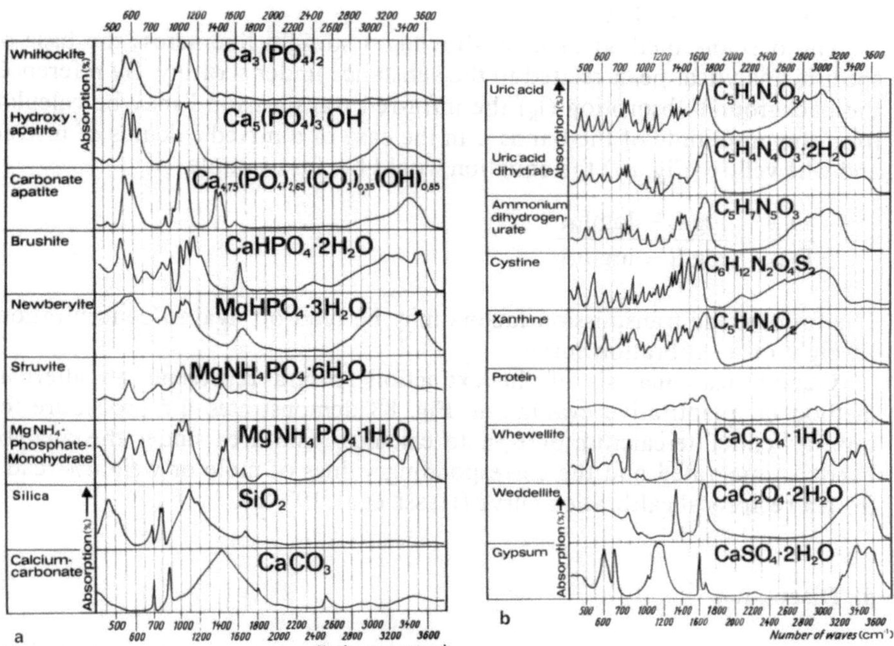

Fig. 86 a, b. Infra-red spectra of the principal urolith components

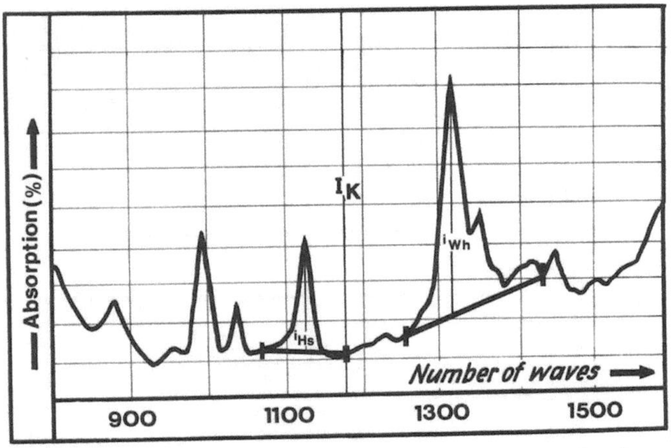

Fig. 87. Quantitative evaluation of absorption spectra showing application of the baseline method to a uric acid/whewellite calculus (HESSE et al. 1974b)

Quantitative analysis is possible by means of an internal standard or by the baseline technique (HESSE et al. 1974b).

A second pen recorder may be used to gain direct information on substance concentration from the amplitude of analytical peaks (HESSE et al. 1973b). This recorder traces extinction lines and thus obviates their computation according to the Lambert-Beer law.

The baseline method involves drawing a straight line across the base of a specific analytical peak related to the substance under scrutiny. By reference to the background absorption (I_k) the infra-red transmission I may be calculated from the amplitude of the bands i. In the case of a mixed calculus of uric acid and whewellite (Fig. 87) the equation would be, for example:

$$\frac{D_{HS}}{D_{Wh}} = \frac{\log I_k - \log I_{HS}}{\log I_k - \log I_{Wh}}.$$

The ratio of the transmission factors may be read off against concentration in %weight on a calibration curve.

Geometrical analysis of the extinction spectra represents an alternative method of quantitative evaluation. Fig. 88 demonstrates the procedure for a mixed weddellite-calcium-phosphate calculus. The area under the analytical bands is integrated and the corresponding values of mole or weight% read off from a reciprocal calibration curve (HESSE et al. 1974b).

d) Discussion

There is a wide divergence of expert opinion on the value of infra-red spectroscopy for urolith analysis.

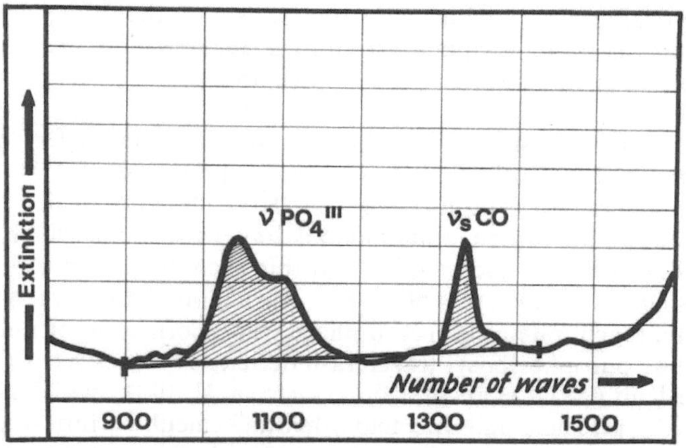

Fig. 88. Quantitative evaluation of extinction spectra for a whewellite/$Ca_3(PO_4)_2$ calculus (60:40% w/w) by integration of the cross-hatched area (HESSE et al. 1974b)

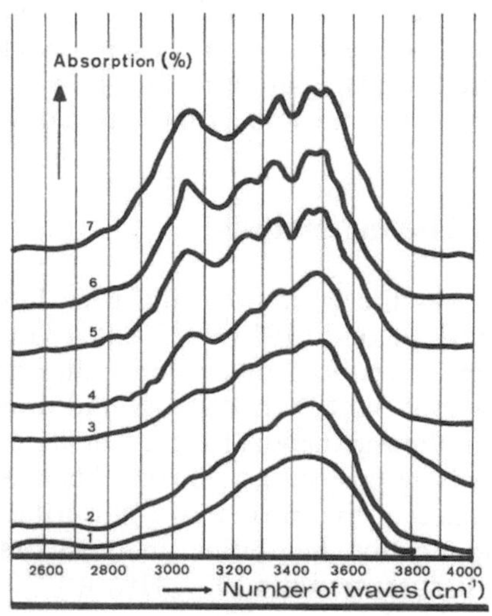

Fig. 89. Characteristic differences of whewellite-OH-band resolution between whewellite and weddellite (HESSE et al. 1972b)

TSAY (1961) considers this new method ideal for rapid accurate analysis of kidney stones. GEBHARDT (1980a), however, found it impossible to distinguish between whewellite and weddellite, uric acid and uric acid dihydrate, ammonium dihydrogenurate and the sodium salt, or between the individual phosphates at a practical level, and it is chiefly for this reason that infra-red spectroscopy has not so far been perfected as the standard technique of urolith analysis (DOSCH, quoted in GEBHARDT 1980a).

On the other hand HESSE et al. (1972b) described impeccable analytical separation of whewellite and weddellite and demonstrate significant differences in the OH-excitation bands (Fig. 89). In their hands (HESSE et al. 1974b) the analytical accuracy achieved by comparison to the reference spectra of serial mixtures is quite adequate for clinical purposes. For research purposes the technique of integrating of the surface area under extinction peaks should be preferred.

Infra-red spectroscopy seems equally suitable for investigating stones of pharmacological causation, e.g. sulfonamide calculi (OTTO and ALLESCH 1969). In a series of 3000 uroliths CIFUENTES DELATTE et al. (1978a) came across 50 sodium dihydrogenurate monohydrate concretions which they characterized by their infra-red spectrogram and thin section appearances. The same group (CIFUENTES DELATTE et al. 1981) also claimed to have detected potassium dihydrogenurate as a urolith phase. An inborn error of purine metabolism (adenine phosphoribosyl transferase deficiency) gives rise to 2,8-dihydroxyadenine calculi (JOOST et al. 1981; SAKOMOTO et al. 1981), which are easily distinguished from uric acid and uric acid dihydrate calculi by infra-red spectroscopy (ASPER and SCHMUCKI 1980; SIMMONDS 1979a, b; SIMMONDS et al. 1981).

DAUDON et al. (1981) have presented a trial series of 150 samples from typical and rare urolith phases analysed by a new method employing an argon laser (green line at 5145 Å). The technique combines molecular spectroscopic features of infra-red and X-ray spectroscopy. Extremely small particles (1 μ) may be analysed with considerable accuracy, particularly in mixtures. At present, the principal disadvantage of the technique lies in its considerable expense and in the inevitable destruction of thermolabile phases (SANTOS et al. 1984).

5. Thermoanalysis

It was the group working with BERENYI (BERENYI et al. 1967; BERENYI et al. 1968; BERENYI 1970, 1973a, 1974; LIPTAY and BERENYI 1967; LIPTAY et al. 1966) who introduced thermal techniques into urolith analysis in the 1960s. As early as 1958 VON PHILLIPSBORN had drawn attention to the advantages of differential thermoanalysis for the classification of uroliths, and calcium oxalate monohydrate has been used for a considerable number of years as a reference substance in thermoanalysis. Nevertheless, the technique has found only limited application in routine analysis, despite reports from a number of countries (BUTHLIASCHWILI 1979; HEIDE 1970, 1979; ROSE and WOODFINE 1976; SCHNEIDER and HEIDE 1971; STRATES and GEORGA-COPOULOU 1969). The following discussion of this technique is mainly derived from the classical descriptions by BERENYI (1974) and HEIDE (1979).

a) Basic Principle

Thermal analysis techniques comprise Differential Thermoanalysis (DTA), Thermogravimetry (TG) and Derivative Thermogravimetry (DTG).

A uniform rise in temperature will bring about changes in most test substances that include loss of the water of crystallization, decomposition, combustion, recrystallization or melting. Differential thermoanalysis is able to iden-

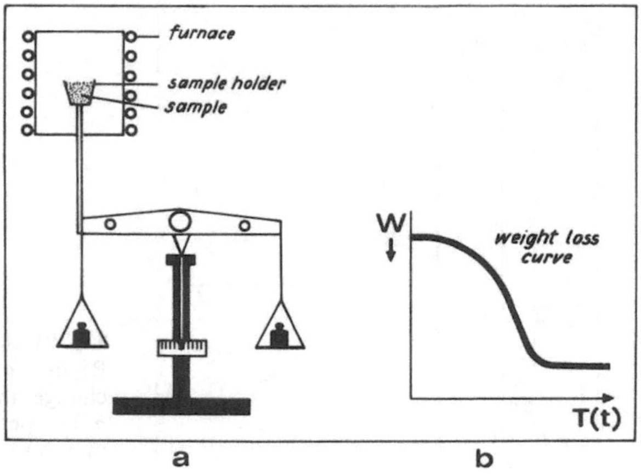

Fig. 90. Diagram of a thermobalance (left) and (right) the relationship between mass deficit and temperature (TG diagram) of an analytical sample

tify any substance undergoing a known phase change at a given temperature. The type of reaction (solid-state reaction, alteration of aggregate state) and whether the substance is crystalline or amorphous are quite immaterial. The key factor for identification is the occurrence of a thermochemical process utilising or generating heat (endothermic or exothermic reaction) or otherwise altering the thermal indices of the sample discontinuously over a narrow temperature range.

The type of reaction, the temperatures at which it occurs and ceases, and the associated changes in weight and enthalpy vary in a substance specific fashion.

DTA is based on measuring the temperature difference occurring between the sample and a thermally inert control during the course of a known reaction. The magnitude of this difference will depend on external factors (weighed in mass, cooling rate, grain size, etc.) and substance specific parameters. The reaction temperature and temperature drop are measured by thermocouples (Fig. 91).

A pair of thermocouples are connected to form a bridge circuit and heated in a furnace, one thermocouple being in the sample and the other in the control substance. The temperature difference between the two is registered on a meter, furnace temperature being controlled by a predetermined linear time-temperature program. The samples are mounted in the furnace either in a single block or in separate sample holders (Fig. 90). Analytical resolving power for small samples may be very substantially improved by the use of separate sample holders (SCHNEIDER et al. 1973b).

Thermogravimetry (TG) depends on continuous measurement by weighing apparatus of mass changes occurring in the sample during controlled linear changes in temperature. Any substance is suitable for phase identification by thermogravimetric analysis that loses mass at a given temperature, e.g. by decomposition or combustion, etc. Where the stoichiometric proportions involved in the reaction are known, the TG curve may be used for quantification of the phase composition.

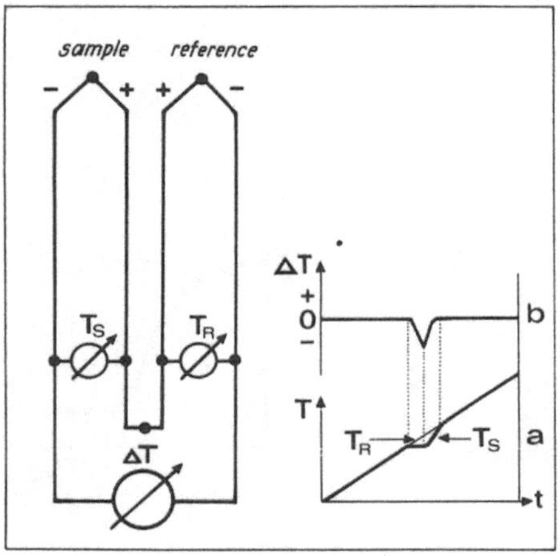

Fig. 91. Left: Circuit diagram for DTA. Right: *a* Time-course of temperature change in specimen and inert substance. *b* Temperature differential between specimen and inert substances as a function of temperature (DTA diagram)

The analytical accuracy is given by the derivative overtime of the TG curve (DTG curve).

DTA is suitable for the qualitative identification of numerous phases both individually and in mixture. By contrast, TG and DTG are able to identify a lesser number of phases but will reveal their quantitative proportions with considerable accuracy.

The advantages of DTA and TG are usually combined in modern thermoanalytical equipment.

b) Sample Processing

One great advantage of thermoanalysis lies in the fact that virtually no preliminary processing of the sample is necessary. The test substance need not be altered by grinding, pounding or pressing prior to the actual analysis. Material from the entire stone or stone domain under scrutiny is simply weighed into the sample holder. Macroanalysis requires 10 – 500 mg and microanalysis approximately 0.1 mg.

c) Data Evaluation

Figure 92 is the original thermogram of a mixed stone showing the stepwise decay measured by DTA and TG. These reactions occur independently of each other, even in mixed calculi, so that stones of multiple crystalline composition may be identified qualitatively with relative ease.

Figure 92 gives a synopsis of the DTA and DTG curves for the most important urolith components. Most urinary calculi are also suitable for quantitative thermoanalysis. If the qualitative composition of the sample is known the quan-

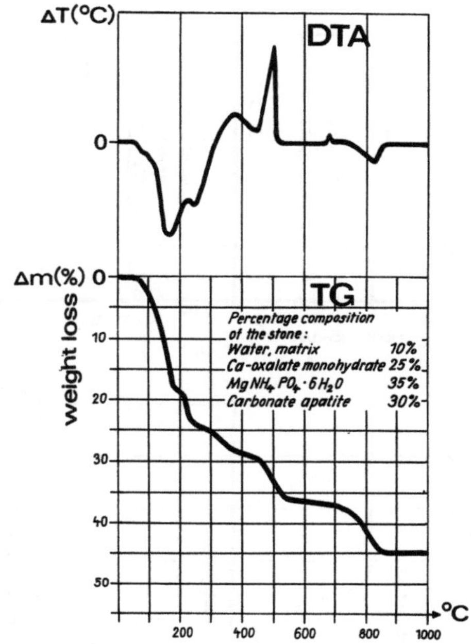

Fig. 92. Actual thermogram of a mixed stone (above – DTA, below – TG)

tities of its principle components may be calculated. Weight loss is read off from the TG curve, and once the fragmentary products of thermal degradation are known (NH_3, H_2O, CO, CO_2), the desired result may be calculated by stoichiometry.

BERENYI (1974) has provided factors which simplify these computations. The quantity of a given compound in mg may be calculated by multiplying mass deficit with the corresponding factor.

Over certain temperature ranges processes of thermal decay may occur in several compounds simultaneously, and such overlap occasionally leads to difficulties of interpretation. The thermal behaviour of a variety of renal calculi has been described in detail by SCHNEIDER et al. (1973b).

Pure *fluorapatite* is unchanged at 1000 °C, and the same is true of *hydroxyapatite,* an uncharacteristic endothermic reaction occurring between 800–900 °C. *Carbonate apatite* may also be difficult to assess, since the endothermic reaction between 800 and 900 °C characteristic of calcite is absent.

Whitlockite is also only indirectly accessible to thermoanalytic identification.

On the other hand *brushite, calcium dihydrogenphosphate, newberyite* and *struvite* are all suitable for thermal identification.

Organic calculi which, from a thermic point of view, include calcium oxalate are usually easy to analyse with accuracy.

They differ from inorganic calculi in the exothermic combustion of carbon compounds.

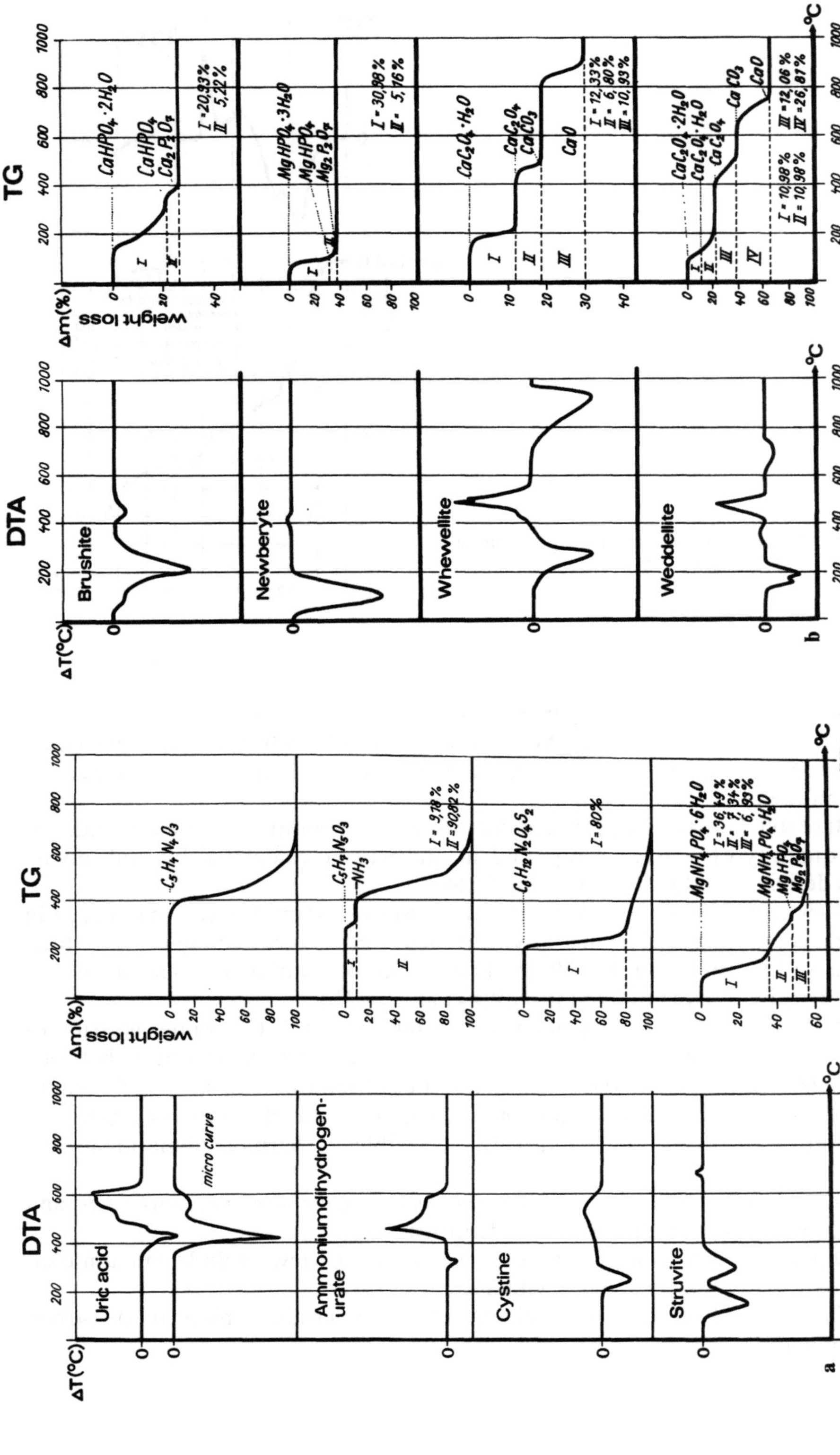

Fig. 93 a, b. Thermograms of principal urolith components (macroanalysis)

Whilst macroanalysis of *xanthine* yields a thermogram barely distinct from that of *uric acid*, microanalysis permits unequivocal distinction (SCHNEIDER and HEIDE 1971). By using very small samples the superimposition of secondary processes (endothermic uric acid and exothermic xanthine degradation) may be largely avoided, and the true reaction becomes manifest.

Calcium oxalate has probably been subjected to more intensive thermoanalysis than any other urolith phase. Its thermal degradation comprises 3 stages (see Fig. 93b).

Weddellite fails to reveal a constant crystallization water content of 2 H_2O as would be suggested by its formula. The water content in fact varies from sample to sample, but once the water has been cleared, degradation proceeds along the same lines as for whewellite (see Fig. 93b).

d) Discussion

Thermoanalysis is a highly suitable technique for the identification of urolith components. For a sensitivity of 0.5 mg the standard error is of the order 10%. The sample escapes any debasement during preliminary processing, and microanalysis is possible on samples of 0.1 – 1 mg. The technique is quantitative for the majority of urolith components, further data being available from microthermoanalysis.

Thermoanalysis is less suitable for the separation of calcium phosphates.

6. Autoradiography

Being relatively costly, auto- and microradiography are less suitable for routine urolith analysis. Nevertheless these techniques, developed by ENGSTRÖM and BELLMANN (quoted in BOSHAMER 1961), may be extremely useful for certain research purposes. LAGERGREN (1956) has examined more than 100 stones in this way and MURPHY and PYRAH (1962) have combined microradiography with polarising microscopy to give precise localisation of calcium. More recent reports have come from MCCONVILLE (1973, 1980).

Thin section of urolith (0.2 – 0.3 mm thickness) are placed directly on fine grain X-ray film and exposed to a primary beam at 20 – 30 cm tube-film distance. Using the softest possible X-rays exposure times of a few seconds will give good pictures, usually requiring photographic enlargement. The coefficients of absorption decrease throughout the series apatite, brushite, whewellite, struvite, cystine and uric acid. Analysis is by comparison to standard absorption values for all known urolith phases, the only precondition being that the exposures were made under identical conditions of section thickness, exposure time, development time and photometer arrangement.

MCCONVILLE and MCCONVILLE (1976) were able to measure the distribution of carbon, oxygen and calcium in a staghorn calculus by means of neutron activation autoradiography. Their calculus contained 10.25% calcium and 27.29% oxalate (Fig. 94).

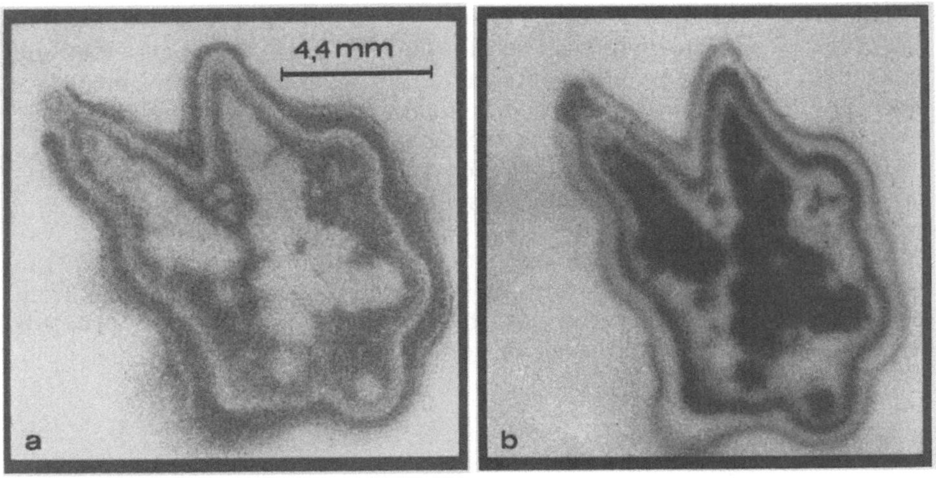

Fig. 94 a, b. Autoradiographs of a staghorn calculus. **a** Carbon, **b** Calcium. Photographs kindly provided by Dr. McCONVILLE, Birmingham

7. Combination Techniques

The power of an individual analytical technique may be assessed by comparing it with the data provided by several authors using different techniques (RODGERS et al. 1982). In one randomised trial two geographically separated workers examined 100 powered urolith samples by quantitative chemistry, by X-ray diffraction, by infra-red spectroscopy and by thermoanalysis (SCHNEIDER et al. 1973). All 4 methods produced correct results for the principal components with an error of 2%. The best correspondence was found between the three physical methods, particularly with regard to components in mixtures, although each individual method had its own specific problems.

KRIZEK et al. (1973) tested 102 calculi chemically identified as cystine and coming from 46 cystinurics by means of X-ray diffraction, infra-red spectroscopy and microthermoanalysis. 85% of the calculi were pure cystine. Mixtures occurred with uric acid and calcium oxalate, in the presence of secondary infection mainly with struvite and carbonate apatite. Cystine was easily recognized by all 3 techniques. Thermoanalysis revealed significant reproducible deviations from the pattern of analytic grade L-cystine for calculi found to be "pure" by X-ray diffraction and infra-red spectroscopy. This difference took the form of a double-reaction at 220 °C and 250 °C, and of unknown causation. Possibly trace quantities of foreign material debase the crystal structure, or alternatively thermal decomposition itself leads to these phenomena.

Overall comparison of the various techniques reveal chemical analysis in the worst and X-ray diffraction in the best light (BEELER et al. 1964; GRIEVE and ZAREMSKI 1973; OTNES and MONTGOMERY 1980; POLLAK and CARLSON 1969).

Combination techniques may be used to establish close correlation between composition and morphology of stones (REVEILLAND et al. 1980). Eight morphological species correspond to 4 types of pure calculus and 6 mixed forms.

FUSS et al. (1976) routinely follow an analytical protocol comprising polarising and phase contrast microscopy with scanning electron microscopy, electron microprobe and X-ray diffraction for the elucidation of cryptocrystalline phases and microcrystals. Because of its considerable expense such a technique can only be advocated in special cases. JOOST and TESSADRY (1983) were able, using the electron microprobe, to detect apatite and struvite in oxalate and cystine stones at levels undetectable by X-ray diffraction studies.

The consistently best results have probably been achieved by combining X-ray diffraction with optical crystallography (FLEROWSKI 1965; HESSE et al. 1981 a; OTNES 1980; RODGERS 1981 b) (see also Section VI, 8 a and d).

Large series employing a combination of microscopy and X-ray diffraction have been reported by HERRING (1962, 10,000 calculi) and PRIEN (1963, 25,000 calculi). BRÖRING et al. (1979) found accurate correspondence between the two methods, notwithstanding which they do not recommend the use of this combination, preferring polarising microscopy alone for quantitative urolith analysis in clinical practice.

A group headed by BRIEN (BRIEN 1982 a, b; BRIEN et al. 1982; BICK and BRIEN 1976; BICK et al. 1974; SCHUBERT 1980) have gone a long way towards the perfection of this method, subjecting powdered samples from 600 calculi to microscopy and X-ray diffraction studies. The former method performed poorly at separating uric acid, uric acid dihydrate and the urates, whilst the latter was unsuitable for calcium phosphates.

Table 18 summarises the results of the two techniques. All uroliths are examined according to the protocol in Table 19.

A series of 3 immersion media are used for the embedding of granular materials. The components are characterised by measuring their refractive indices in relation to that of the immersion medium (see Section VI, 8). Whewellite, weddellite, brushite, struvite and cystine may be recognised with accuracy by

Table 18. Crystallographic and X-ray diffractometric frequency of various urolith phases in a cohort of 600 calculi (BRIEN 1981)

Type of calculus	X-ray diffraction	Polarizing microscopy	Difference
Whewellite	469	475	+ 6
Weddellite	268	272	+ 4
Apatite	179	201	+ 22
Brushite	12	12	–
Struvite	71	79	+ 8
Uric acid	96	96	–
Ammonium hydrogenurate	3	3	–
Cystine	2	2	–
Whitlockite	1	0	1

Table 19. Separation of urolith phases by interference color, refractive index and X-ray diffractometry (Bick et al. 1980)

Polarizing microscopy			*X-ray diffractometry*	
Interference color	Refractive indices	Result	Arc interval (° θ)	Result
Low	$n_\alpha n_\gamma < M_1$	Struvite	N/A	–
Low	$n_\alpha n_\gamma M_1$ → $n_\alpha < M_2$	Weddellite	N/A	–
	$n_\alpha n_\gamma M_1$ → $n_\alpha n_\gamma > M_2$	Brushite	N/A	–
Medium	$n_\alpha n_\gamma > M_1$: $n_\gamma > M_3$	Cystine	N/A	–
High	$n_\alpha < M_1 < n_\gamma$ → $n_\alpha n_\gamma < M_3$	Whewellite	N/A	–
	$n_\alpha < M_1 < n_\gamma$ → $n_\gamma > M_3$	Sodium urate Uric acid dihydrate	4–16	*Sodium dihydrogen urate* *Uric acid dihydrate*
High	$n_\alpha n_\gamma > M_1$ → $n_\alpha n_\gamma < M_3$	Whewellite	N/A	–
	$n_\alpha n_\gamma > M_1$ → $n_\alpha > M_3$	Uric acid & urate group	4–16	*Uric acid* *Uric acid dihydrate* *Ammonium hydrogenurate* *Sodium urate*
Pseudo-isotropic	$n > M_1$	Calcium phosphate group	2 – 18	*Apatite* *Whitlockite* *Octacalcium phosphate*
		Multimineral	4 – 16	% Phase composition
		Whewellite/ Weddellite	6 – 8	% Phase composition

M = immersion media with the refractive indices:
$n_1 = 1.515$, $n_2 = 1.535$, $n_3 = 1.655$

polarising microscopy, so that X-ray diffraction studies are obviated for monomineral calculi. Quantitative data may be obtained from mixed calculi by X-ray diffraction over the range 4–16° of arc, and indeed whewellite-weddellite calculi (33% of all stones) may be adequately diagnosed over the interval 6–8°. Only for the determination of uric acid, urates and calcium phosphates is complete diffractometry required.

8. Microscopy

The principle advantage of microscopic analysis over other techniques is its ability to examine small samples in great detail and to provide adequate or even reliable qualitative data on the phase composition of the most complicated mixtures. Amongst this group of techniques polarising microscopy has proved of particular value, and in recent years its significance in urolith analysis has exceeded that of merely being the method of choice (BICK et al. 1974, 1980; BRIEN 1982; CIFUENTES DELATTE et al. 1973b; HICKING 1979; PRIEN and FRONDEL 1947; PRIEN and PRIEN 1973; SCHNEIDER and SEYFARTH 1980; SEYFARTH et al. 1972; SORGER and BAUSCH 1971; SZABO 1967, 1970, 1974).

For urinary concretions of multimineral composition, combination with X-ray diffraction and infra-red spectroscopy gives improved analytical power (see Section VI, 7, Table 19).

a) Polarizing Microscopy

α) Principle

A detailed description of the technique and various methods of application may be found in EMMONS et al. (1973) and elsewhere. A polarizing microscope is distinguished from an ordinary bench instrument by the addition of 2 polarizing filters (polarizer and analyzer), a λ compensator (Red I) and a rotating stage (Fig. 95).

Both polarizers transmit light in only one plane. In the polarizing microscope measurements are made with these two planes arranged at right angles, so that complete extinction (dark field) normally results. White light from the source is linearly polarized by the polarizer. On passing through an anisotropic crystal such plane-polarized light waves are split into two component rays with their planes of oscillation at right angles (Fig. 95). The birefringence characteristic of every urolith phase consists of these two rays being propagated at different speeds through the anisotropic medium, and thus leaving the crystal with a path length difference dependent on both the thickness of the sample and on its birefringence ($n_\gamma - n_\alpha$).

$$G = d \times (n_\gamma - n_\alpha),$$

G: Path length difference, n_α, n_γ: Minimal and maximal refractive indices of a mineral grain, d: Sample thickness.

The analyzer renders both plane polarized beams coplanar, resulting in the appearance of interference colors. These are generally characteristic of urolith components (for equal sample thickness) and allow an initial assessment of the degree of birefringence (see Michel-Levy tables, Appendix) (HICKING 1979; SCHUBERT 1980; SORGER and BAUSCH 1971; SZABO 1974).

Birefringence values will vary between zero and a maximum characteristic of the individual crystal phase, depending on the plane of section through indi-

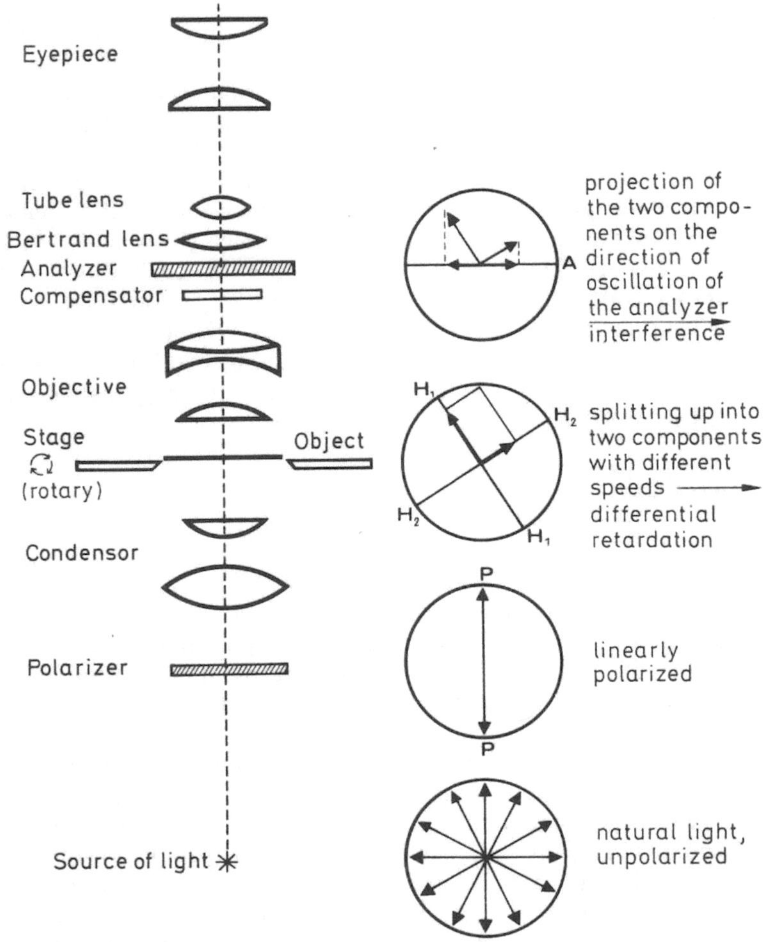

Fig. 95. Basic arrangement and mode of action of the polarizing microscope

vidual grains. The interference colors generated will thus also depend on the direction of light transmission. Contrary to the behaviour of anisotropic grains, isotropic material exhibits no birefringence whatever with crossed polarizers, and extinction is therefore maintained. This is of practical significance for the calcium phosphates, whose extremely low birefringence renders them isotropic or pseudoisotropic (see Table 20). BICK and SCHUBERT (1980) have reviewed the criteria for distinguishing members of the phosphate group by microscopy.

β) Crystallographic Data

As well as the refractive indices and the degree of birefringence along with its associated interference colors, a number of crystallographic parameters may be used for unequivocal characterization of individual grains. These values include the optical axis angle, its *dispersion* and the *optical character*. Together they permit determination of the crystal system and its axis arrangement, as well as the assignation of positive or negative sign (SORGER and BAUSCH 1971; EMMONS et al. 1973). These measurements are made under conoscopic conditions, using an additional lens (BERTRAND lens) and a λ-plate (red I) in the optical pathway. In the main this system sheds further light on problems of phase composition not resolved by refraction studies alone.

Table 20 gives crystallographic data and morphologic characteristics of urolith minerals.

γ) Analytic Protocol for Grain Samples

The following equipment is required:

- Polarizing microscope; 160–200× magnification
- Immersion media

Immersion media	Refractive index
Oxalic diethylester	1.409
Cedar wood oil	1.515
Ethyl iodide	1.516
Ethyl bromide	1.535
Canada balsam	1·535
Monobromobenzene	1.560
Cinnamaldehyde	1.615
Quinoline	1.624
α-monobromonaphthalene	1.658

  By mixing these immersion oils media of any desired refractive index can be made up, the latter being determined with an ABBE refractometer. A synopsis of commonly used immersion media may be found in EISMANN (1980).
- Microscope slides, cover slips, dissection needle, fretsaw and files

Just as for X-ray diffraction and infra-red spectroscopy there is a requirement in urolith microscopy to first break down calculi into very small fragments, whose fracture planes are then assessed by incident light stereomicroscopy, under which microsamples are picked out of nuclear and peripheral zones with a dissecting needle. The grains are then crushed between two slides so as to guarantee a grain size of 10–30 μ. The pulverised stone sample is now dispersed in immersion medium and covered with a cover slip. A whole series of protocols has been described for routine microscopy of uroliths (BICK and BRIEN 1976; SCHNEIDER and SEYFARTH 1980; SORGER and BAUSCH 1971; SZABO 1974), that due to BICK and BRIEN (1976) being given in Fig. 96. An initial morphologic examination is made of individual sample grains with crossed polarizers, at which stage the principle structural and aggregational features of the grain being examined may be determined (see Section V). Following the protocol the interference colors are now assessed, thus subdividing the urolith material into 4 phase groups by estimated refractive index. Refraction behaviour is determined by comparing the refractive index of the crystal with that of

Table 20. Crystallographic data and morphologic description of urinary material (synopsis after PRIEN and FRONDEL 1947, RINGERTZ 1965, SCHNEIDER and SEYFARTH 1980, SHIRLEY 1966, SZABO 1967, WINCHEL and WINCHEL 1967)

Group	Mineral	Crystal system	Refractive index			Birefringence
			n_α	n_β	n_γ	$(n_\gamma - N_\alpha)$
1	Apatite Carbonate apatite Whitlockite	Hexagonal	Variable index 1.52–1.16			Pseudo-isotropic 0.004
2	Struvite	Orthorhombic	1.495	1.496	1.504	0.009
	Brushite	Monocline	1.539	1.545	1.551	0.012
	Weddellite	Tetragonal	1.523		1.544	0.021
3	Cystine	Hexagonal	1.64		1.70	0.06
	Whewellite	Monocline	1.491	1.555	1.650	0.159
4	Uric acid	Monocline	1.588	1.739	1.898	0.210
	Uric acid dihydrate	Orthorhombic	1.508	1.691	1.728	0.220
	Ammonium dihydrogenurate		1.54		1.74	0.200
	Sodium dihydrogenurate	Monocline	1.448	1.750	1.840	0.392

the mounting medium, the condenser being lowered and the position of the Becke line being assessed by eye. This bright fringe of luminance around the grain margins moves into the medium of greater refractive index as the microscope tube is raised. Where the refractive indices of grain and mount are identical the grain margin becomes indistinct. In view of the anisotropic nature of crystals two refractive indices will need to be measured at right angles to each other across the grain. For this purpose the polarizers are first maintained crossed and the crystal grain rotated into a position of complete extinction (optical axis of the grain parallel to the incident beam), the analyzer subsequently being removed from the light path and the refractive index of the

Table 20. (continued)

Interference color (grain thickness $\simeq 20\ \mu$)	Optical character Optical axis angle	Morphologic characteristics
Black (Gray)	Negative Uniaxial	Fine to coarse-grained, vesicular and clustered, hyaline and lamellar aggregates
Gray 1st order	Positive 37°	Large, slipper of coffin-lid shaped crystals, usually coated with dark pigment
1. Order (Gray to pale yellow)	Positive 85°	Micaceous, lanceolate
1st to 2nd order (Gray, red, blue)	Positive Uniaxial	Pyramidal, occasionally trapezoid, triangular, often with characteristic V-markings parallel to crystal margin
Often gray 1. Order, otherwise 2. – 3. Order	Negative Uniaxial	Fragments of hexagonal plates
4. – 6. Order Usually greyish-yellow	Positive 84°	1. Fanning or spherolithic crystals with typical year-ring structure 2. Clear, monocline-prismatic crystals
Often with intensely	Positive 84°	Finely crystalline
colored interference	Negative 40.4°	reddish-yellow, round aggregates,
bands depending on cross-section and		rarely clear prismatic crystals
crystal thickness	Positive Biaxial	

grain compared to that of immersion medium. The stage is then rotated through 90° and the second refractive index determined. The diagram in Fig. 96 shows how initial assessment of refraction values with medium 1 (cedar wood oil) taking due account of interference color, allows approximate separation of urolith components. This recognition process may be further refined by the use of the remaining series of immersion media. Because refractive indices will vary, depending on the angle between optical axis of the microscope and that of the grain, the refractive indices should be determined for a number of grains of similar phase composition, in order to secure statistically significant characterization. The interference colors, and in particular their order number,

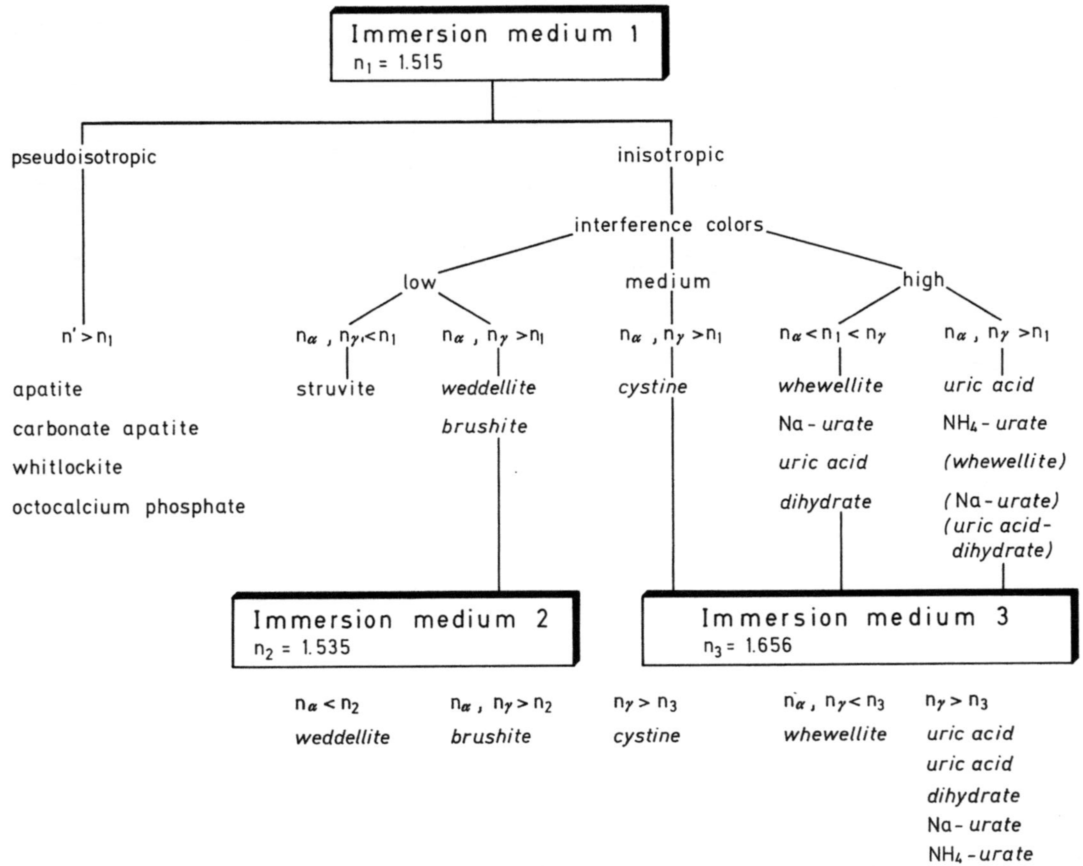

Fig. 96. Protocol for identifying urolith phases (after BICK and BRIEN 1976). The method is based on the refractive indices of the grains and the interference colors generated by them

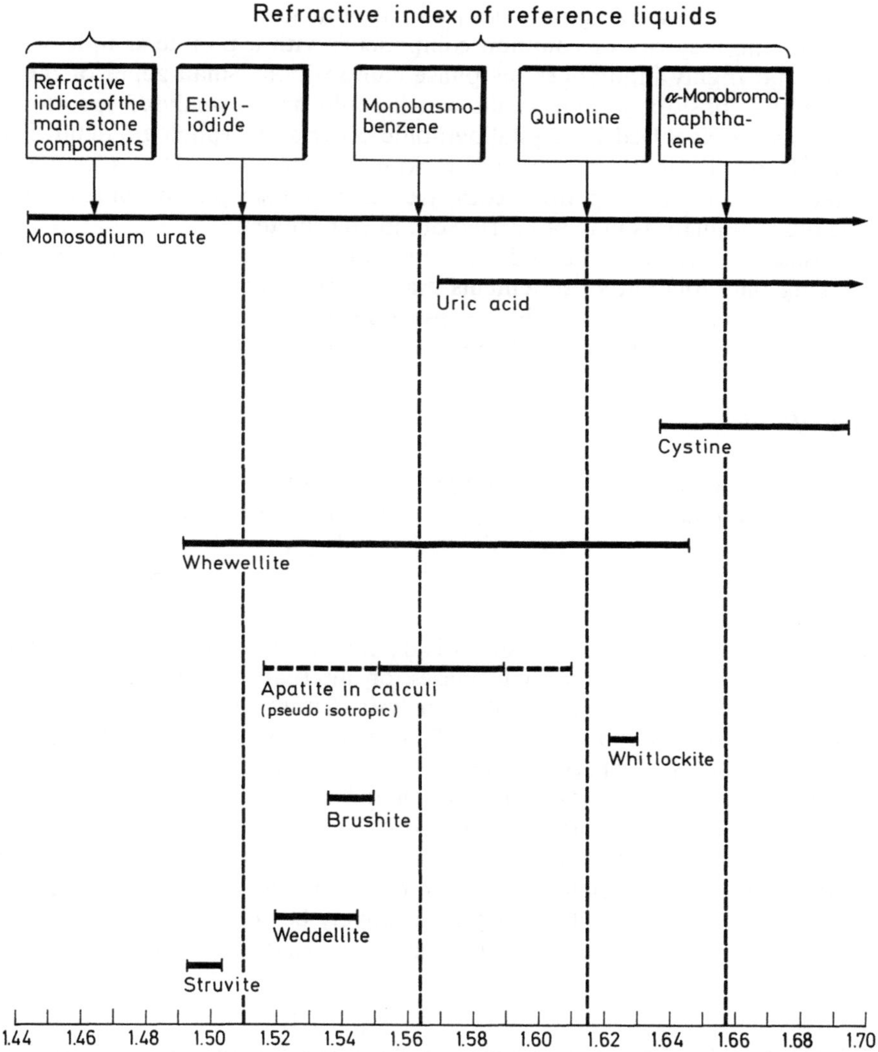

Fig. 97. Refractive indices and birefringence values of principal urolith phases (SZABO 1974)

provide some information on the intensity of birefringence, although the latter may be more accurately determined by means of Michel-Levy tables (see Appendix).

Such morphologic and qualitative analytical data usually provide adequate characterization of uroliths for clinical diagnostic purposes. Conoscopy, or in some cases phase contrast, is also able to provide some separation within the uric acid and phosphate groups (see Section VI, 8c). Figure 97 gives the refractive indices and birefringence of characteristic urolith phases.

Advantages: Polarizing microscopy of urolith grains allows definite recognition of the majority of common components with a minute sample size (μg range) and highly inhomogenous phase composition. Small zones of the concretion and subsidiary components which could not be analysed spectroscopically may be classified by crystallographic criteria. Morphologic detail is also available on the individual phases making up the stone. The investment required is relatively inexpensive compared to spectroscopic equipment. With a little practice analysis may be carried out in 20 minutes.

Disadvantages: The method requires considerable experience. Generally speaking only qualitative statements may be made about phase composition. Representatives of the uric acid and pseudoisotropic calcium phosphate group are inadequately distinguished from one another.

Quantification techniques

Table 21 gives an example in which phase composition has been studied quantitatively, although considerable equipment costs are involved.

δ) Thin Section Studies

In this technique phase composition is determined by assigning observable interference colors to individual phases or alternatively by conoscopy. The method is only rarely used in urolith analysis (CIFUENTES DELATTE et al. 1973b; RODRIGUEZ-MIÑON and CIFUENTES 1976) because of its expense. On the other hand, it provides a representative cross-section through the stone and gives both useful data on its phase composition and clues as to its mode of formation (see Section V, 3). Sections are prepared by embedding the stone in rapid-curing synthetic resin. The stone is then cut and a polished surface attached to a microscope slide with potting resin. Initial coarse grinding brings the section down to 50 μ thickness, which may alternatively be achieved with a microtome saw. The final polish is given with fine grain grinding compound, leaving an

Table 21. Sample calculation for quantitative phase microanalysis of a urolith using the Eltinor integrating device after SCHNEIDER and SEYFARTH (1980)

Qualitatively detectable phases in urolith	Number of grains counted for each phase (a_j)	Phase density (d_j)	$a_j \times d_j$	Quantitative result: phase weight as % total composition
A	23	2	46	19
B	37	2	74	31
C	40	3	120	50
	100		240	100

ultimate thickness of 20 μ. Interference colors appear in sections of 30 – 10 μ thickness. Grinding is discontinued when first and second order interference colors are achieved on individual grains or when print may be read through the section. A drop of synthetic resin and a cover slip are then applied to seal the specimen. A detailed discussion of thin section techniques is given in the literature (EMMONS et al. 1973; HOMRIGHAUSEN 1977; SCHNEIDER and SEYFARTH 1980; SLUKA et al. 1975).

b) Transmitted Light Microscopy

Transmitted light is mainly used to determine grain morphology and is thus of particular descriptive values in the diagnostic examination of urinary sediments. In addition to this BICK and BRIEN (1975) have successfully used transmission microscopy to distinguish between individual types of calcium phosphate grain (whitlockite, octacalcium phosphate, hydroxy- and carbonate apatite).

The incident light method of BERENYI (1981) provides rapid and reliable data on morphology, composition and origin of urolith material both on ground surfaces and in grain samples.

α) Sediment Studies

Urine microscopy provides data on the crystalline components of urinary sediment, and by so doing plays an important role in the diagnosis of urolithiasis, chiefly in terms of morphologic and phase characteristics of individual crystals (ALKEN and SCHÄFER 1978; BERG et al. 1976b, c, 1982b; CATALINA and CIFUENTES DELATTE 1970, 1971, 1974; ELLIOT and RABINOWITZ 1978; ELLIOT et al. 1976; HEINTZ and ALTHOF 1976; KLEEBERG et al. 1981; KRIZEK 1968).

The nature of crystalline urinary sediment furthermore permits early recognition of patients at risk of stone formation, a phenomenon which must be seen in the light of increased concentrations of lithogenic urine components and inadequate activity of crystallization inhibitors. The clinical background for such an increased excretion of lithogenic material may be extremely varied. The frequency and size of sediment crystals are an accurate measure of the crystallization tendency of a given urine (ALKEN and SCHÄFER 1978; BAUMANN 1978; BERG, VAN DEN et al. 1976; BOTHOR and BERG 1980; CATALINA and CIFUENTES DELATTE 1971; CIFUENTES DELATTE 1974; ELLIOT and RABINOWITZ 1976, 1978; ROBERTSON 1978), with particular diagnostic importance attaching to large microliths and crystal aggregates. As a consequence, detailed qualitative and quantitative description of individual sedimentary pictures is important in the diagnosis of urolithiasis.

Sedimentary crystals may be compared with standard grain preparations, and the identification techniques described under VI, 8a, including the production of characteristic interference colors under the polarizing microscope, may thus be used to distinguish between similar crystals of differing phase composition (BERG et al. 1982b; ELLIOT and RABINOWITZ 1978).

X-ray diffractometry, infra-red spectroscopy and scanning electron microscopy combined with the electron microprobe also contribute to the accuracy of phase determination (ASPER and SCHMUCKI 1984; BERG et al. 1982b; CATALINA and CIFUENTES DELATTE 1971; ELLIOT and RABINOWITZ 1976, 1978; FUSS et al. 1976; HESSE et al. 1981a; SEIFERT and GEBHARDT 1984). The microscopic assessment of crystal size distribution may be quantified by means of a measuring eyepiece of known grid interval or by use of a projection microscope (SCHULZ et al. 1980b). The MD-KOVA system offers a diagnostic set of standardised protocols for urine sediment analysis (BAUER et al. 1981).

β) Microchemical Processes

This technique of phase analysis uses transmitted light and is similar to the polarizing microscopy method in its extremely small sample requirement and its high accuracy when applied to samples from critical regions of the stone (nucleus, mantle). For the purpose of examination a grain sample is mounted on a microscope slide. The method perfected by BERENYI and PANOVICS (1980) was originally devised by BERENYI (1973a, b) and depends on the use of suitable reagents to bring about a color change, gas evolution or e.g. recrystallization of the grains or of their immediate locality, in short on evoking a process which may be followed visually under the microscope. When combined with morphologic examination of the grain the various changes which may be brought about in individual urolith components enable qualitative and semiquantitative conclusions to be drawn. It should, however, be said that the analytical interpretation of the color gradations found in stones of heterogeneous composition may require a great deal of experience.

γ) Crystallization Studies

MARCHEK and BURCHARDT (1971) have described a method based on the differential solubility of urolith crystal in solvents from which they will recrystallize in a characteristic fashion. The specific crystal types thus produced are suitable for microscopic diagnosis and may be related in a semi-quantitative fashion to the phase composition of the parent stone. The method is cheap and sensitive but quite unreliable, since individual components may occur in a variety of crystal hibits (e.g. uric acid, whewellite) from which confusion may easily result (DOSCH and ALTROCK 1974).

c) Phase Contrast Microscopy

Grain samples from urolith phases of low birefringence, such as representatives of the calcium phosphate group, may be detected under the polarising microscope by the addition of a phase contrast attachment if the refractive indices of adjacent granules of unequal phase composition constitute a series without overlap. Mineral grains may be detected by a characteristic blue glow if they are mounted in an immersion medium of the same refractive index as the urolith phase (EISMANN 1978; EISMANN et al. 1978). Under positive phase contrast rotation relative to the polarization plane of the light will give rise to a characteristic pale or azure blue tinge with a red border the mirror image of this relationship occurring under negative phase contrast. In practice the color immersion technique is suitable for the detection of weddellite, struvite, brushite and newberyite in urinary calculi, whilst apatite and withlockite still give rise to difficulties, partly because of the varying n_α and n_γ values given in the literature.

d) Scanning Electron Microscopy

Polarizing microscopy and thin section studies enjoy an undisputed pride of place in the application of microscopic technique to the understanding of both the origin of aggregate morphology and the phase composition of uroliths. The parallel application of scanning electron microscopy provides additional morphologic data as well as enabling statements to be made about individual elements, as documented in reports by HESSE et al. (1981 a), LEUSMANN (1981), RODGERS (1981 b), and SCHULZ and BERG (1980). The depth of field is 300× greater than that attainable in light microscopy and allows a three-dimensional spatial appreciation of the most complexly configured objects. Magnification factors may range between 100 and 100,000×.

α) Principle

RIEMER and PFEFFERKORN (1977) give an excellent review of the method of scanning electron microscopy and its applications.

The object is enclosed within the instrument (Fig. 98) under high vacuum ($10^{-5}-10^{-6}$ Torr) and bombarded by an electron beam, the intensity of these so-called primary electrons being controlled by the accelerator voltage U_e (upto 50 kV).

Collision of these primary electrons with a solid body gives rise to a series of interactions (Fig. 99), including:
- Reflected electrons (RE)
- Secondary electrons (SE)
- Absorbed electrons (AE)
- Transmitted electrons (TE)
- Cathode luminescence (CL)
- X-rays (X)

Special detectors may be arranged to intercept this radiation and provide a qualitative and morphologic signal image of the sample.

Conditions: Electrically conductive sample objects require no further processing. By contrast, uroliths and other biological material require vapor deposition on the sample of a very thin film of gold, silver, aluminium or – most frequently – graphite, so as to prevent a steady increase in charge arising from

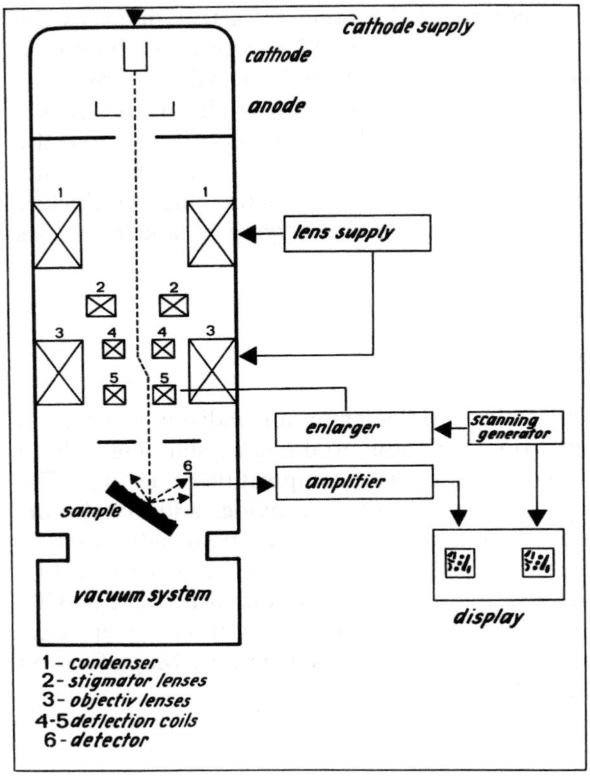

Fig. 98. Basic arrangement and mode of action of the scanning electron microscope

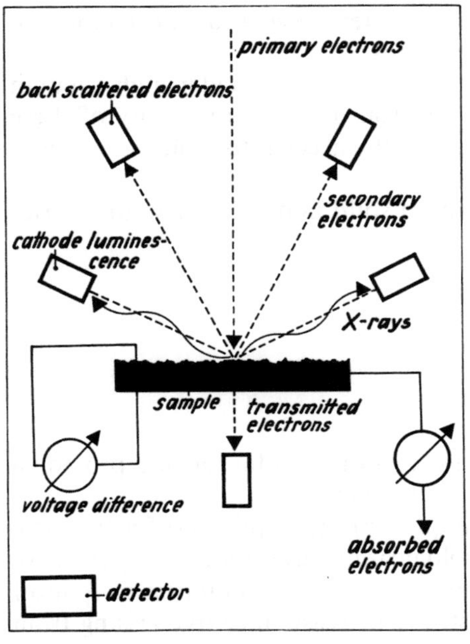

Fig. 99. How primary electrons interact with the sample under the scanning electron microscope

electron bombardment. The sample must be absolutely dry, a condition usually achieved by the CRITICAL POINT method after previous dehydration in serial alcohols.

β) Application

Reflected Electrons

General:
- high energy electrons
- entry angle = exit angle
- maximum resolution approx. 0.4 – 0.6 mm
- great depth of field, as for secondary electrons

Application:
- topographic contrast (better than for secondary electrons)
- material contrast (decreases with the atomic number)

The detected and amplified signal is processed to provide light–dark modulation on a display tube. Simultaneous synchronous phase coherent scanning by the electron beam allows a surface image of the object to be built up. The high contrast rendering available of individual details of the image secures a dominant position for the reflected electron technique among the various forms of scanning electron microscopy.

Secondary Electrons

General:
- most widely used technique
- low energy electrons on parabolic track
- maximum resolution approx. 0.2 nm
- great depth of field

Application:
- topographic contrast
- voltage contrast
- crystallographic orientation

This low energy electron radiation emanates from the object surface under primary bombardment and reproduces details of the specimen (including cavities) not resolvable under the light microscope. Secondary electrons are often employed in combination with primary electrons to provide a spatial and morphologic representation of the specimen surface.

Transmitted Electrons

This technique has its principle application in the imaging of extremely thin specimens, e.g. thin sections (< 1 μ), and is able to provide data on ultrastructure and epitaxial mechanisms. Surface structures can only be imaged in a roundabout fashion by first producing a surface imprint.

Local analytical resolution will depend on the atomic numbers of the principle elements at the point under examination.

High-voltage scanning electron microscopy (800–1000 kV) is reported more and more (EL-SAYED and COSSLETT 1977; SPECTOR et al. 1976; SPECTOR and LILGA 1981) and is distinguished by increased penetrating power of the incident electrons and a related ability to examine thicker urolith sections (> 1 μ). Smaller domains can be examined in detail and there is virtually no danger of destroying the specimen.

X-Rays (Microprobe Technique)

Electron bombardment of the sample excites the emission of more or less element-specific X-radiation. Two approaches are possible in the detection of these X-rays:
- wave length dispersion: sensitivity ranges from boron (atomic number 5) to uranium (atomic number 92)
- energy dispersion: sensitivity ranges from sodium (atomic number 11) to uranium (atomic number 92)

Computer controlled electron microprobe analysis by the energy dispersion technique is gaining increasing importance for phase determination problems. The technique is able to give a percentage distribution for a wide range of elements in minute stone samples (nm range).

The electron microprobe is able to measure distributions of elements on the surface of the object or of thin sections and polished surfaces with an accuracy of < 0.1%. When coupled with a surface imaging technique employing reflected or secondary electrons, he method allows phase distribution details to be characterized which could not allways be interpreted on morphology alone (e.g. apatite–struvite, whewellite–uric acid, urate) and also documents the presence of major and trace elements in individual urolith phases (CIFUENTES DELATTE et al. 1981; GOREW and AGAFONOW 1978; HESSE et al. 1979b, 1981a; JOOST and TESSADRY 1983; KENNOKI et al. 1978; MCCONVILLE and MCCONVILLE 1976; MEYER-JÜRGENS et al. 1981, 1982). As demonstrated by the example of organic matrix or of the presence of phosphorus within the growth centers of calcium oxalate stones, such information may aid our understanding of urolithogenesis (LEUSMANN 1981; MALEK and BOYCE 1972; SPECTOR et al. 1976; ZAREMSKI and GRIEVE 1976). The record consists of point source reflections from the surface of the material (see Figs. 57–60) or of intensity curves.

e) Combined Microscopic Technique – Laser Microspectroanalysis – Polarizing Microscopy – Electron Microprobe

DIMITROV and MARINOV (1976) have reported the use of laser microspectroanalysis for non-destructive measurement of the local element distribution in uroliths. By combining this technique with the electron beam microprobe and with polarizing microscope characterization of thin sections and polished surfaces, its findings may be applied topographically to the overall aggregate (SCHULZ et al. 1980a, 1981).

Figure 100 explains the process. Stones are first split in half and one half ground to a representative polished surface, which is then scrutinised under the polarizing microscope for interesting aggregation details and topographical features. Relevant domains (layering, grains, growth centers and other morphological details) are subsequently bombarded with a laser beam of varying diameter (10 – 100 μ) and the local distribution of elements analysed by spectroscopy of the vaporized material. The points of laser beam attack are easily recognized on cross-section as craters and may thus be identified for further morphologic study under the scanning electron microscope, where further information on their elementary composition may be obtained my means of the electron microprobe, employing wave length or energy dispersion.

Polarizing microscopy of thin sections, either subsequently or in parallel, provides accurate information on phase composition and special morphological features of the aggregate which may be correlated at any time with the trace and major element composition previously elucidated.

f) Computer Tomography

Quantitative CT enables stone composition to be assessed in vivo. In a study of 80 stones uric acid calculi were easily distinguished from all other types of stone and cystine could be told apart from calcium oxalate and brushite. 70% accuracy was achieved in separating cystine from struvite. Struvites with a higher admixture of calcium phosphate could not be distinguished from calcium oxalate or brushite, any more than could these latter two from one another (MITCHESON et al. 1983). DRACH et al. (1983) and RASSWEILER et al. (1985) have presented similar results.

9. Centralising and Standardising Urolith Analysis

a) Centralisation

With the increasing demand for analysis of every urolith, there is not only a steadily rising analytical workload but also a requirement for increasing the accuracy of analytical data. Analyses with wide margins of error are worse than useless. Currently, the method of choice must be X-ray diffraction, although the large investment required demands maximum equipment utilization, and this can only be achieved by centralisation. Under such circumstances the economical cost per sample will be no more than for chemical analysis, and indeed only half that for polarizing microscopy and infra-red spectroscopy. Thermoanalysis is almost 4 times more expensive (ASPER and SCHMUCKI 1980). A further example of centralised urolith analysis lies in its suitability for extensive automation with mechanical sample transport and computerisation, largely re-

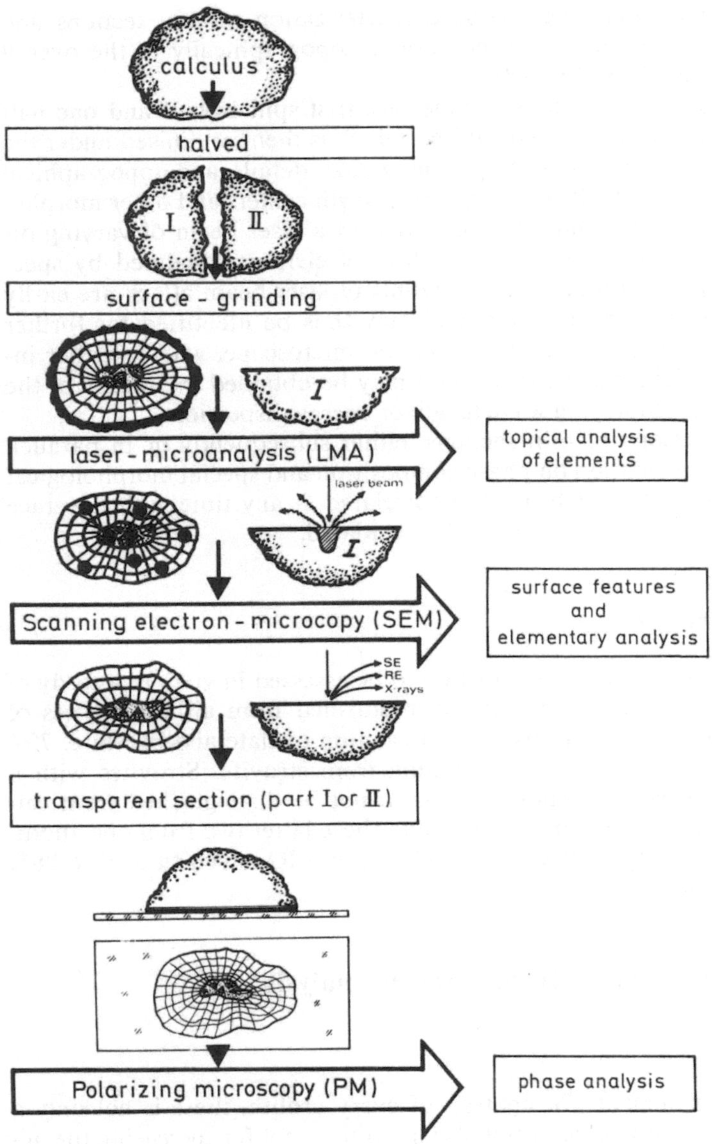

Fig. 100. Schematic protocol for combined microanalysis of urolith phases by element distribution and morphology. Technique combining laser microspectral analysis, scanning electron microscopy and polarizing microscopy

ducing the human workload to 1–2 minutes (sample processing, data evaluation) (DOSCH 1975b). By employing full-time trained laboratory staff the subjective analytical error is further reduced, and the possibility of combined techniques, e.g. X-ray diffraction with polarizing microscopy, may further significantly improve the results.

b) Standardisation

Comparability of results may only be achieved by standardising analytical techniques. Sample preparation, measuring and apparatus parameters for practical analysis and criteria for data evaluation are clearly defined and have already been discussed in Chapter VI, 7.

c) Reporting, Documentation and Data Evaluation

The complexities of urolithogenesis, the requency of urolithiasis and its apparent current increasing trend, together with the still somewhat modest results of conservative treatment, prophylaxis and prevention of recurrence, all point to a pre-requirement for a comprehensive and statistically impeccable data base on which to found any increase in our knowledge.

DOSCH (1975b) has suggested setting up a card index of identification data for the principal crystalline components found in urinary calculi. He gives the example of a weddellite data card comprising the formula, molecular weight, density, crystallographic and optical data, typical X-ray diffraction parameters and infra-red spectroscopy diagrams, the frequency of occurrence and most important accompanying substances. The same author (DOSCH 1975b) has also proposed a questionnaire for the morphologic characterization of uroliths, and this comprises weight, phase composition, number of calculi, configuration, surface structure, color, hardness, space occupation and texture.

Standardised urolith analysis allows the use of a uniform analytical record with all its advantages for data evaluation. The analytical record subserves both documentation and reporting to the source of referral, and it should satisfy the requirements of automatic data processing whilst being simple enough not to add further complexity to medical record-keeping (SCHNEIDER et al. 1974c). The record must contain as much data as possible which can be stored and recalled for subsequent evaluation.

Figure 101 shows an analytical record. It contains personal data on the patient, details of the analytical method and the results of analysis. A tear-off section on the right-hand side serves to communicate the results to the referring physician.

The overall flow of information is shown in Fig. 102: The patient passes the stone to his doctor, who fills the urolith request form and sends it with the stone to his local analytical center. After conclusion of analysis the center will return the tear-off report or indeed pre-empt its contents by telephone. The main analytical record is punched in a computing unit and its contents logged in a cen-

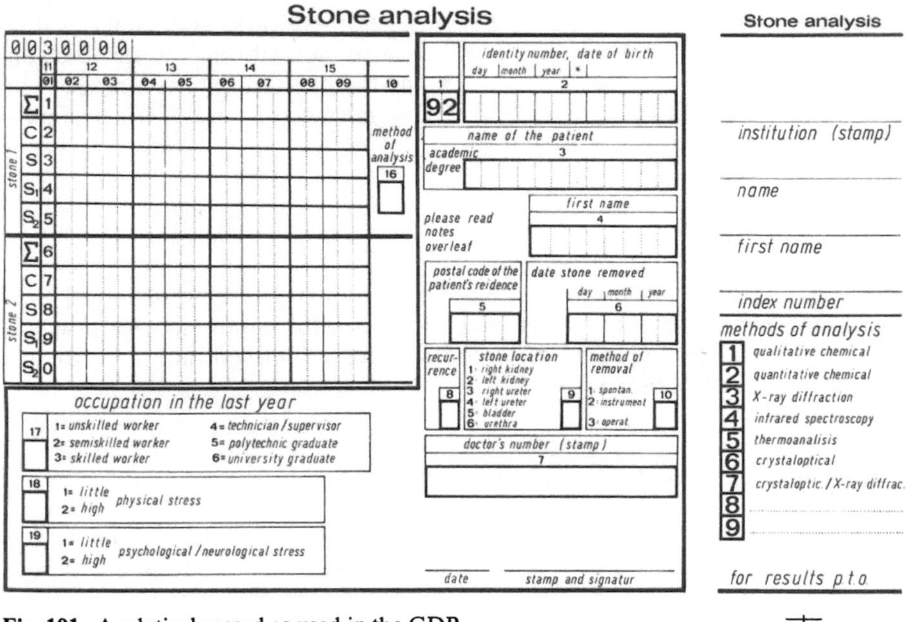

Fig. 101. Analytical record as used in the GDR

tral analytical data bank. Simultaneously, probability studies weed out erroneous material. At the end of this process the original card is returned to the analytical center and stored in a card index.

Data retrieval and processing from the central data base can continue independently of data logging.

The card index may also be used to examine specific problems with a maximum acceptable search requirement in the region of 1000 cards.

The data generated by large numbers has been processed according to programs described in further detail in the section of Epidemiology. Programs include, e.g. distribution of stone type by age and sex, recurrence rate in relation to type of stone, method of removal and data of first presentation.

These data may be linked to other material, e.g. personal identity number, in an attempt to establish relationships to occupation and environment.

Apart from such global evaluation, local factors can also be taken into account. Thus a district physician can obtain the recurrence rate for past years in his district in order to effectively plan local clinical resources.

Such a large quantity of data on both patients and their stones allows epidemiological statements to be made with numerous implications for the causation and clinical course of urolithiasis and for its prevention.

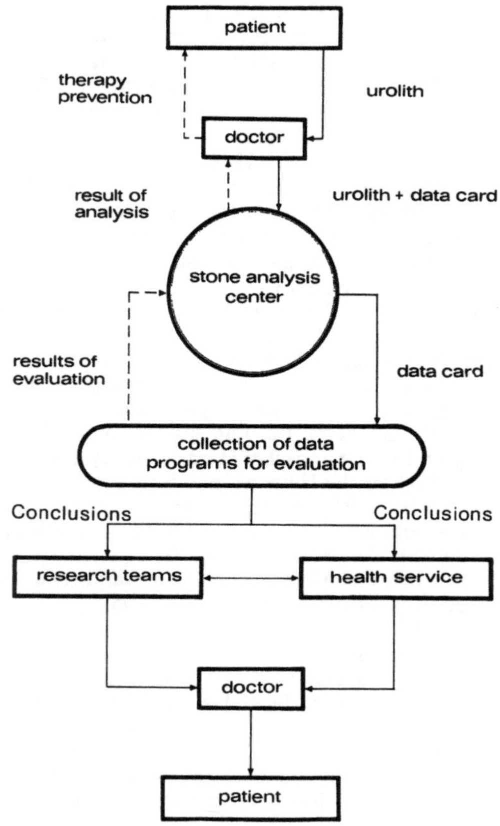

Fig. 102. Information network for centralised stone analysis

References

Adams RG, Harrison JF, Scott P (1969) The development of cadmium-induced proteinuria, renal function and osteomalacia in alkaline battery workers. O J Med 38:425–430

Adrian P (1972) Die Untersuchung von Harnwegskonkrementen mit Hilfe der Infrarotspektroskopie. Beckman-Report 2

Alken CE, Braun J, Bichler K-H, Bressel M, Gaca A, Hohenfellner R, Eisen M, Klosterhalfen H, Burchhardt P, Tamm H, Vahlensieck W (1973) Harnsteinanalyse in der Routinediagnostik. Medical Tribune, Nr 50

Alken P, Schäfer A (1978) Kristallurie bei Cystinsteinpatienten. In: Vahlensieck W, Gasser G (Hrsg) Pathogenese und Klinik der Harnsteine VI Steinkopff, Darmstadt, S 183–191

Alonso J, Somacarrera E (1973) Scanning microscopy in renal lithiasis. In: Cifuentes Delatte L, Rapado A, Hodgkinson A (eds) Urinary Calculi. Karger, Basel, S 256–263

Anke M, Schneider H-J (1973) Die Bedeutung der Spurenelemente in der Pathogenese und Therapie der Urolithiasis. III. Jenaer Harnsteinsymposium. Wissenschaftliche Beiträge der Friedrich-Schiller-Universität, Jena, S 116–126

Armbruster Th (1978) Minerale in menschlichen Harnkonkrementen, Teil 1, Phosphate. Aufschluß 29: 427–433

Armbruster Th (1979) Zum Harnsteinphosphatproblem (II). Die Rolle des „Karbonatapatits" in Harnkonkrementen. In: Gasser G, Vahlensieck W (Hrsg) Pathogenese und Klinik der Harnsteine VII. Steinkopff, Darmstadt S 182–187

Arnold W, Seemann N (1968) Vergleichende infrarot-spektrophotometrische und pathomorphologische Untersuchungen zur Urolithiasis. Dtsch Med Wochenschr 93:1791–1759

Asper R, Schmucki O (1980) Harnsteinanalytik Ther Umschau 37:342–347

Asper R, Schmucki O (1982) Diagnostik und Therapie der 2,8-Dihydroxyadenin-Lithiasis. In: Gasser G, Vahlensieck W (Hrsg) Pathogenese und Klinik der Harnsteine IX. Steinkopff, Darmstadt, S 274–282

Asper R, Schmucki O (1984) Crystal size determination by profile analysis of X-ray diffraction reflexes. In: Schwille PO, Smith LH, Robertson WD, Vahlensieck W (1984) Urolithiasis and Related Clinical Research. Plenum Press, New York-London (in press)

Asslamasow EG (1974) Die Matrix der Nierensteine (russ.) Urol Nefrol (Mosk) 3:59–60

Astm (1971) Radiologic data file powder diffraction file joint comitee on powder diffraction standards. PA, USA

Auermann E, Kühn H (1969) Untersuchungen über den Fluorgehalt von Harnsteinen. Dtsch Ges Wesen 24:565–569

Baba S, Nakazawa K, Odajima K, Fujioka T, Nakamura H (1983) Observation on urinary glycosaminoglycan excretion in patients with urinary calculus in relation to the nature of organic matrix of calculi. Jpn J Urol 74:608–615

Bach D, Gebhardt M, Vahlensieck W (1977) Vergleich zwischen chemischer und röntgendiffraktometrischer Harnsteinanalyse. In: Gasser G, Vahlensieck W (Hrsg) Pathogenese und Klinik der Harnsteine V. Steinkopff, Darmstadt, S 262–267

Bastian HP (1979) Raster-Elektronenmikroskopie. In: Vahlensieck W (Hrsg) Urolithiasis 1; Epidemiologie, allgemeine Kausal- und Formalgenese, Diagnostik. Springer, Berlin Heidelberg New York, S 127–134

Bastian HP, Gebhardt M (1974) The varying composition of the nucleus and peripheral layers of urinary calculi. Urol Res 2:91–95

Bastian HP, Gebhardt M (1975a) Harnsteinwachstum in vitro. In: Gasser G, Vahlensieck W (Hrsg) Pathogenese und Klinik der Harnsteine IV. Steinkopff, Darmstadt, S 30–40

Bastian HP, Gebhardt M (1975b) Möglichkeiten und Erscheinungsformen bei der Auflösung von Harnsteinen. In: Vahlensieck W, Gasser G (Hrsg) Pathogenese und Klinik der Harnsteine III. Steinkopff, Darmstadt, S 143–154

Bastian HP, Gebhardt M (1976) Die Harnsteinanalyse. Therapiewoche 26:5935–5938

Bastian HP, Gebhardt M, Vahlensieck W, Harting R (1976) In: Fleisch H, Robertson WG, Smith LH, Vahlensieck W (eds) Urolithiasis Research. Plenum Press, New York London, P 237–240

Bauer H-W, Haase W, Sieck R (1981) Neue diagnostische Möglichkeiten der Urinsedimentanalyse mit dem MD-KOVA-System. Urologe B 21:295–299

Baumann JM (1978) Wert der Sedimentenuntersuchung bei Kalziumnephrolithiasis. In: Vahlensieck W, Gasser G (Hrsg) Pathogenese und Klinik der Harnsteine VI. Steinkopff, Darmstadt, S 192–195

Bausch WM, Sorger G (1975) Mikrostrukturen von Harnwegkonkrementen Urologe [Ausg A] 14:161–163

Beck CW, Bender MJ (1969) Aragonite, $CaCO_3$, as urinary calculi. J Urol 101:208–211

Beck CW, Mulvaney WP, Rhamy RK, Gibson RI (1974) Monetite as urinary calculi. J Urol 111:673–675

Becker H, Gasteyer KH (1968) Eiweißsteine des Nierenbeckens Int Prax 8:375–378

Beischer DE (1955) Analysis of renal calculi by infrared spectroscopy. J Urol 73:653–657

Bellanato J, Cifuentes Delatte L, Hidalgo A, Santos M (1978) Application of infrared spectroscopy to the study of renal stones. In: Cifuentes Delatte L, Rapado A, Hodgkinson A (eds) Urinary Calculi. Karger, Basel p 237–246

Berenyi M (1970) Thermoanalyse als neue Form der Harnsteinanalyse und eine Zusammenfassung bisheriger Ergebnisse. I. Jenaer Harnsteinsymposium. Symposiumbericht, Jena, S 6–11

Berenyi M (1973a) New methods of stone analysis. In: Cifuentes Delatte L, Rapado A, Hodgkinson A (1973) Urinary Calculi. Karger, Basel, p 209–212

Berenyi M (eds) Vesekõanalizis ultramikro-kemiai modszerrel. Orv Hetil 114:2852–2853

Berenyi M (1974) Thermoanalyse. In: Schneider H-J (Hrsg) Technik der Harnsteinanalyse. Thieme, Leipzig, S 40–50

Berenyi M (1975) Über die Zusammensetzung der Nierensteine in Ungarn Acta Chir Hung 16:73–86
Berenyi M (1981) Urolithiasis-Vesekóbetegseģ. Medicina, Budapest
Berenyi M, Liptay G, Babics A, Erdey L (1967) Thermoanalytische Untersuchung von Nierensteinen I. Steinkomponenten mit Purinstruktur. Urol Nephrol 60:361–368
Berenyi M, Liptay G, Babics A (1968) Thermoanalytische Untersuchung von Nierensteinen II. Kalzium- und magnesiumhaltige Steine. Z Urol Nephrol 61:209–216
Berenyi M, Frang D, Legrady J (1972) Theoretical and clinical importance of the differentiation between the two types of calcium oxalate hydrate. Int Urol Nephrol 4:341–345
Berenyi M, Panovics J (1980) Eigenes mikroskopisch-ultramikrochemisches Analyseverfahren. VI. Jenaer Harnsteinsymposium. Wissenschaftliche Beiträge der Friedrich-Schiller-Universität, Jena, S 91–95
Berg van den CJ, Cahill TM, Smith LH (1976) Crystalluria. In: Fleisch H, Robertson WG, Smith LH, Vahlensieck W (eds) Urolithiasis Research. Plenum Press. New York London. p 365–366
Berg W, Hesse A, Schneider H-J (1976a) A contribution to the formation mechanism of calcium oxalate urinary calculi III. On the role of magnesium in the formation of oxalate calculi. Urol Res 4:161–167
Berg W, Schnapp J-D, Schneider H-J, Hesse A, Hienzsch E (1976b) Crystaloptical und spectroscopical findings with calcium oxalate crystals in the urine sediment. Eur Urol 2:92–97
Berg W, Schneider H-J, Hesse A (1976c) Crystal-optical findings on calcium oxalate of uric concretions. In: Fleisch H, Robertson WG, Smith LH, Vahlensieck W (eds) Urolithiasis Research. Plenum Press, New York London p 241–247
Berg W, Schneider H-J, Vogel E (1976d) Die Oxalatausscheidung im Harn bei oraler Oxalsäure- und Magnesiumzufuhr. In: Schneider H-J, Anke M (Hrsg) Magnesiumstoffwechsel. Wissenschaftliche Beiträge der Friedrich-Schiller-Universität. Jena, S 167–173
Berg W, Hesse A, Schneider H-J (1978a) Gefügebetrachtung und Kristallisationsstudie an Harnsteinen. V. Jenaer Harnsteinsymposium. Wissenschaftliche Beiträge der Friedrich-Schiller-Universität. Jena, S 101–103 (a)
Berg W, Schütt S, Schneider H-J (1978b) Polarisationsmikroskopische Untersuchungen zur Struktur und Genese von Harnsteinen. Jenaer Rundschau 23:188–192
Berg W, Lange P, Bothor C, Rössler D (1979a) Submicroscopic investigations on calcium oxalate stone genesis. Eur Urol 5:136–143
Berg W, Lange P, Rössler D, Bothor C (1979b) Pseudomorphosen in Kalziumoxalat-Harnsteinen. Z Urol Nephrol 72:351–357
Berg W, Schneider H-J, Rössler D, Börner RH (1979c) Krappanthrachinone als wirksame Harnsteinprophylaktika. In: Gasser G, Vahlensieck W (Hrsg) Pathogenese und Klinik der Harnsteine VII. Steinkopff, Darmstadt, S 402–410
Berg W, Rössler D, Bothor C und Lange P (1980) Feinstrukturen an Kalziumoxalatkonkrementen und ihre Interpretation zur Oxalatsteingenese. VI. Jenaer Harnsteinsymposium. Wissenschaftliche Beiträge der Friedrich-Schiller-Universität, Jena, S. 7–11
Berg W, Bothor C, Szabo-Földvari E, Schneider H-J (1982b) El sedimento urinario cristalino y su signification diagnostica para la lithiasis. Arch Esp Urol 35:389–404
Berg W, Bothor C, Erler J, Lange P (1983) Sind Silikate nur Kieselsteine? Z Urol Nephrol 76:319–325
Bernshtam J, Pinto B (1976) Epitaxy mechanism of urinary mucoprotein. In: Fleisch H, Robertson WG, Smith LH, Vahlensieck W (1976) Urolithiasis Research. Plenum Press, New York London p 249–251
Bick C, Brien G (1975) Kristalloptische Untersuchungen an sekundären Harnsteinen (Infektsteine). IV. Jenaer Harnsteinsymposium. Wissenschaftliche Beiträge der Friedrich-Schiller-Universität. Jena, S 73–76
Bick C, Brien UG (1976) Erfahrungen mit der kombinierten kristalloptischen röntgendiffraktometrischen Harnsteinanalytik. Z Med Lab Technik 17:341–348
Bick C, Schubert G (1980) Mikroskopische Differenzierung einiger Phasen der Phosphatgruppe bei Harnsteinen. 3. Berliner Harnsteinmikroskopiewoche. Tagungsbericht. S 21–26

Bick C, Brien G, Braun E (1974) Kristalloptische Untersuchungen an Harnsteinen. Z Urol Nephrol 67:513–521
Bick C, Schubert G, Brien G, Gremske D (1977) Topographische Phasenanalyse von Harnkonkrementen mit kristalloptischen Methoden. Z Urol Nephrol 70:99–105
Bick C, Schubert G, Brien G (1980) Die Kombination von Polarisationsmikroskopie und Röntgendiffraktion in der Harnsteinanalyse. VI. Jenaer Harnsteinsymposium. Wissenschaftliche Beiträge der Friedrich-Schiller-Universität. Jena, S 102–104
Blaschke R, Schmandt W (1978) Kugelförmige Calciumphosphat-Konkremente im Harn und in der Kernzone von Oxalatsteinen. In: Vahlensieck W, Gasser G (Hrsg) Pathogenese und Klinik der Harnsteine VI. Steinkopff, Darmstadt S 84–89
Blomen LJMJ (1981) Anwendung der Rasterelektronenmikroskopie bei der Urolithiasis. In: Vahlensieck W, Gasser G (Hrsg) Pathogenese und Klinik der Harnsteine VIII. Steinkopff, Darmstadt S 216–225
Boer den JNC, Bakker NJ u. Leynse B. Structuranalyse von Nier- en Blaassteinen door Röntgendiffractie, Ned Tijdschr Geneesk. 16:373–377 (1972)
Borgno M, Perolino M (1962) Chemical and crystallographic aspects of calcium oxalate calculi. Minerva Urol 14:1–17
Börner R, Schneider H-J, Berg W (1981) Stabilising factors for uric acid dihydrate – a contribution to the uric acid stone formation. In: Smith LH, Robertson WG, Finlayson B (eds) Urolithiasis: Clinical and Basic Research. Plenum Press, New York London, p 465–468
Boshamer K (1961) Morphologie und Genese der Harnsteine. In: Alken, Dix, Weyrauch, Wildbolz (Hrsg) Handbuch der Urologie, Bd X. Springer, Berlin Göttingen Heidelberg, S 1–171
Bothor C, Berg W (1980) Early stages of intrarenal calcium oxalate crystallization. In: Rose GA (ed) Oxalate in human biochemistry and clinical pathology. Proceedings Oxalate Workshop. London p 153–160
Boyce WH (1968) Organic matrix of human urinary concretions. Am J Med 45:673–677
Boyce WH (1969) Organic matrix of native human urinary concretion. In: Hodgkinson A, Nordin BEC (eds) Renal Stone Research Symposium. Churchill Ltd, London p 93–104
Boyce WH (1973) Ultrastructure of human renal calculi. In: Cifuentes Delatte L, Rapado A, Hodgkinson A (eds) Urinary Calculi. Karger, Basel, p 247–255
Brien G (1981) Erfahrungen mit röntgendiffraktometrischen und kristalloptischen Methoden in der Harnsteinanalytik und Harnsteinforschung. Med. Promot. B.-Arbeit, Berlin
Brien G, Braun E (1973) Röntgenstrukturanalyse von Harnsteinen mit Zählrohrgoniometer. Z Urol Nephrol 66:345–352
Brien G, Bick C, Schubert G (1978) Untersuchungen zur topographischen Phasenverteilung an 4000 Harnsteinen. V. Jenaer Harnsteinsymposium. Wissenschaftliche Beiträge der Friedrich-Schiller-Universität. Jena, S 76–82
Brien G, Schubert G, Bick C (1980) Gefügeuntersuchungen von Harnsteinen in Abhängigkeit von verschiedenen pathogenetischen Bedingungen. VI. Jenaer Harnsteinsymposium, Wissenschaftliche Beiträge der Friedrich-Schiller-Universität. Jena, S 41–47
Brien G, Schubert G, Bick C (1982) Getrennte Untersuchungen von Kern und Schale der Harnsteine – Erfahrungen an 17 000 Analysen. In: Gasser G, Vahlensieck W (Hrsg) Pathogenese und Klinik der Harnsteine IX. Steinkopff, Darmstadt, S 250–254
Brien G, Schubert G, Bick C (1982) 10,000 Analysis of urinary calculi using X-ray diffraction and polarizing microscopy. Eur Urol 8:251–256 (1982)
Bröring S, Bausch W, Bichler KH (1979) Wertigkeit quantitativer Harnsteinanalysen (Polarisationsmikroskopie und Röntgendiffraktion). In: Gasser G, Vahlensieck W (Hrsg) Pathogenese und Klinik der Harnsteine VII. Steinkopff, Darmstadt, S 312–316
Brückner A, Bernheim M (1979) Erfahrungen mit einer halbquantitativen Harnsteinanalyse. Ärztl Lab 25:203–208
Brundig P, Schneider H-J (1980) Zystolithotripsie, ihre Ergebnisse in Beziehung zur Steinart. VI. Jenaer Harnsteinsymposium. Wissenschaftliche Beiträge der Friedrich-Schiller-Universität, Jena, S 247–250
Bühlow H, Klee WE, Hotzel A, Frohmüller H (1977) Zur Frage einer Harnsteinbildung nach Trimethoprim/Sulfamethoxazol-Therapie. In: Gasser G, Vahlensieck W (Hrsg) Pathogenese und Klinik der Harnsteine V. Steinkopff, Darmstadt, S 116–118

Burns JR, Shoemaker BE, Gauthier JF, Finlayson B (1984) Hardness testing of Urinary Calculi. In: Schwille PO, Smith LH, Robertson WD, Vahlensieck W (eds) Urolithiasis and Related Clinical Research. Plenum Press, New York London (in press)
Burr RG (1976) The determination of silicates in urinary calculi. Clin Chim Acta 69:259–265
Burriel Marti F, Alvarez Herrero C, Sandos Rodriguez R (1969) Estudio quimico analitico estructural de calculos en lithiasis humanas. Rev Clin Esp 113:25–34
Buscemi PJ, Warpehoski MA, Finlayson B, Goldberg EP (1980) Surface morphology of calcium oxalate kidney calculi observed by electron microscopy. Fourth Int. Symp. Urolithiasis Res. Williamsburg, USA.
Buthliaschwili NS (1979) Petrographische Studien der Nierensteine der Menschen und der Tiere. Z Urol Nephrol 72:555–562
Carmona P, Garcia-Ramos JV, Gonzalez-Diaz PF, Cifuentes Delatte L, Hidalgo A (1978) Interaction between apatite calciumphosphate and model molecules related to the organic fraction of renal calculi. In: Vahlensieck W, Gasser G (Hrsg) Pathogenese und Klinik der Harnsteine VI. Steinkopff, Darmstadt, S 77–83
Carmona P, Bellanato J, Cifuentes Delatte L (1980) Trimagnesium orthophosphate in renal calculi. Invest Urol 18:151–154
Castro-Mendoza HJ, Cifuentes Delatte L, Rapado Errazti A (1972) Una nueva observacion de xanthinuria familiar. Rev Clin Esp 124:341–352
Catalina F, Cifuentes Delatte L (1970) Calcium Oxalate: Crystallographic analysis in solid aggregates in urinary sediments. Science 169:183–184
Catalina F, Cifuentes Delatte L (1971) Estudio de las cristalurias oxalocaleicas. Arch Esp Urol 24:147–164
Cavero MG (1972) Semejanzas que tienen los calculos con las rocas y con las minerales. Arch Esp Urol 25:135–198
Cavero MG (1973) Calculos, rocas y minerales. Arch Esp Urol 26:115–168
Cavero MG (1981, 1982) Calculos con grandes cristales de oxalatos. Arch Esp Urol 34:199–206, 35:39–46
Cifuentes J, Gonzalez-Diaz PF, Cifuentes Delatte L (1978) Citrate ions on apatite surface. In: Vahlensieck W, Gasser G (Hrsg) Pathogenese und Klinik der Harnsteine VI. Steinkopff, Darmstadt, S 158–162
Cifuentes Delatte L (1974) El Laboratorio del urologa. In: Salvat (ed) S. A., Barcelona, Calciumoxalat p 101–103
Cifuentes Delatte L (1978) Strukturanalyse von Harnsteinen und die Kristallisation von Harninhaltsstoffen. V. Jenaer Harnsteinsymposium. Wissenschaftliche Beiträge der Friedrich-Schiller-Universität, Jena, S 65–70
Cifuentes Delatte L (1981) Historia del estudio microscopico de los calculos del aparato urinario en el siglo XIX. Arch Esp Urol 34:375–384
Cifuentes Delatte L, Castro-Mendoza H (1967) Xanthinuria familiar. Rev Clin Exp 28:244–256
Cifuentes Delatte L, Medina JA (1981) Oolithic structure of milk of calcium sand and milk of calcium stones. In: Smith LH, Robertson WG, Finlayson B (eds) Urolithiasis: Clinical and Basic Research. Plenum Press, New York London, p 917–921
Cifuentes Delatte L, Santos M (1977) Calcified bacteria in renal stones: Electromicroscopic aspects. Eur Urol 3:96–99
Cifuentes Delatte L, Catalina F, Garcia-Vicente J, Estaban B (1967) Electron microscopy and X-ray diffraction of precipitated urinary calcium phosphates Br J Urol 39:450–455
Cifuentes Delatte L, Garcia de la Peña E, Vela Navarrete R, Miñon Cifuentes JR (1973a) Tejido oseo en calculos del aparato urinario. Arch Esp Urol 26:457–480
Cifuentes Delatte L, Hidalgo A, Bellanato J, Santos M (1973b) Polarization microscopy and infrared spectroscopy of thin sections of calculi. In: Cifuentes Delatte L, Rapado A, Hodgkinson A (eds) Urinary Calculi. Karger, Basel, p 220–230
Cifuentes Delatte L, Rapado A, Hodgkinson A (1973c) Urinary Calculi. Karger, Basel
Cifuentes Delatte L, Miñon JLR, Santos M, Troba ML (1976) Ectopic renal ossification as nucleus of urinary stones. J Urol 116:398–401
Cifuentes Delatte L, Carmona P, Bellanato J, Santos M, Hidalgo A (1977) Trimagnesiumphosphates in renal calculi. In: Gasser G, Vahlensieck W (Hrsg) Pathogenese und Klinik der Harnsteine V. Steinkopff, Darmstadt, S 196–202

Cifuentes Delatte L, Bellanato J, Santos M, Hidalgo A (1978a) Brushit in Harnsteinen. In: Vahlensieck W, Gasser G (Hrsg) Pathogenese und Klinik der Harnsteine VI. Steinkopff, Darmstadt, S 153–157

Cifuentes Delatte L, Bellanato J, Santos M, Rodriguez-Miñon JL (1978b) Monosodium urate in urinary calculi. Eur Urol 4:441–443

Cifuentes Delatte L, Medina JA, Santos M, Rodriguez J (1978c) Litiasis urinaria de silice ($SiO_2 \cdot n\ H_2O$) en los animales y en la especie humana. Rev Clin Esp 151:343–346

Cifuentes Delatte L, Santos M, Medina JA (1979) Granatähnliche Struktur in Harnsteinen. Z Urol Nephrol 72:417–425

Cifuentes Delatte L, Medina JA, Juarez M, Bellanato J (1981) Kaliumurat in Harnsteinen. In: Vahlensieck W, Gasser G (Hrsg) Pathogenese und Klinik der Harnsteine VIII. Steinkopff, Darmstadt, S 265–273

Cifuentes Delatte L, Medina JA, Traba ML (1983) Calulò de sulfato calcico de origen renal una observacion homologable? Arch Esp Urol 36:117–123

Cifuentes Delatte L, Medina J, Bellanato J, Santos M (1984) Papillensteine und Randallsche Plaques. In: Vahlensieck W, Gasser G (Hrsg) Pathogenese und Klinik der Harnsteine X. Steinkopff, Darmstadt, S 240–246

Cocco G (1961) Structure Reports SR 26:484 zitiert bei Schubert u. Brien 1978

Corns CM (1983) Infrared analysis of renal calculi: a comparison with conventional techniques. Am Clin Biochem 20:20–24

Crawford D (1984) Electron microscopy of urinary calculisome facts and artefacts. Urol Res 12:17–22

Dalicho WA (1957) Wahrnehmung und Darstellbarkeit von Details im Röntgenbild. Thieme Verlag, Leipzig 1967.

Das S, Joseph B, Dick AL (1979) Renal failure owing to oxalate nephrosis after jejunoilial bypass. J Urol 121:506–509

Daudon M, Protat MF, Reveillaud RJ, Jaeschke-Boyer H (1981) Anwendung des Lasers für die Harnsteinanalyse. In: Vahlensieck W, Gasser G (Hrsg) Pathogenese und Klinik der Harnsteine VIII. Steinkopff, Darmstadt, S 311–321

Deganello S, Kampf AR, Moore PB (1981) The structure of calcium oxalate trihydrate. Symposium on crystallography in the health sciences. Toronto

Denbsky G, Kolb R, Michahelles E (1973) Zur Phosphatbestimmung in Harnkonkrementen. Münch Med Wochenschr 115:1988–1990

Dimitrov G, Marinov M (1976) Laser microspectral analysis of urinary concrements. Medikon 5:5–11

Dimopoulos C, Kyriakidis A, Stokidis D, Karayiannis A, Markopoulos T, Bahioniakis A, Sideris S, Kallistratos G (1983) X-ray diffractometric analysis of L-cystine stones in 12 patients. Eur Urol 9:227–230

Dosch W (1975c) Genese und Wachstum von Harnsteinen In: Vahlensieck W, Gasser G (Hrsg) Pathogenese und Klinik der Harnsteine III. Steinkopff, Darmstadt, S 67–83

Dosch W (1975b) Datensammlung und Vorschläge zur standardisierten Harnsteinanalyse. In: Vahlensieck W, Gasser G (Hrsg) Pathogenese und Klinik der Harnsteine IV. Steinkopff, Darmstadt, S 8–15

Dosch W (1977) Analytik des Harnsteinleidens. In: Gasser G, Vahlensieck W (Hrsg) Pathogenese und Klinik der Harnsteine V. Steinkopff, Darmstadt, S 289–295

Dosch W (1980a) Mineralogische Verfahren zur Strukturanalyse in der Harnsteinforschung. VI. Jenaer Harnsteinsymposium. Wissenschaftliche Beiträge der Friedrich-Schiller-Universität, Jena, S 25–29

Dosch W (1980b) Morphologie von Harnsteinen. VI. Jenaer Harnsteinsymposium. Wissenschaftliche Beiträge der Friedrich-Schiller-Universität, Jena, S 112–115

Dosch W (1980) New crystalline phases in kidney stones. Fourth Int. Symp. Urolithiasis Res., Williamsburg, USA

Dosch W (1981a) Neue Urate I: Vorkommen in Harn- und Prostatasteinen. In: Vahlensieck W, Gasser G (Hrsg) Pathogenese und Klinik der Harnsteine VIII. Steinkopff, Darmstadt, S 241–253

Dosch W (1981b) Neue Urate II: Harnsäure und Harnsäure-Dihydrat. In: Vahlensieck W, Gasser G (Hrsg) Pathogenese und Klinik der Harnsteine VIII. Steinkopff, Darmstadt, S 254–264

Dosch W, Altrock K (1974) Aussagemöglichkeiten und technischer Aufwand verschiedener Methoden der Harnsteinanalyse. In: Vahlensieck W, Gasser G (Hrsg) Klinik und Pathogenese der Harnsteine II. Steinkopff, Darmstadt, S 1–24

Dosch W, Koestel C (1975) Rasterelektronenmikroskopie von Harnsteinen. In: Vahlensieck W, Gasser G (Hrsg) Pathogenese und Klinik der Harnsteine IV. Steinkopff, Darmstadt, S 41–58

Drach GW, Hillmann BJ, Tracey P, Gaines JA (in press) Computed tomographic analysis of the composition of renal calculi. In: Schwille PO, Smith LH, Robertson WD, Vahlensieck W (eds) Urolithiasis and Related Clinical Research. Plenum Press, New York London

Eismann D (1978) Bewährte mikroskopische Verfahren und Gerätekombinationen zur Harnsteinuntersuchung. Jenaer Rundschau 23:193–196

Eismann D (1980) Anforderungen an Immersionsflüssigkeiten für die Harnsteinuntersuchung im mikroskopischen Körnerpräparat. 3. Berliner Harnsteinmikroskopiewoche. Tagungsbericht, S 61–66

Eismann D, Rockstroh H, Hasselbacher K (1978) Einsatzvarianten mikroskopischer Geräte zur Harnsteinuntersuchung in Routine und Forschung. Z Urol Nephrol 71:473–480

Elliot JS (1968) Calcium stones: The difference between oxalate and phosphate types. J Urol 100:687–693

Elliot JS (1973a) Structure and composition of urinary calculi. J Urol 109:82–83

Elliot JS (1973b) Optical analysis of urinary calculi: The value of low power dissection. In: Cifuentes Delatte L, Rapado A, Hodgkinson A (eds) Urinary Calculi. Karger, Basel, p 216–219

Elliot JS, Rabinowitz IN (1976) Crystal, habit, structure and incidence in the urine of a hospital population. In: Fleisch H, Robertson WG, Smith LH, Vahlensieck W (eds) Urolithiasis Research. Plenum Press, New York London, p 257–260

Elliot JS, Rabinowitz IN (1978) Diagnostik der Harnkristalle. Extracta Urologica 1:11–34

Elliot JS, Rabinowitz IN, Silvert M (1976) Calcium oxalate crystalluria. J Urol 116:773–775

El-Sayed K, Cosslett VE (1977) Investigation of the microstructure of kidney stones (oxalate type) by high voltage electron microscopy and electron diffraction. Experientia 33:919–921

Emons H-H, Keyne H, Seyfarth H-H (1973) Chemische Mikroskopie. VEB Deutscher Verlag für Grundstoffindustrie, Leipzig

Ernst G, Rößler D, Lange P, Anke M, Schneider H-J (1980) Kristallstrukturen und feingewebliche Nierenveränderungen bei exogener Oxalose. VI. Jenaer Harnsteinsymposium. Wissenschaftliche Beiträge der Friedrich-Schiller-Universität, Jena, S 123–125

Esteban B, Cifuentes Delatte L, Rapado A, Cortes M (1969) Resultados del analisis quimino cualitativo de 400 calcules del aparato urinario. Arch Esp Urol 22:35–53

Ettinger B, Weil E, Mandel NS, Darling S (1979) Triamterene-induced nephrolithiasis. Ann Intern Med 91:745–747

Ettinger B, Oldroyd NO, Sorgel F (1980) Triamterene nephrolithiasis. Fourth Int. Symp. Urolithiasis Res., Williamsburg, USA

Featherstone JDB, Oldeshaw MD, Shields CP (1981) Modification of structure defects in carbonated-apatites by strontium, zinc and fluoride. Symposium on crystallography in the health sciences. Toronto

Finlayson B, Reid F (1978) The expectation of free and fixed particles in urinary stone disease. Invest Urol 15:442–447

Flach W, Hesse A, Feist H (1978) Aminosäurezusammensetzung der organischen Matrix von Harnsteinen. V. Jenaer Harnsteinsymposium. Wissenschaftliche Beiträge der Friedrich-Schiller-Universität, Jena, S 108–110

Fleisch H, Robertson WG, Smith LH, Vahlensieck W (1976) Urolithiasis Research. Plenum Press, New York London

Flerowski JA (1965) Eine Komplexstudie über die Harnsteinzusammensetzung (russ.) Urol Nefrol (Mosk) 4:3–8

Fornitschew IL (1971) Komplexe Untersuchungen der Steinzusammensetzung der oberen Harnwege (russ.) Urol Nefrol (Mosk) 4:6–11

Frye H, Chan P (1972) Analysis of urinary calculi with attenuated total reflectance infrared spectrophotometry. Invest Urol 10:144–146

Fuss M, Vanlanduyt R, Jedwal J (1976) A routine method for the integrated study of microcrystals in urine; light and scanning electron microscopy, electron microprobe and micro-X-ray diffraction. In: Fleisch H, Robertson WG, Smith LH, Vahlensieck W (eds) Urolithiasis Research. Plenum Press, New York London, p 269–272

Gaca A, Dosch W (1981) Konkremente der Prostata. In: Vahlensieck W, Gasser G. (Hrsg) Pathogenese und Klinik der Harnsteine VIII. Steinkopff, Darmstadt, S 50–56

Garcia de la Peña E, Cifuentes Delatte L (1981) Forms of ammonic urate presentation in urinary calculus of non-infectious and infectious origin. In: Smith LH, Vahlensieck W, Finlayson B (eds) Urolithiasis: Clinical and Basic Research. Plenum Press, New York, London, S 935–942

Garcia-Ramos JV, Bellanato J, Santos M, Cifuentes Delatte L (1984) Spectroscopie studies of the oxalate-phosphate interaction in whewellite calculi. In: Vahlensieck W, Gasser G (eds) Pathogenese und Klinik der Harnsteine X. Steinkopff, Darmstadt S 188–192

Garcia Cuerpo E, Avilla S (1979) Analitical study of urinary calculi from a hospital of spain. XVIII Congres Societe Internationale D'Urologie, Paris

Gardner GL (1975) Nucleation and crystal growth of calcium oxalate trihydrate. J Crystal Growth 30:158–168

Gebhardt M (1974) Harnsteinbildung aus mineralogischer Sicht. In: Vahlensieck W, Gasser G (Hrsg) Pathogenese und Klinik der Harnsteine II. Steinkopff, Darmstadt, S 32–46

Gebhardt M (1975) Unterschiedliche Vorstellungen zur Phosphat- und Oxalat-Steinbildung nach Röntgen- und REM-Untersuchungen. In: Vahlensieck W, Gasser G (Hrsg), Pathogenese und Klinik der Harnsteine III. Steinkopff, Darmstadt, S 84–92

Gebhardt M (1978) Kristallographische Untersuchungen zur Harnsteinbildung unter besonderer Berücksichtigung von Epitaxie und Fixation. V. Jenaer Harnsteinsymposium. Wissenschaftliche Beiträge der Friedrich-Schiller-Universität, Jena, S 54–58

Gebhardt M (1979a) Harnsteinanalyse mittels Röntgendiffraktion. In: Vahlensieck W, Urolithiasis I. Springer, Berlin Heidelberg New York, S 77–121

Gebhardt M (1979b) Problematik und neuere Methoden der Harnsteinanalyse. Therapiewoche 29:2166–2177

Gebhardt M (1980a) Steinanalyse. In: Hautmann R, Lutzeyer W (Hrsg) Harnsteinfibel Deutscher Ärzteverlag, Köln-Lövenich, S 125–137

Gebhardt M (1980b) Harnsteine; Infodienst Deutsche Wellcome GmbH

Gebhardt M, Bastian HP (1975) Problematik der Harnsteingruppierung. In: Vahlensieck W, Gasser G (Hrsg) Pathogenese und Klinik der Harnsteine IV. Steinkopff, Darmstadt, S 1–7

Gebhardt M, Bastian HP (1976a) Harnsteingruppierung und Analysengenauigkeit. Urol Int 31:217–229

Gebhardt M, Bastian HP (1976b) Exact stone analysis – significance for prophylaxis. In: Fleisch H, Robertson WG, Smith LH, Vahlensieck W (Heds) Urolithiasis Research. Plenum Press, New York London, S 273–276

Gebhardt M, Bastian HP, Vahlensieck W (1977) Was kann das Röntgenschattenbild über die Zusammensetzung eines Harnsteins aussagen? In: Gasser G, Vahlensieck W (Hrsg) Pathogenese und Klinik der Harnsteine V. Steinkopff, Darmstadt, S 243–253

Gebhardt M, Bastian HP, Kaufmann J (1978) Experimentelle Untersuchungen zum Wachstum und zur Auflösung von Harnsteinen. In: Vahlensieck W, Gasser G (Hrsg) Pathogenese und Klinik der Harnsteine VI. Steinkopff, Darmstadt, S 233–241

Gibson RJ (1974) Descriptive human pathological mineralogy. Am Mineral 59:1177–1179

Gorew BS, Agafonow NW (1978) Einsatz der Elektronen-Mikrosonde zur mikroanalytischen Untersuchung der Harnsteinzusammensetzung (russ.) 2. Allunionskongreß für Urologie Kiew, Kongreßbericht, S 393–396

Götz W (1974) Zur Präparations- und Aufnahmetechnik der röntgenographischen Harnsteinanalyse. Z Urol Nephrol 67:363–365

Greene ML, Fujimato WY, Seegmiller JE (1968) Urinary xanthine stones – a rare complication of allopurinol therapy. New Engl J Med 280:426–429

Grieve J, Zaremski PM (1973) Infrared spectroscopy in the clinical analysis of renal stones. In: Cifuentes Delatte L, Rapado A, Hodgkinson A (eds) Urinary Calculi. Karger, Basel, p 231–236

Griffith DP (1978) Struvite stones. Kidney Int 13:372–382

Grünberg W (1971) Karbonatharnsteine herbivorer Säugetiere. Zentralbl Veterinar Med 18:767–823
Grünberg W, Preisinger A (1969) Magnesiumhaltiger Calcit in tierischen Harnkonkrementen. Naturwiss 56:518–519
Gusek W, Bode W, Matousckek E, Huber R (1982) Konzentrisch geschichtete Mikrokonkremente im Nierenmark von Harnsteinträgern – Ein Beitrag zur Harnsteingenese. Urologe [AusgA] 21:137–141
Hahne B, Eismann D (1979) Gefügeuntersuchungen an Harnsteinen. 2. Berliner Harnsteinmikroskopiewoche, Tagungsbericht, S 48–54
Hambraeus L, Lagergren C (1962) Biophysical and roentgenological studies of urinary calculi from cystinuric. J Urol 88:826–833
Hawotte Ph (1972) Le calcul mou du rein. Acta Urol Belg 40:47–58
Hazarika EZ, Balakrishna Rao BN (1974a) Spectrochemical analysis of urinary tract calculi. Indian J Med Res 62:776–780
Hazarika EZ, Balakrishna Rao BN, Kapur BML, Misra RK (1974b) Lower urinary tract calculi analysed by X-ray diffraction and chemical methods. Indian J Med Res 62:893–904
He J, Liu G-D, Shen SJ Composition and structure of infected stones. In: Schwille PO, Smith LH, Robertson WD, Vahlensieck W (eds) Urolithiasis and Related Clinical Research. Plenum Press, New York London (in press)
Heide K (1970) Die Mikrothermoanalyse und ihre Vorteile bei der Identifizierung von Harnsteinen. I. Jenaer Harnsteinsymposium. Symposiumbericht Jena, S 16–18
Heide K (1979) Dynamische thermische Analysenmethoden. Deutscher Verlag Grundstoffindustrie, Leipzig
Heide K, Hesse A, Berg W (1978) Zur Keimbildung und Kristallisation im Harn – Untersuchungen an Kalziumoxalat. V. Jenaer Harnsteinsymposium. Wissenschaftliche Beiträge der Friedrich-Schiller-Universität, Jena, S 21–26
Heintz R, Althof S (1976) Das Harnsediment. Thieme, Stuttgart
Heller JF (1860) Die Harnkonkretionen der Menschen. Tendler & Co., Wien
Hering F, Brunner R, Briellmann T, Seiler H, Rutishauser G (1984) Schützt Fluor vor der Kalziumoxalatsteinbildung? In: Vahlensieck W, Gasser G (Hrsg) Pathogenese und Klinik der Harnsteine X. Steinkopff, Darmstadt, S 44–50
Herring LC (1962) Observations on the analysis of ten thousand urinary calculi. J Urol 88:545–562
Hesse A (1972) Infrarotspektroskopische Untersuchungen zur Bedeutung des Hydratwassers am Kalziumoxalatstein. II. Jenaer Harnsteinsymposium. Wissenschaftliche Beiträge der Friedrich-Schiller-Universität, Jena, S 64–67
Hesse (1979) Harnsteinanalyse mittels Infrarotspektroskopie. In: Vahlensieck W (Hrsg) Urolithiasis 1. Springer, Berlin Heidelberg New York, S 70–76
Hesse A (1983) Technik der infrarotspektroskopischen Harnsteinanalyse. J Clin Chem Clin Biochem 20:861–873
Hesse A, Bach D (1982) Harnsteine – Pathobiochemie und klinisch-chemische Diagnostik. In: Klinische Chemie in Einzeldarstellungen Bd. 5. Thieme, Stuttgart New York
Hesse A, Klee WE (1974) Infrarotspektroskopische Analyse. In: Schneider H-J (ed) Technik der Harnsteinanalyse. Thieme, Leipzig, S 51–73
Hesse A, Schneider H-J (1976) Results of the standardization and centralization of stone analysis in the German Democratic Republic. In: Fleisch H, Robertson WG, Smith LH, Vahlensieck W (eds) Urolithiasis Research. Plenum Press, New York London, p 295–298
Hesse A, Schneider H-J, Hienzsch E (1972a) Die infrarotspektroskopische Harnsteinanalyse. Dtsch Med Wochenschr 97:1694–1701
Hesse A, Schneider H-J, Schilling I, Schrumpf G, Hienzsch E (1972b) Infrarotspektroskopische und Röntgenfeinstrukturuntersuchungen an Kalziumoxalat-Harnsteinen. Z Inn Med 27:560–565
Hesse A, Schneider H-J, Hienzsch E (1973a) Stand der Zentralisierung und Standardisierung der Harnsteinanalyse in der DDR. Urol Nephrol 66:341–344
Hesse A, Schneider H-J, Hienzsch E (1973b) Anwendung der Infrarotspektralphotometer UR 10/UR 20 und Specord 71 IR aus Jena für die Harnsteinanalyse. Jenaer Rundschau 18:282–287

Hesse A, Schneider H-J, Weiz, G, Cruse R, Klee WE (1973c) Magnesium ammoniumphosphate monohydrate-A hitherto undetected constituent of urinary calculi. Int Urol Nephrol 5:19–26

Hesse A, Berg W, Schneider H-J (1974a) Experimentelle Untersuchungen zur Bildung farbiger Harnsteine durch Rubia-Präparate. Z Urol Nephrol 67:335–340

Hesse A, Schrumpf G, Schilling I (1974b) Quantitative Bestimmung von Harnsteinkomponenten durch Anwendung der Infrarotspektroskopie. Z Urol Nephrol 67:367–375

Hesse A, Schneider H-J, Berg W, Hienzsch E (1975) Uric acid dihydrate as urinary calculi component. Invest Urol 12:405–409

Hesse A, Berg W, Schneider H-J, Hienzsch E (1976a) A contribution to the formation mechanism of calcium oxalate urinary calculi. I. Stabilising urinary constituents in the formation of weddellite. Urol Res 4:125–128

Hesse A, Schneider H-J, Berg W, Hienzsch E (1976b) A contribution to the formation mechanisms of calcium oxalate urinary calculi. II. In vitro experiments concerning the theory of the formation of whewellite and weddellite urinary calculi. Urol Res 4:157–160

Hesse A, Schneider H-J, Schröder S, Wegner R (1976c) Ergebnisse der AIV-gerechten Auswertung von 10 000 Harnsteinanalysenbelegen. Z Urol Nephrol 69:1–9

Hesse A, Dietze H-J, Berg W, Hienzsch E (1977) Mass spectrometric trace element analysis of calcium oxalate uroliths. Eur Urol 3:359–361

Hesse A, Berg W, Schneider H-J (1978a) Die Bedeutung der Spurenelemente in der Harnsteingenese. Zentralbl Pharm 117:753–756

Hesse A, Lange P, Berg W, Bothor C (1978b) Mikrosondenuntersuchungen an Phosphatphasen von Harnsteinen. V. Jenaer Harnsteinsymposium. Wissenschaftliche Beiträge der Friedrich- Schiller-Universität, Jena, S 98–100

Hesse A, Müller R, Schneider H-J, Taubert F (1978c) Analytische Untersuchungen zur Bedeutung des Fluorgehaltes von Harnsteinen. Urologe [Ausg A] 17:207–210

Hesse A, Berg W, Bothor C (1979a) Scanning electron microscopic investigations on the morphology and phase conversions of uroliths. Int Urol Nephrol 11:11–20

Hesse A, Lange P, Berg W, Bothor C, Hienzsch E (1979b) Scanning electron microscopy and microprobe investigation of phosphate phases in uroliths. Urol Int 34:81–94

Hesse A, Hicking W, Bach D, Vahlensieck W (1980) Investigations for characterising single crystal phases in urinary stones by means of an arrangement of light microscopy in combination with scanning electron microscopy. Abstracts 5th Symp. on Exper. Urology. Urol Res 8:243

Hesse A, Hicking W, Bach D, Vahlensieck W (1981a) Characterization of urinary crystals and thin polished sections of urinary calculi by means of an optical microscopic and scanning electron microscopic arrangement. Urol Int 36:281–291

Hesse A, Röhle G, Voigt U (1981b) Qualitätskontrolle von Harnsteinanalysen – Ergebnisse aus zwei Ringversuchen. In: Vahlensieck W, Gasser G (Hrsg) Pathogenese und Klinik der Harnsteine VIII. Steinkopff, Darmstadt, S 306–310

Hesse A, Ansorge J, Seifert K-F, Vahlensieck W (1984) Polarisationsmikroskopische Untersuchungen zur Klassifizierung von Wachstums- und Umwandlungsgefügen der Kalziumoxalat-Steine. In: Vahlensieck W, Gasser G (Hrsg) Pathogenese und Klinik der Harnsteine X. Steinkopff, Darmstadt, S 160–168

Hicking W (1979) Polarisationsmikroskopische Harnsteinanalyse. In: Vahlensieck W (Hrsg) Urolithiasis 1. Springer, Berlin Heidelberg New York, S 121–126

Hicking W, Hesse A, Vahlensieck W (1981) Comparison of x-ray diffractometric, infrared spectrometric and polarizing microscopic coreshell-analysis of urinary stones. In: Smith LH, Robertson WG, Finlayson B (eds) Urolithiasis: Clinical and Basic Research. Plenum Press, New York London, p 985–991

Hienzsch E, Schneider H-J (1973) Der Harnstein. Gustav Fischer, Jena

Hienzsch E, Hesse A, Berg W, Schneider H-J (1975) Beitrag zur Struktur sekundärer Harnsteine. IV. Jenaer Harnsteinsymposium. Wissenschaftliche Beiträge der Friedrich-Schiller-Universität, Jena, S 30–37

Hienzsch E, Hesse A, Bothor C, Berg W, Roth J (1979) A contribution to the formation mechanism of calcium oxalate urinary calculi IV. Experimental investigation of the intrarenal crystallization of calcium oxalate in rabbit. Urol Res 7:223–227

Hinmann F (1979) Directional growth of renal calculi. J Urol 121:700–705
Hodgkinson A (1971) A combined qualitative and quantitative procedure for the chemical analysis of urinary calculi. J Clin Pathol 24:147–157
Hodgkinson A, Marshall RW (1975) Changes in the composition of urinary tract stones. Invest Urol 13:131–135
Hodgkinson A, Nordin BEC (1969) Renal stone research symposium. Churchill LTD, London
Hodgkinson A, Peacock M, Nicholson M (1969) Quantitative analysis of calcium-containing urinary calculi. Invest Urol 6:549–561
Homrighausen E (1977) Über die Eignung von Epoxin 162 und Laromin C 260 zur Einbettung von Bodenproben. Leitz-Mitt Wiss Techn 8:15–17
Hooft C, van Acker K, Valcke R (1964) Zink en nierensteenvorming. Verh K Acad Geneeskd Belg 26:357–372
Horn G, Hesse A (1972) Eiweißsteine der Harnwege. Methoden ihrer Analyse. Z Urol Nephrol 65:801–813
Ismail SJ, Tawashi R (1980) Effect of the organic matrix on the dissolution of uric acid stones. Eur Urol 6:237–240
Joekes AM, Rose GA, Sutor J (1973) Multiple renal silica calculi. Br Med J 1/5846:146–147
Jones DW, Smith JAS (1962) The structure of brushite, $CaHPO_4 \cdot 2H_2O$. J Clin Soc 16:1414–1417
Joost J, Tessadry R (1983) Combined analysis of kidney stones by X-ray diffraction and electron microprobe. Eur Urol 9:305–311
Joost J, Purtscheller F, Bandtlow K (1978) Prostatasteine. V. Jenaer Harnsteinsymposium. Wissenschaftliche Beiträge der Friedrich-Schiller-Universität, Jena, S 121–123
Joost J, Schabel F, Doppler W (1981) Complete adenine phosphoribosyltransferase deficiency with 2,8-dihydroxyadenine stone formation. In: Sperling O, Vahlensieck W (eds) Uric acid lithiasis. Steinkopff, Darmstadt, p 58–65
Kasantzis G (1979) Some effects of cadmium on the human kidney. In: Anke M, Schneider H-J (eds) Cadmiumsymposium. Wissenschaftliche Beiträge der Friedrich-Schiller-Universität, Jena, p 117–121
Kemoki F, Mizukira V, Konjiki T, Kawai H (1978) Elemental analysis of urinary tract calculi using an electron microscope with electron probe x-ray microanalyzer. Acta Histochem (Jena) 11:387–391
Kerde Ch, Krämer H, Müller Th, Schneider H-J (1980) Gm-Untersuchungen an Nierensteinen. VI. Jenaer Harnsteinsymposium. Wissenschaftliche Beiträge der Friedrich-Schiller-Universität, Jena, S 87–89
Khan SR, Finlayson B, Hackett RL (1983) Agar-embedded urinary stones: A technique useful for studying microscopic architecture. J Urol 130:992–995
Khan SR, Finlayson B, Hackett RL (1984) A microscopic study of the matrix of some calcium oxalate renal stones. In: Schwille PO, Smith LH, Robertson WD, Vahlensieck W (eds) Urolithiasis and Related Clinical Research. Plenum Press, New York London (in press)
Kim KM (1983) Mulberry particles formed by red blood cells in human weddelite stones. J Urol 129:855
Kimura Y, Kisaki N, Ise K (1976) The role of the matrix substance in formation of urinary stones. Urol Int 31:355–367
Kisters R, Terhorst B (1973) Harnsteinanalyse durch Infrarotspektroskopie. Urologe [Ausg B] 13:85–89
Klee WE (1970) Die Infrarotspektroskopie als geeignete Form der routinemäßigen Harnsteinanalyse. I. Jenaer Harnsteinsymposium. Symposiumsbericht, Jena, S 37–45
Kleeberg J (1976) Simplified qualitative chemical analysis for urinary calculi. J Clin Pathol 29:1038–1043
Kleeberg J, Gordon T, Kedar S, Dobler M (1981) Studies on the morphology of human uric acid stones. Urol Res 9:259–261
Koide T, Miyagawa M, Kimoshita K (1977) Matrix stones. J Urol 117:786–787
Koide T, Yokagawa K, Takemoto M, Itatani H, Sagawa S, Sonoda T (1982) Pure calcium carbonate urolithiasis in a human. Eur Urol 8:319–320
Kollwitz AA (1968) Technik und Bedeutung der Harnsteinanalyse Dtsch Med Wochenschr 19:22–28

Kolpakow JS (1971) Zur Frage der Morphologie und Genese der Zentren in den Harnsteinen. Z Urol Nephrol 64:641–645

Kolpakow JS, Gliki VW (1965a) Morphologie und Genese der Harnsteine unter Berücksichtigung der Ergebnisse polarisationsmikroskopischer Untersuchungen von Kalziumoxalat (russ.). Urol Nefrol (Mosk) 2:3–10

Kolpakow JS, Gliki VW (1965b) Morphologie und Genese der Harnsteine nach den Ergebnissen polarisationsmikroskopischer Untersuchungen II. Phosphate (russ.). Urol Nefrol (Mosk) 5:15–21

Kozlovskij JT (1973) Mineralogische Klassifizierung von Harnsteinen (russ.). Urol Nefrol (Mosk) 2:24–26

Kozlovskij JT, Jarygin VI, Sokarev M (1977) Kolloidales Kalziumphosphat (Kollophan) in Harnsteinen (russ.). Urol Nefrol (Mosk) 4:27–32

Krampitz G, Goetz P (1984) Isolierung und teilweise Charakterisierung organischer Komponenten aus Oxalat- und Struvit-Apatit-Harnsteinen. In: Vahlensieck W, Gasser G (Hrsg) Pathogenese und Klinik der Harnsteine X. Steinkopff, Darmstadt, S 225–229

Kreutzmann H, Ecke M (1971) Unsere Erfahrungen mit der qualitativ-chemischen Harnsteinanalyse. Z Urol Nephrol 64:657–661

Krizek V (1968) Das kristalline Harnsediment bei Zystinurie. Therapie Gegenwart 107:1302–1305

Krizek V (1971) Urolithiasis and prostatolithiasis in alcaptonuria with ochronosis. Int Urol Nephrol 3:245–250

Krizek V (1984) Urolithiasis bei der Alkaptonurie. In: Vahlensieck W, Gasser G (1984) Pathogenese und Klinik der Nierensteine X. Steinkopff, Darmstadt, S 73–76

Krizek V, Schneider H-J, Hesse A, Tscharnke J, Heide K (1973) Analytische Untersuchungen zur chemischen Zusammensetzung und Struktur von Zystinsteinen. Urologe [Ausg A] 12:183–187

Krüche A (1979) Über Structur und Entstehung der Uratsteine, Jena 1879. In: Schneider H-J, Doberentz D (Hrsg) Zur Geschichte der Jenaer Harnsteinforschung. Jenaer Reden und Schriften: Friedrich-Schiller-Universität, Jena

Lagergren C (1956) Biophysical investigations of urinary calculi. Acta Radiol [Suppl] (Stockh) 133

Lagergren C (1961) X-ray crystallography of calculi and its diagnostic value Acta Pathol Microbiol Immunol Scand [Suppl] 144:55–57

Lagergren C (1962) Development of silica calculi after oral administration of magnesium trisilicate. J Urol 87:994–996

Larsson L (1980) Kidney stone analysis. In: Danielson BG (ed) Proc. Sympos. Urolithiasis. Scand J Urol Nephrol (Suppl) 53:97–99

Larsson L, Sörbo B, Tiselius H-G, Öhman S (1984) A new method for quantitative wet chemical analysis of urinary calculi and the principles for calculation of results and mass recovery by an algorithm. In: Schwille PO, Smith LH, Robertson WD, Vahlensieck W (eds) Urolithiasis and Related Clinical Research. Plenum Press, New York London (in press)

Laskowski DF (1965) Chemical microscopy of urinary calculi. Anal Chem 37: 1399–1404

Lepage L, Tawashi R (1982) Growth and characterization of calcium oxalate dihydrate crystals (weddellite). J Pharm Sci 71:1059–1069

Leskovar P, Allgayer R (1979) Harnphosphat und das Wachstum von Ca-Oxalat-Kristallen. In: Gasser G, Vahlensieck W (Hrsg) Pathogenese und Klinik der Harnsteine VII. Steinkopff, Darmstadt, S 188–204

Leusmann DB (1981) Erste zusammenfassende Ergebnisse der kombinierten Phasen- und Gefügeanalyse von Harnsteinen mittels Röntgenbeugung und Rasterelektronenmikroskopie. In: Vahlensieck W, Gasser G (Hrsg) Pathogenese und Klinik der Harnsteine VIII. Steinkopff, Darmstadt, S 275–305

Leusmann DB, Tölle E (1984) Häufigkeit und Erscheinungsformen harnsäure- und urathaltiger Harnsteine. In: Vahlensieck W, Gasser G (Hrsg) Pathogenese und Klinik der Harnsteine X. Steinkopff, Darmstadt, S 54–63

Levinson AA, Nosal M, Davidman M, Prien sr EL, Prien jr EL, Stevenson RG (1978) Trace elements in kidney stones from three areas in the United States. Invest Urol 15:270–274

Levison DA, Banim S, Crocker PR, Wallace DMA (1982) Silica stones in the urinary bladder. Lancet I:704–705

Lian JB, Prien EL, Glimcher MJ, Gallop PM (1977) The presence of protein-bound γ-carboxyglutamic acid in calcium-containing renal calculi. J Clin Invest 59:1151–1157

Lilian OM, Hammond WS, Krauss DJ, Elbadawi A, Schoonmaker JE (1981) The microgenesis of some renal calculi. Invest Urol 18:451–456

Liptay G, Berenyi M (1967) Untersuchungen von Harnsteinen mit Hilfe eines neuen analytischen Verfahrens. Z Klin Chem Biochem 5:188–190

Liptay G, Berenyi M, Erdey L, Babics A (1966) Urologiai eredetü kövek derivatografias vizsgalata. Orv Hetil 107:155–158

Lonsdale K (1969a) Nierensteine – Verbreitung und Entstehung. Umschau in Wissenschaft und Technik 69:65–69

Lonsdale K (1969b) Human stones. Science 159:1199–1207

Lonsdale K, Mason P (1966) Uric acid, uric acid dihydrate, and urates in urinary calculi, ancient and modern. Science 152:1511–1514

Lonsdale K, Sutor DJ (1966) Newberyite in ancient and modern urinary calculi. Identification and space group. Science 154:1543–1545

Lonsdale K, Sutor J (1969) X-ray diffraction studies of urinary calculi. In: Hodgkinson A, Nordin BEC (eds) Renal Stone Research Symposium. Churchill, London, p 105–112

Lonsdale K, Sutor J, Wooley S (1968a) Composition of urinary calculi by x-ray diffraction. Collected data from various localities. I. Br J Urol 40:33–36

Lonsdale K, Sutor J, Wooley S (1968b) Composition of urinary calculi by x-ray diffraction. Collected data from various localities II–VI. Br J Urol 40:402–411

MacGregor J, Robertson WG, Nordin BEC (1965) Octocalcium phosphate: the phase governing the solubility equilibrium in apatitic calculi. Br J Urol 37:518–524

Malek RS, Boyce WH (1972) Some observations on the ultrastructure and genesis of urinary calculi. In: van Reen R (ed) Proceedings WHO Regional symposium on vesical calculus disease, Bangkok, p 103–116

Malek RS, Boyce WH (1977) Observations on the ultrastructure and genesis of urinary calculi. J Urol 117:336–341

Mandel G, Mandel N (1981) Composition and growth of renal calculi. Symposium on crystallography in the health sciences, Toronto

Marcet A (1818) Versuch einer chemischen Geschichte und ärztlichen Behandlung der Steinkrankheiten. Johan Georg Heyse. Bremen

Marschek M, Burchardt P (1971) Steinanalysen durch Kristallisationsmethode. Urologe [Ausg A] 10:154–158

Matouschek E, Herrig H (1967) Über Röntgenstrukturanalysen und Lösbarkeitsuntersuchungen von Harnsäure sowie Harnsäuresteinen der harnleitenden Wege. Urol Int 22:193–207

Maurer C (1969) Analysengang zur Beurteilung der quantitativen Zusammensetzung von Harnkonkrementen. Urologe [Ausg A] 8:189–193

Maurer C (1976) Untersuchungen über die Brauchbarkeit von Testkombinationen zur Harnsteinanalyse. Urologe [Aug B] 16:25–29

Maurer C, Götz W (1976) Vergleich verschiedener chemischer und physikalischer Untersuchungsverfahren für die Harnsteinanalyse in der Praxis. Urologe [Ausg B] 16:226–228

Maurer C, Pfitzenmaier N (1976) Evaluation of physical and chemical methods for the analysis of polymineralic urinary calculi. In: Fleisch H, Robertson WG, Smith LH, Vahlensieck E (eds) Urolithiasis Research. Plenum Press, New York London, p 309–312

McConville BE (1973) Activation analysis of renal calculi. In: Cifuentes Delatte L, Rapado A, Hodgkinson A (eds) Urinary calculi. Karger, Basel, p 275–279

McConville BE (1980) Investigations using autoradiographic analysis of urinary stones. Br J Urol 52:243–244

McConville BE, McConville RL (1976) Physical analysis of urinary calculi. In: Fleisch H, Robertson WG, Smith LH, Vahlensieck W (eds) Urolithiasis Research. Plenum Press, New York London, p 313–316

Medina JA, Cifuentes Delatte L (1983) Necrosis papilar calcificada como nucleo de un calculo. Arch Esp Urol 36:154–156

Medina JA, Rodriguez J, Cifuentes Delatte L (1977) Estudio de las cristalizaciones en calculos renales oxalocalcidos mediante microscopia electronica de barrido. Arch Esp Urol 30:11–26

Medina JA, Sanchidrian JR, Cifuentes Delatte L (1981) Silica in urinary calculi. In: Smith LH (ed), Urolithiasis: Clinical and Basic Research. Plenum Press, New York London, p 923 – 929

Medina JA, Rodriguez R, Santos M, Cifuentes Delatte L (1978) Calculo renal de silice en un hombre (undecima observacion mundial). Rev Clin Esp 151:411 – 413

Meyer JL, Bergert JH, Smith LH (1975) Epitaxial relationship in urolithiasis: The calcium oxalate monohydrate-hydroxyapatite system. Clin Sci Mol Med 49:369 – 373

Meyer JL, Bergert JH, Smith LH (1976) The epitaxially induced crystal growth of calcium oxalate by crystalline uric acid. Invest Urol 14:116 – 127

Meyer-Jürgens UB, Blaschke R, Maar K (1981) Neuere elektronenmikroskopische Untersuchungen an calciumphosphathaltigen Sphärolithen in Niere und Harn. In: Vahlensieck W, Gasser G (Hrsg) Pathogenese und Klinik der Harnsteine VIII. Steinkopff, Darmstadt, S 226 – 230

Meyer-Jürgens UB, Blaschke R, Leusmann DB, Maar K (1982) Analyse von Harnkonkrementen im Nierengewebe mittels STEM und ED-RMA. In: Gasser G, Vahlensieck W (Hrsg) Pathogenese und Klinik der Harnsteine IX. Steinkopff, Darmstadt, S 128 – 136

Minami T (1961) Electron microscopic studies of stones of the urinary tract. J Int Coll Surg 36:323 – 333

Miñon Cifuentes L, Santos M (1981) Newberyite in old renal and bladder calculi In: Smith LH, Robertson WG, Finlayson B (eds) Urolithiasis: Clinical and Basic Research. Plenum Press, New York London, p 929 – 934

Mitcheson HD, Zamenhof RG, Bankoff MS, Prien EL (1983) Determination of the chemical composition of urinary calculi by computerized tomography. J Urol 130:814 – 819

Morgenroth K, Backmann R (1969) Vergleichende Untersuchungen an Konkrementen der menschlichen Niere mit dem Rasterelektronenmikroskop. Virchows Arch [A] 347:33 – 43

Morriss RH, Beeler MF (1967) X-ray diffraction analysis of 464 urinary calculi. Am J Clin Pathol 48:413 – 417

Mulvaney WP, Beck CW, Brown RR (1972) Urinary phenazopyridine stones. A complication of therapy. JAMA 221:1511 – 1512

Murphy BT, Pyrah LN (1962) The composition, structure, and mechanisms of the formation of urinary calculi. Br J Urol 34:125 – 159

Nagy Z, Szabo E (1977) Zusammensetzungsveränderungen der Spurenelemente von Rezidivsteinen. Spektralanalytische Untersuchungen. Actas Urol Esp 1:99 – 105

Nagy Z, Szabo E, Kelenhegyi U (1963) Spektralanalytische Untersuchung von Nierensteinen auf metallische Spurenelemente. Z Urol Nephrol 56:185 – 190

Naray-Szabo I, Peter E (1967) Die quantitative Phasenanalyse in der Tonmineralforschung. Acta Geologic Acad Sci Hung 11:347 – 356

Ogbuji LU, Finlayson B (1981) Crystal morphologies in whewellite stones: electron microscopy. Invest Urol 19:182 – 190

Ogbuji LU, Batich CD, Finlayson B (1984) Matrix-mineral configuration in whewellite kidney stones: microchemical analysis. In: Schwille PO, Smith LH, Robertson WD, Vahlensieck W (eds) Urolithiasis and Related Clinical Research. Plenum Press, New York London (in press)

Ohnmacht R, Jobst K (1977) Infrared spectrometric analysis of urinary calculi. Acta Chir Hung 18:49 – 57

Oschurkow AA, Tschesnokow WF, Saburowa AI, Lukoschkowa OF, Orlowa OP (1978) Harnsteinuntersuchung mittels IR-Spektroskopie (russ.). 2. Allunionskongreß für Urologie, Kiew, Kongreßbericht, S 395 – 397

Otnes B (1980) Quantitation in crystallographic stone analysis. In: Danielson BG (ed) Proc. Symposium Urolithiasis. Scand J Urol Nephrol (Suppl) 53:101 – 104

Otnes B (1983) Urinary stone analysis. Methods, materials and values. Scand J Urol Nephrol [Suppl] 71 Almquist a. Wiksell, Oslo

Otnes B, Montgomery O (1980) Method and reliability of crystallographic stone analysis. Invest Urol 17:314 – 319

Otto H, Allesch W (1969) Harnkonkremente nach Langzeitsulfonamiden. Urologe 8:202 – 204

Otto H, Ihmann E (1967) IR(infrarot)-spektrografische Untersuchungen von 700 Harnwegskonkrementen. Frankf Z Pathol 77:262 – 268

PAK CYC (1978) Calcium urolithiasis. Plenum Medical Book Comp., New York London

Perez Castro E (1967) Litolisis en urologia. Arch Esp Urol 20:111 – 123
Phaneuf-Meneault F, Tawashi R (1977) Scanning electron microscopic study of calcium oxalate concretions grown in gel system and calcium oxalate stones. Eur Urol 3:171 – 175
Philipsborn Hv (1950/51) Über Calciumoxalat. Fortschr Min 29/30:393
Philipsborn Hv (1958) Zur Harnsteinbildung aus der Sicht des Mineralogen Urol Int 7:28 – 36
Pinto B (1973) Oxalate binding by the mucoprotein components of renal stones. In: Cifuentes Delatte L, Rapado A, Hodgkinson A (eds) Urinary Calculi. Karger, Basel, p 46 – 52
Pinto B (1976) Litiasis renal. Salvat Editores, S A, Barcelona
Pinto B (1980) Wirkung des Harnmukoproteins auf die Steinnucleation. VI. Jenaer Harnsteinsymposium. Wissenschaftliche Beiträge der Friedrich-Schiller-Universität, Jena, S 75 – 85
Pirlich W, Schwarzer R (1966) Die Urolithiasis bei der Ochronose. Z Ärztl Fortbild (Jena) 60:907 – 909
Pollak SS, Carlson GL (1969) A comparison of X-ray diffraction and infrared technics for identifying kidney stones. Am J Clin Pathol 52:656 – 660
Popelier G, van den Eeckhout E, Dekeyser W (1976) Composition of bladder stone in Rwanda. Br J Urol 48:317 – 322
Prien EL (1949) Studies in urolithiasis; II: Relationship between pathogenesis, structure and composition of calculi. J Urol 61:821 – 840
Prien EL (1955) Studies in urolithiasis; III: Physico-chemical principles in stone formation and prevention. J Urol 73:627 – 652
Prien EL (1963) Crystallographic analysis of urinary calculi. J Urol 89:917 – 924
Prien EL, Frondel C (1947) Studies in urolithiasis; I: The composition of urinary calculi. J Urol 57:949 – 991
Prien EL, Prien EL (1968) Composition and structure of urinary stones. Am J Med 45:654 – 671
Prien EL, Prien EL (1973) Optical crystallographic analysis of urinary stones: A simplified approach. In: Cifuentes Delatte L, Rapado A, Hodgkinson A (eds) Urinary Calculi. Karger, Basel, p 206 – 208
Pyrah LN (1979) Renal Calculus. Springer, Berlin Heidelberg New York
Ramirez CT, Ruiz JA, Gomez AZ, Orgaz RE, Rio Samper del S (1980 a) A crystallographic study of prostatic calculi. J Urol 124:840 – 843
Ramirez CT, Ruiz JA, Gomez AZ, Orgaz R, Rio Samper del S, Martinez Torres JL (1980 b) Calculos renales de nucleo mixto. Arch Esp Urol 33:599 – 610
Ramirez CT, Ruiz JA, Gomez AZ, Rio Samper del S, Fuente Serrano de la A(1980 c) Estudio cristalografico de 804 calculos renales de la provincia de Granada. Arch Esp Urol 33:397 – 406
Rao MVR, Argaval JS (1979) Studies in urolithiasis IV. An electron optical investigation on kinds of crystallization in urinary calculi. Ind J Exp Biol 17:366 – 370
Rao MVR, Argaval JS, Taneja OP (1976) Studies in urolithiasis. II. X-ray diffraction analysis of calculi from Delhi region. Indian J Urol Res 64:102 – 107
Rao MVR, Argaval JS, Taneja OP (1978) Studies in urolithiasis. III. Electron optical investigation on the morphology of the colloidal matrix of urinary calculi. Invest Urol 15:452 – 455
Rapado A, Castro Mendoza HJ, Cifuentes Delatte L (1973) Genetics of xanthinuria. In: Cifuentes Delatte L, Rapado A, Hodgkinson A (eds) Urinary Calculi. Karger, Basel, p 80 – 83
Rapado A, Mancha A, Castrillo JU, Traba LM, Santos U, Cifuentes Delatte L (1976) Etiological classification of renal lithiasis: a study based on 1936 patients. In: Fleisch H, Robertson WG, Smith LH, Vahlensieck W (eds) Urolithiasis Research. Plenum Press, New York London, p 495 – 498
Rassweiler J, Back J, Müller K, Fuchs G (1985) Computertomographische Steindichtemessungen zur Steinanalyse vor extrakorporaler Stoßwellenlithotripsie (ESWL). Akt Urol 16:30 – 35
Rebentisch G, Beyer H (1983) Vorschlag zur Bewertung der röntgendiffraktometrischen Harnsteinanalysenergebnisse an Hand des 5. und 6. DDR-Ringversuches. Z Urol Nephrol 76:303 – 309
Rebentisch G, Braun H, Schroda K-D (1978) Qualitätskontrolle der Harnsteinanalyse. V. Jenaer Harnsteinsymposium. Wissenschaftliche Beiträge der Friedrich-Schiller-Universität, Jena, S 92 – 95

Rebentisch G, Berg W, Schneider H-J (1981 a) Analytische Zuverlässigkeit und diagnostische Aussagekraft der röntgendiffraktometrischen Harnsteinanalyse. Z Med Lab Diagn 22:324 – 332

Rebentisch G, Schneider H-J, Berg W, Yersin A, Göthe W (1981 b) Nachweis und Bestimmung der Komponenten von Harnsteinen. 2. Arzneibuch der DDR. Diagnostische Laboratoriumsmethoden. Akademieverlag, Berlin

Rebentisch G, Schneider H-J, Berg W, Yersin A, Göthe W (1981 c) Kommentar zur Bestimmung der Bestandteile von Harnsteinen; Röntgendiffraktion. 2. Arzneibuch der DDR. Diagnostische Laboratoriumsmethoden. Akademieverlag, Berlin

Redinger L (1970) Halbmikro- und Mikromethoden zur Bestimmung der Hauptbestandteile von Harnkonkrementen. Eine neue Harnsäurebestimmungsmethode. I. Jenaer Harnsteinsymposium. Symposiumsbericht, Jena, S 60 – 63

Reimer L, Pfefferkorn G (1976) Rasterelektronenmikroskopie. Springer, Berlin Heidelberg New York

Reoeillaud RJ, Daudon M (1984) Drug induced stones: detection and diagnosis. In: Schwille PO, Smith LH, Robertson WD, Vahlensieck W (eds) Urolithiasis and Related Clinical Research Plenum Press, New York London (in press)

Resnick M (1984) Substances in urine with affinity to stone forming constituents. In: Schwille PO, Smith LH, Robertson WD, Vahlensieck W (eds) Urolithiasis and Related Clinical Research Plenum Press, New York London (in press)

Resnick ML, Boyce WH (1978) Spherical calcium bodies in stone-forming urine. Invest Urol 15:449 – 453

Reveillaud RJ, Daudon M, Ayrole G (1976) A microscopic, microchemical and infrared spectrometric study of oxalic urinary lithiasis. In: Fleisch H, Robertson WG, Smith LH, Vahlensieck W (1976) Urolithiasis Research. Plenum Press, New York London, p 329

Reveillaud RJ, Daudon M, Protat MF, Ayrole G (1980) Analysis of urinary calculi in adults. Attempt of correlation between morphology and composition. Eur Urol 6:161 – 165

Richter F, Sücker J (1967) Über die Zusammensetzung von Harnsteinen. Urol Int 22:178 – 184

Ringertz H (1965) Optical and crystallographic data of uric acid and its dihydrate. Acta Crystallogr 19:286 – 290

Robertson WG, Morgan DB, Marshall DH, Peacock M, Nordin BEC (1980) Risikofaktoren bei der Kalziumsteinbildung. V. Jenaer Harnsteinsymposium. Wissenschaftliche Beiträge der Friedrich-Schiller-Universität, Jena, p 45 – 52

Rodgers AL (1981 a) Common ultrastructural features in human calculi. Symposium on crystallography in the health sciences. Toronto

Rodgers AL (1981 b) Analysis of renal calculi by x-ray diffraction and electron microprobe: A comparison of two methods. Invest Urol 19:25 – 28

Rodgers AL, Nassimbeni LR, Mulder KJ, Mullins J (1981) Use of a density gradient column in the analysis of urinary calculi. Invest Urol 19:154 – 156

Rodgers AL, Nassimbem. LR, Mulder KJ (1982) A multiple technique approach to the analysis of urinary calculi. Urol Res 10:177 – 184

Rodriguez-Miñon Cifuentes JL (1976) Composition mineral de 244 calculos vesicales antiguos (1913 – 1950). Arch Esp Urol 29:537 – 562

Rolfinck W (1663) Disputatio de renum et vesicae calculo. Jena

Rose GA, Woodfine C (1976) The thermogravimetric analysis of renal stones (in clinical practice) Br J Urol 48:403 – 412

Roth R, Finlayson B (1973) Observations on the radiopacity of stone substances with special reference to cystine. Invest Urol 11:186 – 189

Sakamoto K, Fujisawa Y, Ohmori A, Minoda K, Yamanaka H, Nishioka K (1981) Dihydroxyadenine urolithiasis in children with partial deficiency of adenine phosphoribosyltransferase. Urol Int 36:274 – 280

Santos M, Cifuentes Delatte L, Bellanato J, Hidalgo A, Gonzales-Diaz PF (1976) Prostatic calculi. In: Fleisch H, Robertson WG, Smith LH, Vahlensieck W (eds) Urolithiasis Research. Plenum Press, New York London, p 347 – 350

Santos M, Garcia-Ramos JV, Bellanato J, Carmona P, Cifuentes Delatte L (1984) Application of Raman spectroscopy to the study of urinary calculi. In: Vahlensieck W, Gasser G (eds) Pathogenese und Klinik der Harnsteine X. Steinkopff, Darmstadt, S 405 – 414

Schäfer A, Bausch W (1979) Bedeutung der Spurenelementverteilung in Calciumoxalat-Harnsteinen. In: Gasser G, Vahlensieck W (Hrsg) Pathogenese und Klinik der Harnsteine VII. Steinkopff, Darmstadt, S 236–241
Schäfer A, Dosch W (1975) Das System Calcium-Oxalat-Wasser bei 38 °C. In: Vahlensieck W, Gasser G (Hrsg) Pathogenese und Klinik der Harnsteine IV. Steinkopff, Darmstadt, S 70–82
Schäfer A, Dosch W (1978) Morphologie und Genese von Calciumoxalat-Harnsteinen. In: Vahlensieck W, Gasser G (Hrsg) Pathogenese und Klinik der Harnsteine VI. Steinkopff, Darmstadt, S 110–123
Schmandt W, Blaschke R (1978) Zum Nachweis von Phosphat-Mikrokernen bei der Routineuntersuchung von Harnsteinen. Urologe [Ausg B] 18:83–86
Schneider H-J (1968a) Die anorganischen Bestandteile der Nierensteine und deren Einfluß auf die Steinart. Urologe [Ausg B] 7:347–352
Schneider H-J (1968b) Form und Gestalt der Harnsteine in Abhängigkeit von ihrer Lokalisation im Harntrakt. Med Bild 11:45–49
Schneider H-J (1968c) Form und Gestalt der Harnsteine als Ausdruck ihres strukturellen Aufbaues und der chemischen Zusammensetzung. Med Bild 11:117–121
Schneider H-J (1969a) Die Gesetzmäßigkeiten des Aufbaues anorganischer Nierensteine. Urologe [Ausg B] 8:180–184
Schneider H-J (1969b) Neue Gesichtspunkte zur chemischen Harnsteinanalyse. Urologe [Ausg B] 8:185–188
Schneider H-J (1973a) Form und Gestalt der Harnsteine. In: Hienzsch E, Schneider H-J (Hrsg) Der Harnstein. Gustav Fischer, Jena, S 67–68
Schneider H-J (1973b) Mineralstoffwechsel und Harnsteinleiden. III. Jenaer Harnsteinsymposium. Wissenschaftliche Beiträge der Friedrich-Schiller-Universität, Jena, S 17–28
Schneider H-J (1974a) Technik der Harnsteinanalyse. Thieme, Leipzig
Schneider H-J (1974b) Chemische Harnsteinanalyse. In: Schneider H-J (Hrsg) Technik der Harnsteinanalyse. Thieme, Leipzig, S 10–18
Schneider H-J (1976) Stellungnahme zu der Publikation von C. Maurer „Untersuchungen über die Brauchbarkeit von Testkombinationen zur Harnsteinanalyse". Urologe [Ausg B] 16:183–187
Schneider H-J (1978) Die Harnsteinanalyse in ihrer Bedeutung für Therapie und Metaphylaxe der Urolithiasis. Z Ärztl Fortbild (Jena) 72:380–384
Schneider H-J (1982) What is a urolith and what is a recurrent urolith? J Urol 127:72–74
Schneider H-J, Heide K (1971) Mikrothermische Untersuchungen zur phasenanalytischen Identifizierung von Nierensteinen. Z Urol Nephrol 64:323–329
Schneider H-J, Hesse A (1971a) Spurenelemente in Harnsteinen: Lithium. Z Urol Nephrol 64:759–761
Schneider H-J, Hesse A (1971b) Zur Problematik der Harnsteinanalyse. Zentralbl Pharcol 110:379–392
Schneider H-J, Hesse A (1973) Moderne Methoden der Harnsteinanalyse. Z Med Labortechn 14:3–14
Schneider H-J, Hesse A (1974) Harnsteinanalyse. Z Urol Nephrol 67:145–148
Schneider H-J, Hesse A (1975) Über das System der Zentralisierung und Standardisierung der Harnsteinanalyse in der DDR. Dtsch Gesundheitswes 30:1393–1396
Schneider H-J, Hesse A (1977) Die Harnsteinanalyse und ihre Bedeutung für die Rezidivprophylaxe der Urolithiasis. Polnischer Urologenkongreß, Wisla 1976. Symposiumsbericht
Schneider H-J, Hienzsch E (1970) Bedeutung und Formen der Harnsteinanalyse. Z Ärztl Fortbild (Jena) 64:861–867
Schneider H-J, Seyfarth H-H (1979) Investigations of flow dynamics and microstructure and their contribution to urolith genesis. Eur Urol 5:32–35
Schneider H-J, Seyfarth H-H (1980) Die mikroskopische Harnsteinanalyse. Wissenschaftliche Beiträge der Friedrich-Schiller-Universität, Jena
Schneider H-J, Vahlensieck W (1975) Definition der Harnsteine. IV. Jenaer Harnsteinsymposium. Wissenschaftliche Beiträge der Friedrich-Schiller-Universität, Jena, S 266
Schneider H-J, Hienzsch E, Tscharnke J (1970a) Vorschlag zur Zentralisierung und Standardisierung der Harnsteinanalyse. Dtsch Gesundheitswes 25:1934–1937

Schneider H-J, Hienzsch E, Tscharnke J (1970b) Die Untersuchung von Harnsteinen mit der Röntgenfeinstrukturanalyse nach Debye-Scherrer. Urologe [Ausg B] 9:171–175

Schneider H-J, Straube G, Anke M (1970c) Zink in Harnsteinen. Z Urol Nephrol 63:895–900

Schneider H-J, Hesse A, Wegner R (1972) Vorschlag zur Befundübermittlung und EDV-gerechten Datenspeicherung der Harnsteinanalysenergebnisse. Dtsch Gesundheitswes 27:418–423

Schneider H-J, Berenyi, Hesse A, Tscharnke J (1973a) Comparative urinary stone analysis. Int Urol Nephrol 5:9–17

Schneider H-J, Götz W, Heide K (1973b) Chemische Zusammensetzung und Struktur der Harnsteine; Methoden der Harnsteinanalyse. In: Hienzsch E, Schneider H-J (Hrsg) Der Harnstein. VEB Gustav Fischer, Jena, S 89–182

Schneider H-J, Hesse A, Hienzsch E, Tscharnke J, Schweder P (1974a) Röntgenstrukturuntersuchungen als standardisierte Harnsteinanalyse in der Deutschen Demokratischen Republik (Erfahrungen an 3500 Harnsteinanalysen). Z Urol Nephrol 66:111–119

Schneider H-J, Tscharnke J, Hesse A (1974b) Röntgendiffraktionsanalyse. In: Schneider H-J (Hrsg) Technik der Harnsteinanalyse. Thieme, Leipzig, S 74–137

Schneider H-J, Wegner R, Hesse A (1974c) Dokumentation und Befundübermittlung. In: Schneider H-J (Hrsg) Technik der Harnsteinanalyse. Thieme, Leipzig, S 138–143

Schneider H-J, Hesse A, Berg W (1976) Experimental studies on the effect of different forms of prophylaxis on urolith formation in animals. In: Fleisch H, Robertson WG, Smith LH, Vahlensieck W (eds) Urolithiasis Research. Plenum Press, New York London, p 509–512

Schneider H-J, Berg W, Hesse A (1977a) Morphologische Untersuchungen zur Oxalatsteingenese. Zentralbl Pathol Anat. 121:473–484

Schneider H-J, Hesse A, Berg W, Kirsten J, Nickel H (1977b) Tierexperimentelle Untersuchungen über die Wirkung von Magnesium und Vitamin B_6 auf die Kalziumoxalatnephrolithiasis. Z Urol Nephrol 70:419–427

Schneider H-J, Finke G, Grün U, Anke M (1979) The Cd-concentration of renal calculi in dependence on the kind of stone and the patients' dwelling. In: Anke M, Schneider H-J (Hrsg) Kadmiumsymposium. Wissenschaftliche Beiträge der Friedrich-Schiller-Universität, Jena, S 127–131

Schneider H-J, Rugendorff EW, Dahlke J (1985) Stone analysis – in the doctor's office or in a specialized Laboratory? In: Schwille PO, Smith LH, Robertson WD, Vahlensieck W (eds) Urolithiasis and Related Clinical Research. Plenum Press, New York London (in press)

Scholz R, Walch R (1970) Sulfonamidkonkremente als Harnsteine. I. Jenaer Harnsteinsymposium. Symposiumsbericht, Jena

Schubert G (1980) Die Harnsteinanalyse. Z Med Lab Diagn [Suppl] 21:1–16

Schubert G (1981) Zu einigen Problemen der quantitativen röntgendiffraktometrischen Harnsteinanalyse. Z Med Lab Diagn 22:333–339

Schubert G, Bick C (1978) Kristallographische Untersuchungen zur strukturellen Relation von Whewellit und Weddellit in Harnsteinen. V. Jenaer Harnsteinsymposium. Wissenschaftliche Beiträge der Friedrich-Schiller-Universität, Jena, S 105–107

Schubert G, Brien G (1978a) Untersuchungen zur Umwandlung von Whewellit zu Weddellit in Harnsteinen. In: Vahlensieck W, Gasser G (Hrsg) Pathogenese und Klinik der Harnsteine VI. Steinkopff, Darmstadt, S 124–128

Schubert G, Brien G (1980) Einfluß der Harnzusammensetzung auf Struktur und Gefüge von Harnsteinen. 3. Berliner Harnsteinmikroskopiewoche, Tagungsbericht, S 10–18

Schubert G, Brien G (1981) Crystallographic investigations of urinary calcium oxalate calculi. Int Urol Nephrol 13:249–260

Schubert G, Brien G, Bick C (1980) Der Dehydratationsprozeß in Oxalatharnsteinen – Polarisationsmikroskopische Untersuchungen als Ausgangspunkt für seine kristallstrukturelle Deutung. VI. Jenaer Harnsteinsymposium. Wissenschaftliche Beiträge der Friedrich-Schiller-Universität, Jena, S 14–22

Schubert G, Brien G, Bick C (1983) Separate examinations on core and shell of urinary calculi. Urol Int 38:65–69

Schubert G, Adam K, Uhlmann H (1983) Rasterelektronenmikroskopische Untersuchungen des Gefüges von Kalziumoxalatharnsteinen. Z Urol Nephrol 76:389–397

Schulz E, Berg W (1980) Die Möglichkeiten der Rasterelektronenmikroskopie für die Bestimmung von Harnsteinkomponenten. 3. Berliner Harnsteinmikroskopiewoche, Tagungsbericht, S 44–48

Schulz E, Berg W, Litz E, Lange P, Börner R (1980a) Vergleichsstudie zur Phasen- und Spurenelementverteilung mit LMA, REM und Polarisationsmikroskopie VI. Jenaer Harnsteinsymposium. Wissenschaftliche Beiträge der Friedrich-Schiller-Universität, Jena, S 128–133

Schulz E, Börner R-H, Schneider H-J (1980b) Methode zur differenzierten Analyse des kristallinen Harnsediments. VI. Jenaer Harnsteinsymposium. Wissenschaftliche Beiträge der Friedrich-Schiller-Universität, Jena, S 133–135

Schulz E, Berg W, Litz E, Maier U (1981) Untersuchungen an Harnsteinschliffen mit dem Laser-Mikrospektral-Analysator LM 10 und dem Plangitterspektrographen PGS 2. Jenaer Rundschau 26:97

Schwille PO, Smith LH, Robertson WD, Vahlensieck W (1984) Urolithiasis and Related Clinical Research. Plenum Press, London New York (in press)

Scott R, East BW, Janczyszyn J, Boddy K, Yates AJ (1980) Concentration and distribution of some minor and trace elements in urinary stones: A preliminary study. Urol Res 8:167–169

Seegmiller JE (1968) Xanthine stone formation. Am J Med 45:780–783

Seifert KF, Gebhardt M (1979) Quantitative röntgenographische Harnsteinanalyse mittels Guinierdiffraktometer. In: Gasser G, Vahlensieck W (Hrsg) Pathogenese und Klinik der Harnsteine VII. Steinkopff, Darmstadt, S 275–284

Seifert KF, Gebhardt M (1984) Röntgenbeugungsuntersuchungen zur Texturbestimmung der Kristalle in Harnsteinen. In: Vahlensieck W, Gasser G (1984) Pathogenese und Klinik der Harnsteine X. Steinkopff, Darmstadt, S 399–404

Seyfarth H-H, Hahne B (1978) Mikroskopische Untersuchungen von Harnsteinen. Jenaer Rundschau 23:182–187

Seyfarth H-H, Schneider H-J (1978) Strömungsmechanische Untersuchungen an Mikrogefügeanalysen und ihre Aussage zur Harnsteingenese. V. Jenaer Harnsteinsymposium, Wissenschaftliche Beiträge der Friedrich-Schiller-Universität, Jena, S 59–62

Seyfarth H-H, Schneider H-J (1980) Mikroskopische Gefügeanalysen von Harnsteinen und ihre Aussage zur Steingenese. VI. Jenaer Harnsteinsymposium. Wissenschaftliche Beiträge der Friedrich-Schiller-Universität, Jena, S 32–37

Seyfarth H-H, Anger G, Hahne B (1972) Mikroskopische Phasenanalyse von Nierensteinen. Münch Med Wochenschr 114:670–674

Seyfarth H-H, Hahne B, Pitschel A, Sluka G, Eismann D (1974) Mikroskopische Gefügeanalyse von Harnsteinen. Münch Med Wochenschr 116:2169–2174

Seyfarth H-H, Hahne B, Rostek FP, Sluka G, Eismann D (1975) Mikroskopische Untersuchung der Teilschritte von Auflösungsvorgängen an Harnsteinen. Münch Med Wochenschr 117:1841–1844

Shaker YM, El Hawary MFS, Zahran MM, Mostafa SO (1983) Urine and calculus amino acids in the different types of urolithiasis. Urol Int 38:51–54

Shirley R (1966) Uric acid dihydrate: Crystallography and identification. Science 152:1512–1515

Shirley R, Sutor DJ (1967) Science 159:544, zitiert bei Dosch (1981b)

Simmonds HA (1979a) Harnsteine bei Kindern. Differentialdiagnose und Therapie eines neu entdeckten Defekts der Adenin-Phosphoribosyltransferase. Münch Med Wochenschr 121:1654–1656

Simmonds HA (1979b) 2,8-Dihydroxyadeninuria – or when is a uric acid stone not a uric acid stone. Clin Nephrol 12:195–197

Simmonds HA, van Acker KJ, Dillon MJ, Barrat TM, Potter CE, Sahota A, Cameron JS (1981) 2,8-dihydroxyadeninuria: or when is a uric acid stone not a uric acid stone? In: Smith LH, Robertson WG, Finlayson B (eds) Urolithiasis: Clinical and Basic Research. Plenum Press, New York London, p 125–130

Singh SM, Chally R, Subramanian KA (1969) Observations on the chemical analysis of 117 urinary calculi. Indian J Med Sci 23:607–609

Sluka G, Hahne B, Seyfarth H-H, Hasselbacher K, Eismann D (1975) Verfahren zur Dünnschliffherstellung von Harnkonkrementen. Z Urol Nephrol 68:43–49

Smith LH, Robertson WG, Finlayson B (1981) Urolithiasis: Clinical and Basic Research. Plenum Press, New York London
Smith LH, Jenkins AD, Wilson JWL, Werness PG (1984) Is hydroxyapatite important in calcium urolithiasis. In: Vahlensieck W, Gasser G (Hrsg) Pathogenese und Klinik der Harnsteine X. Steinkopff, Darmstadt, S 193–197
Somacarrera E, Alonso J (1977) La ultramicroscopia electronia en la lechada calculos. In: Problemas actuales de urologia. Salvat Editores, S A Barcelona, p 225–259
Sorger G, Bausch W (1971) Die kristalloptische Bestimmung von Harnwegskonkrementen. Urologe [Ausg A] 10:151–154
Spector M, Lilga JC (1981) High voltage electron microscopy in urinary calculi. In: Smith LH, Robertson WG, Finlayson B (eds) Urolithiasis: Clinical and Basic Research. Plenum Press, New York London, p 997–1001
Spector M, Garden NM, Rous SN (1976) Ultrastructural features of human urinary calculi. In: Fleisch H, Robertson WG, Smith LH, Vahlensieck W (eds) Urolithiasis Research. Plenum Press, New York London, S 355–359
Spector M, Garden NM, Rous SN (1978) Ultrastructure and pathogenesis of human urinary calculi. Br J Urol 50: 12–15
Spector M, Magura CE, Lilga J (1981) Prostatic calculi. In: Smith LH, Robertson WG, Finlayson B (eds) Urolithiasis: Clinical and Basic Research. Plenum Press, New York London, p 943–948
Sterling C (1965) Crystal structure analysis of weddellite, $CaC_2O_4 \cdot (2+x)H_2O$. Acta Cryst 18:917–921
Strates B, Georgacopoulou C (1969) Derivatographic thermal analysis of renal tract calculi. Clin Chem 15:307–312
Sücker J (1963) Harnsteinanalyse mit Hilfe physikalisch-chemischer Methoden, speziell Infrarotspektroskopie. Ärztl Lab 9:260–269
Sutton RAL, Walker VR, Drance SM (1984) Renal calculi and acetazolamide therapy. In: Schwille PO, Smith LH, Robertson WD, Vahlensieck W (eds) Urolithiasis and Related Clinical Research. Plenum Press, New York London (in press)
Sutor DJ (1968a) Difficulties in the identification of components of mixed urinary calculi using the X-ray powder method. Br J Urol 40:29–34
Sutor DJ (1968b) Newberyite. Its formation in human urinary calculi. Nature 2218:295
Sutor DJ (1972) Ammonium acid urate and its role in the pattern of stone composition. In: van Reen R (ed) Proceedings WHO. Regional symposium on vesical calculus disease, Bangkok, p 206–213
Sutor DJ (1975) Constituents of urinary calculi containing struvite. Br J Urol 47:585–587
Sutor DJ, O'Flynn JD (1973) Matrix formation in crystalline material in vivo. In: Cifuentes Delatte L, Rapado A, Hodgkinson A (eds) Urinary Calculi. Karger, Basel, p 280–284
Sutor DJ, Scheidt SE (1968) Identification standards for human urinary calculus components using crystallographic methods. Br J Urol 40:22–28
Sutor DJ, Wooley SE (1969) Composition of urinary calculi by X-ray diffraction. Collected data from various localities VII. Br J Urol 41:397–400
Sutor DJ, Wooley SE (1970) Composition of urinary calculi by x-ray diffraction. Collected data from various localities VIII. Br J Urol 42:302–305
Sutor DJ, Wooley SE (1971) Composition of urinary calculi by x-ray diffraction. Collected data from various localities IX–XI. Br J Urol 43:268–274
Sutor DJ, Wooley SE (1972a) Composition of urinary calculi by x-ray diffraction. Collected data from various localities XII–XIV. Br J Urol 44:287–291
Sutor DJ, Wooley SE (1972b) The structure and formation of urinary calculi. I. Oriented crystal growth. Br J Urol 44:532–536
Sutor DJ, Wooley SE (1974a) Composition of urinary calculi by x-ray diffraction. Collected data from various localities XV–XVII. Br J Urol 46:229–232
Sutor DJ, Wooley SE (1974b) The crystalline composition of prostatic calculi. Br J Urol 46:533–535
Sutor DJ, Wooley SE (1975) Some data on urinary stones which were passed. Br J Urol 47:131–135
Sutor DJ, Wooley SE, Křižek V (1970) The composition of calculi from patients with alcaptonuria. Br J Urol 42:386–388

Sutor DJ, Wooley S, MacKenzie KR, Wilson R, Scott R, Morgan HG (1971) Urinary tract calculi – a comparison of chemical and crystallographic analysis. Br J Urol 43:149–153
Sutor DJ, Wooley SE, Illingworth JJ (1974) A geographical and histological survey of the composition of urinary calculi. Br J Urol 46:393–407
Szabó E (1967) Über die mikroskopische Analyse von Nierensteinen. Z Urol Nephrol 60:474–486
Szabó E (1970) Die mikroskopische kristalloptische Harnsteinanalyse. I. Jenaer Harnsteinsymposium. Symposiumsbericht, Jena, S 20–25
Szabó E (1973) Polarizing microscopic studies on the fine structure of renal stones. In: Cifuentes Delatte L, Rapado A, Hodgkinson A (eds) Urinary Calculi. Karger, Basel, S 213–215
Szabó E (1974) Kristalloptische Harnsteinanalysen. In: Schneider H-J (Hrsg) Technik der Harnsteinanalyse. Thieme, Leipzig, S 19–39
Szabó E (1978) Struktur und Aufbau der Harnsteine im Kindesalter. In: Vahlensieck W, Gasser G (Hrsg) Pathogenese und Klinik der Harnsteine VII. Steinkopff, Darmstadt, S 94–97
Szabó E, Modis L (1980) Histochemische Untersuchungen der Matrix kalziumhaltiger Harnsteine anhand topo-optischer Reaktionen. Z Urol Nephrol 73:879–885
Szabó E, Modis L (1981) Über die Anwendung der polarisationsmikroskopischen Untersuchungsmethoden bei der strukturellen Erforschung der Harnsteinmatrix. Jenaer Rundschau 26:89–92
Szabó E, Berg W, Hesse A, Schneider H-J (1976a) Experimentelle und kristalloptische Betrachtungen zur Kalziumoxalatsteingenese. Akt Urol 7:325–330
Szabó E, Orszagh E, Nagy Z (1976b) Chemische Zusammensetzung und Struktur magnesiumhaltiger Harnsteine. In: Schneider H-J, Anke M (Hrsg) Magnesiumstoffwechsel. Wissenschaftliche Beiträge der Friedrich-Schiller-Universität, Jena, S 118–121
Szabó E, Nagy Z, Orszagh E, Jeney F (1979) Spurenelemente in den kalziumhaltigen Harnsteinen. In: Gasser G, Vahlensieck W (Hrsg) Pathogenese und Klinik der Harnsteine VII. Steinkopff, Darmstadt, S 233–235
Szabó-Földvari E, Modis L (1984) Polarisationsmikroskopische Untersuchungen der Harnsäuresteinmatrix. In: Vahlensieck W, Gasser G (Hrsg) Pathogenese und Klinik der Harnsteine. Steinkopff, Darmstadt, S 267–269
Szederkenyi Gy, Jósza L (1968) Untersuchung des Sacchariden- und Eiweißzuckergehaltes von Nierensteinen. Z Urol Nephrol 61:289–300
Takasaki E (1975) An observation on the composition and recurrence of urinary calculi. Urol Int 30:228–236
Terhorst B (1969) Xanthinsteine und Xanthinurie. Ein kasuistischer Beitrag. Z Urol Nephrol 62:37–44
Thomas J, Rodrigue E, Levillain A, Henry R, Cherleit J, Thomas E, Steg A (1978) Calculs phosphatiques coralliformes. Donnees fournies par differentes techniques physiochemiques d'analyse. J Urol (Paris) 84:773–786
Thomas WC (1976) Renal calculi. A guide to management. CC Thomas, Springfield/Ill.
Toggenburg H, Bandhauer K (1980) Der Harnstein als Infektionsquelle. Akt Urol 11: 345–349
Tomazič BB, Nancollas GH (1979) A study of the phase transformation of calcium oxalate trihydrate-monohydrate. Invest Urol 16:329–335
Tozuka K, Konjiki T, Sudo T (1983) Study of passed stones by means of X-rays, infrared and thermal analyses. J Urol 130:1119–1124
Try K (1981) The composition of urinary stones analysed by infrared spectrophotometry and the precipitation of calcium phosphates from saturated solutions. Scand J Urol Nephrol 15:263–267
Tsay YC (1961) Application of infrared spectroscopy to analysis of urinary calculi. J Urol 86:838–854
Tscharnke J, Hesse A, Schneider H-J (1972) Farbige Harnsteine. Akt Urol 4:99–101
Unni Mooppan, Hong Kim, Wax H (1979) Pattern of urolithiasis in Brooklyn, New York. Urology 14:482–486
Vahlensieck W (1979) Urolithiasis 1. Springer, Berlin Heidelberg New York
Vizkelety J (1965) Harnsteinanalyse durch Mikroschnellverfahren. Z Urol Nephrol 58:345

Wachter PW, Matouschek E (1977) Über die Mikrohärte von Harnsteinen. In: Gasser G, Vahlensieck W (Hrsg) Pathogenese und Klinik der Harnsteine V. Steinkopff, Darmstadt, S 224 –230

Warpehoski MA, Buscemi PJ, Osborn DC, Finlayson B, Goldberg EP (1980) Organic matrix distribution in kidney stones. Fourth Int. Symp. Urolithiasis Res., Williamsburg, USA

Warpehoski MA, Buscemi PJ, Osborn DC, Finlayson B, Goldberg EP (1981) Distribution of organic matrix in calcium oxalate renal calculi. Calif Tissue Int 33:211–222

Watanabe T (1972) Histochemical studies on mucosubstances in urinary stones. Tohoku J Exp Med 107:345–357

Westbury EJ (1974) Some observations on the quantitative analysis of over 1000 urinary calculi. Br J Urol 46:215–227

Westbury EJ, Omenogor P (1970) A quantitative approach to the analysis of renal calculi. J Med Lab Technol 27:462–474

Whiteside N, Bowyer RC, Henderson G, Brockis JA (1983) Composition of stone matrix. 2. Int. Urinary Stone Conference, Singapore

Williams G, Sallis D (1981) The sources of phosphocitrate and its influential role in inhibiting calcium phosphate and calcium oxalate crystallization. In: Smith LH, Robertson WG, Finlayson B (eds) Urolithiasis: Clinical and Basic Research. Plenum Press, New York London, p 569 –578

Willnow U, Strauch G (1967) Histochemische Untersuchungen von Kolloidkörperchen in Säuglingsnieren bei Nephrolithiasis. Frankfurt Z Pathol 76:149–155

Winchel AN, Winchel G (1967) Optische Eigenschaften synthetischer Minerale (russ.). Verlag Mir, Moskau

Witten FR, Morgan JM, Foster JG, Glenn JF (1983) 2,8-dihydroxyadenine urolithiasis: Review of the literature and report of a case in the United States. J Urol 130:938–942

Yong GO K, Börner RH, Berg W, Schneider H-J (1980) Stabilisierungsfaktoren für Harnsäuredihydrat – ein Beitrag zur Harnsäuresteingenese. VI. Jenaer Harnsteinsymposium. Wissenschaftliche Beiträge der Friedrich-Schiller-Universität, Jena, S 71–74

Zaremski PM, Grieve J (1976) Analysis of urinary stones using infrared spectroscopy and scanning electron microscopy. In: Fleisch H, Robertson WG, Smith LH, Vahlensieck W (eds) Urolithiasis Research. Plenum Press, New York London, p 371–374

Zechner O, Loebenstein Th, Pflüger H, Legenstein E, Brandstätter F, Kurat G (1984) Harnsteinwachstum in vitro. In: Vahlensieck W, Gasser G (Hrsg) Pathogenese und Klinik der Harnsteine X. Steinkopff, Darmstadt, S 147–150

Epidemiology of Urolithiasis

H.-J. SCHNEIDER

In many European countries urolithiasis has a higher incidence than any other disease of the urinary tract. At a frequency of 15 per 10,000 of the population it is the commonest urological cause for inpatient admission (RUHLE et al. 1972) and calculus patients constitute over ⅓ of all urological outpatient material (SCHNEIDER 1979).

Working days are frequently lost (by 68% of male patients and 100% of women) and the death rates of 4.7 men and 3.6 women per 100,000 population are the highest in the field of urology (DAHM 1974). One-third of all patients with a recurrent stone may be expected to lose a kidney (MALEK 1977).

In the absence of appropriate treatment the recurrence rate is in the region of 60%, a very considerable figure supplemented by an apparently steady year-on-year increase in the number of new cases. If one takes into account that 12% of the population of the U.S.A. will suffer at least one bout of stone-related illness during their lifetime (SIERAKOWSKI et al. 1978), it can be no surprise that total U.S.A. treatment costs for this disease are estimated at 47.3 million dollars a year (MALEK 1977).

The causes governing calculus formation are manifold and in individual cases often obscure. They range from excessive food intake in the absence of exercise to malnutrition in endemic areas and may represent biochemical change in response to anything from simple stress reactions to psychopathological events. All in all, however, such causes are only clinically or biochemically detectable in 30–50% of stone patients. The remainder we label as 'idiopathic' (MALEK 1977 = 70–80%, RAPADO et al. 1976 = 53%, MARSHALL et al. 1975 = 87%, BENABE et al. 1979 = 62%).

"The 'stone former' is identified as one who forms stones, and there are only a few rather tenuous characteristics which may distinguish him from his fellows who do not form stones. Characterization of the 'stone former' is at best an imprecise assessment derived by selection of the most plausible explanation for urinary crystallization and attainable only by a detailed metabolic evaluation." (BOYCE 1979).

In every case of urinary stone it is probable that both extrinsic (environmental and socio-economic) factors and intrinsic (congenital and acquired) factors are involved. Recent historical and geographical studies have yielded valuable understanding of their relative importance (ANDERSEN 1972).

I. Historical Overview

Examination of archeological urolith material demonstrates both that urolithiasis was recognised in antiquity and that despite considerable changes in nutrition and living conditions over the millennia there has been little change in the composition of urinary calculi (KRIZEK 1973; KRIZEK and SCHNEIDER 1974). All stones examined have consisted of uric acid, calcium oxalate and a variety of phosphates.

Excavations by E. SMITH in 1901 at El Amrah in Egypt brought to light a bladder calculus of uric acid and calcium phosphate within the pelvis of a young man. This oldest known urolith dates to approximately 4800 BC. A stone found by WILLIAMS in the mummy of a boy in North Arizona proved to be 3000 years old. This calculus weighed 32 g and consisted of calcium phosphate and carbonate-(apatite). A calcium oxalate and struvite kidney stone was found in a Late Bronze Age burial mound on the Hungarian plain. Little is known of the frequency of urolithiasis in antiquity. Certainly there is no mention of urolithiasis of its treatment in the Smith, Ebers or Brugsch papyri (DOBERENTZ 1976). Nevertheless, the Egyptians in all probability knew of the existence of urinary stone disease, giving it the name "wrmjt" (BLOOMEN, 1982).

Historical documentation is uniformly concerned with bladder stones (BLACKLOCK 1979). The first written mention of lithotomy is to be found in the Susrutan Agur Veda, a collection of ancient Indian materia medica dating to 500 BC. AULUS CORNELIUS CELSUS (25 BC–45 BC) gives a detailed description of perineal lithotomy in his book "De re medicina" (NÖSKE 1974).

The Papal encyclic Ecclesia Abhoret Sanguine, issued by Pope INNOCENCE III in 1214, prohibited any clerical involvement in surgical procedures. Thus began the age of wandering lithotomists, of whom few were expert or successful. The ensuing disasters engendered popular scepticism which resulted in frequent home surgery. Thus the young Dutchman JAN DE DOOT employed a large knife and the assistance of his brother to excise a stone from his bladder in 1651, and in the period 1735–1800 in Lucknow in India a certain COLONEL MARTIN filed away 10–12 times daily at his own bladder calculus by means of a transurethral probe, resulting in its complete destruction and spontaneous passage after 6 months.

Although DOMENICO DE MARCHETTI is reputed to have successfully excised a kidney stone from an English consul to Venice, called HOPSON, as early as 1663, nephrolithotomy was a late development, not practised until some time after nephrectomy had been pioneered by SIMON in Heidelberg in 1869.

An instrument was demonstrated by FRANZ VON GUITHUISEN in Munich in 1813, which enabled bladder calculi to be trapped in a noose and subsequently drilled. It was however JEAN CIVIALE (1793–1867) who ushered in the era of litholapaxy.

Operations and instrumentation were so hazardous that attempts were soon made to dissolve stones by conservative means. The concepts and procedures employed were occasionally highly imaginative. Fluid regimes and dietary control were popular even in antiquity, as were a variety of medicines and concoctions. JOANNA STEPHENS rose to fame by selling the formula for her stone-dissolving potion to the English parliament for £ 5,000, although it was subsequently proved ineffective.

A number of theories of urolithogenesis had an influence on conservative treatment. HIPPOCRATES described a defective mixing of juices as the cause of stone formation, an excess of heat and wind being favored by AVICENA, whilst PARACELSUS considered it to result from disharmony of humoral functions. SEYDENHAM and EBSTEIN introduced the concept of a stone-forming diathesis, rephrased by MECKEL VON HEMSBACH as a stone-forming 'catarrh'. From the 19th Century onward views on urolithogenesis become subdivisible into crystallization theories and matrix theories.

A number of experiments were designed to expand or confirm current knowledge. In 1723 NUCK implanted wooden spheres in the bladder of a dog to

Table 1. Historical data on urolithiasis (SCHNEIDER 1979)

Year	Country	
4800 BC	Egypt	Bladder calculus found at El Amrah
1728 – 1686	Mesopotamia	Treatment of bladder calculi documented on the Hammurabi tablets
500	India	Susruta-Samhita, operative and conservative treatment of bladder calculi
460 – 377	Greece	Hippocrates; diagnosis and treatment of kidney and bladder calculi
150	Alexandria	Ammonius "lithotomos", crushing of large stones prior to operation
30 AD	Rome	Celsus, detailed description of the lateral approach to bladder calculi
100		Ruphus of Ephesos, recognises urolithiasis as a chronic disease
129 – 199	Rome	Galen, recognises relationship between urolithiasis and gout
1214	Rome	Lateran council prohibits operative procedures by clerics
1556	France	Colot teaches lithotomy
1561	France	Pierre Franco, suprapubic lithotomy
1651 – 1714	France	Frère Jacques, famous French lithotomist appears at fairs
1663	Naples	Domenico de Marchetti, first operation for kidney stones
1665	Netherlands	Hooke, describes crystalline urinary sediment
1695	Netherlands	Loewenhoek, structural studies on uroliths and gouty tophi
1732	Germany	Nuck, experimental foreign body stones in dogs
1739	England	Joanna Stephens, sells a litholytic formula to parliament for £ 5,000.
1776	Germany	Scheele, recognises uric acid as a component of calculi
1780	England	Wollaston, discovery of oxalic acid
1824	France	Jean Civiale, first litholapaxy on live patients

simulate foreign bodies, and in 1720 JOHANN ADOLPH WEDEL described in his doctoral thesis at Jena University attempts to dissolve marble balls in decoctum corticis querus (SCHNEIDER and DOBERENTZ 1979).

It was soon realised that stones were not of a single type, and the distinction was made between hard and soft calculi. The principal components, uric acid (SCHEELE), oxalic acid (WOLLASTON) and cystine (BERZELIUS) were discovered in the 18th Century, resulting in the emergence of detailed chemical analytical protocols (MARCET 1817; HELLER 1860; ULTZMANN 1812). KRÜCHE (Jena, 1879) was the first to insist on microstructure studies of thin sections (Table 1). The extensive urolithiasis literature of the 19th Century revealed considerable differences in the age, sex and social distribution, as well as in the overall frequency of stone disease.

At that time children in the age range 5–15 and adult in the 5th–7th decade provided the bulk of patients. According to CIVIALE (quoted by EBSTEIN 1884) 56% of 5,376 stone patients were younger than 20. Bladder calculi continue to occur with a similar frequency among children in a number of countries, as a result of incorrect or inadequate nutrition and of a lack of hygiene (Chapter VIII).

Throughout this period it was generally accepted that the poor had phosphate calculi and the rich urate stones, the latter as a complication of gout and the former resulting from recurrent infection. The vast majority of bladder stone patients were drawn from the poorer classes and consisted mainly of children. The statement is however misleading, since bladder calculi were far more frequently diagnosed. Even allowing for analytical errors there is a significantly high incidence of uric acid and urate stones.

Table 2 summarises the incidence of various types of calculus in England (London, Norwich, Manchester, Bristol), Denmark (Copenhagen) and Germany (Suabia).

JEDINY (1972) also found a considerably higher proportion of uric acid calculi among bladder than kidney stones (Table 3). Extensive studies by SUTOR and colleagues (1974) have, however, revealed that this high proportion of uric acid is found only among bladder calculi from the so-called developing countries and from British museums (collections from the previous century).

Table 2. Distribution of stone types in various countries during the first half of the 19th Century (by principal component) (PROUT 1843)

Stone type	England	Denmark	Germany	Total	%
Uric acid and urate	847	228	70	1145	70
Cystine	5	–	–	5	0.3
Calcium oxalate	300	4	3	307	19
Phosphate	144	23	8	175	11
Total	1296	255	81	1632	100

Table 3. Distribution of stone types among kidney and bladder stones in %

Stone type	Bladder stones	Kidney stones
Uric acid	63	7
Phosphate	30	34
Calcium Oxalate	7	59

II. The Frequency of Urolithiasis

On a worldwide scale there is considerable variation in the incidence of urolithiasis, both from country to country and from one age to another. All the available explanations remain hypothetical. Any review of the literature must also take account of varying terms of reference (hospital patients, surgical statistics, demoscopic studies, etc.).

In epidemiological terms the prevalence of a disease is the number of subjects who have the condition at a given time and the incidence is found by discovering the number of subjects who develop the condition in the population at a suitable interval after the prevalence figure is determined (SCOTT et al. 1977).

As early as 1966 ALKEN had drawn attention to an unequivocal increase in the incidence of urolithiasis (LENKO and POLITOWSKI 1970).

There appears to have been a dramatic increase in the U.S.A. (BOYCE 1979). Whilst in 1952 there were 9.5 stone patients per 10,000 of the population, that figure had risen to 16.4 in 1974. In the area around Rochester (USA) the figure for males alone rose over 25 years from 7.9 to 12.4, remaining relatively static at 3.6 for women (JOHNSON et al. 1979).

SIERAKOWSKI et al. (1978) have calculated that approximately 12% of the U.S. population will suffer from a urinary calculus at least once in their life.

In America alone 14.7 million working days are lost through urolithiasis (DAVIS et al. 1978).

Unfitness for work due to urolithiasis increases with age and reaches a higher total for women than for men (Table 4).

Despite a steady decrease in the death rate in our country from urolithiasis, urinary tract calculi still represent one of the chief causes of death in urological practice. In fact 0.3% of all deaths in 1970 were attributed to this cause (DAHM 1974).

In Italy the mean population risk of stone disease rose from 7% in 1954 to 13% in 1974 (PAVONE-MACALUSO and MIANO 1979). DE VRIES et al. (1979) give the following figures for Israel: in 1958 11.8% of a population of 30,000 inhabitants suffered from urolithiasis, whilst in 1961 the figure had risen to 24%, although these figures apply only to the south of the country.

An authorative study by SCHMINCKE and LENGWINAT (1968) conducted in the Zittau district (GDR), which has a population of 108,000, documented a

Table 4. Unfitness for work due to urolithiasis in the GDR 1970 (SCHNEIDER and HESSE 1976)

Age in years	Men			Women		
	Cases	Cases per 10,000 employees	Days per case	Cases	Cases per 10,000 employees	Days per case
<25	1258	25	15	1651	31	18
Up to 30	2152	54	14	1255	36	24
Up to 40	5835	75	16	2816	42	26
Up to 50	5393	101	19	2589	40	28
Up to 60	4160	97	24	1988	40	30
Up to 65	2274	82	31	484	28	32
>65	968	39	34	171	14	28

stone morbidity of 0.11% for men and 0.05% for women. It should be noted, however, that the proportion of stone patients among 25 to 55-year-old men was as high as 2.2% (see also RUHLE et al. 1972). In the meantime, the overall prevalence in the GDR has also risen to 1 – 2% (HIENZSCH 1973; HESSE et al. 1977b; SCHNEIDER and HESSE 1976). In Berlin this figure is still higher at 3.6% (HÜTTNER and WIESNER 1971).

In 1974 23,000 people underwent inpatient treatment for urolithiasis, but HEDENBERG (1951) suggested that this would only be 20% of all patients meriting treatment, and this could correspond to an overall morbidity of 1%. In 1974 the inpatient urolithiasis rate was 0.12% (RUHLE and WINTER 1976), a definite decrease on the 1969 figures. This may reflect an improvement in outpatient care. According to ALMBY et al. (1976) about 0.1% of the total population are likely to require hospital admission because of urinary tract stones. According to LJUNGHALL (1984) 10% of stone patients are treated in hospital, 60 as outpatients and 30% not at all.

Other countries have experienced a similar increase in the urolithiasis rate. On the other hand ROBERTSON (1984) has reported a decreasing incidence in Leeds, the first such report in recent years.

A representative survey in a small Tyrolean community of 1,804 inhabitants resulted in a figure of 4.8% stone patients (JOOST et al. 1980). A similar urolith prevalence (4 – 5%) is given by VAHLENSIECK et al. (1980, 1982) for the Federal Republic of Germany.

The Sedish group headed by LJUNGHALL has investigated the epidemiology of urolithiasis most thoroughly, (LJUNGHALL 1978; LJUNGHALL and HEDSTRAND 1975; LJUNGHALL and WAERN 1977; LJUNGHALL et al. 1977). 8.9% of 35 to 53-year-old men and 3.2% of women in the same age group fell ill with urinary calculi during the period 1970 – 75, i.e. they had their first attack during this period. In the 49 to 50 age group 13.7% had already suffered one episode, and this figure was 18% for 60-year-olds. In one Swedish town 5% of 38 to 60-year-old women gave a history of kidney stones (BENGTSSON et al. 1980).

Over a 5-year period LARSEN and PHILIP (1962) found a stone rate of 12% for male Danish doctors and 7% for female, although only 2% is reported for the CSSR (KOHLICEK 1963). In Norway the frequency has risen from 2.2 to 3.3‰ for men and from 0.5 to 0.8‰ for women (NORLIN et al. 1976). Hungary has also suffered only a slight increase between 1976–78, the number of new cases rising by only 0.15% (ROSDY 1979). On the other hand TOTH (1978) gives an incidence of 1.25% for Central Hungary, the equivalent figure for Budapest being calculated by BALOGH et al. (1979) as over 2%. In the Granada area of Spain VIVALDI et al. (1979) recorded a prevalence of 2.95%. A randomised study by SCOTT et al. (1977) gave a prevalence of 3.83% (Table 5).

The wide variations between the figures given by these authors demonstrate not only a variability in the incidence of urolithiasis but also considerable difference among population at the outset. In particular, the number of patients missed by these surveys is usually unknown. At autopsy the urolithiasis rate lies between 1–3% (GERSHOFF 1964; SCHUMANN 1963).

VAN GEUNS (1978) examined 2,038 persons over the age of 12 years in one Dutch community. He found a prevalence of 4.4%, with 1% so-called silent stones only being detected by special investigations, e.g. radiography. It thus appears that the incidence figures quoted are generally too low, since most studies made no attempt to estimate silent stones.

Both BIBUS (1939) and KNEISE and BEYER (1933) described a fluctuating pattern in European stone frequency. After a massive peak in 1927 there was a rapid and continuous decrease up to the Second World War, only reversed by an increase in 1948. Postmortem statistics for 1913–1958 at the St. George Institute of Pathology in Leipzig revealed the effect of world wars on urolith frequency (Fig. 1).

Table 5. Occurrence rates of stones in selected countries

Author	Year	Country	Occurrence rate (%)	
LARSEN	1962	Denmark	4.5	(Medical practitioners)
KOHLICEK	1963	Czechoslovakia	2.0	
BLACKLOCK	1969	England	3.5	(Sailors)
DE VRIES	1971	Israel	24.0	
HÜTTNER	1972	GDR	3.6	
BOYCE	1974	USA	0.16	(Hospital patients)
NORLIN	1976	Norway	0.3	
TAKASAKI	1977	Japan	1.0	(Electricity workers)
SCOTT	1977	Scotland	3.8	
GEUNS	1978	Holland	4.4	
TOTH	1979	Hungary	1.25	
LJUNGHALL	1979	Sweden	9.0	
VIVALDI	1979	Spain	2.95	
PAVONE	1979	Italy	13.0	
JOOST	1980	Austria	4.8	
VAHLENSIECK	1980	FRG	5.0	
ROBERTSON	1984	England	3:8	(Men in Leeds)

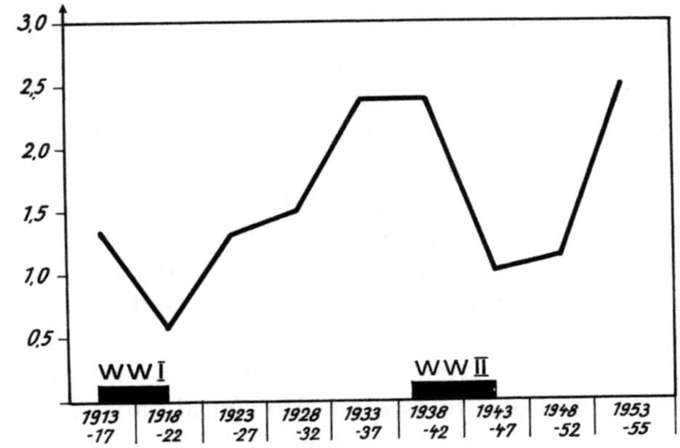

Fig. 1. Frequency of urolithiasis in postmortem material, 1915–1958 (SCHUMANN 1963)

These inroads during war years into the frequency of stone disease were also noted by ANDERSEN (1973) in Norway and by INADA et al. (quoted in BLACKLOCK 1976a) in Japan. They are generally thought to be connected with a change in nutrition and particularly with a marked reduction in sugar consumption during the relevant years (BLACKLOCK 1976b). SCHÖLL (1978) has drawn attention to a recurrent increase in stone frequency in Austria with a period of 21 years (1927, 1948, 1970). According to this study a further peak should occur in 1990.

This varying frequency of urinary calculi and the distribution of various types of stone from country to country may depend on a variety of factors, e.g. lifestyle, nutrition, climate, race, etc.

Maps of endemic areas in Europe published many years ago are now barely valid. Territorial variations continue to decrease so that an overall rate of around 5% may be assumed for central Europe with less than 0.1% new cases per year. There remain a number of endemic areas in which children are chiefly affected.

Dagesthan (Soviet Union) is one such endemic area in which the year-on-year increase represents 2%. Iodine deficiency is generally considered to be the cause (MARTYNENKO 1974).

PAVONE-MACALUSO and MIANO (1979) have documented a marked North-South distribution. In North-Eastern Italy the frequency was only 0.25%, yet 0.44% in the South. In Northern Sardinia 0.7% of the population required in-patient treatment for urolithiasis (BO et al. 1978). Urinary calculi are common in Turkey and the rate is steadily increasing (GÜNALB 1979).

In Africa, however, urolithiasis is not common overall. The central laboratory of Nigeria has analysed only 50 calculi from the entire country in the past 3 years. These were mainly infective calculi related to some urinary tract obstruction (ESHO 1978; ESHO and AMAKU 1979). The cause of this extremely low incidence are considered to lie in a low drinking water calcium content, very low dairy product consumption and in a physically active lifestyle.

A study carried out in the Sudan shows an equal distribution of bladder, kidney and ureteric calculi. The former mainly affect children, 95% of them boys (KAMBAL et al. 1979). Ureteric calculi, on the other hand, seem to be far rarer than in Europe (PERQUIS et al. 1969). As in Europe, about 30% of all urologic patients in Egypt have stones (SAWAT et al. 1979).

SIERAKOWSKI et al. (1978) have drawn attention to some marked variations in the calculus rates in the U.S.A. About 2000 questionnaires sent to and returned by hospitals were analysed by computer. Washington D.C. had the highest calculus rate at 4.5% (of the hospital population), the lowest being in Wyoming. Most states reported a 74% increase in the last 22 years.

In Europe stone patients constitute 7–30% of all hospital patients, the equivalent figure for Latin America being 9–18% (MATOUSCHEK and HUBER 1981).

Stone disease is also far commoner in the South of China than in the North, 30–59% of urologic patients in the former region suffering from urolithiasis (WU CHIEH-P'ING 1979).

This ratio is reversed in India (MELIDIRATTA 1972). In the North there were 211 stone patients per 10,000 of the population, yet only 23 in the South. Most of these calculi are in the bladder, particularly in boys under the age of 6 of poor social background (RAO et al. 1976; THIND and NATH 1969).

Endemic bladder calculi were discussed in great detail at a symposium in Bangkok (VAN REEN 1972). Authors reported on the situation in India, Laos, Thailand, Pakistan, Iran, Indonesia and other countries, generally stating that 90% of patients are under the age of 5 (SINGH 1972; WESTERMEYER 1971; JAECK et al. 1979).

Inadequate nutrition, based mainly on rice and extremely low quantities of animal protein, may represent the chief cause for such bladder stone formation (BROCKIS et al. 1981; HALSTEDT and VALYASEVI 1972). This would also provide an explanation for the sevenfold excess prevalence of bladder calculi among village children in the North of Thailand compared to city dwellers in the same country (VALYASEVI and DHANAMITTA 1972).

Most of these calculi consist of calcium oxalate, ammonium dihydrogenurate being a common component (RAHMAN and VAN REEN 1972; SHANJEHAN and RAHMAN 1971). In 80% of cases the urine is sterile (SINGH 1972). This of course represents a considerable contrast to juvenile bladder stones occurring in Europe, where they are nearly always related to a urinary outflow obstruction and secondary infection. Consequently they are composed chiefly of phosphate.

Bladder calculi are also endemic in Iran, occurring mainly in boys between the age of 2 and 10 from large, poor families (KADIVAR 1972; SADRE et al. 1972).

III. Type Distribution of Calculi

1. Geographic Distribution

Classification of almost 100,000 urinary calculi from all over the GDR according to their principal components results in the analysis given in Table 1, Chapter A, where both absolute numbers, percentages and sex ratios are given for each type of calculus.

The causes for the type distribution of calculi in various countries and indeed within an individual country are numerous, and it is impossible to mention all of them. Table 6 summarises the overall distribution given in the literature (SCHNEIDER and HEINZSCH 1979). The experience of GEBHARDT and BASTIAN (1984) provides a good example of the scale of differences that may be encountered within a single country. Whereas in Hamburg 79% of stones contained whewellite, only 58% did so in Bavaria. Workers under the leadership of LONSDALE (SUTOR and WOOLEY 1969, 1970, 1971, 1972, 1974; LONSDALE et al. 1968a, b; SUTOR et al. 1974) have undertaken extremely precise X-ray diffraction studies on calculi from a variety of countries and from regions of England, and they have given an interesting discussion of their results.

Calcium oxalate calculi are in the overwhelming majority, representing 60–90% of calculi in virtually all countries. The whewellite to weddellite ratio ranges from 4:1 to 10:1. Most calcium oxalate calculi both phases.

Uric acid stones are relatively common in Bulgaria, CSSR, Italy and Austria. In Czechoslovakia they constitute ¼ of all stones (HRADEC et al. 1969), in Israel this figure is ⅓ (DE VRIES et al. 1972; FRANK et al. 1970) and in the Sudan over one-half (IBRAHIM 1979). In the series reported from the Soviet Union by TIKTINSKI (1979) 71% of calculi consisted of uric acid and urates.

Ammonium dihydrogenurate is relatively rare in Europe, occurring mainly in bladder calculi from endemic areas. Among 170 such calculi ARMBRUSTER (1979) came across this substance only 13 times. In every case the calculi came from children of Turkish extraction (ARMBRUSTER 1978).

BORDEN and DEAN (1979) have described 5 pure ammonium dihydrogenurate calculi in Navajo children.

The proportion of so-called infective calculi of struvite and carbonate apatite lies at a mean of 5–10%. In Nigeria the figure is particularly high at 40%, but Japan at 22% and England at 15–32% are also above average. Such calculi occur more commonly in the bladder than in the kidney. At electrohydraulic litholapaxy BORGMANN et al. (1980), KAMBAL et al. (1979) and BRUNDIG and SCHNEIDER (1980) recorded the composition of bladder calculi given in Table 7.

Crystallographic analysis of 244 bladder calculi by RODRIGUEZ-MINON CIFUENTES (1976) showed 78% to contain ammonium dihydrogenurate, 67% carbonate apatite, 59% struvite, yet only 25% uric acid. The value of 22% is given for newberyite, which must have arisen by metamorphosis of struvite.

There are obvious differences between these figures and the composition of renal and ureteric calculi, among which 5% were struvite, 4.3% apatite, 14% uric acid and 73% calcium oxalate calculi (Table 1, Chapter A).

Cystine calculi account for only 1% of all uroliths. In England the proportion of homozygous cystinurics is 1:20,000, in Sweden 1:10,000 (WILLIAMS et al. 1980) and in Czechoslovakia 1:75,000 (KRIZEK 1981). Among the series of 206 homozygous cystinurics reported by KRIZEK the actual incidence of stone disease was 82%. By 1981 KRIZEK had accumulated a cohort of 255 cystinurics, of whom 83% had stones.

In most countries of the world calcium oxalate stones are increasing whilst the proportion of uric acid and infective calculi is decreasing. There is a similar juxtaposition between bladder and renal calculi (PAVONE-MACALUSO and MIANO (1979) showed this quite clearly for Sicily over a period of 40 years, see Fig. 2).

We have been able to document a similar development over just 10 years (Table 8).

Between 1965 and 1973 HODGKINSON and MARSHALL (1975) recorded an increase of oxalate and a corresponding decrease of phosphate calculi. There was little alteration in the sex ratio (2.98 to 2.76).

In Finland there was an increase in the proportion of calcium oxalate from 4.8% in 1970 to 60% in 1954 (SALLINEN, quoted by ANDERSEN 1969). There was a corresponding decrease of phosphate calculi.

2. Age and Sex of Stone Patients According to Type of Calculus

The relationship between calculus rate and age and sex of patients in the GDR is given in Fig. 3. Children and young people are rarely affected but there is a sharp increase fom the 20th year onwards, with a broad low plateau for women between the age of 40 and 70. The peak occurring in the 5th decade has also been reported by SCHWILLE et al. (1980).

25% of GIBBAS' (1969) urolithiasis patients were over the age of 60, and in the series of KLINGENBERG et al. (1971) 3.1% were over 70.

Among the younger patients in the cohort of LJUNGHALL et al. (1977) 3.2% had had their first stone before their 30th year, whereas this figure was only 1.4% for the older patients. The authors therefore suggest that there has been a cumulative increase in the incidence of uroliths in recent years. The peak age of first episode lies between the 2nd and 4th decade of life (WILLIAMS 1969).

It is of some interest to compare the age and sex incidence of calculi in the GDR and Japan (Fig. 4a, b).

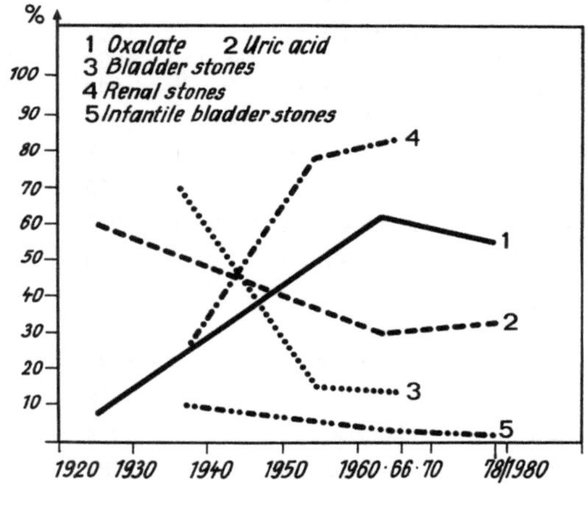

Fig. 2. Patterns of stone disease in Sicily, 1920–1980 (PAVONE-MACALUSO and MIANO 1979)

Table 6. Urolithiasis in various countries of the world

Country	Author	Year	Total stones	Sex ratio ♂ : ♀	Children %	Uric acid	Urates	Cystine	Xanthine
Belgium	Fuss et al.	1978	377	2	–	5.3	–	1.1	–
FRG	Kisters and Terhorst	1973	1 000	–	–	15	1.3	1.3	–
	Gebhardt and Bastian	1975	1 237	–	–	11	2.3	1.3	–
	Kallistratos	1978	3 390	1.8	1.56	10	–	0.7	0.02
	Scholz et al.	1979	709	1.2	–	17	–	1	–
Bulgaria	Budevski[a]	1975	5 930	1.7	–	38 ♂ 25 ♀	–	0.8	–
Czechoslovakia	Mates and Krizek	1955	3 340	2	–	34	–	–	–
GDR	Hesse et al.	1972	2 000	1.9	–	19	0.9	0.5	–
	Schneider et al.	1975	17 344	1.9	–	15	0.7	0.4	–
	Schneider	1980	95 780	1.9	1.4	14	0.2	0.4	–
	Brien et al.	1984	168 000	–	1.3	13.6	0.4	0.7	–
England	Westbury	1974	1 022	3	–	8	–	3	–
	Rose and Woodfine	1976	502	–	–	3	–	1	–
Finland	Oravisto[a]	1978	323	1.9	–	4	–	0.3	–
Italy	Lombardi	1969	1 120	2	–	30	–	–	–
Yugoslavia	Janca[a]	1978	–	1.9	–	6	1.6	3.9	–
Netherlands	Donker[a]	1978	1 610	2	1.8	7	–	0.3	0.1
Portugal	Reis-Santos	1984	1 320	1.1	–	19	–	0.9	–
Austria	Schöll	1978	2 700	–	–	22	–	–	–
Turkey	Ayder[a]	1978	500	1.9	18.8	11	3	0.2	–
USSR	Koslowski	1973	101	–	–	14	–	2	1
	Jediny	1972	–	–	–	7	–	–	–
Hungary	Berenyi	1975	2 300	1.4	6.2	20	–	1.1	–
	Toth[a]	1978	550	1.6	1	19	–	–	–
	Szabo[a]	1978	–	1.5	2.5	10	2	0.3	–
Spain	Matouschek and Huber	1981	–	–	–	14	–	1.3	–
USA	Herring	1962	9 895	–	–	7.6	0.15	0.9	–
	Gershoff	1964	1 000	–	–	–	6	3	–
	Griffith	1978	7 194	–	–	6.7	0.4	0.3	–
(New York)	Unni Moppan et al.	1979	261	3.3	–	15	–	–	–
(Rochester)	Johnson et al.	1979	347	2.3	–	6	0.6	–	–
	Keefe and Smith	1981	1 034	–	–	5	–	0.2	–
Canada	Oreopolus[a]	1978	120	3	–	20	–	1.6	–
Puerto Rico	Rivera and Isales	1970	128	0	–	6	–	–	–
Israel	Zaidmann and Pinto	1976	1 000	–	–	13	–	0.5	–
Thailand	Hodgkinson	1975	20	–	–	4	2	–	–
Sudan	Kambal	1979	78	3.1	49	7	–	–	–
Nigeria	Esho	1978	50	6	–	8	–	–	–
Japan	Takasaki	1975	735	2.6	–	2.2	1.8	1.0	–
Korea	Jong Go[a]	1978	–	1.6	3	10	–	3	–
Taiwan	Hsien et al.	1979	–	2.8	1.3	8	–	–	–
Brasil	Matouschek and Huber	1981	–	–	–	18	–	–	–
Mexico	Matouschek and Huber	1981	–	–	–	26	–	–	–
Argentina	Goldschmidt et al.	1984	200	–	–	48	–	2	–

Types of calculus according to principal component (%)							Type of analysis
Oxalate	Whewellite	Weddellite	Phosphates	Struvite	Carbonate apatite	Calcium phosphate	
61.6	–	–	–	13.5	–	15.6	Chemical
45	34	11	19.4	14.3	–	5.1	IR
59	37	22	25.6	10.4	–	15.2	X-ray diffr.
61.4	–	–	26	12.8	–	13.2	IR
66	–	–	–	2	–	8	Microscopy
42	–	–	7 ° 12 °	–	–	–	Chemical
50	–	–	16	–	–	–	Chemical
59	49	10.5	18	8.8	6.8	2.4	X-ray diffr.
64	52	12	11	7.3	1.9	1.8	X-ray diffr.
71	57	14	–	5.1	3.5	2	X-ray diffr.
73.3	60.2	13.1	–	4.6	3.4	1.7	X-ray diffr.
60	–	–	–	15	–	13	Chemical
59	53	6	–	32	–	–	IR
69	–	–	–	11	–	16	Chemical
53	–	–	17	–	–	–	Chemical
46	27	19	–	2	14	24	X-ray diffr.
63	–	–	–	9	–	20	Chemical
64.5	–	–	–	14	–	–	X-ray diffr.
70	–	–	–	8	–	–	Chemical
62	57	5	–	11	0.6	12	Chemical
57	47	10	27	13	14	–	Chemical
59	–	–	34	–	–	–	Chemical
59	44	15	14	12.5	1.6	–	Therm.
50	34	16	30	–	–	–	Chemical
54	43	11	28	–	–	3	Microscopy
75	–	–	–	0.1	–	2	X-ray diffr., IR
73	31.7	41.3	17.5	9.2	4.5	3.9	X-ray diffr.
67	–	–	–	19	–	5	Chemical
77	61	16	–	3.7	–	15.4	–
76	70	6	–	6	–	–	Microscopy
86	–	–	–	–	–	8	Chemical
68	–	–	–	13	–	3	X-ray diffr.
23	–	–	–	4	–	–	–
86	–	–	–	6	–	1	Microscopy
75	–	–	–	5	–	6	Chemical
61	–	–	–	12	–	8	Chemical
88	–	–	–	6	–	–	Chemical
28	–	–	–	40	–	24	Chemical, microscopy
60	–	–	–	22	–	13	Chemical
60	–	–	25	–	–	–	Chemical
78	–	–	–	14	–	–	Chemical
50	–	–	–	–	–	7	Chemical
37	–	–	–	30	–	–	Chemical
40	–	–	–	10	–	–	Chemical

Table 7. Composition of bladder calculi

Type of stone	% Total		
	BORGMANN et al.	KAMBAL et al.	BRUNDIG and SCHNEIDER
Struvite	18	24	33
Apatite	39		5
Uric acid	25	29	39
Calcium oxalate	24	43	22
Cystine	–	4	1

Table 8. Occurrence rate for principal types of urolith in the years 1971–1979 (in %)

Type of calculus	To 1970	1971	1972	1973	1974	1975	1976	1977	1978	1979
Uric acid and uric acid dihydrate	19.8	18.4	17.3	16.1	15.8	15.7	13.9	13.9	13.7	13.2
Whewellite and weddellite	63.9	61.7	65.6	69.3	68.3	71.2	72.6	75.3	75.4	75.9
Carbonate apatite	3.5	4.4	4.6	4.6	3.8	3.3	3.5	3.0	3.4	3.9
Struvite	8.1	9.3	8.3	6.3	7.0	5.9	4.9	4.7	4.6	4.2

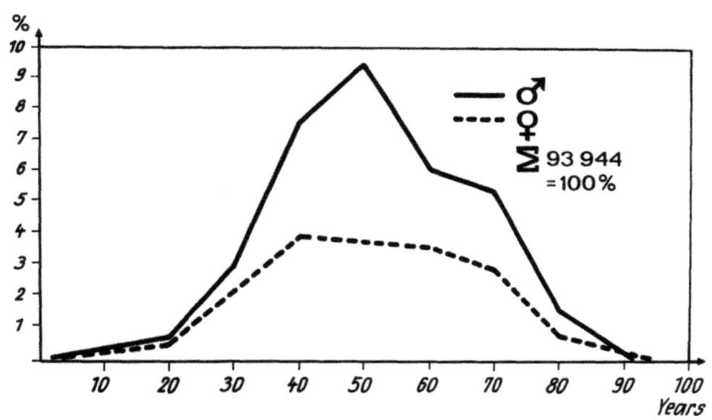

Fig. 3. Occurrence rate of stones by age and sex

The peak frequency for Japan occurs almost 20 years earlier in both men and women than in our country. The sharp among 30-year-old women must give particular cause for concern.

In most countries the mean sex ratio among stone patients is 2:1 (men to women). In bygone years this ratio was considerably more asymmetric (20:1) and is continuing to approach 1:1 (ZIELINSKI 1979). Age and sex ratios vary from stone type to stone type. Calcium oxalate calculi are the typical stones of men and phosphate stones occur mainly in women (OTNES 1980; WESTBURY 1979). Men have a 4–5 times greater likelihood of developing idiopathic cal-

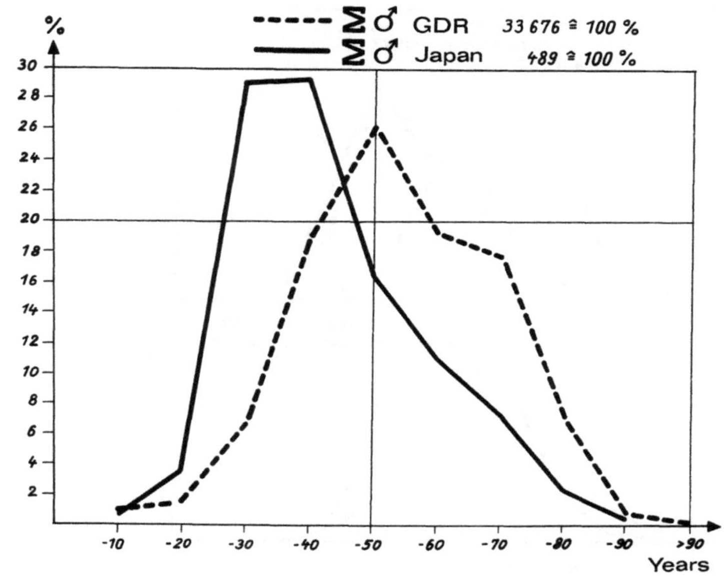

a

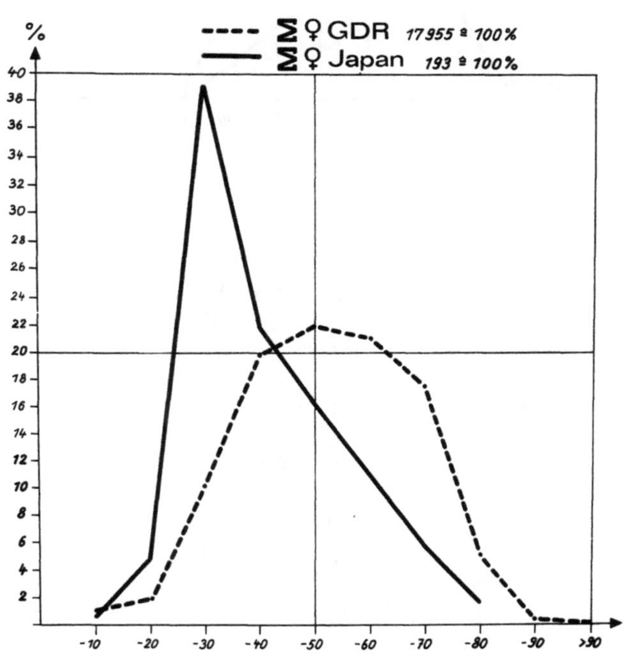

b

Fig. 4. a, b. Age and sex distribution among urolith patients in Japan and the GDR **a** Men, **b** Women (TAKASAKI 1975, SCHNEIDER and HIENZSCH 1979)

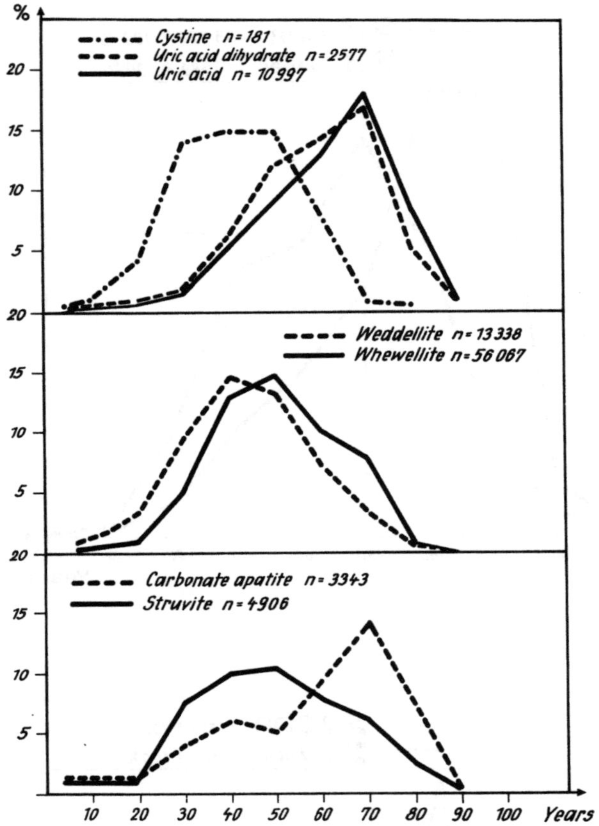

Fig. 5. Occurrence rates for various types of calculus by age group

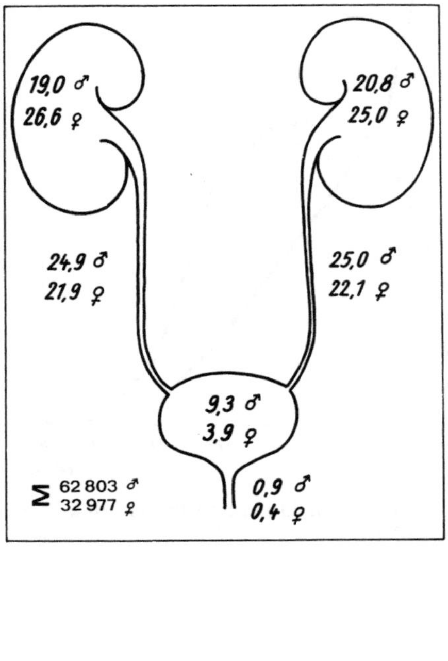

Fig. 6. Distribution of stones within the urinary tract

cium calculi than women (ROBERTSON et al. 1980). Among our own data the sex ratio varies from 0.6 for whitlockite and hydroxyapatite to 2.6 for uric acid.

An INFAS questionnaire sent to 10,130 persons over the age of 18 revealed a prevalence of 1.8% men and 2.2% women suffering from calculi (VAHLENSIECK et al. 1981). A further increase of the stone rate may be expected among women, perhaps in connection with a change in lifestyle.

Figure 5 gives the age distribution for various types of calculi based on just under 100,000 analyses. Uric acid and carbonate apatite calculi increase with age, peaking in the 7th decade (GIBBA 1969); weddellite peaks 15 years before whewellite calculi, and there is a rapid decrease in cystine stones after the 5th decade. Struvite stones occur in a broad flat peak between the 30th and 60th year. This latter substance is nearly always associated with urinary tract infection by urea-splitting bacteria, giving rise to the staghorn calculi of young women (FRANG et al. 1979).

The prevalence of uric acid stones peaks earlier in men than in women, the reverse being true of struvite and carbonate apatite calculi (HORN 1973).

3. Distribution of Calculi in the Urinary Tract

Figure 6 gives the overall distribution of stones within the urinary tract. Kidney stones are commoner among than men. The relatively higher number of ureteric calculi found in men corresponds to an increased tendency to spontaneous passage. The high proportion of bladder stones among males must of course be causally related to the bladder neck obstruction of older men (Table 9).

A previously reported side preference (also documented by SHABAD 1975, for women) can no longer be demonstrated (HESSE et al. 1975, 1977a).

There are specific variations in the frequency of individual types of calculus within the urinary tract (Fig. 7).

Table 9. Bladder calculi in men and women of varying age (n = 6,994)

Age	Men		Women	
	Absolute	%	Absolute	%
1 – 10	50	0.7	19	0.3
11 – 20	66	0.9	21	0.3
21 – 30	116	1.7	54	0.8
31 – 40	215	3.1	128	
41 – 50	422	6.0	179	2.6
51 – 60	720	10.3	260	3.7
61 – 70	1813	25.9	285	4.1
71 – 80	2041	29.2	211	3.0
81 – 90	341	4.9	38	0.5
> 90	12	1.7	3	0.04

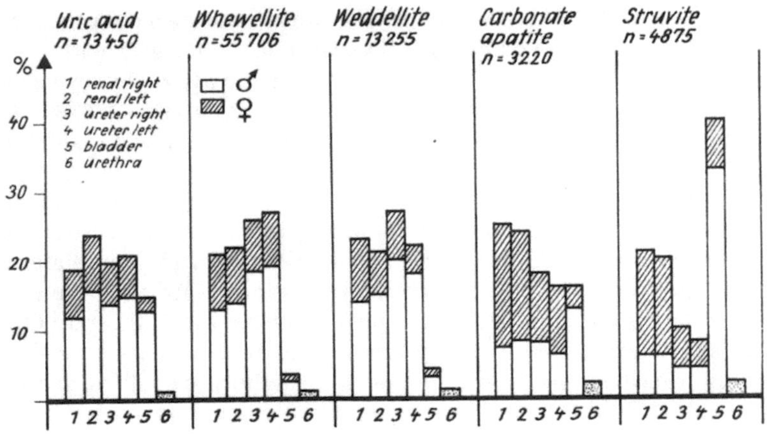

Fig. 7. Occurrence rates for various types of stone within the urinary tract

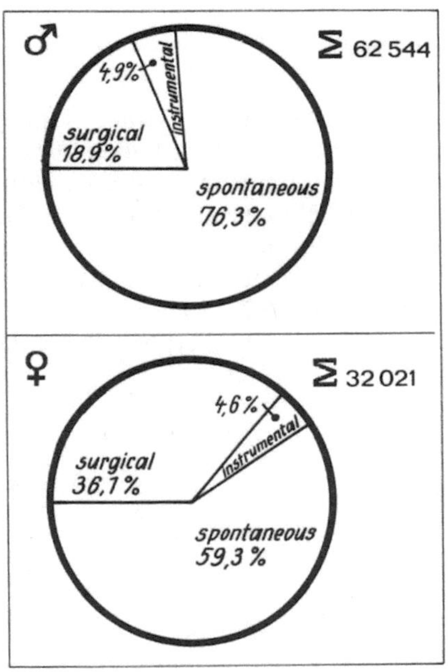

Fig. 8. Route of stone elimination for men and women

Whewellite is commoner in the ureter than in the kidney. Struvite is the chief component of bladder calculi.

Two-thirds of all uroliths, approximately 80% of ureteric calculi, pass spontaneously (MERCZ and BOGA 1978), but one-third of calculi still require surgical removal, despite all advances in litholysis and in recurrence prevention. Once again there is some variation between the figures for men and women (Fig. 8). Such variations occur even between individual types of calculus, their locali-

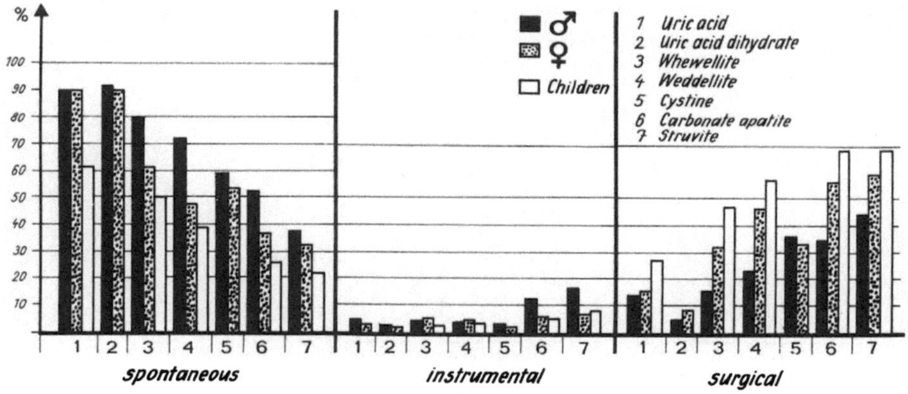

Fig. 9. Influence of stone type on stone elimination for men and women

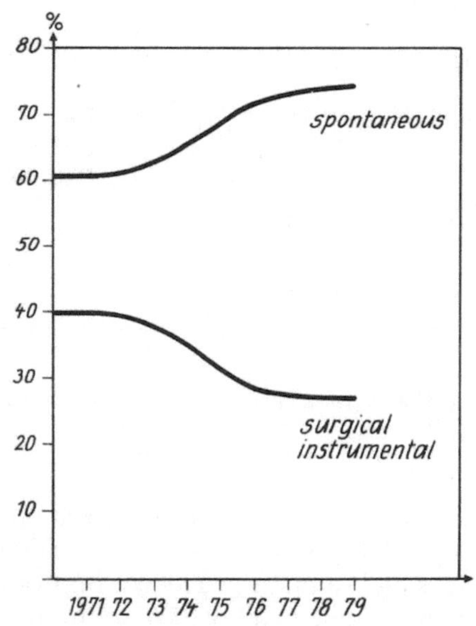

Fig. 10. Proportions of operatively removed and spontaneously passed calculi, 1971 – 1979

sation and the probable means of removal (Fig. 9). In women 65% of infective calculi require operative removal.

There has been a steady decrease in the proportion of stones removed by surgery in the years 1971 – 1979 (Fig. 10).

IV. Seasonal Variations in Incidence of Recurrent and de novo Stone Disease

A hot climate per se would not appear to have a decisive influence on the incidence of stone disease if there is proper acclimatization. In hot countries such as

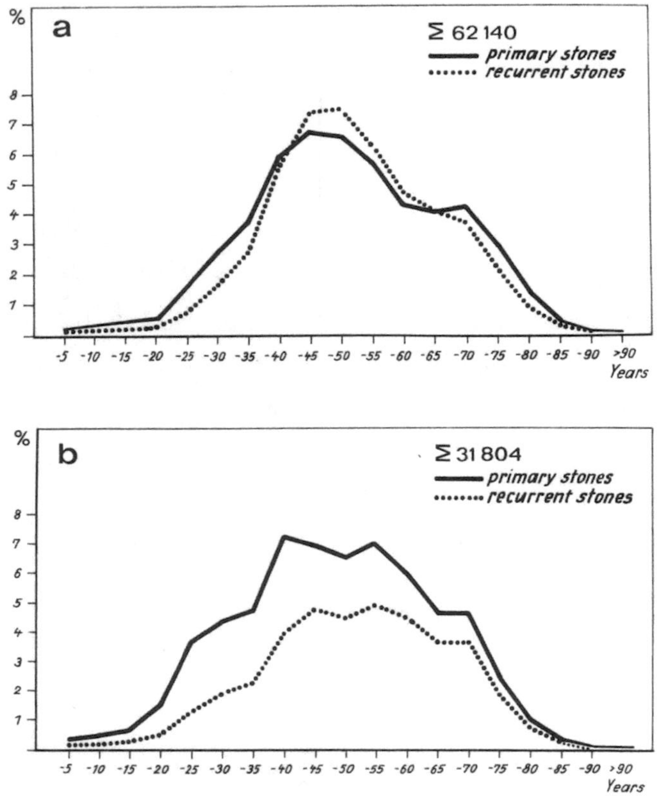

Fig. 11 a, b. Initial and recurrent stones in man **a** and women **b** by age

Ecuador and in the North of Peru urolithiasis is indeed exceptionally rare (PYRAH 1979). On the other hand soldiers spending prolonged periods in hot regions have a higher incidence of urolithiasis than at home, as was demonstrated by the German and British armies in North Africa in the Second World War. In one region of Israel, the overwhelming majority of 622 stone patients were of European extraction (FRANK et al. 1970).

A number of workers have documented an increase in the spontaneous passage of stones during the summer months (ATSMON et al. 1963; BATESON 1973; ELLIOT et al. 1975; HESSE et al. 1977a). In Kuwait twice the number of renal colics occur during the summer months, when temperatures may reach 50 °C, than do in the rest of the year. It is of particular interest that 73% of these colic patients are foreigners (SALEM 1969).

In contrast to an earlier study, our 10-year survey has been unable to demonstrate any preference for individual months, either for calculi as a whole or for whewellite or uric acid stones individually.

According to AL-DABBAGH and FAHADI (1977) the majority of calculi occur during the autumn in Iraq. These authors assume that the calculi are formed during the hotter months and subsequently pass as diuresis increases during the following cooler period. GLUZEK et al. (1978) measured a peak in calcium excretion occurring in July (224 mg/day) and a trough during December (122 mg/day). Similar results were arrived at by HALLSON and ROSE (1977) and by HALLSON et al. (1977). July and August were characterised by high crystalluria rates, mainly in the nocturnal urine, and by a marked increase in oxalate excretion. Despite variations in the stone rate between Scotland (0.2%) and the South Coast of England (1.1%) differences in urine composition were minimal despite a general oxaluria peak in the summer months (ROSE and WESTBURY 1979).

It is assumed that both a rising temperature load and an increase in fruit and vegetable consumption with its concomitant urinary oxalate excretion together favor crystallization and microlith formation.

GALOSY (1981) comes to a different conclusion. He was able to confirm seasonal variations in a study based on 141 patients and 34 controls, but found the lowest urinary oxalate concentration in summer and the highest in winter.

On the other hand, SCHÖLL (1979) also found a peak among his urolith patients in July, but also 3 further (smaller) subpeaks in January, April and October, on the basis of which he considers a 3-month rhythm to be at work. In Japan ureteric colic is commonest on hot days with low barometric pressure (FUJITA 1979a, b).

My own data on recurrence rates and new cases is always given in terms of the definition in Chapter A. Every new stone throughout a patient's life is therefore counted as a recurrence, irrespective of the type and localisation. Such a method results in a relatively high recurrence rate. LJUNGHALL (1978) gives a value of 77%, WILLIAMS (1969) 75%, TAKASAKI (1975) 41%, BONO et al. (1979) 30%. 74% of 538 patients with recurrences have had more than one recurrence (WILLIAMS 1969). In the cross-sectional study by VAHLENSIECK et al. (1980) 40% of patients had had one or more recurrence, the sex ratio for 1 or 2 stones being 1 : 1 and only rising in favor of men in multiple stone cases. 11% of male and 2.5% of female patients with recurrent stone disease had suffered more than 10 recurrences (VAHLENSIECK et al. 1984). People who suffer their first stone before their 30th year are twice as likely to suffer a recurrence as those who pass their first stone after 30 (LJUNGHALL et al. 1980).

There is good agreement between the INFAS material of VAHLENSIECK et al. (1980) and our own data (Table 10).

The likelihood of recurrence decreases continuously from the time the first stone is passed (MARSHALL et al. 1975). Figure 12 represents recurrence rates for the first 8 years and the first 6 months after passage of a first stone.

Among a collection of 95,780 uroliths 43,018 (45%) were recurrences. On the other hand only 25% were from patients who passed their first stone in the years 1971/72.

Patients with a family history of urolithiasis are more likely to suffer a recurrence than those without (Fig. 13).

If one assumes 70 – 80% of all stones occurring in our country come to analysis in the central laboratories, one arrives at a figure for new cases of 0.1% of the population (HESSE et al. 1977b).

Table 10. Number of patients with recurrent calculi (VAHLENSIECK et al. 1980, n = 202, own data, n = 983, first episode after 1971)

Number of recurrences	SCHNEIDER		VAHLENSIECK	
	Absolute	%	Absolute	%
1	540	55	112	55
2	202	21	47	23
3	100	10	21	10
4	56	6	6	3
5	24	2	4	2
6 – 12	61	6	12	6

Table 11. Proportion of recurrent stones among individual stone types

Type of stone	Total	Recurrent	%
Uric acid	10 997	6 406	58
Uric acid dihydrate	2 577	1 685	65
Ammonium hydrogenurate	372	198	53
Cystine	181	115	64
Whewellite	56 067	23 738	42
Weddellite	13 338	5 686	43
Apatite	1 409	553	39
Carbonate apatite	3 343	1 355	40
Brushite	243	150	62
Struvite	4 906	1 903	39

Table 12. Route of stone elimination by stone type in new and recurrent cases (in %)

Type of stone	Spontaneous		Instrumental		Operative	
	New	Recurrent	New	Recurrent	New	Recurrent
Uric acid	70.6	91.4	5.3	2.4	24.1	6.2
Whewellite	58.5	76.2	5.4	5.2	35.1	18.6
Weddellite	61.6	79.4	3.8	2.8	34.7	17.7
Struvite	41.1	47.5	13.0	6.7	45.9	45.8
Carbonate apatite	40.6	55.5	7.1	6.5	42.3	38.0

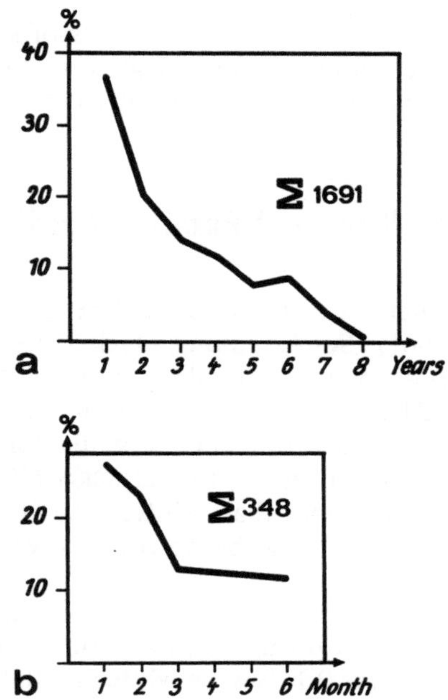

Fig. 12. Recurrence rate and interval after first episode (**a** in years, **b** in months)

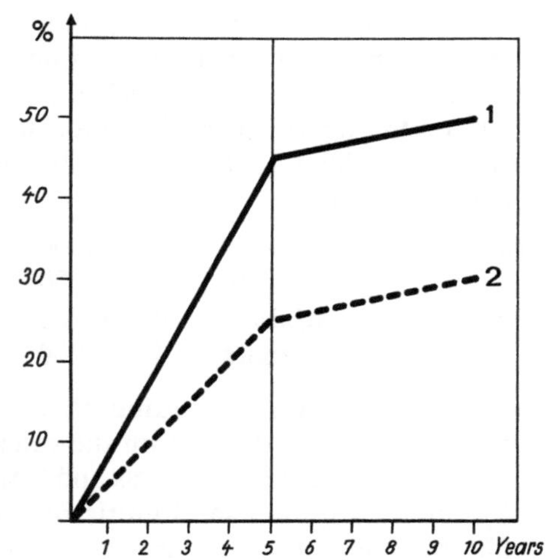

Fig. 13. Frequency of recurrences in relation to observation period in subjects with (1) or without (2) a family history of renal stone disease (LJUNGHALL 1980)

The proportion of recurrent stones is also dependent on the type of calculus (Table 11).

Uric acid dihydrate, cystine and brushite recur the most commonly. Oxalate and apatite most rarely.

Table 12 shows how the method of stone extraction may depend on the type of calculus involved, both in new patients and in recurrent cases. Recurrent stone far more rarely require operative removal, passing in 80–90%, with the exception of infection stones of struvite or carbonate apatite. A series of 675 operations for stone disease included 175 nephrectomies. In 76% of cases the stones were of struvite. (ANDROULAKIS et al. 1982).

V. Race and Familial Predisposition

There are no racial differences in susceptibility to urolithiasis (BOSHAMER 1961). Solely among black races does there appear to be a reduced predisposition to form kidney stones. GOETZEE (1963) examined 162,000 Africans and 12,000 Indians during an 8-year period in South Africa. The Indians had a urolithiasis rate of 0.2%, whilst for Africans it was only 0.01%.

According to EICKENBERG (1978) colored Americans are less likely to develop stones than whites, and Bantus equally less likely than colored Americans. It should be noted, however, that considerable territorial differences are involved.

Of a population of 231,000 in North Carolina there were 0.2% urolith patients requiring hospitalisation. 0.36% were white and 0.1% were colored males, whereas 0.14% were white and 0.03% colored women (SCHEY et al. 1979). A variety of mechanisms are postulated to account for the lower overall frequency among Africans, including the protective function of skin pigment preventing vitamin D activation, reduced protein intake, reduced urinary calcium excretion, the absence of urinary uromucoid, etc. (KEUTEL 1975; MODLIN 1969). Note, however, that BICHLER (1975) takes precisely the opposite view to that of KEUTEL on the significance of uromucoid.

In New Zealand 1,000 adult urolith patients were drawn from the general population as follows:

Europeans	Male	58/100,000
	Female	19/100,000
Polynesians	Male	19/100,000
	Female	14/100,000

Environmental factors inculding changes in lifestyle and nutrition certainly have a more profound effect on the calculus rate and the distribution of stone types than do racial factors (FUSS and SIMON 1979).

Cystinuria, familial xanthinuria or congenital oxalosis are typical examples of inherited stone-forming disease, a pattern not seen in the vast majority of urolithiasis patients. On the other hand it is a common experience of clinical practice that numerous urolith patients will give a family history of urolithiasis (LJUNGHALL 1979 = 30%; DE VRIES et al. 1972 = 46%; PAVONE-MACALUSO and MIANO 1979 = 35%; CHURCHILL et al. 1980 = 38%; VENDL 1975 = 25%; GÜNALP 1979 = 14%; BOYCE 1979 = 3 times the frequency of healthy people; MATES and KRIZEK 1958 = 13%; BURCH and DAWSON 1969).

We have taken the family history of over 1,000 urolith patients 29% (165 men, 135 women) new of blood relatives who suffered from stone disease (Table 13).

Table 13. Stones found in relatives of 1,000 stone patients

Relationship	
Parents	169
Sibs	97
Grandparents	28
Other blood relatives (children, uncles, etc.)	68

Of the blood relatives of 97 pediatric stone patients there was a 7.6% prevalence of urolithiasis, whereas a control group contained only 2.5%. One notable feature was a high percentage (43%) of consanguinous marriages among blood relatives of this pediatric cohort. Again, the control group reached only 8% (DZHAVAD-ZADE and GAMZAEVA 1980). In the form in which they are reported these results suggest a latent familial predisposition to form stones, yet they do not permit formal relationship to individual types of stone to be constructed.

Urolith patients with a positive family history are at increased risk, although genuine genetic causes are difficult to prove (GIUGLIANI and FERRARI 1981. Women from stone-forming families are less at risk than men (RESNICH et al. 1968).

No doubt this familial accumulation of urolithiasis has strong environmental and nutritional causes. Indeed WHITE et al. (1969) noted that spouses of stone-formers had a higher urinary calcium excretion than those of controls.

VI. Occupation and Lifestyle

There can be little doubt that a multitude of circumstances of every day life exert an influence on the current prevalence of urolithiasis all over the world. As the scientific-technological revolution proceeds an ever increasing number of people are engaged in primarily mental rather than physical occupations.

Furthermore, persons who take inadequate physical exercise frequently indulge in over- or incorrect nutrition. A large proportion of stone patients is of sedentary occupation (STEG et al. 1979).

There is a higher incidence of urolithiasis among sailors than in the rest of the population (CHMIELEWSKI et al. 1974), and in the Royal Navy this affects chiefly officers, administrators and cooks, but rarely deckhands, marines or engine room personnel (BLACKLOCK 1969).

MATES (1969) has also produced some interesting figures. Among patients at the Marienbad spa, senior officials and others of sedentary occupation yielded the highest proportion of stone sufferers, agriculturalists the least (Table 14).

Table 14. Urolithiasis rates by occupation among patients at Marienbad (in %) (MATES 1969)

	Population (13,607,000) %	Stone sufferers %
Housewives	31	8
Workers	17	16
Pensioners	16	5
Agriculturalists	13	1
Clerical workers	9	23
Other sedentary occupations	6	24
Teachers	1	5
Nurses and Auxiliaris	1	4
Transport workers	0.9	9

Table 15. Occupation, prevalence and recurrence rate of stones (in %) (VAHLENSIECK et al. 1980)

Occupation	Prevalence	Recurrence rate
Self-employed	4	50
Employees	3	66
Officials	6	17
Skilled workers	4	15
Unskilled	5	60
Housewives	5	60
Pensioners	9	44

Of the 5,000 urolith patients that formed the subject of our own sociologic survey, 32% were production workers (irrespective of physical exertion) and 33% officials and professionals with college qualifications (SCHNEIDER et al. 1973). The mean age of the latter group was 20 years less than that of the production workers. There was a marked excess of motor transport drivers in our sample. The GÖTZENS study (JOOST et al. 1980) likewise showed a considerably lower prevalence of urolithiasis among manual workers than among academics and officials.

Table 15 summarizes the relationship between occupation and the prevalence and recurrence rate of stones.

In MATES' (1969) study the lowest stone frequency occurred in border regions with purely agricultural economy and the highest in industrial cities.

In Egypt urban stones were predominantly uric acid, whilst those of rural peasants tended to be infective (SAFWAT et al. 1979). For the GDR we have compared the distribution of various types of stone in rural areas and small towns with industrial zones and in large conurbations (Table 16).

There do not appear to be serious variations, although the large conurbations and industrial areas yielded relatively more uric acid and fewer struvite calculi than did small towns and country areas.

Among the data of VAHLENSIECK et al. (1980) the stone incidence increased with the size of town, whereas the recurrence rate decreased. In our own data there was also some territorial variation in the route of stone extrusion. Fewer stones pass spontaneously in large cities and industrialised areas (Table 17).

Over the years we have come to the conclusion that our traditional view on occupational risk factors among urolith patients require some revision. For example, we investigated steel plant workers on a three-shift system with high heat exposure and compared them to administrative personnel at the some works (FRANK et al. 1975). Of 650 persons with high heat exposure, 1.22% suffered from urolithiasis, yet among 484 clerical workers there were 3.67%. ZIELINSKI (1972) also failed to find an increased incidence of stones among 1,276 heat-exposed workers compared to a control group of 2,000 student nurses. Nevertheless, the fact that 11 out of 45 Israeli swimming pool attendants suffer from kidney stones is usually attributed to the heat and sun exposure of their occupation (KEDAR et al. 1979).

Table 16. Distribution of stone types in industrialised and agricultural areas, and in large and small towns (in %)

Stone type	Schwerin and Neubrandenburg area		Small towns		Halle and Karl-Marx-Stadt area		Large cities		Berlin	
Uric acid	8.2		8.2		12.3		9.9		8.0	
		10.4		11.0		14.5		12.4		10.5
Uric acid dihydrate	2.2		2.8		2.2		2.5		2.5	
Whewellite	62.3		59.8		62.1		62.2		59.9	
		74.8		73.6		74.2		75.5		73.6
Weddellite	12.5		13.8		12.1		13.3		13.8	
Apatite	3.3		3.0		0.6		2.1		1.1	
Carbonate apatite	2.3		2.5		2.6		1.9		6.2	
Struvite	6.0		6.1		4.8		5.0		5.0	

Table 17. Geographical variations in the route of stone elimination (in %)

Route of elimination	Schwerin and Neubrandenburg area	Small towns	Halle and Karl-Marx-Stadt area	Large cities	Berlin
Spontaneous	66.2	65.7	73.2	71.7	74.3
Instrumental	5.9	6.9	4.6	4.2	3.3
Operative	27.9	27.4	22.2	24.1	22.4

Both BRUNDIG et al. (1980, 1981a, b) and SCHMUCKI and ASPER (1979, 1977) have drawn attention to the effect of stress on urolithogenesis. This would explain the abnormally large proportion of drivers among stone patients and the high rate of kidney stones among flight crew. Pilots have twice the urolith rate of the population at large and in the Israeli airforce this proportions is said to reach 25%, compared to 4,2% among non-fying airforce personnel (PÖNISCH et al. 1973). Thus the 10-fold excess of stones among Danish doctors (PLANZ 1962) may also be explained both by their increased exposure to stress and their socio-economic grouping (ROBERTSON et al. 1979).

TOGGENBURG et al. (1981) have given some particularly interesting data on stress factors and urolithogenesis. Not quite 20% of patients in their clinical material are immigrant workers from Italy, Spain, Turkey, etc. who are usually manual or household workers. 81% suffered their first stone symptoms after arriving in Switzerland. Only 12% gave a history of urolithiasis, yet the recurrence rate after immigration reached 7%. Only 17% had an abnormality in their 24-hour urine that could be classed as a risk factor. There was a definite increase in the incidence of stone disease during the first two years after their arrival. Together, this marked incidence peak in the first and second year, the proponderance of calcium oxalate stones and the ureter as the dominant site of occurrence (80%) suggest that the social stress of moving to a new society represents a significant causal factor.

The best data on occupational intoxication as a cause of nephrolithiasis has been gathered in relation to long-term cadmium exposure (ANKE and SCHNEIDER 1979; AXELSON 1963; FRIBERG et al. 1974; SCOTT et al. 1979, 1982).

The pathophysiology of this condition is hypercalciuria due to renal damage.

Nutrition would appear to play an important part in urolithogenesis. ROBERTSON et al. (1978a, 1978b, 1979, 1984), KNEBEL (1982), ULSHÖFER (1984), ZECHNER and SCHEIBER (1981a) were able to establish a direct relationship between income, expenditure on food, protein intake and urolith frequency. Large quantities of alcohol have also been said to be a risk factor (ZECHNER 1982; ZECHNER and SCHEIBER 1981b).

ASPER and SCHMUCKI (1984) have reviewed 200 publications describing 250,000 calculi from 50 countries, demonstrating that the distribution of stones in Europe in the last century by age, sex, type and anatomical site corresponds to the pattern in the developing countries of today. This pattern is quite significantly different to that seen nowadays in Europe, the USA and Japan. Although no causal relationship is postulated, socioeconomic development seems to go hand in hand with a falling proportion of childhood urolithiasis, bladder stones, phosphate-, uric acid- and urate stones. By contrast, the proportions of stones found in women and composed of calcium oxalate both rise.

Table 18 presents a comparative study of stone type distribution and dietary habits in three different countries (GOLDSCHMIDT et al. 1984).

A connection between the composition of drinking water and the incidence of urolithiasis has often been looked for. Thuringia with its extremely hard water has traditionally been regarded as an area with a high urolithiasis rate, although stone disease was in fact always quite rare. There is in fact no relation-

Table 18. Dietary practice and stone composition

	Major type of lithiasis	Major food source
Alsace (France)	Calcium oxalate (58.5%)	Lipids (168 g/day)
Buenos Aires (Argentina)	Uric acid (48%)	Protein (104 g/day)
Vientiane (Laos)	Calcium oxalate (57%)	Glucose (392 g/day)

ship (or perhaps even a weak inverse one) between the hardness of drinking water and the incidence of nephrolithiasis (Bo et al. 1978; DEREZIC et al., DONALDSON et al. 1979; SIERAKOWSKI et al. 1979; ROSE and WESTBURY 1975). The same is true of the magnesium content of water (SCHNEIDER and ANKE 1976; ILLIEVSKI and ILLIEVSKI 1984). GOLUBCHANSKAJA (1976), however, has drawn attention to a connection between the major and trace element composition of water in relation to that found in uroliths.

VII. Constitution, Psychological Factors and Concomitant Disease

We have analysed the general constitution, the psychological profile, the symptoms and typical concomitant illnesses of 500 urolith patients (SCHNEIDER et al. 1979, 1980). 70% of patients were obese, indeed 90% of those with uric acid stones. KRIZEK (1968) and HORN et al. (1980) also pointed to a high rate of obesity among stone patients (JARROV and BOEDECKER 1984).

Morphometric classification according to KRETSCHMAR revealed a marked proponderance of the pyknic type among women. The men were chiefly of athletic habit. In the GRÖNINGER (1962) series there was an excess of pyknics among both sexes. Pyknic women are twice as likely to suffer from uric acid stones as are athletic or leptomorphic women.

KRIZEK (1968) investigated the relationship between eye pigmentation and type of calculus in 3,073 patients. Calcium oxalate stones coincide most commonly with brown eyes and uric acid stones with blue.

Half of all urolith patients may be shown to be hypertensive, and MAURER and VAHLENSIECK (1967) also found 109 urolith patients among 253 renal hypertensives. In an individual case it may be difficult to decide whether hypertension is the cause or the consequence of stone disease. The diabetic morbidity was equally impressive at 5.1% among urolithiasis patients, a figure considerably in excess of that for the general population. 10% of female uric acid patients and 6% of males suffered from diabetes mellitus, suggesting a powerful correlation between these two metabolic disorders. On the other hand TSCHOEPE et al. (1984) were unable to demonstrate an increased risk of stone disease (non-infective stones) among diabetics. Almost half of all patients with uric acid stones gave a history of rheumatic symptoms and of frequent ingestion of analgesics. One may assume this group to contain a large proportion of latent or manifest gout sufferers (THEILE et al. 1983). Primary urolithiasis is without any significant effect on the risk of developing renal tuberculosis, but the latter is associated in 8% of cases with secondary stone formation (STRAUSS 1982).

Renal tubular acidosis, on the other hand, is much more commonly linked with recurrent stone disease.

Our data confirms that of LOMBARDI (1969) and conflicts with that of GÜNALP (1979) in showing a random distribution of blood groups.

A symptom-orientated questionnaire has enabled an approximate psychologic assessment of our patients in respect of neurotic conditions (SCHNEIDER et al. 1980). The results show that the majority of female kidney stone patients belong to the group of 'possible neurotic' whilst the males tend to be 'without neurosis'. Since these are broad-peaked distributions one may assume a relatively large proportion of neurotic women among stone sufferers. Results of an MMPI-based study by WOCHNIK and SCHNEIDER (1972) suggest that autonomic nervous disorders resulting from psychological stress may represent an important etiological factor in urolithogenesis.

We have also employed an adapted INR (introversion, rigidity, neuroticism) score according to BÖTTGER. This questionnaire provides data on current circumstances and response to professional and social demands. It also assesses weighting factors including the effects of discrepancies between expectation and achievement. 30% of female patients have above average INR scores, only 5–10% are at the lower end of the range. Interestingly enough there are marked variations between the whewellite and weddellite groups. These data would tend to confirm the characteristics suggested by PFLÜCKER (1950) and MATES and KRIZEK (1955) for patients suffering from uric acid, calcium oxalate and phosphate calculi. Men with calcium oxalate stones are frequently dissatisfied with their occupation, timid, irritable, indecisive and frequently suffer from psychological conflicts. By way of contrast, uric acid stones occur more frequently among manual workers who are content with their work, tending to be neither egoistic, irritable nor timid, although they are frequently rather melancholic.

VIII. Urinary Calculi in Children

In contrast to the last century and to areas of endemic urolithiasis, children in most European countries and in America are nowadays rarely affected by urinary calculi. The figures available in the literature are based on highly variable clinical material. According to MEHNERT and HOKO (1978) 5.6 per 100,000 children underwent inpatient treatment for urolithiasis in 1974, whereas KAPLAN et al. (1979) report 0.1%, NORONA et al. (1979) 0.1% and LOUTFI et al. (1972) 0.8%.

In one (admittedly endemic) area of Turkey there were 8 stone patients per 1000 children of school age (REMZI et al. 1979).

According to FRICK and BARTSCH (1979) children constitute 4–5% of all urolith patients, and in one area of Yugoslavia this figure was 2.5% (JANCA et al. 1978). 10% of all children undergoing surgery in the Cairo children's hospital over a period of 20 years had urinary stones (LOUTFI et al. 1972). WILLNOW (1967) found stones in the urinary tract of 1.1% of about 8000 children examined at postmortem in the University Department of Pathology, Leipzig.

COHEN (1979) discusses the frequency and causation of neonatal nephrolithiasis. One half of all children had a family history of stone disease (NOE et al. 1983).

A questionnaire sent by BOKAI (1895) to all medical practitioners in Hungary brought to light 1,621 children with urinary stones, and in 1912 he extended this study (1,836 children). Stones occurred most commonly in the region of the Danube and the Theis. The varying distribution of childhood stones is not clearly understood. Environmental factors and unsuitable nutrition would appear to have an important influence. The majority of children with urolithiasis were of poor family background and had bladder or urethral calculi.

In 1976, 91 children aged 0–12 years were treated for urinary calculi in 16 children's clinics in the GDR (Fig. 14). This represents unselected clinical material derived from a population of 200,000 children, from which a morbidity of 0.5% may be calculated. In 1976 and 1977 one new case of urolithiasis was diagnosed per 10,000 children years, with three times more new cases among school age than pre-school children (OTTO-UNGER 1978). ZVARA et al. (1979) have documented a decrease in the initial stone rate in one large city from 20 to 7 per 100,000 children. Nevertheless, the overall urolithiasis rate among children rose during the same period (1965–1974) from 3.6 to 59.

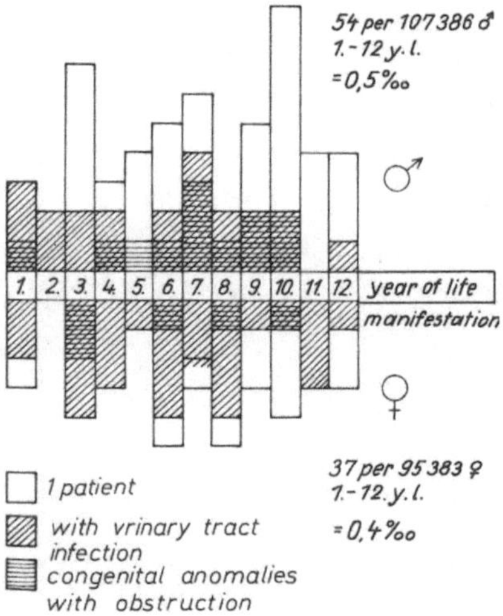

Fig. 14. 91 children with urolithiasis – unselected clinical material from a defined population area (SCHNEIDER and OTTO-UNGER 1978)

Table 19. Sex ratio among juvenile stone patients (various authors)

Author	Year	Sex ratio ♂:♀
BOKAI	1895	26
VALYASEVI	1979	10
BUDEVSKI et al.	1978	2.6
MARQUARDT and NAGEL	1977	2.0
WILLNOW	1962	1.4
DDR-Statistics	1981	1.4
VENDL	1975	1.2
MEHNERT and HOKO	1978	1.1
CHURCHILL et al.	1980	1.0

Table 20. Frequency distribution by stone type in childhood (n = 1,366) compared to the overall distribution (n = 95,788) (n = 100%)

Type of stone	Male		Female	
	Total	Children	Children	Total
Uric acid	12.5	2.2	1.1	9.2
Uric acid dihydrate	2.6	0.5	0.2	2.8
Ammonium dihydrogenurate	0.4	1.4	1.1	0.4
Cystine	0.1	0.8	0.2	0.3
Whewellite	59.8	29.7	32.8	55.0
Weddellite	14.9	32.0	32.8	11.8
Apatite	0.9	3.0	2.1	2.5
Carbonate apatite	2.3	9.3	6.3	5.7
Brushite	0.2	2.2	1.9	0.2
Struvite	4.2	13.4	12.5	6.8
Artefacts	1.1	3.8	6.5	3.6

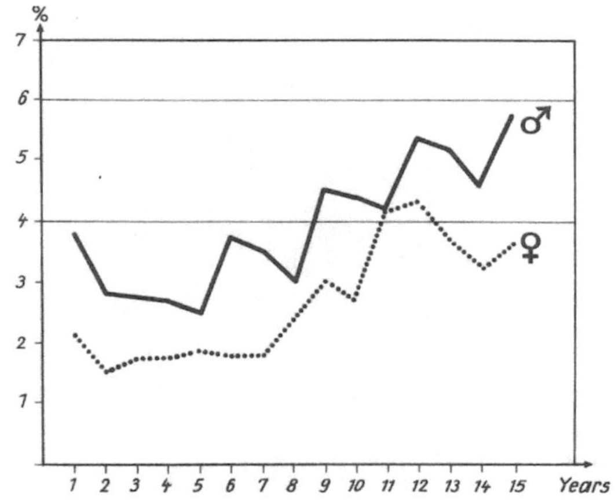

Fig. 15. Age distribution of uroliths among boys and girls (n = 1,366)

Among 95,780 uroliths analysed in the GDR, 1,366 were from children under the age of 15, i.e. 1.4%. With a ratio of 1.4 the sex distribution is more equal than in the general population (Table 19).

In the series of ZVARA et al. (1978) girls outnumbered boys, although this data relates only to schoolchildren. Although BOKAI (1895) and VALYASEVI (1979) found an excess of boys, it should be pointed out that their material consists predominantly of bladder and urethral stones (GHARIB 1970).

In our own series the distribution was equal only among 11-year-old boys and girls (Fig. 15).

Although VAHLENSIECK (1978) found a falling age distribution among 94 children with uroliths, our own data suggests a steady rise after an initial fall between the first and fifth years, with a peak occurring at the age of 12. There are wide variations in the data given in the literature. VAHLENSIECK (1978) failed to find any age-related peak, ECKSTEIN (1965) and HELBIG and GHARIB (1969) found the greatest prevalence among 2 to 5-year-olds. CHURCHILL et al. (1980), MEHNERT and HOKO (1978) and JANCA et al. (1978) found the same of 9 to 14-year-olds.

These variations in the age distribution of stones are mirrored in the distribution of stone types by age, a distribution widely at variance with that among adults (HODGKINSON 1977) (Table 20).

The majority of authors are agreed on the rarity of uric acid stones among children. Only in Bulgaria is a figure of 19% quoted (BUDEVSKI et al. 1978). Ammonium dihydrogenurate calculi are more common in children than in adults. The reverse is true of the whewellite–weddellite ratio: weddellite is equally common or perhaps commoner (SZABO 1978).

Infective calculi of struvite or carbonate apatite are considerably commoner in children (up to 3 times more frequent in boys) (JOOST and MORBERGER 1982; MAZEMAN et al. 1983; REVEILLAND and DAUDON 1984). Struvite calculi have their peak occurrence in 3-year-olds (Fig. 16). On the other hand whewellite predominates in the first year of life. Its occurrence decrease rapidly, only to

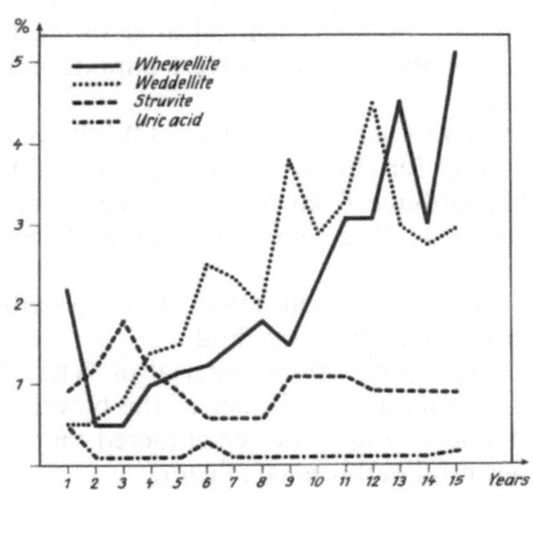

Fig. 16. Distribution of juvenile stone types by age

rise again steadily from the 4th year of life to become the principal type of calculus at the age of 13. Weddellite is the most common phase between the 5th and 12th year.

BARRADT and GHAZALI (1977) have devided children with uroliths into three etiological groups.

1. Endemic calculi: chiefly ammonium dihydrogenurate stones, mainly in the Far East.
2. Urinary tract infection: struvite calculi related to Proteus infections (commonest cause in Europe).
3. Rare metabolic disorders and calcium oxalate stones.

Urinary tract infection, not uncommonly related to anatomical anomalies, appear to be the commonest cause of urinary calculi, particularly among infants.

60–80% of urolithiasis is considered to be associated with infection, organisms of the Proteus and Coliform group predominating (FINN and SAUPE 1981; MARQUARDT and NAGEL 1977; MAZEMAN et al. 1978, 1983; NORONA et al. 1979; REMZI 1980; SINNO et al. 1979; TURKYILMAZ 1976). Approximately ¼ of children with urolithiasis have an anatomical abnormality of the urinary tract (HOMANN et al. 1977), and according to BORGMANN and NAGEL (1980, 1982) the related outflow and urodynamic disorders are of great importance in childhood urolithogenesis.

Metabolic disorders are a relatively rare cause of stones in childhood. Figures vary between 14% (SINNO et al. 1979) and 6% (SCHNEIDER and OTTO-UNGER 1979; VAHLENSIECK 1978). Such disorders include hypercalciuria, found by CHURCHILL et al. (1980) in 38% of their pediatric urolithiasis patients, more rarely disorders of purine metabolism or primary hyperoxaluria and mainly cystinuria.

Of 250 cystine patients from 190 cystinuric families 42 suffered their first manifestation during childhood (KRIZEK 1978). Indeed 15 had their first calculus episode during the first year of life. Among younger children boys are mainly affected (4:1), the sex ratio becoming almost even by the age of 15.

A series of 148 children undergoing surgery for urolithiasis in Teheran contained 6 with cystine and 3 with xanthine stones on X-ray diffraction, polarising microscopy and chemical analysis (KHERADPIR and ARMBRUSTER 1984). The vast majority of stones were a mixture of whewellite and ammonium hydrogen urate.

SCHOENBERGER et al. (1983) followed up patients operated on ten years previously for childhood kidney stones. 11% had had a true recurrence and 20% had suffered from residual stones, more than half of which had passed spontaneously. The commonest cause of recurrence was persistent urinary tract infection.

DE VOOGT et al. (1973) have described a xanthine stone occuring in a 10-year-old xanthinuric child.

The postmortem material of WILLNOW (1962) yielded a figure of 73% for inflammatory conditions of the bowel among children with urolithiasis, but it should of course be remembered that the concomitant dehydration must be a powerful pathogenetic factor.

Table 21. Recurrence rates for various stone types in children compared to overall rates

Type of stone	Total	Recurrent	Percent recurrence rate	
			Children	Total
Uric acid and uric acid dihydrate	29	11	38	58
Cystine				
Whewellite	423	83	20	42
Weddellite	442	108	24	43
Apatite	36	8	22	39
Carbonate apatite	110	43	39	40
Brushite	29	14	48	62
Struvite	178	52	29	39

Bladder and urethral stones are even rarer in children than in adults. A sole exception is constituted by endemic areas (LOUTFI 1981; REMZI 1980; VALYASEVI 1979; VAN REEN 1972). The latter type of stone is nearly always ammonium dihydrogenurate (HSIEN et al. 1973). In Europe and North America bladder calculi occur mainly in children with anatomical abnormalities or who have been immobilised for a long time. Their stones consist of struvite and carbonate apatite (AURORA et al. 1970; FRICK and BARTSCH 1972; GHAZALI et al. 1973; HERTKENS and VÖLZ 1970; HESSE and SCHNEIDER 1978; REINER et al. 1979).

In our own studies there were 332 recurrent stones, i.e. 24.3%. Compared to the figure of 45% for our total data this figure is remarkably low.

The following figures may be found in the literature: KAPLAN et al. (1979) = 6.5%, MINKOW (1978) = 12%, ZVARA et al. (1978) = 11.4%, SCHNEIDER et al. (1978) = 25%, REETZ (1980) = 15%, VENDL (1975) = 24%, ABERLE (1968) = 23%, STROHMENGER and MELLIN (1970) = 22%, BORGMANN and NAGEL (1980) = 21%, GOSALBEZ et al. (1981) = 30%.

Table 21 gives the recurrence rate for various types of calculus compared to the overall recurrence rate. With the exception of brushite and carbonate apatite virtually all types of stone show only half the general recurrence rate in children.

Stones are also eliminated differently to those of adults. VAHLENSIECK (1978) pointed out that 80% of adult ureteric stones are passed spontaneously, against only 25% of juvenile stones. Figure 17 depicts the ratio of spontaneous passage, operative and instrumental removal. For adults these ratios are 70:25:5, and for children 40:56:4.

"Studies on the epidemiology of stone formation have shown that many factors appear to be involved in the pathogenesis of the disorder. Apart from the traditional epidemiological factors such as age, sex, occupation, geographical localisation and climate, other variables reported to influence the risk of stones

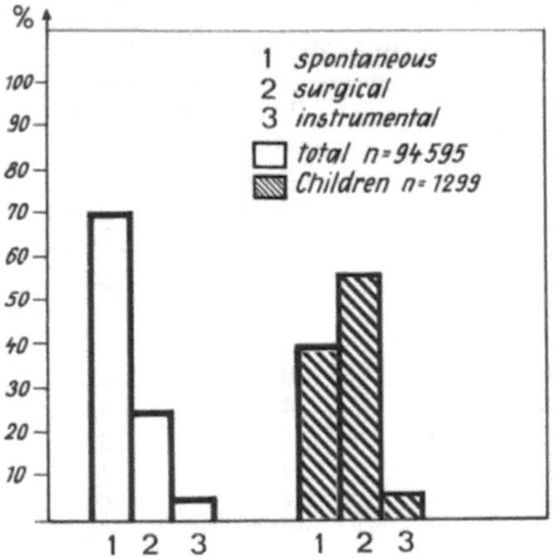

Fig. 17. Modes of stone elimination in adults and children

include social class, dietary and fluid intake and genetic factors. Stone formation is a multifactorial disorder of some complexity. Ultimately the task of the researcher must be to fit all the pieces of the puzzle together to provide a unifying theory which explains why and how stones form in the urinary tract" (ROBERTSON et al. 1979).

References

Aberle B (1968) Die Nierensteinkrankheit beim Kind. Urologe 7:279–283
Ahlstrand Chr, Tiselius H-G (1981) Renal stone disease in a Swedish district during one year. Scand J Urol Nephrol 15:143–146
Ál-Dabbagh T, Fakadi K (1977) Seasonal variations in the incidence of ureteric colic. Br J Urol 49:269–275
Almby B, Meirik O, Schönbeck J (1975) Incidence, morbidity and complications of renal and ureteral calculi in a well defined geographical area. Scand J Urol Nephrol 9:249–253
Androulakakis P, Frangoulis E, Lefkidis C, Varkarakis M, Deliveliotis A (1982) Kidney damage in recurrent renal lithiasis. Eur Urol 8:261–264
Aplas G, Schrott KM, Böwing B (1981) Ursachen, Therapie und Verlauf der Urolithiasis im Kindesalter (Eine Analyse von über 170 Fällen). XXXIII. Kongreß der Deutschen Gesellschaft für Urologie Köln
Alken CE (1966) Gedanken zur Klinik der Nephrolithiasis. Urologe 5:161
Andersen DA (1969) Historical and geographical differences in the pattern of urinary stones considered in relation to possible aetiological factors. In: Hodgkinson A, Nordin BEC (eds) Renal stone research symposium. Churchill LTD, London, p 7–31
Andersen DA (1972) History of bladder stone disease. In: van Reen R (ed) Proceedings WHO. Regional Symposium on vesical calculus disease. Bangkok, p 1–16
Andersen DA (1973) Environmental factors in the aetiology of urolithiasis. In: Cifuentes Delatte L, Rapado A, Hodgkinson A (eds) Urinary calculi. Karger, Basel, p 130–144
Anke M, Schneider H-J (Hrsg) (1979) Kadmium-Symposium. Symposiumsbericht. Wissenschaftl. Beiträge der Friedrich-Schiller-Universität, Jena
Armbruster Th (1979) Ammonium acid urate in human urinary calculi. Naturwissenschaften 66:115
Asper R, Schmucki O (1984) Epidemiology and socioeconomic aspects of urolithiasis. Urol Res 12:1–5

Atsmon A, de Vries A, Frank M (1963) Uric acid lithiasis. Elsevier, Amsterdam
Aurora AL, Taneja OP, Gupta DN (1970) Bladder stone disease of childhood. I. An epidemiological study. Acta Paediatr Scand 59:177–184
Axelson B (1963) Urinary calculus in long term exposure to cadmium. Int Congr Occup Health 14:939–946
Balogh F, Tóth Cs, Berényi M (1979) Epidemiological problems of the care of patients with urinary stone disease. XVIII. Congres Societe Internationale d'Urologie, Paris
Barratt TM, Ghazali S (1977) The etiology of renal stones in children. Postgrad Med J [Suppl] 53:35–40
Bateson EM (1973) Renal tract calculi and climate. Med J Aust 2:111–113
Benabe J, Martinez-Maldonado M (1979) Some characteristics of recurrent calcium stone formers in Puerto Rico. Urology 14:13–17
Bengtsson C, Lennartsson J, Lindquist O, Noppa H (1980) Renal stone disease – Experience from a population study of women in Gothenburg, Sweden. In: Danielson BoG (ed) Proced Sympos Urolithiasis. Scand J Urol Nephrol [Suppl] 53:39–43
Berenyi M (1975) Über die Zusammensetzung der Nierensteine in Ungarn. Acta Chir Acad Sci Hung 16:73–86
Bibus B (1939) Zur Frage der Harnsteinwelle. Z Urol 33:37–43
Bichler K-H (1975) Diskussionsbemerkung zum Uromukoid. IV. Jenaer Harnsteinsymposium. Wissenschaftl. Beiträge der Friedrich-Schiller-Universität, Jena, S 136–137
Bichler K-H, Ideler V (1977) Uromukoidausscheidung bei Negern. In: Gasser G, Vahlensieck W (Hrsg) Pathogenese und Klinik der Harnsteine V. Steinkopff, Darmstadt, S 107–108
Blacklock NJ (1969) The pattern of urolithiasis in the Royal Navy. In: Hodgkinson A, Nordin BEC (eds) Renal stone research symposium. Churchill LTD, London, p 33–47
Blacklock NJ (1976) Epidemiology of urolithiasis. In: Williams, Chisholm (eds) Scientific Foundations of Urology, Vol. 1, Heinemann, London, p 235–243
Blacklock NJ (1976a) Dietary content of refined carbohydrate: An explanation for the "stone wave" and apparent immunity to renal stones. In: Fleisch H, Robertson WG, Smith LH, Vahlensieck W (eds) Urolithiasis Research. Plenum Press, New York London, p 413–416
Blacklock NJ (1979b) Epidemiology of renal lithiasis. In: Wickham JEA (ed) Urinary calculous disease. Churchill Livingstone, Edinburgh London New York, p 20–39
Blomen L (1982) Growth and agglomeration of calcium oxalate monohydrate crystals. Habilitationsschrift, Leiden
Bo G, Maida A, Muresu E, Pisani E (1978) Epidemiology of urinary calculuresis in Sassari province. Eur Urol 4:431–432
Bocancea D (1981) Diagnosis and treatment of recurrent lithiasis in children. Eur Urol 7:136–138
Bokay J v (1895) Die Lithiasis des Kindesalters in Ungarn. Jahrb Kinderheilk 40:32–38
Bokay J v (1912) Über die infantile Lithiasis in Ungarn. Z Kinderhk 4:365–371
Bono AV, Rogia A, Benvenuti C, Comeri GC, Gianneo E, Santoro G (1979) Statistic investigation on a great number of calculous people. Urol Int 46:136–144
Borden ThA, Dean WM (1979) Ammonium acid urate stones in Navajo indian children. Urology 14:9–12
Borgmann V, Nagel R (1980) Analyse von 171 Fällen von Urolithiasis im Kindesalter. Z Kinderchir 29:48–56
Borgmann V, Nagel R (1982) Urolithiasis in childhood. A study of 181 cases. Urol Int 37:198–204
Borgmann V, Salim SA, Nagel R (1980) Ergebnisse der elektrohydraulischen Lithotripsie von Harnblasensteinen mit dem Urat I. Acta Urol 11:421–426
Boshamer K (1961) Morphologie und Genese der Harnsteine. In: Alken, Dix, Weyrauch, Wildbolz (Hrsg) Handbuch der Urologie. Bd X: Die Steinerkrankungen. Springer, Berlin Göttingen Heidelberg
Boyce WH (1979) Epidemiology of lithiasis in the United States. XVIII Congres Societe Internationale d'Urologie, Paris. Kongreßbericht, Tome 1, p 79–86
Brockis JG, Bowyer RC, Ryan G, Taylor TA, Kamardi T, Rizal A (1981) Endemic bladder stones in Indonesia. In: Smith LH, Robertson WG, Finlayson B (eds) Plenum Press, New York London, p 329–332

Brundig P, Schneider H-J (1980) Zystolithotripsie, ihre Ergebnisse in Beziehung zur Steinart. VI. Jenaer Harnsteinsymposium. Wissenschaftl. Beiträge der Friedrich-Schiller-Universität, Jena, S 247–250

Brundig P, Schneider H-J (1981) Streßinduzierte Veränderungen der Magnesiumausscheidung und der Magnesiumkonzentration im Urin bei Kalziumoxalatsteinpatienten und bei Normalpersonen. IV. Hohenheimer Magnesiumsymposium 1980. Magnes Bull 3:69–73

Brundig P, Schneider H-J, Berg W (1981a) Streß und Harnsteinbildungsrisiko. I. Der Einfluß von Streß auf lithogene Harnsubstanzen. Urol Int 36:199–207

Brundig P, Schneider H-J, Berg W (1981b) Streß und Harnsteinbildungsrisiko. II. Der Einfluß von Streß auf litholytische Harnsubstanzen. Urol Int 36:265–273

Brueziere J, Roubach L (1981) Urinary lithiasis in children. Eur Urol 7:134–135

Budewski G, Mincov N, Konstantinov D, Tabanska T (1978) Die Zusammensetzung der Harnsteine im Kindesalter. V. Jenaer Harnsteinsymposium. Wissenschaftl. Beiträge der Friedrich-Schiller-Universität, Jena, S 235–236

Burch PRJ, Dawson JB (1969) Aetiological implications of the sex- and age-distributions of renal lithiasis. In: Hodgkinson A, Nordin BEC (eds) Renal Stone Research Symposium. Churchill LTD, London, p 71–84

Chmielewski J, Tomaszewski R, Renke W (1974) Urolithiasis in seamen. Biul Inst Med Morsk Gdansku 25:228–232

Churchill DN, Maloney CM, Nolan R, Gault MH, Winsor G (1980) Pediatrie urolithiasis in the 1970s. J Urol 123:237–238

Coe FL (1978) Nephrolithiasis, Pathogenesis and treatment. Year Book Medical Publishers, Chicago London

Cohen R (1979) 115 cases of neonatal renal lithiasis. Study and etiological investigation. Rev Pediatr 15:291–300

Diaz E, Lopez Rodriguez LM, Francia Bengoechea A (1981) Epidemiologia de la litiasis renoureteral en la provincia de Toledo. Arch Esp Urol 34:115–132

Dahm I (1974) Untersuchungen zur Morbidität in der DDR. Eine prognostisch orientierte Studie. Verlag Volk und Gesundheit, Berlin

Danielson BoG (ed) (1980) Proceedings of the Symposium on Urolithiasis. Scand J Urol Nephrol [Suppl] 53

Davis GK, Cummings NB, Finlayson B, Meyer JL, Smith MJV (1978) Urolithiasis. In: Geochemistry and the invironment. Natl Acad Sci, Washington, p 133–138

Derezic D, Zebec M, Cecuk Lj, Kulcar Z (1979) Different rate of nephrolithiasis in coastal and inland part of Croatia and possible relation to water hardness. XVIII Congres Societe Internationale D'Urologie, Paris

De Voogt H-J, van de Kamp JJP, van Gelderen H (1973) A xanthine calculus in a child with xanthinuria. Notes on a rare inborn error of metabolism. Med Tijdschr Geneeskd 117:976–979

De Vries A, Sperling O, Frank M (1972) Uric acid lithiasis in Israel. In: van Reen R (ed) Proceeding WHO. Regional symposium in vesical calculus disease. Bangkok, p 41–44

Doberentz D (1976) Das Harnsteinleiden im Spiegel der Schriften Jenaer Ärzte des 19. Jahrhunderts. Med Dipl-Arbeit, Jena

Donaldson D, Pryce JD, Rose GA, Tooly JE (1979) Tap water calcium and its relationship to renal calculi and 24 h urinary calcium output in Great Britain. Urol Res 7:273–276

Dzhavad-Zade MD, Gamzaeva ZK (1980) Klinisch-geneologische und biochemische Untersuchungen bei Kindern in Asserbaidschan (in Russian). Urol Nefrol (Mosk) 1:13–17

Ebstein W (1984) Die Natur und Behandlung der Harnsteine. Wiesbaden

Eckstein HB (1965) Harnsteine im Kindesalter. Z Kinderchir 4:451–459

Eickenberg H-U (1978) Urolithiasis bei Negern. In: Vahlensieck W, Gasser G (Hrsg) Pathogenese und Klinik der Harnsteine VI. Steinkopff, Darmstadt, S 75–76

Elliot JP, Gordon JO, Evans JW, Platt L (1975) A stone season. A 10-year retrospective study of 768 surgical stone cases with respect to seasonal variation. J Urol 114:574–577

Elomaa I, Karonen S-L, Kairento A-L, Pelkonen R (1981) Seasonal variation of urinary calcium and oxalate excretion, serum 25 $(OH)D_3$ and albumin level in relation to renal stone formation. In: Vahlensieck W, Gasser G (eds) Pathogenese und Klinik der Harnsteine VIII. Steinkopff, Darmstadt, S 120–126

Entrup M, Leusmann DB, Blaschke R, Schmandt W (1984) Rate and composition of recurrent urinary concrements. In: Schwille PO, Smith LH, Robertson WD, Vahlensieck W (eds) Urolithiasis and Related Clinical Research. Plenum Press, New York London (in press)

Esho JO (1978) Analysis of urinary calculi formed by Nigerians. Eur Urol 4:288–291

Esho JO, Amaku EO (1979) Epidemiological survey of urinary calculous disease in Nigeria. XVIII Congress Societe Internationale D'Urologie, Paris

Ferguson AF, Morrison RBI (1979) Urinary calculi in new Zealand Experience with 1000 Patients. XVIII Congress Societe Internationale D'Urologie, Paris

Finn H, Saupe A (1981) Aus der Arbeit eines kindernephrologischen Dispensaires. Dtsch Gesundh-Wesen 36:59–61

Frang D, Götz F, Verebelyi A, Nagy Z (1979) Epidemiology of urolithiasis. XVIII Congress Societe Internationale D'Urologie, Paris

Friberg L, Piscator M, Nordberg GF, Kjellström T (1974) Cadmium in the environment, 2. Ed. CRC-Press, Cleveland, p 106–107

Frank M, Lazebnik J, de Vries A (1970) Uric acid lithiasis. A study of six hundred and twenty two patients. Urol Int 25:32–46

Frank D, Schneider H-J, Hesse A (1975) Untersuchungen zum Harnsteinleiden bei Hitzearbeitern. Dtsch Gesundh-Wesen 30:716–720

Frick J (1969) Steinleiden im Kindesalter. Wien Klin Wochenschr 81:802–804

Frick J, Bartsch G (1972) Nachbetreuung harnsteinoperierter Kinder aus der Sicht des Urologen. II. Jenaer Harnsteinsymposium. Wissenschaftliche Beiträge der Friedrich-Schiller-Universität, Jena, S 186–194

Fujita K (1979a) Weather and the incidence of urinary stone colic. J Urol 121:318–319

Fujita K (1979b) Epidemiology of urinary stone colic. Eur Urol 5:26–28

Fuss M, Simon J (1979) Renal stone composition in 768 Belgian Patients. XVIII Congress Societe International D'Urologie, Paris

Fuss M, Simon J, Verbeelen D, Weiser M, van Landuyt P, Elskens I (1978) Chemical analysis of renal stones from 377 Belgian patients by using qualitative or quantitative methods. Eur Urol 4:90–93

Galosy R (1981) Oxalatausscheidung der Niere bei Urolithiasis. Extracta Urol 4:38–40

Gebhardt M, Bastian HP (1984) Epidemiologische Untersuchungen zur Harnsteinzusammensetzung. In: Vahlensieck W, Gasser G (Hrsg) Pathogenese und Klinik der Harnsteine X. Steinkopff, Darmstadt, S 15–22

Gershoff StN (1964) The formation of urinary stones. Metabolism 13:875–882

Geuns H von (1978) Urinary tract calculi. A population survey in a Dutch community (Hasselt) on the occurrence and consequences of "silent stone disease". Van Gorcum, Assen the Netherlands

Gharib R (1970) Lithiasis in the urinary system of children. General reviews based on observations in 167 affected Iranian children. Clin Pediatr (Phila) 9:157–164

Ghazali S, Barratt TM, Williams DI (1973) Childhood urolithiasis in Britain. Arch Dis Child 48:291–295

Gibba A (1969) Consideraziani clinico statistiche sulla calcolosi urinaria nelleta avanzata. G Geront 17:133–158

Gingell JC, Gaches CGC (1981) A review of urinary calculi in children in the Bristol clinical area. Eur Urol 7:122–125

Giugliani R, Ferrari I (1981) Some observations on genetic factors in urolithiasis. Urology 17:33–38

Gluzek J, Raszeja-Wanic B, Grajek S, Kwias Z, Ratajczak T, Smarsz C (1978) Seasonal variations in urinary excretion of calcium and magnesium in healthy subjects and patients with renal calculus and chronic renal failure. Int Urol Nephrol 10:147–152

Goetze Th (1963) Urinary calculi in the Indian and African in Natal. S Afr Med J 1092–1095

Goldschmidt P, Jaeck D, Francone A, Saenz N, Bollack C (1984) Urinary stones and dietary practice: A comperative study based on 600 stones in Alsace, Argentina and Laos. In: Vahlensieck W, Gasser G (eds) Pathogenese und Klinik der Harnsteine X. Steinkopff, Darmstadt, S 23–26

Golubchanskaja AV (1976) Urolithiasis in der Novosibirsker Region (in Russian). Urol Nefrol (Mosk) 3:43–44

Gosalbez R, Garat JM, Piro C, Martin J-A (1980) Lithiase urinaire chez l'enfant. J Urol (Paris) 86:665–670

Green NA, Shaw AB (1981) Bladder stones in children. The Norwich school of lithotomy. Eur Urol 7:126–131

Gröninger KH (1962) Urolithiasis und Konstitution. Z Urol Nephrol 55:129–135

Günalp I (1979) The epidemiological aspects of urolithiasis in Turkey. XVIII Congress Societe International D'Urologie, Paris

Hallson PC, Rose G (1977) Seasonal variations in urinary crystals. Br J Urol 49:277–284

Hallson PC, Kasidas GP, Rose GA (1977) Seasonal variations in urinary excretion of calcium and oxalate in normal subjects and in patients with idiopathic hypercalcuria. Br J Urol 49:1–4

Halstead SB, Valyasevi A (1972) Current epidemiology of bladder stone disease studies in the Thailand endemic area. In: van Reen R (ed) Proceedings WHO, Regional Symposium on vesical calculus disease. Bangkok, p 17–22

Hautmann R, Lutzeyer W (Hrsg) (1980) Harnsteinfibel. Deutscher Ärzteverlag, Köln

Hedenberg I (1951) Renal and ureteral calculi, a study of recurrence in Sweden during 1911–1938 with some notes of geographical distribution. Acta Chir Scand 101:17–36

Helbig D, Gharib M (1969) Ein klinischer Beitrag zu den Problemen der Urolithiasis im Kindesalter. Z Kinderchir 7:463–469

Heller F (1860) Die Harnkonkretionen, ihre Entstehung, Erkennung und Analyse. Tendler u. Co, Wien

Herring LC (1962) Observations on the analysis of ten thousand urinary calculi. J Urol 88:545–562

Hertkens HJ, Völz B (1970) Beobachtungen an kindlichen Harnsteinträgern in den Jahren 1957 bis 1967. Paediatrie 9:333–352

Hesse A, Schneider H-J, Schröder S, Wegner R (1975) Ergebnisse der AIV-gerechten Auswertung von 10 000 Harnsteinanalysenbelegen. Z Urol Nephrol 69:1–9

Hesse A, Schneider H-J, Hienzsch E (1977a) Zu einigen Fragen der Harnsteinerkrankung. Z Gesamte Inn Med 32:222–225

Hesse A, Schneider H-J, Schweder P, Flach W, Rebentisch G, Suntheim L, Webert C, Taubert F, Köhler H, Klemm D (1977b) Das Harnsteinleiden in der DDR. Untersuchungen zur altersabhängigen und territorialen Verteilung. Dtsch Gesundh-Wesen 32:900–904

Hiatt RA, Friedman GD (1982) The frequency of kidney and urinary tract diseases in a defined population. Kidney Int 22:63–68

Hienzsch E (1973) Harnsteinprophylaxe, Notwendigkeit und Wirklichkeit. II. Jenaer Harnsteinsymposium. Wissenschaftliche Beiträge der Friedrich-Schiller-Universität, Jena, S 106–116

Hodgkinson A (1977) Composition of urinary tract calculi in children of different ages. Br J Urol 49:453–455

Hodgkinson A (1979) Composition of urinary tract calculi from some developing countries. Urol Int 34:26–35

Hodgkinson A, Marshall RW (1975) Changes in the composition of urinary tract stones. Invest Urol 13:131–135

Homann W, Mellin P, Kersting D, Bachmann HJ (1977) Harnsteine im Kindesalter. Urologe [Ausg A] 16:279–282

Horn H-D (1973) Morphologische, biochemische und therapeutische Grundlagen des Harnsteinleidens. In: Alken-Staehler (Hrsg) Klinische Urologie. Thieme, Stuttgart, S 164

Horn G, Weiß K-B, Kaszubowski U (1980) Wert der Diätetik und allgemeiner Ernährungsrichtlinien in der Harnsteinmetaphylaxe. Z Urol Nephrol 73:539–547

Hradec E, Petrik R, Sramek E, Simon V (1969) Uratsteinleiden in Böhmen. Urologe 8:193–198

Hsien Yu-Fu, Chiang W-S, Hsu T-Ch (1973) Urinary calculi among the children in Taiwan. XVI. Int. Urologenkongreß Amsterdam. Tome 2/3, S 583–584

Hsienh YF, Hsu TC, Tsai CC, Chiang CP (1979) Urolithiasis in Taiwan. XVIII Congress Societe Internationale D'Urologie, Paris

Hüttner H, Wiesner G (1971) Gesundheit 71. Akad ärztl Fortb DDR. Berlin

Hüttner I (1972) Soziologische Merkmale und Gesundheitsverhalten des Harnsteinträgers. II. Jenaer Harnsteinsymposium. Wissenschaftliche Beiträge der Friedrich-Schiller-Universität. Jena, S 144–151

Ibrahim A (1979) Urinary lithogenesis in Sudanese patients: A study on 125 stone formers. J Urol 121:572–574

Illievski P, Illievski S (1984) Drinking water quality and urolithiasis. In: Schwille PO, Smith LH, Robertson WD, Vahlensieck W (eds) Urolithiasis and related clinical research. Plenum Press, New York London (in press)

Jaeck D, Sicard D, Vannareth T, Chelius Ph, Zech P (1979) Frequence et particularites de la lithiase urinare au Laos. XVIII. Congres Internationale D'Urologie, Paris

Janca K, Petrovic S, Stojkov J (1978) Einige Aspekte der Urolithiasis im Kindesalter in einer multinationalen Provinz Jugoslawiens. V. Jenaer Harnsteinsymposium. Wissenschaftliche Beiträge der Friedrich-Schiller-Universität, Jena, S 164–165

Jarrar K, Boedecker RH (1984) Häufigkeit der Begleiterkrankungen bei Harnstein-Patienten und ihre Verteilung je nach Steinart. In: Vahlensieck W, Gasser G (Hrsg) Pathogenese und Klinik der Harnsteine X. Steinkopff, Darmstadt, S 33–37

Jaruszewski H, Tredt H-J, Zenker K (1975) Nephrologie. Wissenschaftliche Grundlagen und Epidemiologie, Klinik und Therapie in der Praxis. Volk und Gesundheit. Berlin

Jediny YuG (1972) Nichtoperative Methoden zur Therapie und Metaphylaxe der Urolithiasis (russ.) Harnsteinsymposium Kiew. Symposiumsbericht, S 38–43

Johnson CM, Wilson DM, O'Fallon WM (1979) Renal stone epidemiology: A 25 year study in Rochester. Kidney Int 16:624–631

Joost J (1981) Metabolische Ursachen der Urolithiasis im Kindesalter. Z Urol Nephrol 74:838–845

Joost J, Marberger H (1982) Urolithiasis im Kindesalter. Urologe [Ang A] 21:133–136

Joost J, Egger G, Hohlbrugger G, Marberger H (1980) Epidemiologie des Nierensteinleidens in Tirol. Oest Ärtzetg 35:1016–1020

Juuti M, Heinonen OP (1980) Incidence of urolithiasis and composition of household water in southern Finland. Scand J Urol 14:181–187

Juuti M, Heinonen OP, Alhava EM (1981) Seasonal variation in urinary excretion of calcium, oxalate, magnesium and phosphate on free and standard mineral diet in men with urolithiasis. Scand J Urol 15:137–141

Kadivar R (1972) Studies of vesical calculi in Shivaz, Iran. In: van Reen R (ed) Proceedings WHO. Regional symposium in vesical calculus disease. Bangkok, p 45–52

Kambal A (1981) The relation of urinary Bilharziasis to vesical stones in children. Br J Urol 53:315–317

Kambal A, Wahab EMA, Khattab AHH (1979a) The pattern of urolithiasis in the Sudan. Br J Urol 50:376–377

Kambal A, Wahab EMA, Khattab AHH (1979b) The composition of urinary stones in the Sudan. Br J Urol 51:342–344

Kambal A, Wahab EMA, Khattab AHH, Zaki J (1981) Urolithiasis in the Sudan. Studies in a stone-prone and stone-free population. Br J Urol 53:7–12

Kaplan CW, Lamm D, Walther PC (1979) Urolithiasis in children: A ten year review. XVIII Congress Societe Internationale D'Urologie, Paris

Kedar SS, Shabtai M, Haimovitz C, Better OS (1979) Increased incidence of nephrolithiasis in LIFEGUARDS in Israel. XVIII Congres Societe Internationale D'Urologie, Paris

Keefe WE, Smith MJV (1980) Calculi in Richmond, Virginia. An x-ray diffraction study. Fourth Int Symp Urolith Research, Williamsburg/USA

Keutel H-J (1975) Uromukoidkomplex als ein Faktor der Harnsteinbildung bei bakterieller Infektion. IV. Jenaer Harnsteinsymposium. Wissenschaftl. Beiträge der Friedrich-Schiller-Universität, Jena, S 38–44

Khan RS, Finlayson B, Hackett RL (1984) Microstructure of calcium oxalate foreign-body stones produced in rat bladder. In: Schwille PO, Smith LH, Robertson WD, Vahlensieck W (eds) Urolithiasis and Related Clinical Research. Plenum Press, New York London (in press)

Kheradpir MH, Armbruster Th (1984) Childhood urolithiasis in Iran: A study of urinary calculi using X-ray diffraction, polarizing microscopy, chemical analyses. In: Schwille PO, Smith LH, Robertson WD, Vahlensieck W (eds) Urolithiasis and Related Clinical Research. Plenum Press, New York London (in press)

Knebel L (1982) Experimentelle und epidemiologische Untersuchungen zur Morbidität und Metaphylaxe der Urolithiasis. Habilitationsschrift, Mannheim Heidelberg

Kisters R, Terhorst B (1973) Harnsteinanalyse durch Infrarotspektroskopie. Urologe [Ausg B] 13:85–89

Klingenberg J, Czecholinski AU, Hirth KE (1971) Das Harnsteinleiden bei über 70jährigen. Z Gerontol 4:274–284

Kneise O, Beyer G (1933) Die Harnsteinwelle in Mitteldeutschland. Z Urol 27:1–20

Kohlicek J (1969) Urolithiasis. Konferenz der Urologischen Sektion. Marienbad

Koslowski YuG (1973) Mineralogische Klassifizierung von Harnsteinen (in Russian) Urol Nefrol (Mosk) 2:24–27

Krizek V (1968) Iris colour and composition of urinary stones. Lancet, I:1432a

Krizek V (1968) Körpergewicht und Übergewicht bei Urolithiasis mit verschiedener Zusammensetzung der Konkremente. Z Inn Med 23:86–91

Krizek V (1973) Zur Geschichte des Harnsteinleidens. III. Jenaer Harnsteinsymposium. Wissenschaftliche Beiträge der Friedrich-Schiller-Universität, Jena, S 241–249

Krizek V (1974) Manifestation des Harnsteinleidens bei Zystinurikern in Abhängigkeit vom Alter. Z Urol Nephrol 67:491–494

Krizek V (1981) Epidemiologische und genealogische Studien der Zystinurie und Zystinsteinkrankheit anhand von 255 Fällen. In: Vahlensieck W, Gasser G (Hrsg) Pathogenese und Klinik der Harnsteine VIII. Steinkopff, Darmstadt, S 61–67

Krizek V, Schneider H-J (1974) Älteste Harnsteinfunde. Zur Geschichte des Harnsteinleidens. I. Älteste Harnsteinfunde, Urania 50:8–10; II. Harnsteinzertrümmerung – uralt? Urania 50:74–75

Krizek V, Vendl L (1978) Urolithiasis cystinurica bei Kindern. V. Jenaer Harnsteinsymposium. Wissenschaftliche Beiträge der Friedrich-Schiller-Universität, Jena, S 195–199

Krüche A (1879) Structur und Entstehung der Uratsteine. Neuenhahn, Jena

Larsen JF, Philip H (1962) Studies on the incidence of urolithiasis. Urol Int 13:53–64

Lenko J, Dec W, Politowski L (1970) Renal lithiasis in patients at the urological department of the army medical academy (pol). Biuletyn Wojskowej Academii Medyczney XIII, p 591–595

Ljunghall S (1978) Incidence and natural history of renal stone disease and its relationship to calcium metabolism. Eur Urol 4:424–430

Ljunghall S (1979) Family history of renal stones in a population study of stone-formers and healthy subjects. Br J Urol 51:249–252

Ljunghall S, Hedstrand H (1975) Epidemiology of renal stones in a middle aged male population. Acta Med Scand 197:439–444

Ljunghall S, Waern AU (1977) Urinary electrolytes in urinary stone formers and healthy subjects. A population study of 60 year old men. Scand J Urol Nephrol [Suppl] 41:55–60

Ljunghall S, Christensson T, Wengle B (1977) Prevalence and incidence of renal stone disease in a health-screening programme. Scand J Urol Nephrol 41:39–45

Ljunghall S, Backman U, Danielson BG, Fellström B, Johansson G, Wikström B (1980) Epidemiological aspects of renal stone disease in Scandinavia. In: Danielson BG (ed) Proc Sympos Urolithiasis. Scand J Urol Nephrol [Suppl] 53:31–36

Ljunghall S (1984) Stone incidence in western countries. In: Schwille PO, Smith LH, Robertson WD, Vahlensieck W (eds) Urolithiasis and Related Clinical Research. Plenum Press, New York London (in press)

Lombardi R (1969) Considerazioni clinico – statistiche e terapeutiche su 1120 osservaziani di calcolosi reno-ureterale. Urologia 36:325–336

Lonsdale K, Sutor J, Wooley S (1968a) Composition of urinary calculi by x-ray diffraction. Collected data from various localities I. Br J Urol 40:33–36

Lonsdale K, Sutor J, Wooley SE (1968b) Composition of urinary calculi by x-ray diffraction. Collected data from various localities II–VI. Br J Urol 40:402–411

Loutfi AH (1980) Renal calculi in children in Egypt. Fourth Int Symp Urolith. Research, Williamsburg/USA

Loutfi A, Abdel Hamid G, Francis M, Abdel Salam I (1972a) Study of urinary tract calculi in Egyptian children. J Egypt Med Ass 55:805–812
Loutfi A, Abdel Hamid G, Francis M, Abdel Salam I (1972b) Study of urinary tract calculi in Egyptian children. In: van Reen R (ed) Proceedings WHO, Regional Symposium on vesical calcules disease. Bangkok, p 34–40
Malek RS (1977) Renal lithiasis: A practical approach. J Urol 118:893–901
Marcet A (1818) Versuch einer chemischen Geschichte und aerztlichen Behandlung der Steinkrankheiten. JG Heyse, Bremen
Marquardt H, Nagel R (1977) Urolithiasis in childhood. Urology 9:627–629
Marshall V, White RH, de Saintonge MC, Tresidder GC, Blandy JP (1975) The natural history of renal and ureteral calculi. Br J Urol 47:117–124
Martynenko NG (1974) Distribution of urolithiasis in Daghestan and factors conditioning its endemicity (in Russian). Urol Nefrol (Mosk) 5:34–38
Marya RK, Dadoo RC, Sharma NK (1981) Genetic predisposition to renal stone disease in the first degree relatives of stone-formers. Urol Int 36:245–247
Mateos Antòn FM, Puig JG, Gaspar G, Martines ME, Ramos T, Pineiro JAM (1984) Renal tubular acidosis in recurrent renal stone formers. Eur Urol 10:55–59
Mates J (1969) External factors in the genesis of urolithiasis. In: Hodgkinson A, Nordin BEC (eds) Renal Stone Research Symposium. Churchill LTD, London, p 59–64
Mates J, Krizek V (1958) Urolithiase. Prag, p 33
Matouschek E, Huber RD (1981a) Ergebnisse einer internationalen kooperativen Studie über das Harnsteinleiden. In: Vahlensieck W, Gasser G (Hrsg) Pathogenese und Klinik der Harnsteine VIII. Steinkopff, Darmstadt, S 23–32
Matouschek E, Huber RD (1981b) Urolithiasis. Pathogenese – Diagnostik – Therapie. Schattauer, Stuttgart New York
Mazeman E, Wemeau L, Foissac MC, Riquet R, Triboulet JP (1978) Urinary lithiasis in children. A review of 155 cases. Eur Urol 4:157–161
Mazeman E, Biserte J, Foissac MC, Francke B, Wemeau L (1983) Lithiase urinaire de l'enfant. Anm Pediatrie 30:35–44
Maurer H-J, Vahlensieck W (1967) Bluthochdruck bei Nierensteinkranken. Med Welt 18:632–637
Mehdiratta KS (1972) Study on vesical calculus disease in India. In: van Reen R (ed) Proceeding WHO. Regional symposium on vesical calculus disease. Bangkok, p 79–83
Mehnert P, Hoko EJE (1978) Die kindliche Urolithiasis in der DDR im Jahre 1974. V. Jenaer Harnsteinsymposium. Wissenschaftliche Beiträge der Friedrich-Schiller-Universität, Jena, S 169–171
Mercz L, Boga G (1978) Betreuung von Steinkranken in urologischer Fachambulanzen. Urol Nephrol Szle [Suppl] 5:224–227
Mincov N (1978) Zur Frage der Ätiopathogenese der Urolithiasis im Kindesalter. V. Jenaer Harnsteinsymposium. Wissenschaftliche Beiträge der Friedrich-Schiller-Universität, Jena, S 148–151
Mioli V, Lombardo E, Figus S (1981) Reno-ureteral lithiasis: Regional epidemiologic survey. II. Int Symp on Advances in metabolic physico-chemical and therapeutic aspects of urolithiasis. Turin
Moderova M, Kocvara R, Louzensky G, Smuglerova J (1982) Metabolische Störungen bei an Nierensteinkrankheit leidenden Kindern. VII. Jenaer Harnsteinsymposium. Wissenschaftliche Beiträge der Friedrich-Schiller-Universität, Jena, S 190–195
Modlin M (1969) Renal calculus in the Republic of South Africa. In: Hodgkinson A, Nordin BEC (eds) Renal Stone Research Symposium. Churchill LTD, London, p 49–58
Noe HN, Stapleton FB, Jerkins GR, Roy Sh (1983) Clinical experience with pediatric urolithiasis. J Urol 129:1166–1170
Nöske HD (1974) Zur Entwicklung des Blasensteinschnittes. Muench Med Wochenschr 116:1783–1788
Norlin A, Lindell B, Granberg P-O, Lindvall N (1976) Urolithiasis. A study of its frequency. Scand J Urol Nephrol 10:150–153
Norona RFX, Gregory JG, Duke JJ (1979) Urolithiasis in children. J Urol 121:478–479
Otnes B (1980) Sex differences in crystalline composition of stones from the upper urinary tract. Scand J Urol Nephrol 14:51–56

Otto-Unger G (1978) Pädiatrische Aspekte zum Harnsteinleiden des Kindes. V. Jenaer Harnsteinsymposium. Wissenschaftliche Beiträge der Friedrich-Schiller-Universität, Jena, S 129–135
Pak CYC, McGuire J, Peterson R, Britton F, Harrod MJ (1981) Familial absorptive hypercalciuria in a large kindred. J Urol 126:717–719
Pavone-Macaluso M, Miano L (1979) Epidemiology of urolithiasis in Italy XVIII. Congres Societe Internationale d'Urologie, Paris. Kongreßbericht, Tome 1, p 113–137
Perquis P, Muret G, Fillaudeau G (1969) La lithiase urinaire du noir african. A propos de 100 observations. Med Trop (Mars) 29:576–583
Pflücker L (1950) Diskussionsbeitrag zum Steinproblem. Z Urol (Sonderheft) S 166
Pflanz M (1962) Sozialer Wandel und Krankheit. Enke, Stuttgart
Pönisch G, Richter E, Schur W (1973) Nephrolithiasis und Flugtauglichkeit. Z Militärmed 6:329–334
Prout W (1843) Über das Wesen und die Behandlung der Krankheiten des Magens und der Harnorgane. Leipzig
Pyrah LN (1979) Renal calculus. Epidemiology of urolithiasis. Springer, Berlin Heidelberg New York, p 3–17
Rahman MA, van Reen R (1972) Current investigations of vesical lithiasis in Pakistan. In: van Reen R (ed) Proceedings WHO. Regional symposium on vesical calculus disease. Bangkok, p 57–67
Rao MVR, Agarwal JS, Taneja OP (1976) Studies in urolithiasis: II. X-ray diffraction analysis of calculi from Delhi region. Indian J Med Res 64:102–107
Rapado A, Maneha A, Castrillo JM, Traba LM, Santos M, Cifuentes Delatte L (1976) Etiological classification of renal lithiasis: a study based of 1936 patients. In: Fleisch H, Robertson WG, Smith LH, Vahlensieck W (eds) Urolithiasis Research. Plenum Press, New York London, p 495–498
Reen R van (ed) (1976) Proceedings of WHO Regional Symposium on vesical calculus disease. Bangkok 1972, Washington
Reen R van (ed) (1977) Idiopathic urinary bladder stone disease. Washington
Reetz H (1980) Urolithiasis im Kindesalter (unter besonderer Berücksichtigung des Kleinkind- und Säuglingsalters). Z Kinderchir 30:225–238
Reiner RJ, Kroovand RL, Perlmutter AD (1979) Unusual aspects of urinary calculi in children. J Urol 121:480–481
Reis-Santos JM (1984) Urolithiasis-Epidemiological data from the south of Portugal. In: Schwille OP, Smith LH, Robertson WD, Vahlensieck W (eds) Urolithiasis and Related Clinical Research. Plenum Press, New York London (in press)
Remzi D (1980) Urolithiasis in infancy. Urology 15:248–250
Remzi D, Cakmak F, Erkan I (1979) A study on the urolithiasis incidence in turkish schoolage children. XVIII. Congres Societe Internationale D'Urologie. Paris
Resnick M, Pridgen DB, Goodman HO (1968) Genetic predisposition to the formation of calcium oxalate stones. N Engl J Med 278:1313–1318
Reveillaud RJ, Daudon M (1984) Struvite stone analysis by IR-spectrophotometry in adults and children. In: Schwille PO, Smith LH, Robertson WD, Vahlensieck W (eds) Urolithiasis and Related Clinical Research. Plenum Press, New York London (in press)
Rivera JV, Isales LM (1970) Urinary calculi in Puerto Rican males. I. Chemical composition. Bol Asoc Med PR 62:317–319
Robertson WG (1984) Influence of dietary components. In: Schwille PO, Smith LH, Robertson WD, Vahlensieck W (1984) Urolithiasis and Related Clinical Research. Plenum Press, New York London (in press)
Robertson WG, Peacock M, Heyburn PJ, Speed R, Hanes F (1978b) The role of affluence and diet in the genesis of calcium containing stones. In: Vahlensieck W, Gasser G (eds) Pathogenese und Klinik der Harnsteine VI. Steinkopff, Darmstadt, S 5–14
Robertson WG, Peacock M (1982) The pattern of urinary stone disease in Leeds during the period 1960–1980. In: Gasser G, Vahlensieck W (eds) Pathogenese und Klinik der Harnsteine IX. Steinkopff, Darmstadt, S 8–14
Robertson WG, Morgan DB, Marshall DH, Peacock M, Nordin BEC (1978) Risikofaktoren bei der Kalziumsteinbildung. V. Jenaer Harnsteinsymposium. Wissenschaftliche Beiträge der Friedrich-Schiller-Universität, Jena, S 45–53

Robertson WG, Peacock M, Heyburn PJ, Marshall RW, Hanes F, Speed R, Rutherford A (1979) Practical implications for urologists from epidemiological studies on stone formation. XVIII. Congres Societe Internationale d'Urologie, Paris. Kongreßbericht, Tome 1, S 138–162
Robertson WG, Peacock M, Heyburn PJ, Hanes FA (1980) Epidemiological risk factors in calcium stone disease. In: Danielson BoG (ed) Proc. Symposium on Urolithiasis. Scand J Urol Nephrol [Suppl] 53:15–28
Robertson WG, Peacock M, Baker M (1984) Epidemiological studies on urinary stone disease in men in Leeds. In: Vahlensieck W, Gasser G (eds) Pathogenese und Klinik der Harnsteine X. Steinkopff, Darmstadt, p 15–22
Rodriguez-Minon Cifuentes JL (1976) Composition mineral de 244 calculos vesicales antiguos (1913–1950). Arch Esp Urol 29:537–562
Rosdy E (1979) Observations on the epidemiology of nephrolithiasis in some districts of Budapest. XVIII. Congress Societe Internationale d'Urologie. Paris
Rose GA, Westbury EJ (1975) The influence of calcium content of water, intake of vegetables and fruit and other food factors upon the incidence of renal calculi. Urol Res 3:61–66
Rose GA, Westbury EJ (1979) Seasonal and geographic variations in urinary composition in England, Scotland and Wales. Urol Res 7:235–240
Ruhle G, Winter P (1976) Das Gesundheitswesen DDR 2.9.2. Urologische Erkrankungen, S 158–160
Ruhle G, Winter P (1978) Häufigkeit und Verteilung urologischer Erkrankungen in Berlin 1969 und 1974. Z Arztl Fortbild (Jena) 72:389–393
Ruhle G, Winter P, Kreuz B (1972) Häufigkeit und Verteilung urologischer Erkrankungen in Berlin 1969. Z Arztl Fortbild (Jena) 66:290–303
Sadre M, Bastanfar M, Ziai M (1972) Urinary calculi in Iran. Hospital experience over a three-year period, 1968–1971. In: van Reen R (ed) Proceedings WHO. Regional symposium on vesical calculus disease. Bangkok, p 53
Salem SN (1969) Die Häufigkeit von Nierenkoliken und Harnsteinen in Kuweit. Eine epidemiologische Untersuchung. Lab Med J 747–751
Safwat M, Attwa I, Abdel-Kader M, Hegazy A (1979) The geographical distribution of stones in Egypt. XVIII. Congress Societe Internationale d'Urologie, Paris
Schey HM, Corbett WT, Resnick MI (1979) Prevalence rate of renal stone disease in Forsyth Country, North Carolina during 1977. J Urol 122:288–291
Schmincke H, Lengwinat A (1968) Beitrag zur Erforschung der allgemeinen Morbidität. Verlag Volk und Gesundheit, Berlin
Schmucki O, Asper R (1977) Qualitative und quantitative Urin- und Serumuntersuchungen unter Extrembedingungen. In: Gasser G, Vahlensieck W (Hrsg) Pathogenese und Klinik der Harnsteine V. Steinkopff, Darmstadt, S 35–40
Schmucki O, Asper R, Weihe WH (1979) Streßinduzierte Veränderungen der Elektrolytkonzentrationen im Urin bei der Ratte. In: Gasser G, Vahlensieck W (Hrsg) Pathogenese und Klinik der Urolithiasis VII. Steinkopff, Darmstadt, S 126–134
Schneider H-J (1979) Epidemiologische Aspekte der Urolithiasis. Urologe [Ausg B] 19:54–61
Schneider H-J, Anke M (Hrsg) (1976) Magnesiumstoffwechsel. Wissenschaftliche Beiträge der Friedrich-Schiller-Universität. Jena, Symposiumsbericht
Schneider H-J, Bauerschmidt L (1973) Alters- und Geschlechtsverteilung beim Harnsteinleiden unter besonderer Berücksichtigung der Steinart. Z Altersforsch 26:415–421
Schneider H-J, Doberentz W (1979) Zur Geschichte der Jenaer Harnsteinforschung. Jenaer Reden und Schriften, Jena
Schneider H-J, Hesse A (1976) Zur Epidemiologie des Harnsteinleidens. Therapiewoche 26:5881–5899
Schneider H-J, Hienzsch E (1979) Epidemiologie der Urolithiasis. XVIII. Congress Societe Internationale d'Urologie, Paris. Kongreßbericht, Tome 1, S 87–112
Schneider H-J, Otto-Unger G (1978) Das Harnsteinleiden im Kindesalter. Z Arztl Fortbild 72:1164–1169
Schneider H-J, Heyne S, Dittrich G, Riedel E (1973) Untersuchungen zur soziologischen Struktur der Harnsteinpatienten. Z Arztl Fortbild 67:735–740
Schneider H-J, Schweder P, Flach W, Rebentisch G, Suntheim L, Webert C, Taubert F, Köhler H, Klemm D (1978) Das Harnsteinleiden in der DDR II. Untersuchungen zur Zusam-

mensetzung und Rezidivquote von Harnsteinen im Kindesalter. Dt Gesundh-Wesen 33:655–658

Schneider H-J, Janetzky H, Schüler G (1979) Somatische Parameter bei Harnsteinpatienten und ihre Beziehung zu Alter, Geschlecht und Steinart. Z Urol Nephrol 72:315–321

Schneider H-J, Schüler G, Janetzky H (1980) Psychosomatische Parameter bei Harnsteinpatienten und ihre Beziehungen zu Geschlecht und Steinart. Untersuchungen mit einem modifizierten Fragebogen. Z Urol Nephrol 73:523–530

Schneider H-J, Dedek W, Grahl R, Mothes B, Uhlemann J, Schwarz H, Schwachulla G, Reuter H, Möhring M (1983) Studies of the persorption of large particles from radio-labelled cation exchangers. Urol Int 38:116–120

Schöll H (1978) Über periodische Harnsteinhäufigkeit und Beziehungen zur Steinart im Laufe von 10 Jahren. Wien Med Wochenschr 128:46–49

Schöll H (1979) Der typische Jahresverlauf der Häufigkeit von Harnsteinerkrankungen in Beziehung zur chemischen Steinart. Ergebnisse einer 10-Jahres-Studie. Wien Med Wochenschr 129:679–681

Schoenberger A, Kehrer B, Glinz B, Lustenberger FX (1983) Residuen und Rezidive kindlicher Harnsteine. Akt Urol 14:175–178

Scholz D, Schwille PO, Ulbrich D, Bausch WM, Sigel A (1979) Composition of renal stones and their frequency in a stone clinic: relationship to parameters of mineral metabolism in serum and urine. Urol Res 7:161–170

Scholz D, Schwille PO, Sigel A (1980) zur metabolischen Klassifikation und Metaphylaxe der häufigsten Lithiasisformen. Erfahrungen einer Harnstein-Poliklinik. Urologe [Ausg A] 19:202–206

Schumann HJ (1963) Die Häufigkeit der Urolithiasis im Sektionsgut des Pathologischen Instituts. St. Georg, Leipzig. Zentralbl Allg Pathol 105:88–94

Schwille PO, Scholz D, Sigel A (1980) Urolithiasis – ein Überblick zur Pathophysiologie, Diagnostik und Therapie. Wien Klin Wochenschr 92:411–420

Scott R, Freeland R, Mowat W, Gardiner Mary, Hawthorne V, Marshall RM, Ives JGJ (1977) The prevalence of calcified upper urinary tract stone disease in a random population – Cumbernauld Health Survey, Br J Urol 49:589–593

Scott R, Paterson PJ, Burns R, Fell GS, Ottoway JM (1979) The effects of treatment of the hypercalciuria of chronic cadmium poisoning. Urol Res 7:285–289

Scott R, Cunningham C, McLelland A, Fell GS, Fitzgerald-Finch OP, McKellar N (1982) The importance of cadmium as a factor in calcified upper urinary tract stone disease – a prospective 7-year study. Br J Urol 54:584

Shabad AL (1975) On the increase of the percentage of females among patients with infectious and calculous renal diseases and on its possible causes. Int Urol Nephrol 7:179–185

Shahjehan S, Rahman MA (1971) Studies on the etiology of urolithiasis in Karachi. Am J Clin Nutr 24:32–37

Sierakowski R, Finlayson B, Landes RR, Finlayson CD, Sierakowski N (1978) The frequency of urolithiasis in hospital discharge diagnoses in the United States. Invest Urol 16:438–441

Sierakowski R, Finlayson B, Landes R (1979) Stone incidence as related to water hardness in different geographical regions of the United States. Urol Res 7:157–160

Singh SM (1972) Studies on vesical calculus disease in India. In: van Reen R (ed) Proceedings WHO. Regional symposium on vesical calculus disease. Bangkok, p 68–78

Sinno K, Boyce WH, Resnick MI (1979) Childhood urolithiasis. J Urol 121:662–664

Smith GE, Dawson WR (1972) Egyptian Mummies. Allen & Unwin, London

Steg A, Landier JF, Teyssier P, Champagnae A, Thomas J (1979) XVIII. Congress Societe Internationale d'Urologie, Paris. Kongreßbericht, Tome 1, S 163–178

Strauss, Ingrid (1982) Kombination von Nierentuberkulose und Nierensteinbildung. Pharmakotherapie 5:88–94

Strohmenger P, Mellin P (1970) Harnsteine im Kindesalter. Med Welt 21:1610–1616

Sutor DJ, Wooley SE (1969) Composition of urinary calculi by x-ray-diffraction: Collected data from various localities VII. Br J Urol 41:397–400

Sutor DJ, Wooley SE (1970) Composition of urinary calculi by x-ray-diffraction. Collected data from various localities VIII. Br J Urol 42:302–305

Sutor DJ, Wooley SE (1971) Composition of urinary calculi by x-ray-diffraction: Collected data from various localities IX–XI. Br J Urol 43:268–272

Sutor DJ, Wooley SE (1972) Composition of urinary calculi by x-ray-diffraction. Collected data from various localities XII–XIV. Br J Urol 44:287–291

Sutor DJ, Wooley SE (1974) Composition of urinary calculi by x-ray diffraction. Collected data from various localities XV–XVII. Br J Urol 46:229–232

Sutor DJ, Wooley SE, Illingworth JJ (1974) A geographical and historical survey of the composition of urinary calculi. Br J Urol 46:393–407

Szabo E (1978) Struktur und Aufbau der Harnsteine im Kindesalter (Kalziumoxalat-Steine). In: Vahlensieck W, Gasser G (Hrsg) Pathogenese und Klinik der Harnsteine VI. Steinkopff, Darmstadt, S 94–97

Takasaki E (1975) An observation on the composition and recurrence of urinary calculi. Urol Int 30:228–236

Takasaki E, Maeda K (1977) A population study of urolithiasis. Dokkyo J Med Sciences 4:88–92

Takasaki E, Murohashi I, Nagata M (1979) A four-year-retrospective study of urolithiasis. Dokkyo J Med Sci 6:120–125

Theile U, Böcking B, Krauß G (1983) Empirische Belastungsziffern bei Gicht und Hyperurikämie – Ergebnisse einer Familienuntersuchung. Dtsch Ärztebl 80:35–49

Thind SK, Nath R (1969) Chemical analysis of urinary calculi in Chandigarh area. Indian J Med Res 57:1790–1801

Tiktinsky OL (1979) On the pathogenesis of stone formation in stone-eliminating patients. Eur Urol 4:22–25

Toggenburg H, Horica Ch, Bandhauer K (1981) Das Harnsteinleiden bei Gastarbeitern – eine epidemiologische Studie. In: Vahlensieck W, Gasser G (Hrsg) Pathogenese und Klinik der Harnsteine VIII. Steinkopff, Darmstadt, S 15–19

Torres RC, Navarro A, Zuluaga A, Aguilar J, Espejo E, Abad F (1981) Influencias estacionales de lá edad, sexo y composicion del agua beleida sobre los calicos nefriticos. Arch Esp Urol 34:273–288

Toth C (1978) Persönliche Mitteilung

Tschöpe W, Ritz E, Haselbeck M, Mehnert H, Wesch H (1981) Prevalence and incidence of renal stone disease in a German population sample. Klin Wochenschr 59:411–412

Tschöpe W, Ritz E, Haselbeck M, Mehnert H, Deppermann D (1984) Epidemiology of urolithiasis and calcium metabolism in human diabetes mellitus. In: Schwille PO, Smith LH, Robertson WD, Vahlensieck W (eds) Urolithiasis and Related Clinical Research. Plenum Press, New York London (in press)

Turkyilmaz R (1976) Childhood urolithiasis in Cukurova area. Cukurova Univ Tip Fak Derg 1:291–294

Ulshöfer B (1984) Epidemiological aspects of urolithiasis in the Federal Republic of Germany. In: Schwille PO, Smith LH, Robertson WD, Vahlensieck W (eds) Urolithiasis and Related Clinical Research. Plenum Press, New York London (in press)

Ulshöfer B, Paar G, Cramer B (1982) Harnsteinmanifestation und Streß. In: Gasser G, Vahlensieck W (Hrsg) Pathogenese und Klinik der Harnsteine IX. Steinkopff, Darmstadt, S 46–51

Ultzmann R (1882) Die Harnkonkretionen des Menschen. Tendler u. Co., Wien

Unni Mooppan MM, Kim Hong, Wax SH (1979) Pattern of urolithiasis in Brooklyn, New York. Urology 14:482–486

Vahlensieck W (1977) Epidemiologie und Klinik der Urolithiasis. Akt Ernährungsmed 3:76–81

Vahlensieck W (1978) Therapie und Rezidivprophylaxe des kindlichen Harnsteinleidens. V. Jenaer Harnsteinsymposium. Wissenschaftliche Beiträge der Friedrich-Schiller-Universität, Jena, S 136–144

Vahlensieck W (1979) Urolithiasis 1. Springer Verlag, Berlin Heidelberg New York, Epidemiol, S 1–8

Vahlensieck W (1980) Epidemiologie und Pathogenese des Harnsteinleidens. Dtsch Med Wochenschr 105:799–804

Vahlensieck W, Bastian HP (1976) Clinical features and treatment of urinary calculi in childhood. Eur Urol 2:129–134

Vahlensieck W, Hesse A, Bach D (1980) Zur Prävalenz des Harnsteinleidens in der Bundesrepublik Deutschland. Urologe [Ausg B] 20:273–276

Vahlensieck W, Hesse A, Bach D (1981) Inzidenz, Prävalenz und Mortalität des Harnsteinleidens in der Bundesrepublik Deutschland. In: Vahlensieck W, Gasser G (Hrsg) Pathogenese und Klinik der Harnsteine VIII. Steinkopff, Darmstadt, S 1–5

Vahlensieck W, Hirth R, Bach D, Hesse A (1984) Epidemiological Determinations with 377 recurrent stone formers. In: Schwille PO, Smith LH, Robertson WD, Vahlensieck W (eds) Urolithiasis and Related Clinical Research. Plenum Press, New York London (in press)
Vahlensieck W, Bach D, Hesse A (1982) Incidence, prevalence and mortality of urolithiasis in the German Federal Republic. Urol Res 10:161 – 164
Valyasevi A (1979) Epidemiology of idiopathic bladder stone disease in children. XVIII. Congres Societe Internationale d'Urologie, Paris. Kongreßbericht, Tome 1, p 179 – 197
Valyasevi A, Dhanamitta S (1972) Clinical and field studies in Thailand. In: van Reen R (ed) Proceedings WHO. Regional symposium on vesical calculus disease. Bangkok, p 84 – 97
Vendl L (1975 a) Rezidivierende Urolithiasis im Kindesalter. Urologe [Ausg A] 14:164 – 167
Vendl L (1975 b) Harnsteinleiden im Kindesalter. Urologe [Ausg A] 14:168 – 171
Vivaldi J, Godoy J, Gámiz A, Berjon F, Cohen JS (1979) Epidemiology of renal lithiasis in Granada. XVIII. Congres Societe Internationale d'Urologie, Paris. Tome 2
Westbury EJ (1974) Some observations on the quantitative analysis of over 1000 urinary calculi. Br J Urol 46:215 – 227
Westermeyer JJ (1971) Urinary calculi in Laos. JAMA 217:82 – 83
White RW, Cohen RD, Vince FP, Williams G, Blandy J, Tresidder CG (1969) Minerals in the urine of stone formers and their spouses. In: Hodgkinson A, Nordin BEC (eds) Renal stone research symposium. Churchill, LTD, London, p 289 – 296
Williams, DI, Chisholm GD (eds) (1976) Scientific foundations of urology, Bd I: Urolithiasis. W. Heinemann Medical Books LTD, London, p 245 – 331
Williams G, Chandary M, Castro JE (1980) Cystine stones. Urology 16:339 – 342
Williams RE (1969) The natural history of renal lithiasis. In: Hodgkinson A, Nordin BEC (eds) Renal Stone Research Symposium. Churchill, LTD, London, p 65 – 70
Willnow U (1962) Zur Steindiathese im Kindesalter. Helv Paediatr Acta 17:472 – 485
Willnow U (1967) Nephrolithiasis im Säuglings- und Kindesalter. Dtsch Med Wochenschr 92:1668 – 1673
Wu Chieh-p'ing (1979) Urolithiasis in China. XVIII. Congres Societe Internationale d'Urologie, Paris
Zaidman JL, Pinto N (1976) Studies on urolithiasis in Israel. J Urol 115:626 – 627
Zechner O (1981) Richtlinien zur Rezidivprophylaxe von Harnsteinen. Wien Klin Wochenschr 93:619 – 624
Zechner O (1982) Epidemiologische und metabolische Aspekte des Harnsäuresteinleidens. In: Vahlensieck W, Gasser G (Hrsg) Pathogenese und Klinik der Harnsteine VIII. Steinkopff, Darmstadt, S 76 – 79
Zechner O, Scheiber V (1981 a) The role of affluence in recurrent stone formation. In: Smith LH, Robertson WG, Finlayson B (eds) Urolithiasis: Clinical and Basic Research. Plenum Press, New York London, p 309 – 314
Zechner O, Scheiber V (1981 b) Alcohol as an epidemiological risk in urolithiasis. In: Smith LH, Robertson WG, Finlayson B (eds) Urolithiasis: Clinical and Basic Research. Plenum Press, New York London, p 315 – 320
Zechner O, Pflüger H, Scheiber V (1982) Idiopathic uric acid lithiasis: Epidemiologic and metabolic aspects. J Urol 128:1219 – 1223
Zielinski J (1972) Epidemiologie und klinisch-chemische Zusammenhänge des Harnsteinleidens in Oberschlesien. II. Jenaer Harnsteinsymposium. Wissenschaftliche Beiträge der Friedrich-Schiller-Universität, Jena, S 100 – 102
Zielinski J, Nowak A, Patalong A (1979) Changes concerning nephrolithiasis in Silesia during the past 25 years. XVIII. Congres Societe Internationale d'Urologie, Paris
Zvara V (1979) Epidemiological and clinical significances of urolithiasis in childhood. XVIII. Congres Societe Internationale d'Urologie, Paris
Zvara V, Revusova V, Hornak U, Landsmannova L, Páyer J (1978) Die epidemiologische und klinische Bedeutung der Urolithiasis bei Kindern. V. Jenaer Harnsteinsymposium. Wissenschaftliche Beiträge der Friedrich-Schiller-Universität, Jena, S 160 – 162
Zvara V, Revusova V, Hornak M, Landsmannova L, Payer J, Badalik L (1979 a) Epidemiological and clinical significances of urolithiasis in childhood. Urol Int 34:36 – 45
Zvara V, Hornak M, Karlikova L, Borosova M, Kridl J (1982) Langfristige Ergebnisse bei der Behandlung von Kindern mit Urolithiase in Bezug zur komplexen Diagnostik. VII. Jenaer Harnsteinsymposium. Wissenschaftliche Beiträge der Friedrich-Schiller-Universität, Jena, S 289 – 295

Pathogenesis of Urolithiasis

W. G. ROBERTSON and M. PEACOCK

"No stretch of chemical or physical imagination will permit so heterogeneous a group of compounds (as renal stones) to be ascribed to a common origin, or their disposition in the kidney, urether, or bladder to be uniformly charged to an identical cause" – Howard Kelly.

I. Introduction

Urinary stone disease is one of the oldest and most ubiquitous diseases known to man. The earliest evidence of this disorder is a bladder stone, dating back to about 4800 BC, found among the pelvic bones in the tomb of a young predynastic Egyptian (SHATTOCK 1905). Other stones from that era have been reported although, out of 9000 mummies examined, only 4 had positive evidence of calculi, so that the prevalence of the disorder must have been fairly low, at least among upper class Egyptians. Stones have also been found in North America in the graves of early Indians (ca 1500 BC) (WILLIAMS 1926; BECK and MULVANEY 1966) but in South America stone disease appears to have been rare amongst the indigenous population until after the Spanish Conquest (BUTT 1956). In India, references to stone-formation can be located in early Sanskrit documents written between 3000 and 2000 BC (DESNOS 1914) and stones were well-recognised in Classical times by Hippocrates in Greece (ADAMS 1939) and by Celsus in Rome (DESNOS 1914).

Since that time the pattern of stone disease has changed with fluctuation both in the geographical distribution and in the type and composition of stones formed (ANDERSEN 1969, 1973; BLACKLOCK 1976). Over the centuries the incidence appears to have been generally increasing, particularly amongst the more industrially developed nations, although there are reports of "troughs" and "waves" in the incidence pattern during and after the two World Wars (ANDERSEN 1969, 1973; BLACKLOCK 1976, 1979). The stone most commonly found today in North America, Europe and Australia consists mainly of calcium oxalate occurring with or without calcium phosphate (PEACOCK and ROBERTSON 1979). This contrasts with the composition of stones in countries where endemic bladder stones are still common among children, particularly boys, and where the stones consist mainly of calcium oxalate and/or ammonium acid urate (LONSDALE 1968a; SUTOR 1976; THALUT et al. 1976). Renal stones composed of magnesium ammonium phosphate, usually in conjunction with calcium phosphate, are common throughout the world and occur in patients with certain urinary tract infections involving urea-splitting organisms. The relative incidence of this type of stone appears to have been decreasing in recent years at least in the United Kingdom (HODGKINSON and MARSHALL 1975) and is presumably related to better clinical diagnosis and treatment of urinary tract infection. Upper urinary tract stones consisting of uric acid or cystine are relatively uncommon in most parts of the world although certain areas such as Israel (ATSMON et al. 1963), central Europe (SUTOR 1976) and parts of South America (SCHNEIDER and HIENZSCH 1979; MATOUSCHECK and HUBER 1981) do have a traditionally high incidence of uric acid stones. There is some evidence that uric acid stones were becoming more common in many of the more industrially developed countries up till about 1970 (MAY and SCHINDLER 1973; SCHNEIDER and HIENZSCH 1979) but thereafter the incidence appears to have been falling (SCHNEIDER and HIENZSCH 1979; ROBERTSON and PEACOCK 1982) in response to the effect of inflation on the standard of living of the populations of these countries. In the last few years, however, in the U.K., the incidence of uric acid stones has again been increasing (Fig. 1). Figure 1 shows that the incidence of calcium-stone formation has followed a similar pattern to that of uric acid stones. This is almost entirely due to fluctuations in the number of "pure" calcium oxalate stones, with no obvious pattern of change in the number of "mixed" calcium oxalate/calcium phosphate stones (ROBERTSON and PEACOCK 1982). The overall pattern of stone incidence in the U.K. has followed very closely that of the economic situation and its effect on animal protein consumption over the last 25 years (ROBERTSON et al. 1979a, b, c; 1981b).

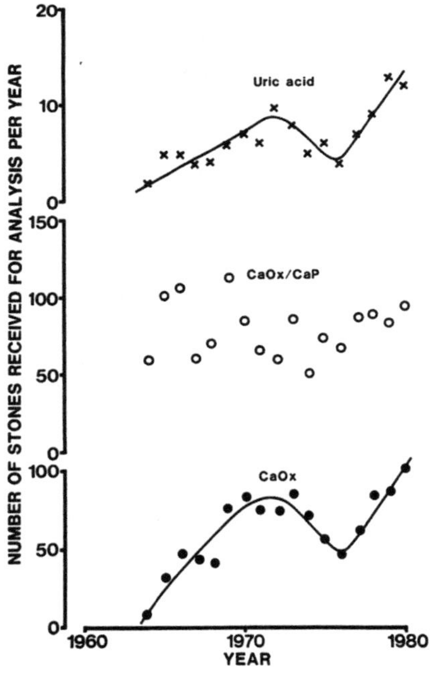

Fig. 1. The annual number of urinary stones received for analysis from the Leeds area during the period 1964–1980: top – uric acid stones; middle – "mixed" calcium oxalate/calcium phosphate stones (*CaOx/CaP*); bottom – "pure" calcium oxalate stones (*CaOx*)

II. Theories of Stone-Formation

Many theories have been advanced to account for the formation of stones in the urinary tract, but none has evolved which completely explains why certain individuals form stones whereas others do not. The main problem is that only in a few instances can the cause of the stone be attributed to one factor; in the majority of patients, the disorder appears to be multifactorial in origin.

The essential features of a complete theory of stone-formation are that it should account for the formation and retention within the urinary system of some critical nucleus which then accretes in size by the processes of crystal growth and agglomeration until it produces the clinical symptoms associated with the disorder, namely, renal colic, dysuria and haematuria. The final stone may range from a few milligrams to several grams in weight (HODGKINSON et al. 1969).

Broadly two groups of theories have emerged. Firstly, there are those which attempt to explain the initiation of stones in terms of an *intracellular* or *interstitial* process involving some localised lesion within the kidney tissue, followed by eruption of the nucleus into the urinary collecting system and growth into a stone. The second group of theories, on the other hand, describes stone-formation as being essentially an *extracellular* or *intratubular* phenomenon, i.e. the whole process takes place within the lumen of the urinary tract. Stone-formation is considered to take place in four stages: firstly, a nucleation phase during which crystal embryos are formed in the urinary tract; secondly, a period during which the initially formed embryos grow and aggregate to form larger particles; thirdly, the retention of one of these secondary particles which has become large enough to be trapped at some narrow point in the urinary tract; and finally, the growth of this trapped particle into a stone.

1. Localised Lesions in the Kidney

Several theories have evolved in this category derived mainly from histological and radiographic studies on kidney tissue removed at operation or at autopsy from patients with and without clinical evidence of stone disease.

a) Randall's Plaques

In the late 1930s, RANDALL (1937, 1940) published a series of reports describing the presence of papillary calcifications which he suggested might be precursors of renal stones. These were observed in 19.6% of 1154 pairs of kidney examined at autopsy. In 65 individuals a primary renal stone was observed growing upon and attached to a papilla (RANDALL 1940). Two types of lesion were identified. Type I, the more common of the two, consists of subepithelial plaques of a calcium salt measuring 1 to 2 mm in diameter located in the interstitial tissue of the papillae. Sometimes there are several such plaques on the

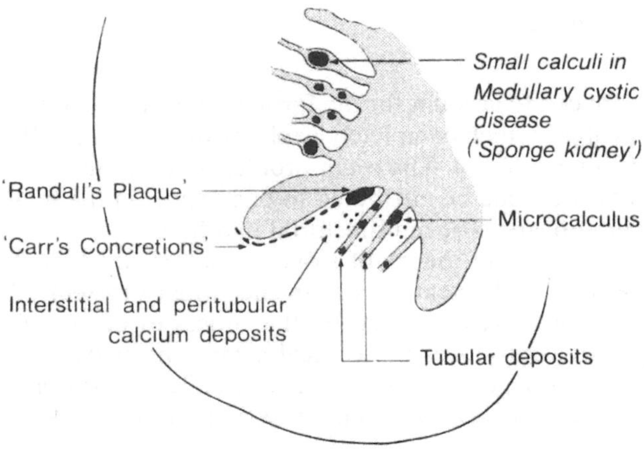

Fig. 2. Medullary calcification: showing the various types of precipitates formed (ANDERSON 1979; with the permission of the author and publishers)

same papilla and several papillae on the same kidney may be involved (Fig. 2). RANDALL postulated that these plaques, which first appear in the basement membrane of the cells of the collecting tubulus, act as foci for further mineral deposition and that they eventually ulcerate and expose themselves to calyceal urine. Microchemical analysis of these foci has shown that they are usually composed of calcium phosphate, less commonly of calcium oxalate and extremely rarely of uric acid (POSEY 1942; RESNICK and BOYCE 1979a).

A second, but less common, pre-calculus lesion (Type II) was also described by RANDALL. This was characterised by intratubular inspissation by calcium salts of the terminal portions of the collecting ducts (Fig. 2) and was associated with hyperexcretory disorders such as primary hyperparathyroidism, vitamin D poisoning and urinary infection.

Subsequent studies on renal tissue have supported (ROSENOW 1940; POSEY 1942; VERMOOTEN 1941, 1942; BRUWER 1979) and contradicted (KJØLHEDE and LASSEN 1942; ANDERSON 1969; HAGITT and PITCOCK 1971) RANDALL's observations. VERMOOTEN (1956) eventually concluded that papillary calcification is a fairly normal physiological process. Furthermore, as pointed out by PRIEN (1975), examination of RANDALL's original data shows that there is a major discrepancy between the age incidence pattern of plaque-formation and that of stone-formation. The former tends to be most common in subjects more than 60 years old whereas the peak in the latter occurs some 3 decades earlier. It would appear that this form of calcification may be simply some function of the ageing process. Indeed the concensus amongst most researchers in the field over the last decade is that, whereas a few stones probably originate by this mechanism, this lesion is not a major cause of renal stone-formation (ANDERSON 1969, 1979; RESNICK and BOYCE 1979a).

There are, however, some observations on small ureteral calculi which lend some support to RANDALL's hypothesis. Optical studies reveal that, although many have no regularity of structure, some do, and this often allows a nucleus to be identified. This is usually found at the focal point of the concentric growth layers of the stone. In the majority of such stones the nucleus is centrally situated, consistent with the hypothesis that they originate by *expulsion* from the papillary ducts of nuclei which develop into free-growing stones in the pelvo-calyceal space (Fig. 3a). However, according to PRIEN (1955, 1975), about 15% of all laminated stones have an *eccentric* nucleus, such as would come about if the growth phase took place while the stone embryo (growing on a RANDALL's plaque Type I) was attached to the renal papilla (Fig. 3b). In support of this mechanism, stones have been found with small smooth concavities (PRIEN 1955; ELLIOT 1973), often containing pedicle-like structures of apatite or calcium oxalate or even small pieces of papillary tissue, suggesting that they may have been the points of mural attachment (PRIEN 1949, 1955). The Type II lesion described by RANDALL may be considered to produce stones as suggested in the scheme in Fig. 3c. According to PRIEN this is identical to the calcium infarct described by older pathologists and may produce the "snow-capped" papillae described by VERMOOTEN. In this lesion the papillary ducts become ob-

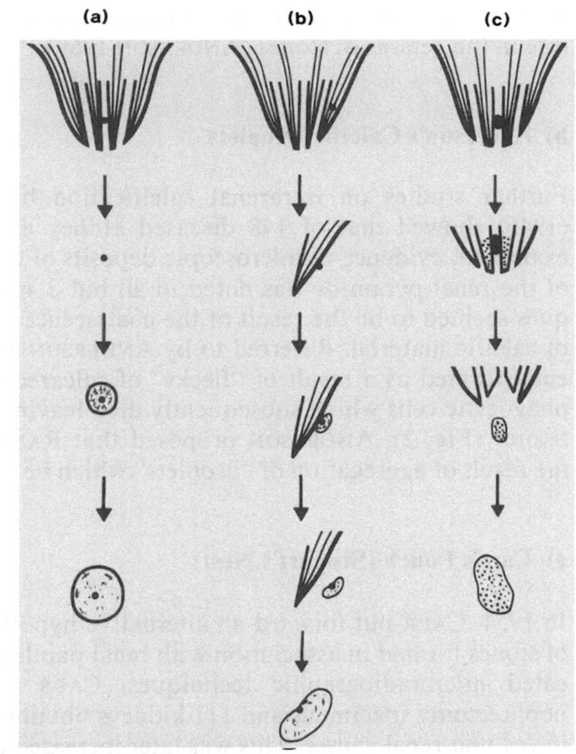

Fig. 3a–c. Diagrammatic representation of the renal papilla depicting the development of calculi: **a** "free-particle" stone-formation in the pelvo-calyceal space; **b** formation of a stone with an eccentric nucleus (starting on a Randall's plaque (Type I) attached to the papilla); **c** obstruction of a papillary duct by a stone salt followed by anaemic infarction and sloughing of the adjacent peritubular tissue (Type II lesion). (Adapted from the diagram of PRIEN 1975)

structed by impacted crystals. This is followed by anaemic infarction, necrosis and sloughing of the adjacent peritubular tissues. Eventually the stone embryo separates from the papilla and is passed in the urine or becomes lodged at another point in the urinary system. According to PRIEN (1975), however, such calculi are quite uncommon.

Some support for the possibility of precipitation of calcium salts in the renal papillae comes from studies on the calcium and oxalate concentration gradients across the kidney. Both in the rat (WRIGHT and HODGKINSON 1972) and in man (COOKE 1971, 1973; HAUTMANN et al. 1980; HAUTMANN and OSSWALD 1983) calcium and oxalate concentrations in renal tissue increase from cortex through the medulla to the papillae. This may explain the presence of precipitates in the tissues in this region.

In summary, papillary lesions of the type described by RANDALL do exist but there is no evidence that they differ in any way from other forms of renal focal calcification – nor does RANDALL himself appear to have considered them so. It is their vulnerability to exposure to pelvic urine which makes them unique. Although they may be a rare cause of stone-formation, their overall importance in the aetiology of stone disease has not yet been elucidated. At this point in time the majority of evidence suggests that they do not play a major role in the genesis of stones (ANDERSON 1969).

b) Anderson's Calcific Droplets

Further studies on intrarenal calcification by ANDERSON and MCDONALD (1946) showed that of 148 diseased kidney and 20 normal autopsy kidneys examined, evidence of microscopic deposits of calcium salts in the parenchyma of the renal pyramids was noted in all but 3 specimens. These interstitial plaques seemed to be the result of the coalescence of innumerable microspherules of calcific material. Referred to by ANDERSON as "droplets", they were apparently formed as a result of "flecks" of calcareous material being taken up by phagocytic cells which subsequently died leaving the deposits in the interstitial tissues (Fig. 2). ANDERSON proposed that RANDALL's plaques were probably the result of aggregation of "droplets" which he himself had described.

c) Carr's Pouch (Stewart's Nest)

In 1954, CARR put forward an alternative hypothesis to explain the occurrence of stones formed in association with renal papillae (CARR 1954). Using sophisticated microradiographic techniques, CARR initially examined 98 partial nephrectomy specimens and 111 kidneys obtained at autopsy from patients dying of non-renal causes. This was later increased to 250 specimens (CARR 1969). In almost every kidney from patients over the age of 9 years, small concretions could be demonstrated which were just visible to the naked eye. There were usually only one or two such radio-opaque bodies in each kidney but occasionally as many as twelve. CARR noted that these microscopic concretions were primarely located in three specific areas of the kidney; firstly, and most commonly, just outside the calyceal fornices, secondly, in the corticomedullary junction zone and, thirdly, immediately beneath the renal capsule. Since these areas correspond to the anatomical positioning of the renal lymphatic system, CARR suggested that, by analogy with the lungs, particulate matter formed in the upper urinary tract under conditions of excessive supersaturation may be drained away, not only in the urinary stream itself, but also via the lymphatic network. When the latter system ceases to function adequately, either because of overloading with excessive numbers of crystals or because of inflammatory changes produced by infection, blockage occurs at the mouth of the fornix (or fornices) concerned. These trapped crystals may accrete in size and eventually, in the form of a small concretion, erupt into the calyceal lumen. There in contact with supersaturated calyceal urine, it may then act as a nucleus for the formation of a true stone.

CARR and his surgical colleague STEWART so consistently found small concretions in the region of the fornices that they introduced the terms "Carr's pouch" (CARR 1969) and "Stewart's nest" (STEWART 1955) to describe this critical area of the kidney which they considered to be a potential nidus for the initiation of stones. In support of this, CARR cites the evidence that a partial nephrectomy which removes "Stewart's nest" prevents the patients from having further stone episodes (STEWART 1960; CARR 1969; PAPATHANASSIADIS and SWINNEY 1966) and this has been supported by later data (ROSE and FOLLOWS 1977). However, the operation has been condemned by others who consider it unsuitable for the majority of renal stones since it involves loss of renal tissue without proven benefit to the patient (ANDERSON 1974; MARSHALL et al. 1975). Furthermore ANDERSON (1979) considers that despite the striking clarity of CARR's microradiographs, it has not been proven conclusively that the concretions are in the lymphatics rather than in or around tubules. Like RANDALL's theory, CARR's has yet to be completely refuted or confirmed.

d) Anderson-Carr-Randall Progression

Recently an attempt has been made by BRUWER (1980) to bring together the observations of ANDERSON, CARR and RANDALL into a composite hypothesis of stone-formation. He proposes that primary renal calculi result, under certain defined circumstances, from the migration of calcium-containing deposits from the inside to the surface of renal papillae through a sequence of events which he terms "Anderson-Carr-Randall morphologic progression". According to this hypothesis the process begins with the formation of ANDERSON's "droplets" within the parenchyma of the renal pyramids, an observation confirmed by other workers (COOKE 1970; HAGGITT and PITCOCK 1971; WELLER et al. 1972). These deposits are said to be localised in the collagen bundles of the connective tissue around the loops of Henle (WELLER et al. 1972). The second stage of the progression is claimed to involve movement of ANDERSON's droplets from a locus within the substance of the papilla to a subepithelial position near to or at the surface of the papilla prior to removal of the deposits via the lymphatic sys-

Table 1. Incidence of histological calcification and radio-opaque micro-calculi in recurrent stone-formers and male non-stone-formers (ANDERSON 1969) (With the permission of the author and publishers)

Type of case	Number	Histological calcification present	Radio-opaque microcalculi present
Stone-formers	45	29 (64%)	41 (91%)
Non-stone-formers	108	32 (30%)	8 (7%)

tem as suggested by CARR. The final stage would then be eruption of the deposit through the papillary epithelium and contact with pelvic urine as proposed by RANDALL. This composite hypothesis of the initiating process in renal stone-formation remains to be confirmed.

In contrast to these findings, the studies of ANDERSON (1969, 1976, 1979) suggest that, although histologically detectable foci of calcification (> 20 μm in diameter) are indeed more common in the renal tissue of stone-formers than in that of non-stone-formers, they are absent in more than one third of patients with stones and present in one third of those without stones. On the other hand, microcalculi consisting of deposits of calcium phosphate or calcium oxalate up to 2 mm in diameter are present in all but a handful of stone patients and almost completely absent in non-stone-formers (Table 1). They usually occur in the terminal collecting ducts and are easily detected by serial contact radiography. Whatever the calcium salt forming the concretions, there is also a variable amount of matrix material present which ANDERSON (1979) considers to be a co-precipitate. ANDERSON's (1976) overall conclusion is that calcium stone-formation is essentially a matter of precipitation from supersaturated solution and that nephrocalcinosis is largely a by-product of precipitation rather than a primary cause of stones. He claims that intrarenal calcification is undoubtedly the cause of some stones but that the vast majority are due to biochemical abnormalities in the urine of stone-formers.

e) Intranephronic Calculosis

The process of stone-formation within the nephron has been termed "intranephronic calculosis" and was first described by OLIVER et al. (1966) in the kidneys of magnesium-depleted rats. The deposits observed in these studies consisted of structurally organised microcalculi generally lodged in the thin limb of Henle's loop. These were composed essentially of a mucopolysaccharide matrix of PAS(periodic-acid-Schiff)-positive substances and calcium phosphate occurring in a periodic pattern simulating that of Liesegang rings. OLIVER considered the formation of these microcalculi to be the first step in the genesis of stones. Similar spherular bodies have been since observed in the tubules of the squirrel monkey (DRACH and BOYCE 1972; RESNICK et al. 1978).

In man, examination of renal biopsy tissue from patients with stones and normal subjects has shown that idiopathic calcium oxalate stone-formers all had intranephronic calculi present and the number of these bodies in an individual kidney was directly related to the severity of the disorder in that patient (BOYCE et al. 1973; MALEK and BOYCE 1973, 1977). Non-stone-formers and patients with infection stones, uric acid stones or crystine stones, on the other hand, did not appear to have these microliths (MALEK and BOYCE 1973). Examination of the retentate after ultrafiltration of 24-hour urines from stone-formers and non-stone-formers showed that, in 24 out of the 26 stone-formers' urines studied, there were microscopic spherical bodies containing calcium, phosphorus and proteinpolysaccharide complexes. These were found in only 3 out of 15 urines from non-stone-formers (RESNICK and BOYCE 1978). No crystalline elements were detected and it may be that these bodies are precursors of the so-called intranephronic calculi.

It is not known whether or not intranephronic calculi form within the lumen of the renal tubule or are derived from deposits actually extruded by the tubular cells (RESNICK and BOYCE 1979a). Laminated spherules of hydroxyapatite-mucosubstance complexes are known to be associated with disruption of the mitochondria of the renal tubular cells under a variety of conditions in animals and in man. Extrusion of these spherules into the lumen of the nephron and further mineralization may represent the initial stage of intranephronic calculosis (MALEK and BOYCE 1977). However it may be that the whole process takes place in the lumen following precipitation of salts under the highly supersaturated conditions existing in the loop of Henle (WRIGHT and HODGKINSON 1972; HAUTMANN et al. 1980).

As with the other hypotheses which invoke localised lesions within the kidney as being the cause of stone disease, further studies are clearly required to confirm or refute these suggestions.

2. Hyperexcretion-Crystallization Theory

a) General Principles

The simplest theory to account for urinary stone-formation is based on the principle that it is simply due to the increased excretion of sparingly soluble substances in urine leading to spontaneous precipitation of these salts independently of a pre-formed matrix or of inhibitors of crystallization. This is supported to the extent that in most forms of the disorder stone-formers tend to have higher excretions of one or more of the constituent ions of the salt or acid concerned (see Section III). Since all the stone-forming salts and acids are sparingly soluble under normal urinary conditions, any increase in the saturation of urine with these increases the risk of precipitation and crystalluria. Persistent crystalluria of this nature may eventually result in the formation of some large crystal or aggregate of crystals which may become trapped in a narrow portion of the urinary tract. Alternatively, blockage may occur by a "log-jamming" mechanism in a urinary stream overcrowded with crystals (VERMEULEN et al.

1964, 1966, 1967; ROBERTSON et al. 1969). Further crystal growth and aggregation on the trapped particle, together with adsorption of urinary mucoprotein on the growing crystal faces, is thought to produce a fully developed stone. (See section II.5(b) on "Free-particle" theory.) In support of this hypothesis it has been shown that periods of spontaneous crystalluria may trigger off stone-formation in animals (VERMEULEN et al. 1966) and in man (SENGBUSCH and TIMMERMANN 1957; ROBERTSON et al. 1969, 1971; ETTINGER and KOLB 1971; CIFUENTES DELATTE et al. 1973; VALYASEVI and DHANAMITTA 1974). It has also been shown that the severity of the disease in a given individual, as measured by his stone episode rate is proportional to the percentage of large crystals and aggregates in his urine (ROBERTSON et al. 1981 d).

b) Solubility Concept

It was recognised by the early crystallographers that crystals will not develop in just-saturated solutions. Indeed, a high level of supersaturation is often necessary before spontaneous precipitation will take place. This phenomenon is due to the existence of a zone of metastable supersaturation lying, in the case of a salt, between the classical solubility product and the empirically defined formation product of the salt (Fig. 4). The solubility product is the saturation level at which a solution of a given salt is in equilibrium with excess crystals of the salt. The formation product is the so-called upper limit of metastability and is defined as the level of supersaturation at which spontaneous crystallization of the salt takes place. At saturation levels below the solubility product, a solution is undersaturated with respect to the salt concerned, and any crystal of that salt added to the solution will dissolve. Within the metastable region a solution may exist for long periods without precipitation taking place spontaneously. If, however, any nucleating material is added to such a solution, heterogeneous nucleation, followed by crystal growth or epitaxial growth, may take place (ROBERTSON et al. 1972a; ROBERTSON 1973; COE et al. 1975; MEYER et al. 1975, 1976;

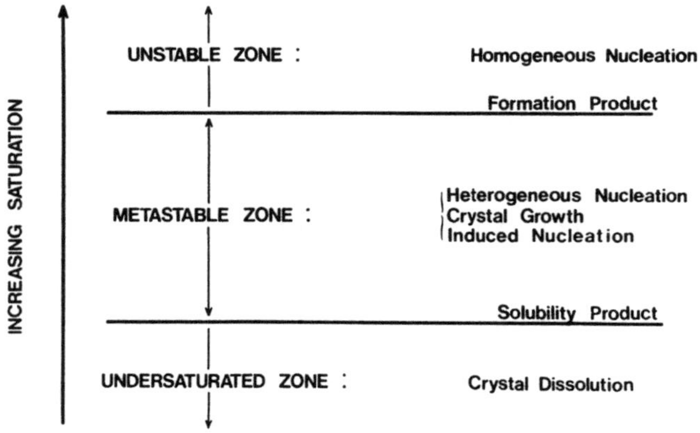

Fig. 4. Diagram of the various regions of saturation

MEYER and SMITH 1975a; PAK and ARNOLD 1975; PAK et al. 1976). A feature of such a process is the limited number of crystals which it produces compared with the vast numbers of new crystals generated by homogeneous nucleation (WALTON 1967; FINLAYSON 1978).

c) Saturation of Urine

The saturation of a solution of a given salt (CA), which dissociates to according to the equilibrium $CA \rightleftharpoons C^+ + A^-$, is defined by its activity product ({AP}) under a given set of conditions, where $\{AP\} = \{C^+\}\ \{A^-\} = [C^+]\ f_C \times [A^-]\ f_A$. In these expressions, { } represents the *chemical activity* of the enclosed ion and [ ] represents its *concentration*. The activity coefficients of the cation (C^+) and anion (A^-) are represented by f_C and f_A respectively. Thus, instead of measuring the activities of the ions which constitute the stone-forming salts (an impossible task at present), it is possible to measure the free (ionized) concentrations of the ions (in this case $[C^+]$ and $[A^-]$) and to calculate the activity coefficients (f_C and f_A) from some form of the Debye-Hückel equation (DEBYE and HÜCKEL 1923).

Several procedures have been developed for calculating activity products of the main stone-forming salts, namely, calcium oxalate (CaOx), calcium phosphate (CaP) and magnesium ammonium phosphate (MAP) (RAAFLAUB 1963; ROBERTSON et al. 1968; ROBERTSON 1969a, c; FINLAYSON and MILLER 1969; PAK 1969; SMALES 1972; ACHILLES et al. 1976; LESKOVAR 1979) and also for the minor constituents of stones, namely, cystine, uric acid, ammonium acid urate and sodium acid urate (MARSHALL and ROBERTSON 1976; PAK et al. 1976).

Rigorous calculation of the activity products of these various salts and acids in urine involves measuring the concentrations of all the main ionizing species in urine and calculating their free (ionized) concentrations from the extent to which they interact with one another to form soluble complexes and ion-pairs. For CaOx, CaP and MAP this requires the measurement in urine of pH and the total concentrations of calcium, magnesium, sodium, potassium, ammonium, phosphate, oxalate, citrate, chloride and sulphate. For cystine and the various urates, the calculation requires the additional meausrement of the total concentrations of uric acid and cystine. A computer program is used to calculate the ionized concentrations of calcium, magnesium, ammonium, sodium, phosphate, oxalate, urate and cystinate and the mean activity coefficients for monovalent, divalent and trivalent ions. The activity products are then obtained by multiplying the relevant free ion concentrations and activity coefficients according to the following equations:

For calcium oxalate: $K_{CaOx} = [Ca^{2+}]\,[Ox^{2-}]\,(f_2)^2$

For octocalcium phosphate: $K_{OCP} = [Ca^{2+}]^4\,[H^+]\,[PO_4^{3-}]^3\,f_1(f_2)^4\,(f_3)^3$

For brushite: $K_{DCP} = [Ca^{2+}]\,[HPO_4^{2-}]\,(f_2)^2$

For magnesium ammonium phosphate: $K_{MAP} = [Mg^{2+}]\,[NH_4^+]\,[PO_4^{3-}]\,f_1f_2f_3$

For uric acid: $K_{UA} = [H^+][U^-](f_1)^2$

For ammonium acid urate: $K_{NH_4U} = [NH_4^+][U^-](f_1)^2$

For sodium acid urate: $K_{NaU} = [Na^+][U^-](f_1)^2$

For cystine: $K_{Cys} = [H^+]^2[Cys^{2-}](f_1)^2 f_2$

To check the validity of these calculations of free ion concentrations it has been necessary to develop methods for measuring ionized calcium in urine. Several techniques have been reported based on the precipitation of calcium salts (NORDIN 1959; LIGHT et al. 1973), colorimetry using murexide (WALSER 1960; NORDIN and TRIBEDI 1962; MODLIN 1967a) or tetramethylmurexide (RAAFLAUB 1962; HUNT and KING 1963; ROBERTSON 1969a), ion-exchange (ACHILLES et al. 1977) and ion-selective electrodes (ROBERTSON 1969a; JACOBSON et al. 1979a, b). The last three of these techniques have proved useful for research purposes, but only under limited conditions. Both colorimetric methods and the electrode method are influenced by differences in sodium concentration and ionic strength so that standards containing the same concentration of sodium and ionic strength as the sample being measured have to be prepared for each urine. If murexide is used as the ionized calcium-sensitive dye, variations in urinary pH must also be taken into account. Calcium electrodes too are sensitive to hydrogen ion concentration in the low urinary pH range (<5.3).

The main problem, however, in the determination of ionized calcium in whole urine is that many urines are so supersaturated with calcium salts that these may precipitate spontaneously thereby altering the original level of ionized calcium. The resultant value for ionized calcium measured in the supernatant of urine is of little use to the researcher for estimating the risk of precipitation of stone-forming salts, since after precipitation this value may bear no relationship to that of ionized calcium in the original urine. However, by comparing the calculated value of ionized calcium in the *crystal-free supernatant of urine* with the measured value in the same fluid it is possible to utilise this comparison to check the validity of the computer calculation, at least for determining the concentration of ionized calcium in urine. Using both tetramethylmurexide (RAAFLAUB 1962, 1963; ROBERTSON 1969a) and the calcium-selective electrode (ROBERTSON 1969a; JACOBSON et al. 1979a, b, 1983) methods there is reasonably good agreement between the calculated and the measured values of ionized calcium (ROBERTSON 1969a). Thus the calculation of free ion concentrations in urine, although essentially an indirect technique, appears to be valid at least in the case of calcium.

Since the measured values of ionized calcium in whole urine containing crystals of calcium salts are of little use to the research worker, most studies in this area have relied on calculating the theoretical concentration of ionized calcium *which would have been achieved assuming that all the calcium had remained in solution*. Analysis in this way shows that on average about 40% to 50% of total calcium in urine would be in the free ionized form, although the range is very broad (30% to 70%) (RAAFLAUB 1962, 1963; ROBERTSON et al. 1968; JACOBSON 1979a). Of the bound fraction, about 25% is bound to citrate, 12% to sulphate,

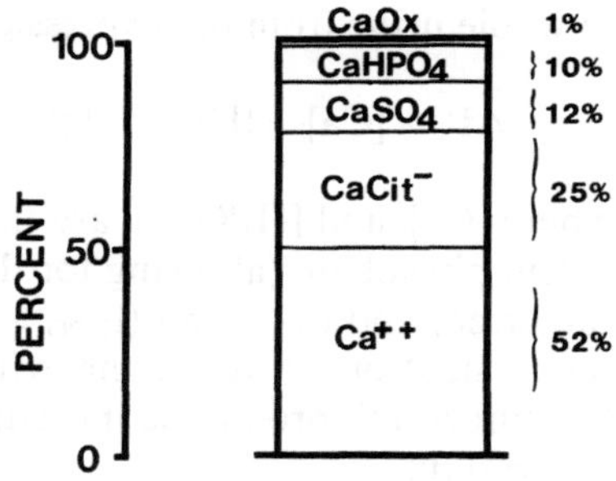

Fig. 5. The various fractions of calcium in urine which contains no crystals

10% to phosphate and about 1% to oxalate (Fig. 5) (ROBERTSON and NORDIN 1969a; FINLAYSON 1977; JACOBSON 1979a).

A simpler procedure has been described for estimating the saturation of urine with the above constituents by using a set of nomograms. This technique reduces the number of chemical estimations necessary to a minimum. For the saturation of urine with calcium salts, the estimations required are those of pH and the concentrations of calcium, oxalate and phosphate; for the saturation of infected urines – pH, calcium, phosphate, magnesium and ammonium; for the saturation of urine with the various urates – pH, urate, sodium and ammonium ion; and for the saturation of urine with cystine – pH and cystine (MARSHALL and ROBERTSON 1976).

From a knowledge of the activity products of the stone-forming salts in urine it is a simple matter to determine the relative saturation of urine with respect to each constituent by comparing the activity products with the relevant solubility (K_{sp}) and formation (K_{fp}) products (ROBERTSON et al. 1968; MARSHALL and ROBERTSON 1976; FINLAYSON 1977a). The values may be expressed in two ways, either on an absolute scale i.e. as $-\log_{10}$ (activity products), or on a $\log_{10}$ (relative supersaturation) scale, where the latter is defined either as $\log_{10}$ (activity product/K_{sp}) as used by FINLAYSON (1977a) or as $\log_{10}$ (activity product/K_{sp}/$\log_{10}(K_{fp}/K_{sp})$) as used by ROBERTSON et al. (1976c).

On both these latter scales, a urine, whose activity product for a particular salt is at its solubility product, has a $\log_{10}$ (relative supersaturation) value of 0. A negative value indicates that the urine is undersaturated with the salt and should re-dissolve any pre-existing crystals of it and a positive value indicates that the urine is supersaturated. On the scale of ROBERTSON et al. (1976c) a value between 0 and 1 indicates that the urine is in the metastable region of supersaturation and, therefore, is able to support further growth and aggregation of pre-existing crystals, but will not allow the spontaneous formation of new crystals in the absence of a nucleating agent. A value greater than 1 indicates that spontaneous precipitation of the salt will occur.

As an alternative to the above computer and nomogram techniques, PAK and CHU (1973) have proposed a semi-empirical approach to the determination of relative supersaturation. Instead of measuring all the ions in urine necessary for the calculation of the activity product by computer program, PAK and CHU determine the initial activity product (AP_i) (for example, of brushite) in whole urine from the expression:

$$AP_i = [Ca]_i \times [HPO_4^{2-}]_i (f_{Ca})_i (f_{HPO_4})_i$$

where $[Ca]_i$ and $[HPO_4^{2-}]_i$ are the initial concentration of total calcium and divalent phosphate (allowing for the dissociation of phosphoric acid at the pH of the urine) and $(f_{Ca})_i$ and $(f_{HPO_4})_i$ are the corresponding activity coefficients. After incubation of the urine with crystals of brushite ($K_{sp} = 1.86 \times 10^{-7}$) the "equilibrium" product is measured in the supernatant and calculated from the expression:

$$AP_f = [Ca]_f \times [HPO_4^{2-}]_f (f_{Ca})_f (f_{HPO_4})_f$$

where the subscript f refers to the final concentrations and activity coefficients of calcium and divalent phosphate. The activity product ratio (APR) of initial to final activity product, it is claimed, provides a measure of the relative saturation of the urine under study. In practice, the initial and final activity coefficients are not significantly different and so cancel out in the expression for ARP which essentially reduces to (PAK 1969):

$$APR = ([Ca]_i \times [HPO_4^{2-}]_i)/([Ca]_f \times [HPO_4^{2-}]_f)$$

The APR for calcium oxalate (based on the equilibration of urine with crystals of calcium oxalate monohydrate and a thermodynamic $K_{sp} = 2.2 \times 10^{-9}$) may be calculated from a similar expression (PAK and HOLT 1976). The APRs for uric acid, sodium acid urate, potassium acid urate and ammonium acid urate may also be obtained after allowing for the dissociation of uric acid at the pH of the urine under study (PAK et al. 1977 b, 1980 a, b).

Comparison of the various techniques for measuring saturation shows that, in terms of the absolute activity product of brushite in urine at equilibrium with that salt, the calculated value of ROBERTSON (1969 a) is almost identical with the thermodynamic K_{sp} (PAK et al. 1977 a), whereas the estimates of FINLAYSON and MILLER (1969) and PAK (1969) are somewhat higher. Since, however, the corresponding activity products of brushite in whole urine *before* equilibration are also in the order $AP_{Robertson} < AP_{Finlayson} < AP_{Pak}$, when the relative saturation value is expressed as the ratio of the initial to the final activity product, the values given by the three methods are almost identical. Thus, in relative terms the semi-empirical method of PAK and CHU is as good as the more rigorous methods of ROBERTSON and of FINLAYSON and MILLER.

In terms of the absolute calcium oxalate activity products of urine at equilibrium with that salt, the calculated values are said by PAK et al. (1977 a) to be 1.5 to 15 times higher than the thermodynamic K_{sp} of calcium oxalate monohydrate. One possible explanation for this is that in the calculation of the free-ion concentrations of calcium and oxalate, some, as yet unidentified, factor(s) which bind one or both of these ions have been ignored (NICAR et al. 1980; HODGKINSON 1980). Indeed, there is some evidence that about 12% of oxalate and 10% of calcium may be bound to urinary macromolecules (SHEINFELD et al.

1978). However, in another study, the equilibrium saturation levels were found to be almost identical with the K_{sp} of calcium oxalate (ROBERTSON et al. 1972a). One of the differences between the studies of PAK et al. (1977a) and ROBERTSON et al. (1972a) is the longer equilibration time and higher slurry density of crystals used by the latter group which might have allowed "true" equilibrium to be reached in a given time period by supplying a greater surface area of crystals for growth. Ironically, this observation is supported by a study of PAK et al. (1975b) which showed that in the presence of ethane-1-hydroxy-1,1-diphosphonate (a well-known inhibitor of crystal growth), a large excess of calcium oxalate crystals is required to allow equilibration to the thermodynamic K_{sp} to be reached even in simple aqueous solution. This suggests that the measured solubility product after equilibration in PAK's semi-empirical system represents only a "pseudoequilibrium state" and that it is greater than the true K_{sp} because of the presence of various crystal growth inhibitors which effectively block active growth sites on the crystal surface and thereby reduce the effective surface area available for growth. Thus, in terms of relative saturation the semi-empirical APR method of PAK would be expected to give lower values than the relative saturation values of ROBERTSON et al. (1976c) and of FINLAYSON (1977a) which are both based on the ratio of the activity product to the true K_{sp}, since PAK is employing a denominator which is higher than the true thermodynamic K_{sp}. This is what is observed (PAK et al. 1977a). However, when relative saturation is expressed as an APR in each of the three techniques, the values again come very close together, at least in urines whose total calcium and oxalate concentrations are less than 5 mmol/l and 0.5 mmol/l respectively (PAK et al. 1977a). In urines where either the total calcium concentration > 5 mmol/l or the total oxalate concentration > 0.5 mmol/l, the semi-empirical estimate of APR of PAK overestimates the saturation of urine compared with the APR derived from ROBERTSON's or FINLAYSON's programs. In spite of these problems with the semi-empirical method, PAK and others (FINLAYSON 1978; COE 1978; PYLYPCHUK et al. 1979) have concluded that, in general, it is the most useful practical method of estimating the propensity of the calcium salts in urine to grow on seed crystals of the appropriate salt.

It is clear from the above discussion, however, that the semi-empirical estimate of the APR (particularly of calcium oxalate) must be more than a simple function of urine saturation as the *thermodynamic driving force* towards crystal growth, since the denominator of the expression used to calculate the APR is affected by the concentration of inhibitors of crystallization. If the APR is a function of the concentration of inhibitors in urine relative to the defined amount of crystals (and therefore surface area) added to obtain equilibrium, then it must also influence the *kinetics* of the approach to equilibrium. In practical terms, therefore, it may be that the semi-empirical estimation of APR may be a better indicator of the *overall* risk of crystal growth in a given urine since it is a function of both saturation and inhibitory activity. A critical evaluation of this hypothesis has not yet been made.

An alternative semi-empirical approach to the measurement of urinary saturation with respect to calcium oxalate has been suggested by GILL et al. (1974) and GILL and ROMA (1976). The method differs from that of PAK and

CHU's (1973) in that an oxalate tracer is added to the system and only changes in oxalate concentration are measured. The main drawback to this method is that there is appreciable exchange and solid state diffusion of ^{14}C-oxalate into the crystals of calcium oxalate. The method only becomes completely valid in the absence of seed crystals. In the presence of small amounts of seed crystals the method is reasonably satisfactory, although there is the same intrinsic objection to the measurement of the pseudo-equilibrium activity product as with the method of PAK and CHU (1973). Comparison of the method of GILL et al. (1974) with that of FINLAYSON yields a correlation coefficient of 0.86 (ERWIN et al. 1976).

There are now several data on the relative saturation of urine with respect to the various stone-forming salts and acids. These are discussed later in the relevant sections on the different types of stone-formation (Section III).

d) Crystal Nucleation

Nucleation is the initial event in the transformation of a substance from the solution phase to the solid phase. Classically there are two main types of nucleation, homogeneous and heterogeneous. The term "*homogeneous nucleation*" is used to describe the first stage in the *spontaneous precipitation* of a salt. Theoretically it occurs without the assistance of any catalytic forces (such as heterogeneous nucleating material, temperature changes, physical shock, etc.) and usually at a very high level of supersaturation known as the formation product of the salt (Fig. 4). The latter is not a true constant but an empirically observed upper limit of metastable supersaturation.

Below the formation product, i.e. within the metastable region of supersaturation, urines may exist for some time without precipitation taking place spontaneously. If, however, some nucleating material is added to such a solution "heterogeneous nucleation" followed by crystal growth may take place at levels well below the formation product. A feature of this process is the limited number of crystals produced compared with the vast numbers of new particles generated by homogeneous nucleation ($> 10^6$ nuclei/ml) (WALTON 1967).

Because urine is rich in cellular debris (TRUMP et al. 1972) and possibly crystals of other salts which may cause heterogeneous nucleation to occur, and because extremely high levels of supersaturation are necessary to produce homogeneous nucleation (80 to 100 times the K_{sp} for calcium oxalate), in the view of some workers it is extremely unlikely that the spontaneous formation product of any of the stone salts will ever be attained in urine (FINLAYSON 1978; FINLAYSON and REID 1978). These workers claim that virtually all nucleation in urine is heterogeneous in nature. If FINLAYSON's data and calculations are correct regarding the unlikelihood of homogeneous nucleation being achieved in urine, then it must be concluded that the estimates of the "formation product" made in simple salt solutions and in urine 10 to 15 minutes after mixing are a measure of the onset of rapid *heterogeneous* nucleating and not, as previously suggested, homogeneous nucleation (ROBERTSON et al. 1968, 1972a; ROBERTSON 1973; PAK et al. 1975b). The value of this empirical formation product for cal-

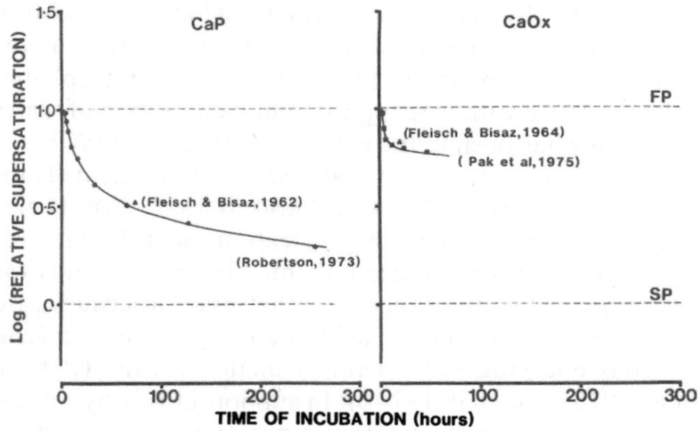

Fig. 6. The formation products of calcium phosphate (*CaP*) and calcium oxalate (*CaOx*) plotted against time of incubation taken from various sources in the literature. The data are shown in relation of the 10-minute formation products (*FP*) of ROBERTSON et al. (1968)

cium oxalate corresponds to a supersaturation ratio of about 19 (ROBERTSON et al. 1976c). It is time-dependent (ROBERTSON 1973; PAK et al. 1975b) such that at long time periods (> 1 day) the critical level falls to values well down in the metastable region. Thus the values for the formation product reported by FLEISCH and his co-workers (FLEISCH and BISAZ 1962a, b, 1964) at 1 day and 3 days are considerably lower than those quoted by ROBERTSON or PAK at shorter time periods down to 10 to 15 minutes (Fig. 6).

More recent studies, however, suggest that, as far as calcium oxalate is concerned, FINLAYSON may have been grossly overestimating the level of supersaturation necessary to attain homogeneous nucleation (SCURR and ROBERTSON 1984). Indeed, the relative supersaturation value of 22 at which spontaneous precipitation occurs with $>10^6$ nuclei/ml, is almost identical with that originally published by WALTON (1963) and ROBERTSON et al. (1976c). The question then of whether or not homogeneous nucleation of calcium oxalate is possible in urine has still to be answered.

Studies on the appearance of crystals in urine both in vitro (ROBERTSON et al. 1972b, 1981d) and in vivo (ROBERTSON et al. 1971, 1972b) show that significant crystalluria of both calcium phosphate and calcium oxalate becomes observable at or around the 10-minute empirical formation product of these two salts as defined both in urine and in simple aqueous solutions (ROBERTSON et al. 1968; ROBERTSON 1973). Moreover, the volume of crystals of calcium salts produced is proportional to the level of oversaturation of urine above the point of spontaneous precipitation (ROBERTSON et al. 1971, 1972b). This is compatible with a homogeneous nucleation mechanism.

Based on FINLAYSON's calculations that homogeneous nucleation of calcium oxalate is not likely in urine, other workers have sought potential heterogeneous nucleators of this salt in urine. It was first suggested that crystals of brushite were the initiators of calcium oxalate crystallization (PAK et al. 1971; PAK 1969, 1981). If this were true, however, calcium oxalate stone disease could be prevented by maintaining urinary pH at values of about 5.6 or less, since calcium phosphate crystals would not form in such an environment and, indeed, existing crystals of any of the known calcium phosphates would dissolve. Clinical experience with treating calcium oxalate stone-formers by simply acidifying their urine has been to the contrary (FINLAYSON 1977a).

It has also been shown that crystals of uric acid (HARTUNG et al. 1980) or of sodium acid urate (PAK and ARNOLD 1975; COE et al. 1975; PAK et al. 1976) may cause heterogeneous nucleation of calcium oxalate crystals in vitro although this has not been confirmed in another study (MEYER 1981). These observations led to the suggestion that hyperuricosuria, by increasing the risk of uric acid and/or sodium acid urate crystalluria, might stimulate the heterogeneous nucleation of calcium oxalate in urine (PAK and ARNOLD 1975; COE et al. 1975; PAK et al. 1977b). In support of this hypothesis, it has been shown in several clinical trials that recurrence of calcium oxalate stone-formation can be markedly reduced by treatment with allopurinol (COE and RAISEN 1973; COE and KAVALICH 1974; SMITH 1977; SCOTT et al. 1980). The rationale behind this

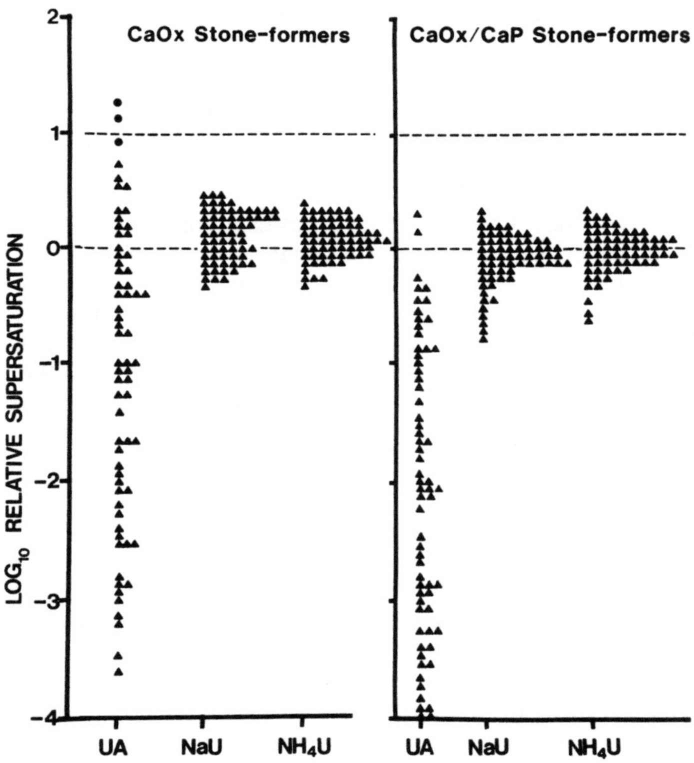

Fig. 7. The saturation of urine from "pure" calcium oxalate and "mixed" calcium oxalate/calcium phosphate stone-formers with respect to uric acid (*UA*), sodium acid urate (*NaU*) and ammonium acid urate (*NH_4U*). On this scale the formation products have a value of 1 and the solubility products a value of 0

approach is that lowering the excretion of total urate with allopurinol reduces the risk of precipitation of uric acid or sodium acid urate in urine thereby removing the potential source of heterogeneous nucleation of calcium oxalate. This hypothesis has been challenged, however, on the grounds that, first, crystals of uric acid (although fairly common in urine of hyperuricosuric individuals) are not very active nucleators of calcium oxalate crystallization (PAK and ARNOLD 1975; HALLSON et al. 1982b) and secondly, that urine (even in hyperuricosuric individuals) never becomes sufficiently supersaturated with sodium acid urate to allow spontaneous precipitation of that salt (Fig. 7) (ROBERTSON et al. 1976b; TAK et al. 1980a, b; LABEEUW et al. 1980). Thus although crystals of sodium acid urate may be good heterogeneous nucleators of calcium oxalate crystallization in vitro, urine may never become sufficiently supersaturated with the salt to produce crystals spontaneously.

It would appear from the above discussion that the role of heterogeneous nucleation in stone-formation, although theoretically possible, is not likely to be a major one. Further studies in this area are clearly necessary.

Apart from homogeneous and heterogeneous nucleation there are other nucleation processes by which crystallization may be initiated. These include "epitaxial nucleation" and "secondary nucleation". The former is thought to occur on surface defects of crystals which are able to catalyze nucleation; the latter is due to collisions of crystals with a second solid object which produce one or more nuclei. Little has been done in the stone field, however, on these aspects of nucleation.

e) Crystal Growth

Crystals grow either by a diffusion-controlled process or by a surface-controlled process or by a combination of the two. For most salts occurring in stones, the process appears to be surface-controlled and the growth rate equation may be written in the form:

$$-dC/dt = k\,(C - C_0)^m$$

where C is the concentration of the precipitating salt, k is the rate constant for the system, and m is the order of reaction. In the case of the seeded growth of calcium oxalate, for example, the reaction has been shown to obey 2nd order kinetics for the monohydrate salt (NANCOLLAS and GARDNER 1974; MEYER and SMITH 1975a; LIGABUE et al. 1979; TOMAZIC and NANCOLLAS 1980a), for the dihydrate salt (WERNESS et al. 1979; TOMAZIC and NANCOLLAS 1980a) and for the trihydrate salt (GARDNER 1975; TOMAZIC and NANCOLLAS 1980a). An alternative kinetic model to that described above has recently been proposed by BLOMEN and WILL et al. (1979, 1983) based on the concept of "growth affinity" as the driving force for the crystallization of sparingly soluble salts (VAN LEEUWEN 1979).

Parallel studies have examined the rates of transformation of the higher hydrates of calcium oxalate to the more stable monohydrate (GARDNER 1976;

Tomazic and Nancollas 1979, 1980b). These transformations may be important in that the initial precipitate of calcium oxalate formed in urine may not consist of the most stable salt under the conditions prevailing in that urine. Conversion to a more stable (and more insoluble) form may take place with time. The significance of this phenomenon was, in fact, recognised by the early workers in the field (Hammarsten 1929; Tovborg-Jensen 1941).

Studies on the crystal growth of the other main constituents of stones have also been carried out. In the case of calcium phosphate, there is a vast literature on the crystal growth of brushite and of hydroxyapatite. The reader is referred to only a few of these (Marshall and Nancollas 1969; Nancollas and Tomazic 1974; Meyer and Eanes 1978; Koutsoukos and Nancollas 1981; Moreno and Varughese 1981; Brown and Chow 1981). In the cases of cystine (Ettinger and Kolb 1971), uric acid (Lam et al. 1978) and magnesium ammonium phosphate (Johnson 1959), however, there are few good data on crystal growth.

One of the disadvantages of the standard seeded crystal growth technique employed in most of the above studies is that the level of supersaturation of the salt concerned decreases with time and the reaction becomes slower and slower as equilibrium is approached. More recently, however, a modification of this technique has been developed in which the level of supersaturation is maintained at a fixed value throughout the study. This so-called "constant composition method" has been applied to the study of growth rates of calcium phosphates (Koutsoukos et al. 1980a) and of calcium oxalate (Sheehan and Nancollas 1980; Lanzalaco et al. 1982). The main advantage of this technique is that it allows the growth rate and the effect of inhibitors on it to be measured within 30 minutes. Moreover, whereas the simple seeded growth system requires growth rates to be measured at a series of dilutions in order to estimate an "inhibitor unit" (Meyer and Smith 1975a, b), the constant composition method requires measurement to be made at only one dilution.

Crystal growth rates may also be obtained from a variant of the constant composition system which employs the "continuous crystallizer" principle. Continuous crystallizers are widely used by chemical engineers for the controlled production of crystals of a specific size and type on a commercial scale. In this system a crystallization chamber continously receives a supersaturated solution of constant composition and ejects a slurry of precipitated particles in their partially depleted mother liquor. Measurement of the particle size distribution in the effluent suspension yields information on both nucleation and particle growth rates. In the absence of aggregation (a necessary feature of the system if the data are to be analysed according to the continuous crystallizer theory (Randolph and Larson 1971)), the calculated growth rates correspond to true linear crystal growth rates. Finlayson (1972) has argued that the continuous crystallizer more closely reproduces the conditions existing in the kidney. To date a number of reports on the crystallization of calcium oxalate have been published using this technique (Randolph and Larson 1971; Finlayson 1972; Miller et al. 1977; Nyvlt 1978; Rodgers and Garside 1981; Randolph and Drach 1981a; Drach et al. 1982a, b; Robertson et al. 1984).

One other feature of crystal growth, which may be relevant to stone-formation, is the phenomenon of epitaxial over-growth of crystals of one salt on top of those of another. This may result when the atomic arrangement of a substrate surface is similar to that of the material overgrowing on it, so that the crystal lattices of the substrate and the growing material are aligned with respect to each other.

The possible significance of this in stone-formation, where admixtures of two, and sometimes more, salts are frequent findings in stones, was first emphasised by LONSDALE (1968a, b). In her papers, she pointed out the near geometrical fits between a number of the salts and acids found in urinary stones. This has recently been re-emphasised by MANDEL and MANDEL (1981). However, although epitaxy between certain stone constituents appears to be theoretically possible, only a few examples of true epitaxial growth have so far been reported. Thus calcium oxalate monohydrate may be grown on crystals of anhydrous uric acid (MEYER et al. 1976; KOUTSOUKOS et al. 1980b), sodium acid urate (KOUTSOUKOS et al. 1980b), hydroxyapatite (MEYER et al. 1975; KOUTSOUKOS et al. 1981) and brushite (MEYER et al. 1977a). Conversely, brushite (but not hydroxyapatite (MEYER et al. 1975; KOUTSOUKOS et al. 1981)) may be grown on crystals of calcium oxalate monohydrate (MEYER et al. 1977a). Hydroxyapatite, on the other hand, may be grown on crystals of calcium oxalate trihydrate (KOUTSOUKOS et al. 1981), uric acid or sodium acid urate (KOUTSOUKOS et al. 1980b).

In spite of this in vitro evidence of epitaxial growth between certain of the stone-forming salts and acids, there is no substantial evidence to support the suggestion that epitaxy plays a major role in the genesis of stones. The crystals in stones that have well defined radial growth patterns (such as calcium oxalate monohydrate, uric acid and brushite) often have a common crystal axis oriented radially with the other two axes oriented randomly (CARR 1953). Conceivably, this radial orientation could be due to epitaxy (LONSDALE 1968a). However, there is an alternative possible explanation. If a stone surface is randomly and densely populated with seed crystallites, the predominant growth will be on the fastest-growing faces, particularly on those faces which are parallel to the seeded surface. Radial orientation could then be due to preferential growth on a common crystal face. According to FINLAYSON (1974) this interpretation is consistent with observation on the relation between radial stone-growth orientation and the composition of urine (MURPHY and PYRAH 1962).

Many stones appear, on careful examination, to have identifiable nuclei (HERRING 1962; PRIEN and PRIEN 1968; TAKASAKI 1971) and it has been postulated that they may be instrumental in the genesis of urinary stones by causing either heterogeneous nucleation or epitaxial growth of a second constituent on top of the first. However, most stones constituents tend to be associated with each other (FINLAYSON 1974) and it is well-recognised that stone materials will grow on a variety of unconnected substrates including rubber catheters, hair grips, silk sutures, glass thermometers, ball-point pen refills, etc. This suggests that almost any surface can act as a nucleus for any of the common stone-forming salts without epitaxy being a necessary factor for the process to occur.

f) Crystal Aggregation

One of the few points of agreement among stone research workers is that stones essentially consist of aggregates of smaller particles (CARR 1953; LAGERGREN 1956; MURPHY and PYRAH 1962; HERRING 1962; LONSDALE 1968a; PRIEN and PRIEN 1968; BOYCE 1969a; MEYER et al. 1971; SUTOR 1972). Indeed, the smallest stones (~ 1 mg in weight) appear to be no more than polycrystalline aggregates. Such aggregates are common findings in the urines of patients with stone disease but not in those of normal subjects (SENGBUSCH and TIMMERMANN 1957; VALYASEVI and DHANAMITTA 1974; SMITH 1976; WERNESS et al. 1981; HERING et al. 1981).

The possible importance of aggregation in the initiation of stone-formation is that it constitutes the most rapid and effective mechanism for increasing particle size within a given time period. It is, therefore, a more potent risk factor than the slower process of crystal growth for the production (within the transit time of urine through the kidney) of a particle large enough to be trapped even at the narrowest portions of the urinary tract. Indeed, FINLAYSON has calculated that, even at high levels of supersaturation, the probability of a single crystal growing sufficiently (within the urinary transit time through the collecting system) to be trapped at the ducts of Bellini is extremely remote (FINLAYSON 1974, 1977b; FINLAYSON and REID 1978). Thus for trapping to occur by a "free particle" mechanism (Section II, 5(b)), aggregation must almost certainly be invoked.

There are six basic mechanisms by which aggregates may be held together (RUMPF and SCHUBERT 1977; FINLAYSON 1978). In order of increasing energy they are electrostatic attraction < van der Waal forces < liquid bridge < capillarity < viscous binding < crystal bridge. Since the crystals in urine are totally immersed, liquid bridge and capillary forces are not likely to play a major role in the aggregation phenomena occurring therein. Electrostatic binding may take place between two growing crystals of near neutral charge or between two crystals of opposite charge. As far as calcium oxalate crystals are concerned, however, the electrostatic forces will be generally repulsive since there is usually a net negative zeta potential due to adsorption of negatively charged macromolecules (glycosaminoglycans, glycoproteins, RNA etc.) on the surface. Solid bridges can occur only after particle-to-particle apposition has already taken place due to other adhesive forces. Viscous binding involves inter-particle bridging by a polymeric material, such as mucoprotein, which can bind separately to the surfaces of at least two crystals thereby linking them together.

Qualitatively, then, in urine the following equation may be written:

the force of adhesion = van der Waal forces + viscous binding forces − electrostatic forces.

Most of the elements of this equation can be measured and some preliminary studies have already been carried out on viscous binding forces (LEAL and FINLAYSON 1977) and on electrostatic forces (CURRERI et al. 1979; ROBERTSON et al. 1984). Van der Waal forces, however, have not yet been determined between the crystals of the various stone-forming salts.

Aggregation, and the effects of various crystallization inhibitors on the process, may be readily measured in vitro by means of a Coulter Counter (ROBERTSON 1969b; ROBERTSON and PEACOCK 1972; ROBERTSON et al. 1973a, b; RYALL et al. 1981a, c; HERING et al. 1981; FÜREDI-MILHOFER et al. 1981) or by differential filtration (FLEISCH and MONOD 1973). Essentially these measure the particle size distributions of crystals and their aggregates. Provided there is no nucleation of *new* crystal formation during the incubation period, the data may be analysed to yield information on the rate and degree of aggregation and on the rate of crystal growth separately (MARKOVIC and KOMUNJER 1979; RYALL et al. 1981a, c; ROBERTSON et al. 1981d; SCURR et al. 1981).

Some workers, however, are skeptical of the importance of aggregation in the stone-forming process. According to FINLAYSON (1978), if aggregation constitutes a significant step in the initiation of stone-formation, it might be anticipated to take place according to the theory of Smoluchowski agglomeration. Indeed, from the early published data on the number of calcium oxalate crystals excreted per unit volume of fresh urine (ROBERTSON 1969b; ROBERTSON et al. 1969) it can be calculated that significant aggregation would be unlikely. However, these early data only included crystals greater than 3.8 µm in diameter (ROBERTSON 1969b). By counting down to particle diameters of about 1 µm much greater numbers of crystals could be found (> 10^6/ml) (ROBERTSON, unpublished results). At this level of crystalluria, aggregation could become highly significant.

More recent studies (SCURR and ROBERTSON 1984) show that the Smoluchowski equation may grossly underestimate the true degree of aggregation of newly generated calcium oxalate crystals under a number of situations, in particular when the oxalate/calcium ratio of the precipitating solution is reduced from the normal urinary ratio of about 10 to 1. Clearly, further studies in this area are required to elucidate the true importance of aggregation in the stone-forming process.

3. Matrix Theory

a) General Principles

Since it was first demonstrated in 1684 by VON HEYDE that renal stones contain an organic phase (referred to by SCHADE 1928), it has been an attractive hypothesis to suggest, by analogy with what some workers believe to be the initiating factor in bone formation, that the matrix plays an active role in the nucleation and growth of the mineral phase around it (PAK 1978). Only within the last 25 to 30 years, however, has the nature of the organic material been elucidated. Normally the proportion by weight of matrix to mineral in stones is small. It was on average about 2.5% (range 2.0 to 3.2%) in a series of 264 mixed stones analyzed by BOYCE and GARVEY (1956). In cystine stones, however, the percentage of matrix may be as much as 10% (BOYCE 1969a) and in so-called "matrix calculi" the organic phase constitutes 62% (BOYCE and KING 1959; BOYCE 1969a) or more (BOMMER et al. 1979) of the total weight of the stone. These "jelly-like stones" are usually found in patients with low or sub-normal urinary calcium levels, which may be as low as 0.5 to 1.2 mmol/day (BOYCE and KING 1959; ALLEN and SPENCE 1966; BOMMER et al. 1979). They are often associated with a urinary tract infection (WILLIAMS 1963; MOGG 1964; ALLEN and SPENCE 1966; BOMMER et al. 1979). Under these conditions the saturation of urine with calcium salts is almost certainly too low to allow spontaneous precipitation of either calcium phosphate or calcium oxalate, so the low mineral content of these calculi is perhaps not surprising.

Early microscopic studies of decalcified urinary stones by CARR (1953, 1956) and by BOYCE and GARVEY (1956) demonstrated the presence of regular concentric laminations composed of densely arranged amorphous matrix material. Radial striations of fibrous matrix were also present in most stones occurring at right angles to the concentric laminations (BOYCE et al. 1958 b). These observations were confirmed by MURPHY and PYRAH (1962) and by WATANABE (1972). In general, calcium phosphate was found in association with fibrous matrix, magnesium ammonium phosphate with amorphous matrix, calcium oxalate monohydrate in both and calcium oxalate dihydrate in the interlaminar zones (BOYCE and KING 1959; BOYCE 1969 a). Later studies, however, have differentiated further morphological forms of matrix (RAO et al. 1978) although the significance of these is not yet clear.

Scanning electron microscopy of a calcium oxalate stone demonstrated the presence on some areas of the surface of alternating electron dense and light fibrils while in other areas a more amorphous granular material was present (BOYCE 1973). The fibrils were noted by BOYCE to assume a parallel orientation over the stone surface although others (ALONSO and SOMACARRERA 1973; SPECTOR et al. 1978) have not found this. Transmission electron microscopy showed that the "nuclei" of stones consist of organized spherules of matrix and crystallites as in intra-nephronic calculosis (Section II.1(e)) rather than of single crystals or aggregates of crystals (BOYCE 1973). The highly organized structure of the organic matrix, the intimate relationship between the organic and crystalline phases and the mere fact of its presence in all stones have led BOYCE and KING (1959) and others (WICKHAM 1976; HALLSON and ROSE 1979; ROSE and SULAIMAN 1982) to put forward the hypothesis that the observed architecture could only result from deposition or trapping of crystals upon or within a preformed matrix, thus attributing to the matrix a primary role in the genesis of stones.

The chemical analysis of stone matrix shows it to consist essentially of a series of protein-carbohydrate complexes (mucoproteins) (BOYCE and GARVEY 1956; KING and BOYCE 1957). However, the relative proportion of the individual components of matrix differs from that of similar macromolecular species in urine (Fig. 8) (BOYCE 1968, 1969 b; WICKHAM 1976). The constituent amino acids and carbohydrate moieties have been identified and reported by BOYCE and SULKIN (1956).

Immunological studies of stone matrix have consistently shown the presence of albumin, α_1- and α_2-globulins and occasionally γ-globulins. Tamm-Horsfall mucoprotein (TAMM and HORSFALL 1950) and its closely related mucoprotein complex, uromucoid, form a constant but small fraction of matrix. By far the

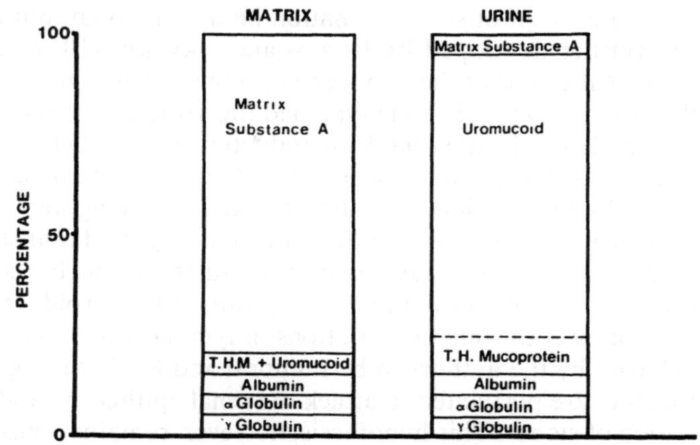

Fig. 8. The relative proportions of the various macromolecular constituents of stone matrix and urine. (Adapted from WICKHAM 1976)

most prominent antigenic constituent of matrix, found in all calculi, is a protein-polysaccharide called by the authors "matrix substance A" (BOYCE et al. 1962; KING and BOYCE 1963a). It may account for as much as 85% of the mucosubstance content of matrix (BOYCE 1969a).

Matrix substance A has been shown to consist of two-thirds protein, the remainder being made up of the carbohydrate sugars, galactose, mannose, methyl pentose, glucosamine and galactosamine with an overall molecular weight of 30,000–40,000 daltons (BOYCE and KING 1963). It originates from the renal parenchyma and has not been detected in the serum of stone-formers, nor in the serum or urine of persons with normal renal function (BOYCE et al. 1962; KING and BOYCE 1963a; BOYCE 1968).

The hypothesis that the presence of matrix substance A in urine is essential for the formation of stones was later weakened, however, by the observation that it was present in the urine of a variety of hospitalized patients – not all of whom had had stones (KEUTEL and KING 1964). Out of 104 patients studied, 70 were stone-formers of whom only 20 (29%) produced detectable amounts of matrix substance A in their urine; whereas of the remaining 34 non-stone-formers, 18 (53%) were found to excrete this mucosubstance. On the whole, the presence in the urine of matrix substance A was associated with infection of the urinary tract, particularly with the microorganisms *E. Coli*, *Klebsiella* and *Aerobacter aerogenes* (SENECA et al. 1964; KEUTEL and KING 1964). It was also noted in diseases involving renal injury and repair, an observation confirmed, in part, by FIDALGO and CHORDI (1964). To weaken further the hypothesis that matrix substance A promotes stone-formation, it has been shown recently that the fraction of matrix which contains matrix substance A actually *inhibits* the crystal growth of calcium oxalate rather than promotes it (GJALDBAEK and ROBERTSON 1980). Thus, although it is the main component of stone matrix, the precise role of matrix substance A in the genesis of stones is far from clear.

The concept of stone-formation being due to an immunological mechanism was further developed by BURCH and DAWSON (1969). Studying the age- and sex-distributions of the incidence of renal lithiasis in various parts of the world, they found that each stone type had the same age-of-onset pattern, the only difference being in the length of induction period before the onset. The implication was that there was a single underlying cause of stone-formation and that the induction period may be shortened or lengthened by infection or environmental factors. The authors further suggested that stone-formation is initiated in genetically predisposed individuals by a forbidden-clone of cells which synthesizes "autoantibodies", the growth of the forbidden-clone being triggered by spontaneous somatic mutations in lymphoid stem cells. The autoantibodies, believed by the authors to be humoral and likely to migrate in the α_2- globulin fraction, are postulated to attack the renal epithelium and act as foci for the initiation of stones. This hypothesis, however, remains untested.

The chemical analysis of urine shows that the main macromolecule is not matrix substance A but the so-called uromucoid group of mucoproteins (Fig. 8) which may include the mucoprotein of TAMM and HORSFALL (1950) or a condensation product of other unidentified mucoproteins with Tamm-Horsfall mucoprotein (WICKHAM 1976). This complex appears to originate from the normal renal cortex. MAXFIELD (1963) has pointed out that the conditions in urine are ideal for the induction of mucoprotein aggregation and that high concentrations of Tamm-Horsfall mucoprotein would be likely to coalesce readily with other macromolecules into a definable stone matrix.

Tamm-Horsfall mucoprotein has been shown to occur in two forms (TAMM and HORSFALL 1950; MAXFIELD 1959, 1960; KEUTEL et al. 1964; CORNELIUS et al. 1965). In the polymerized state, it is insoluble in 0.58 molar sodium chloride and in buffer solutions over the pH range 4.5 to 8.6. In the non-polymerized form it is soluble under these conditions. Later studies by MCQUEEN and ENGEL (1966) showed that lowering pH within the physiological range, addition of electrolytes and increase in magnesium concentration all produced aggregation. Similar aggregation was observed when urine flow rate fell below 25 ml/h (HAUGEN et al. 1980).

The evidence that uromucoid promotes stone-formation is largely circumstantial. First, although it has been inferred (but never proven) that uromucoid is the main precursor of the mucoprotein of stone matrix (MALEK and BOYCE 1973), it is itself only a minor constituent of stone matrix (KEUTEL et al. 1964). In this connection, however, MALEK and BOYCE (1973) note that sialic acid (which is frequently reported to be the terminal unit of the carbohydrate fraction of mucoproteins and is a moderate complexor of calcium (JAQUES et al. 1980)) is found regularly in the uromucoid complexes of urine but is virtually absent from stone matrix (KEUTEL et al. 1964; MALEK and BOYCE 1973). They go on to suggest that under the action of the urinary enzyme, sialidase (N-acetylneuraminidase), the terminal neuraminic acid group is removed, thereby converting uromucoid into the major constituent of matrix, inferred to be matrix substance A. Conclusive evidence of this conversion, however, has never been produced. Furthermore, more recent data indicate that, in fact, sialic acid residues do occur in stone matrix in significant quantities (MELICK et al. 1980).

The second point about uromucoid is that it is the most important constituent of hyaline casts (McQueen 1962, 1966), thought by some to be important for the trapping and gluing together of crystals (von Hemsbach 1856; Hallson and Rose 1979; Rose and Sulaiman 1982). Others, however, have found no significant relationship between cast formation and uromucoid concentration (Haugen et al. 1980) and large numbers of such casts have never been shown to increase the risk of stones (King 1967).

Thirdly, although it has been claimed by some that uromucoid excretion is increased in the urine of uninfected calcium stone-formers (Boyce et al. 1954a; Gale et al. 1966), other workers have not been able to confirm this observation (Thomas et al. 1960; King 1967; Bichler et al. 1976; Samuell 1979; Sophasan et al. 1980). Indeed, there are two reports that calcium stone-formers actually excrete less Tamm-Horsfall mucoprotein than do normal subjects (Wilkström and Wieslander 1981; Robertson et al. 1984).

Fourthly, it has been pointed out by the proponents of the uromucoid matrix theory that racially pure Negroes (who as an ethnic group are known to form stones less commonly than Caucasians) have little or no uromucoid in their urine (Keutel et al. 1964). There may, however, be other reasons why Negroes have fewer stones than Whites including differences in level of affluence and composition of the diet (Robertson et al. 1979c, 1980a, 1981b).

Finally, in vitro studies on the crystallization of calcium phosphate have been claimed to show that, in the presence of uromucoid derived from normal urine, the amount of precipitation is proportional to the concentration of uromucoid in the crystallizing solution (Boyce et al. 1954b). Similar studies on calcium oxalate apparently show that crystallization is enhanced in the presence of uromucoid and decreased in its absence (Hallson and Rose 1979). However, the uncertainty concerning what other materials might be added to or removed from urine in this study casts doubt on the authors' conclusions. Indeed, other workers have not been able to confirm the promotive role of uromucoid in the crystallization of calcium oxalate (Sophasan et al. 1980; Kitamura and Pak 1982; Kitamura et al. 1982) and other still have actually found it to be an inhibitor rather than a promoter of crystallization both of calcium oxalate (Robertson et al. 1981d, 1984; Scurr et al. 1981) and of uric acid (Sperling et al. 1965), but only when in its non-polymerized form (Scurr and Robertson 1984). In the polymerized form it promotes crystal agglomeration (Robertson 1985).

Antagonists of the matrix theory have accumulated evidence against uromucoid being important in the genesis of stones. First, as mentioned above, it is only a minor constituent of stone matrix (Keutel et al. 1964) and there is no direct evidence to suggest that its presence in stones is other than adventitious (Vermeulen et al. 1965). Indeed, simulated stones may be grown in urine in vitro, even when all the urinary colloids have been removed by dialysis (King and Boyce 1963b; Vermeulen et al. 1965). Under these circumstances the presence of colloids appears only to modify the crystal habit and texture of stones (McDonald et al. 1964). Second, the association of mucoprotein with mineral in the composite stone may be largely accounted for in terms of simple adsorption (Leal and Finlayson 1977). Indeed, uromucoid has been shown to coat crystals growing in its presence (MAXFIELD 1963). This has also been shown to occur in in vivo studies of stone induction both in rats (FINLAYSON et al. 1961) and in humans (SUTOR and O'FLYNN 1973). Third, since uromucoid originates from kidney tissue (KEUTEL et al. 1964), probably in the cells of the loop of Henle, distal convoluted tubules and collecting ducts (POLLAK and ARBEL 1969), it is possible that its increased production in certain stone-formers, particularly those with urinary tract infections may be the result of inflammation of the urinary tract either from the infecting organism itself or from the irritation caused by the crystals produced by the persistent increased excretion of one of the stone-forming salts. Indeed, it is still far from clear which comes first – the crystals or the organic matrix.

Finally, it has been reported by several groups that children excrete higher concentrations of Tamm-Horsfall mucoprotein in their urine than do adults (GALE et al. 1966; HAUGEN et al. 1978; MEBERG et al. 1979). Since 25 to 30% of children also have levels of calcium oxalate supersaturation as high as those of stone-formers and their mean calcium oxalate supersaturation level is as high as that of normal adults (ROBERTSON, unpublished results), it would be anticipated on the basis of their excretion of Tamm-Horsfall mucoprotein that children would have an incidence of idiopathic calcium stones at least as high as, if not higher than, that of adults. On the contrary, there is an extremely low incidence of such stones in this section of the population (GHAZALI et al. 1973; BENNET and COLODNY 1973; PURI et al. 1975; MALEK and KELALIS 1975; VAHLENSIECK and BASTIAN 1976, SINNO et al. 1979; CHURCHILL et al. 1980). Thus the hypothesis, that uromucoid is a possible promoter of stone disease is greatly weakened. The probable reasons for the low incidence of idiopathic stones in children are discussed in more detail in Section III 4(d).

Stimulated by the work of BOYCE and his colleagues, subsequent workers have gone on to shown that there are certain urinary polyelectrolytes, smaller than those considered by BOYCE, which interact specifically with calcium ions (ANDERSON et al. 1960; CHOW et al. 1968; SHEINFELD et al. 1978; RESNICK and BOYCE 1979b). A recent study has demonstrated that the molecular weight of these calcium-binding molecules is less than 50,000 daltons and that the calcium-binding activity in the urine of active calcium oxalate stone-formers is greater than that in the urine of both inactive stone-formers and normal control subjects (RESNICK et al. 1980).

It has also been demonstrated that stone-forming urine has a higher degree of sulphated mucopolysaccharides (MPS) than non-stone-forming urine although the quantity of total MPS was the same in the two groups. The sulphate MPS of the stone-formers formed insoluble calcium salts whereas those from normal urines generally remained soluble in the presence of calcium ions (FOYE et al. 1976). It is not known, however, whether or not these various calcium-binding polyelectrolytes are present in stone matrix.

Acid protein-containing macromolecules which are likely to have a high affinity for calcium have been identified in the matrix of stones. These proteins contain a high proportion of aspartic and glutamic acids (SPECTOR et al. 1976). In other studies, γ-carboxyglutamic acid (Gla), a constituent of vitamin K-dependent blood-clotting protein (NELSESTUEN and SUTTIE 1973), has been identified both in bone (Hauschka et al. 1975; Price et al. 1976) and in the matrix of calcium-containing stones (Lian et al. 1977). Gla has also been identified in urine (Joost et al. 1981 a) and it has been shown that calcium oxalate stone-formers excrete more of this in their urine than do normal subjects (Joost et al. 1981 b). The presence of Gla in both bone and stone-matrix has led Pak (1978) to suggest a positive role for this amino acid in the process of mineralization. Indeed, it is well documented that acidic proteins, similar to those found in stone matrix, are associated with mineralization in other biological systems (Glimcher and Krane 1964; Veis and Perry 1967; Travis et al. 1967).

In spite of 30 years work on the macromolecular constituents of stone matrix and of urine, however, the question still remains – is stone matrix a non-specific adsorbant onto pre-formed crystals or does it form a framework for nucleation and/or crystal growth and agglomeration?

b) Crystal Nucleation

Several mechanisms have been suggested by which some suitable component of the organic matrix of stone might initiate or promote the formation of urinary stones. The first of these involves the possible role of organic molecules as nucleating agents for the precipitation of calcium salts. Studies have shown, for example, that Formvar grids impregnated with the strong calcium-binding agent, ethylenediamine-N,N,N′,N′-tetraacetate (EDTA), are better nucleators of calcium phosphate deposition than are uncoated grids (Schwartz 1967), presumably because they produce a high local concentration of calcium. Similarly, Glimcher and Krane (1964) have shown that serine phosphate, a constituent of enamel protein and chelator of calcium ions, is a good nucleator of calcium phosphate. Since some of the macromolecular constituents of both stone and urine are claimed to be good complexors of calcium, it was suggested, by analogy, that such molecules may trigger off the crystallization of calcium in the urinary tract (Boyce et al. 1954b, 1955). In a later study, Spector et al. (1976) speculated that the predominance of acidic amino acids in stone matrix and the fact that stones of particular mineral composition have a fairly high specific amino acid composition together indicated that the organic matrix might play a role as a nucleating agent.

An alternative nucleating mechanism has been proposed (Pinto 1973; Bernshtam and Pinto 1976; Paternain et al. 1980) according to which a mucoprotein component of stone matrix nucleates the crystallization of calcium salts through two types of binding site, one specific for calcium and one for phosphate. The authors claim that the latter may also bind oxalate via phosphate bridges of the type:

mucoprotein – phosphate – oxalate – oxalate ------

It is difficult, however, to conceive chemically of such a bridging between anions without a cation such as calcium or magnesium being involved as an intermediate. There has, as yet, been no corroboration of this hypothesis.

A third possibility has been recently proposed by Drach et al. (1980) from their study on the effect of urinary macromolecules on the crystallization kinetics of calcium oxalate in a continuous crystallizer system. This showed that when diluted urine (5% v/v) filtered through a 3 μm pore filter was added to synthetic urine, the growth rate of calcium oxalate crystals generated in the crystallizer was lower than that in the synthetic urine alone. On the other hand, the nucleation rate in the presence of urine was much increased. The decrease in growth rate and increase in nucleation rate were greater in the presence of 5% stone-forming urine than 5% normal urine. Since uromucoid (at a concentration of approximately 1/20 that in normal urine) produced the same order of changes in growth and nucleation rates as did 5% urine, the authors concluded that it was the macromolecular constituents of urine which were responsible for these observed changes. If true, this would imply that stone-formers would have more crystals of calcium oxalate in their urine than normal subjects but that they would be smaller. This prediction, however, is not consistent with the observation from studies on crystalluria in fresh, warm urine which generally have shown that the crystals of calcium oxalate in stone-forming urine tend to be larger and more aggregated than those found in normal urine (SENGBUCH and TIMMERMANN 1957; ROBERTSON et al. 1969; ROBERTSON and PEACOCK 1972; VALYASEVI and DHANAMITTA 1974; ADAMTHWAITE 1983). This discrepancy has not yet been reconciled.

Other studies have shown, however, that macromolecules may not influence the nucleation stage of crystallization in *whole* urine. First, there is no evidence that there is any difference either in the type of crystallization or in the precipitability of urinary salts in whole urine from normal as compared with stone-forming subjects (BOYCE et al. 1954c; LIGHT and ZINSSER 1961; ROBERTSON and NORDIN 1969). Nor is there any difference in the level of supersaturation at which both calcium oxalate and calcium phosphate nucleate in simple inorganic solutions compared with the levels at which these salts precipitate in whole urine (ROBERTSON et al. 1972a). It would seem unlikely, therefore, that the crystallization of calcium salts is triggered off preferentially in stone-forming urine by heterogeneous nucleation since spontaneous crystallization would be observed to commence at a lower level of supersaturation than that found in inorganic solutions.

c) Crystal Aggregation

The second possible mechanism by which urinary macromolecules may promote stone-formation is through the "gluing" together of crystals which have already formed in a more proximal portion of the urinary tract. According to this model, the matrix may be considered as providing a framework on which crystals may be trapped or which itself may act as a bridge between crystals. As mentioned earlier, the trapping theory dates back over a century to VON HEMSBACH (1856) although this concept has been recently revived (HALLSON and ROSE 1979; HALLSON et al. 1981). The bridging theory (WATANABE 1972) rests on no solid evidence. On the contrary, there is evidence to suggest that crystal bridging can take place in urine in the absence of macromolecules FINLAYSON et al. 1961; KING and BOYCE 1963b; MCDONALD et al. 1964; VERMEULEN et al.

1965). To complicate matters, however, SCURR et al. (1981) have recently shown that there is a weak-to-moderate promoter of calcium oxalate crystal aggregation in the EDTA-insoluble residue from urine and also a very strong promoter of aggregation in the EDTA-insoluble fraction of stone matrix. On the other hand, when these fractions were re-mixed with the main macromolecular constituents of urine and of stone matrix in the same relative proportions as in whole urine or matrix, the net reaction of both mixtures is strongly inhibitory. It has also been suggested from studies on feeding hydroxyproline in the diet that this amino acid might stimulate crystal aggregation (VALYASEVI et al. 1973). More detailed examination of the data, however, shows that, during the period of hydroxyproline feeding, the urinary excretion of oxalate doubled. Since an increase in urinary oxalate markedly increases calcium oxalate crystal growth and aggregation (ROBERTSON and PEACOCK 1980) and is probably the most important risk factor in the formation of calcium oxalate stones (ROBERTSON et al. 1978), it seems that this is a more likely explanation of the effect of feeding hydroxyproline than any effect of the amino acid per se in urine.

The most likely mechanism by which a polyelectrolyte such as uromucoid or a glycosaminoglycan might stimulate aggregation is one involving reduction of the surface potential on the crystal. Normally the stability of a hydrophobic colloid or suspension (such as a spontaneously crystallizing system) is maintained when the resultant force of attraction due to the combination of van der Waal's forces and viscous binding forces and the repulsion due to the surface potential of the particles is greater than the kinetic energy of the particles (FINLAYSON 1978). The surface potential of a particle is represented by the charge of the ionized layer adsorbed on this surface (Stern's layer).This is measurable experimentally as the ζ-potential (zeta potential). Calcium oxalate crystals in synthetic urine (in the absence of polyelectrolytes) have a net positive ζ-po-

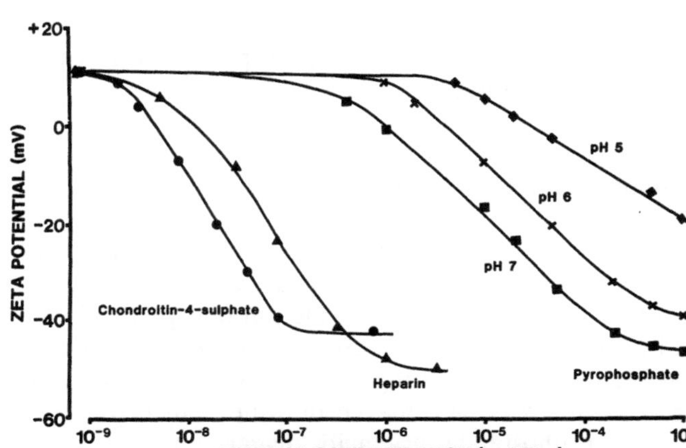

Fig. 9. The effect of various polyanionic inhibitors of aggregation on the zeta potential associated with crystals of calcium oxalate monohydrate (MARSHALL and ROBERTSON, in preparation)

tential of about + 10 to + 20 mV (CURRERI et al. 1979; ROBERTSON et al. 1984). Addition of polyanions such as heparin, sodium alginate, chondroitin-4-sulphate and the glycosaminoglycan inhibitory fraction from urine negates the positive ζ-potential in a dose-response manner (Fig. 9). At the mean concentrations of the polyelectrolytes generally found in urine there is a net negative ζ-potential of − 15 to − 30 mV and so the crystals repel each other (ROBERTSON et al. 1984). At these concentrations the polyelectrolytes are inhibitors of aggregation (see Section II. 4 (d)). If, however, these polyanions are added at lower concentrations than found in normal urine, a ζ-potential is established which is close to zero. Under these conditions the crystals may aggregate much more readily. Such a phenomenon has been observed in a study of the effect on the sedimentation rate of calcium carbonate suspensions in the presence of sodium alginate, stone matrix substance, albumin and chondroitin-4-sulphate (KIMURA et al. 1976). Thus a reduced amount of inhibitors of aggregation in urine may be worse than having no inhibitors at all as this may produce a situation in which aggregation is actually stimulated.

d) Crystal Adhesion to Cell Walls

From a consideration of the kinetics of crystallization and urinary flow (FINLAYSON 1977b; FINLAYSON and REID 1978) it has been calculated that there must be crystal-to-membrane adhesion before stone-formation can occur in the renal tubules or in the renal pelvis (the so-called "fixed particle theory"which is discussed in more detail in Section II.5 (c)). Basically, this requires crystals formed in the renal tubules (or pelvis) to be actively sequestered to the cell walls of some part of the renal system. Scanning electron micrographs of calcium oxalate crystals apparently attached to tubule walls by strands of organic material have been demonstrated in a patient with primary hyperoxaluria (MORGENROTH et al. 1968) and in rats given large intraperitoneal injections of sodium oxalate (KHAN et al. 1979; DYKSTRA and HACKETT 1979). No evidence of this phenomenon has so far been produced, however, in patients with idiopathic urinary stones.

e) Inhibition of Crystal Dissolution

It has been shown that as much as 70% of the surface of urinary crystals of calcium oxalate may be coated by adsorbed proteins and mucoproteins (LEAL and FINLAYSON 1977). Crystals of calcium phosphate (HANSEN et al. 1976) and uric acid (SPERLING et al. 1965) are also known to adsorb macromolecules. It seems possible that such a coating might limit the rate of re-dissolution of the salt concerned which may be achieved in urine. This is theoretically possible in the case of calcium phosphate, uric acid, magnesium ammonium phosphate and cystine crystals but is less likely to be achieved for calcium oxalate. There is evidence that the rate of dissolution of both calcium-containing stones (ROBERTSON, unpublished results) (Fig. 10) and uric acid stones (ISMAIL and TAWASHI 1980) is

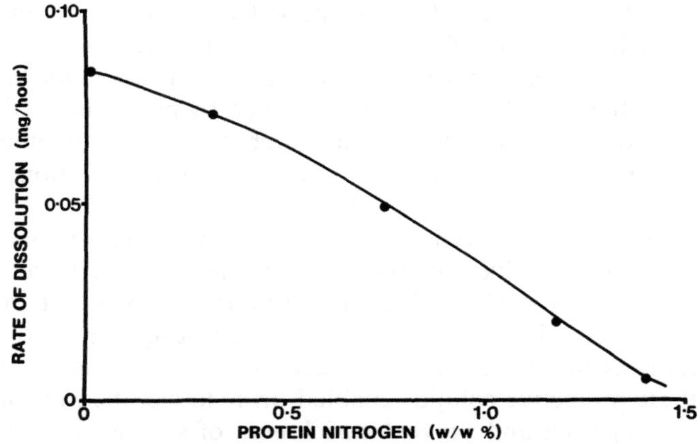

Fig. 10. The effect of increasing matrix content of calcium phosphate stones (expressed as protein nitrogen w/w%) on the rate of dissolution of the stone in saline buffered at pH 6

inversely proportional to the matrix content of the stone. Thus the matrix may act as a barrier for dissolution of the mineral associated with it. Indeed, it has been shown recently that crystals in stones are surrounded by a matrix skin (KHAN et al. 1983). Although perhaps not the primary function of the matrix, it may be an important factor both during the initiation phase of the stone (when any process hindering the re-dissolution of the critical particle before it has become established as the nucleus of a stone must be considered as an additional hazard to the patient) and during treatment (where optimal conditions are necessary to re-dissolve the stone).

4. Inhibitor Theory

a) General Principles

As an alternative to the matrix theory, a diametrically opposite, but equally attractive hypothesis was put forward which primarily attributes the disorder, not to the presence of excessive amounts of macromolecules in the urine of stone-formers, but to an absence on deficiency in their urine of certain protective agents. These are considered to inhibit one or more of the various processes of crystallization of stone-forming salts, much in the same way as water-conditioners prevent the formation of boiler-scale in water pipes in hard water areas. According to this hypothesis, normal urine is postulated to contain sufficient of these "crystal poisons" to protect the individual against the formation of crystals and stones in the urinary tract, whereas urine from stone-formers is deficient in protective inhibitors.

Over the years many constituents of urine have been invoked to account for the relative stability of normal urine to precipitation. The first reference to the presence of crystal modifiers came as early as 1879 in a book by ORD entitled

"On the Influence of Colloids upon Crystalline Form and Cohesion". In it ORD described the modifying effects of certain organic colloids on the crystal habit of calcium oxalate, calcium carbonate and uric acid. In particular, he emphasized the globular form often assumed by precipitates of these salts in the presence of such colloids and suggested that this phenomenon might have some bearing on the formation of stones. Similar observations were made by SCHADE (1928) and LICHTWITZ (1944).

Another observed property of the hydrophilic colloids in urine was their ability to stabilize precipitating salt solutions which were themselves still in the colloidal state. This led LICHTWITZ and ROSENBACH (1909) to suggest that protective colloids were essential to preventing supersaturated urine from crystallizing out. It was also suggested that, by lowering the surface tension of urine, these protective colloids enabled urine to wet the mucous membrane lining the urinary tract and prevent enrichment of salts at the urinary-mucosal interface (SPITZER and HILLKOWITZ 1924).

The concept of protective colloids was later re-emphasized by BUTT (1952). He postulated that stone-formation was initiated either by the growth of crystals of the stone-forming salts from highly concentrated urines or by the coagulation of dispersed colloidal solutions of these salts owing to a reduction (or removal) of the zeta potential on the colloid particle surface. BUTT suggested that if sufficient charged colloids were present, these might be adsorbed on to the particle surface and possibly prevent both growth and coagulation of the sol taking place. In a further study (BUTT 1956) it was claimed that normal urine had more of this protective material than stone-forming urine.

Several workers have since refuted the suggestion that protective colloids are important for the prevention of stone-formation. Firstly, it was shown that the solubilities of calcium oxalate, uric acid and the alkaline earth phosphates are not enhanced by various hydrophilic colloids (NEWCOMB 1930; SISK and TOENHART 1937; DULCE 1958a, b, c), although this would not be anticipated to be the main effect of macromolecular inhibitors since their concentration in urine is insufficient to complex enough calcium to increase the solubility of calcium salts to any significant degree (SHEINFELD et al. 1978). The second objection to the protective colloid hypothesis comes from early studies (GOLDBERG 1934). These suggested that normal urine did not, in fact, reduce the rate of coagulation of calcium oxalate suspensions although more recent research has provided convincing evidence that the degree of aggregation of seed crystals of both calcium oxalate (ROBERTSON et al. 1973a, 1976a, 1981d; FELIX et al. 1977; BAUMANN et al. 1977; BOWYER et al. 1979; RYALL et al. 1981c; SCURR et al. 1981) and calcium phosphate (HANSEN et al. 1976) may be inhibited by a macromolecular constituent of urine. Furthermore, the macromolecular constituents of urine decrease the adhesion between crystals and glass surfaces (GILL et al. 1977). The importance of macromolecular weight inhibitors will be dealt with in more detail in a later section.

After the initial objections to the protective colloid hypothesis, attention was directed to the lower molecular weight constituents of urine following the observation of VERMEULEN et al. (1958) that there was an unidentified, dialyzable (and therefore non-colloidal) substance which inhibited the precipitation of calcium phosphate in vitro. HOWARD and THOMAS (1958) (and THOMAS and HOWARD 1959) confirmed these findings using the technique developed by YENDT et al. (1955). Likening stone-formation on an organic matrix to the calcification of cartilage, HOWARD showed that if poorly mineralized cartilage from rachitic rats is incubated in urine from normal subjects, calcification will not readily take place, even in the presence of high concentrations of calcium and phosphate. On the other hand urine from stone-formers frequently, but by no means always, induced mineralization of the cartilage. Urines which failed to mineralize the cartilage were referred to as "good" and those which induced calcification as "evil" (HOWARD 1962). The difference was attributed to the presence of an inhibitor of crystallization in "good" urine and its absence in "evil" urine. From their observations, HOWARD and his colleagues suggested that it was a phosphopeptide (HOWARD et al. 1962). Further studies led to the belief that there were at least three acidic peptides in urine (HOWARD et al. 1967; SMITH and MCCALL 1969) which had the ability to inhibit both the mineralization of rachitic rat cartilage and the spontaneous precipitation of calcium phosphate in vitro using the system devised by SOLOMONS and NEUMAN (1960). although some were later considered to be artefactual (SMITH et al. 1973a).

The technique of studying inhibitors by observing their effect on the mineralization of rachitic rat cartilage has been heavily criticised by FLEISCH (1978) on the basis that the cartilage contains many active enzymes which may destroy some of the inhibitors being tested but not others. Furthermore, the test substance or urine may influence the activity of such enzymes thereby altering the precipitation of calcium phosphate by a mechanism unrelated to that by which crystal growth inhibitors are thought to act.

During the investigations on "good" and "evil" urine, it was noted that magnesium conferred a marked inhibitory effect on the mineralization of rachitic rat cartilage (MUKAI and HOWARD 1963; JETHI and WADKINS 1971) although it could no account for all the inhibitory activity in this system. Magnesium was also found to inhibit the re-hardening of tooth enamel (FEAGIN et al. 1969), the nucleation and crystal growth of hydroxyapatite (BACHRA and FISCHER 1969; BISAZ et al. 1978), and the conversion of amorphous calcium phosphate to crystalline hydroxyapatite (EANES and POSNER 1968; TERMINE et al. 1970; BOSKEY and POSNER 1974; NANCOLLAS et al. 1976). It has only a small effect, however, on the aggregation of hydroxyapatite crystals (HANSEN et al. 1976).

Magnesium has also been claimed to inhibit the in vitro precipitation of calcium oxalate (HAMMARSTEN 1929; DULCE 1958a, b, c; DESMARS and TAWASHI 1973) although subsequent studies have not confirmed this (SUTOR 1969; WELSHMAN and MCGEOWN 1972; ROBERTSON et al. 1973b; MEYER and SMITH 1975b; FETNER et al. 1978) except at concentrations of magnesium sufficiently high to increase the complexing of oxalate (ROBERTSON et al. 1973b; MEYER and SMITH 1975b; FELIX et al. 1977; RYALL et al. 1981b; HALLSON et al. 1982a).

This emphasises one of the problems of studying the effect of magnesium on the crystallization of calcium salts, namely that at the concentrations necessary to produce an observable effect on the rates of crystal nucleation, growth or aggregation, magnesium complexes significant amounts of the precipitating anion concerned. This reduces both the saturation level of the crystallizing solution with respect to the salt concerned and, consequently, the rate of crystallization. Whether or not magnesium acts as a "crystal poison" in its own right is not clear, although in one study on factors affecting the crystal growth of calcium oxalate, there appeared to be no significant inhibition of growth after the complexing of oxalate with the added magnesium had been taken into account (MEYER and SMITH 1975 b).

In vivo studies in which urinary magnesium has been increased by oral administration of magnesium supplements have also failed to influence significantly the in vitro crystallization of either calcium phosphate or calcium oxalate when added to the urines concerned (HODGKINSON and MARSHALL 1972; FETNER et al. 1978), although dietary magnesium supplementation has been claimed to have a marked beneficial effect on the rate of calcium stone recurrence in multiple stone-formers (MOORE and BUNCE 1964; DANIELSON et al. 1979; JOHANSSON et al. 1980 a, 1981). There are, however, several puzzling features about the latter observation. First, if a high urinary magnesium is important for the prevention of calcium stone-formation, then it might be anticipated that a low urinary magnesium excretion would increase the risk of stone disease. Indeed, some studies claim to show that stone-formers, as a population, have a lower urinary excretion of magnesium (SUTTON and WATSON 1968; OREOPOULOS et al. 1968; HODGKINSON 1974; TISELIUS et al. 1978) or a lower magnesium/(calcium × oxalate) concentration ratio (TAKASAKI and SHIMANO 1967) than normal subjects. Since, however, urinary magnesium falls with age in both sexes and since males excrete more magnesium than females (ROBERTSON 1976 a; JOHANSSON et al. 1980 b), it is vital to match the populations being compared for these factors. Indeed, when care is taken to match stone-formers and controls for both age and sex, the difference in the urinary magnesium between the two groups is eliminated (ROBERTSON et al. 1968; ZECHNER and LATAL 1978; JOHANSSON et al. 1980 b; BACH et al. 1981; ROBERTSON et al. 1984). For example, the effect of age on magnesium excretion (ROBERTSON 1976 a) almost certainly explains the apparent difference in urinary magnesium of about 1 mmol/day between stone-formers (mean age 46 years) and normal controls (mean age 35 years) as reported by HODGKINSON (1974). It may also account for the apparent differences reported by other workers since there is a tendency in many studies to use laboratory staff as controls which may result in the selection of a control population whose mean age is at least 10 years less than that of a randomly selected group of stone-formers.

The urinary inhibitor which undoubtedly has commanded most attention is pyrophosphate (FLEISCH and NEUMAN 1961). This was first identified in urine by FLEISCH and BISAZ (1962 a) and shown to be a potent inhibitor of both calcium phosphate (FLEISCH and BISAZ 1962 a, b; FLEISCH et al. 1966, 1968) and calcium oxalate precipitation (FLEISCH and BISAZ 1964). However, it requires almost 10 times the concentration of pyrophosphate to inhibit calcium oxalate precipitation as that to inhibit calcium phosphate precipitation. Furthermore, pyrophosphate does not influence the precipitation of the other main constituents of stones, namely, magnesium ammonium phosphate and uric acid (FLEISCH et al. 1967).

Since the initial work of FLEISCH's group there have been many reports confirming the potency of pyrophosphate as an inhibitor of the crystallization of calcium phosphate (LEWIS et al. 1966; FRANCIS 1969; FEAGIN et al. 1969; MARSHALL and NANCOLLAS 1969; TERMINE et al. 1970; ROBERTSON 1973; SMITH et al. 1973b; SUTOR et al. 1978; LEGEROS and MORALES 1973; MEYER et al. 1974; HANSEN et al. 1976; BISAZ et al. 1978; EVANS et al. 1980) and of calcium oxalate (SUTOR 1969; WELSHMAN and MCGEOWN 1972; ROBERTSON et al. 1973b; NANCOLLAS and GARDNER 1974; MEYER and SMITH 1975b; GARDNER 1975, 1976, 1978; FELIX et al. 1977; DOREMUS et al. 1978; DRACH et al. 1978), although others have not confirmed this latter observation (SARIG et al. 1973; LEGEROS and MORALES 1973).

In spite of the potency of pyrophosphate as an inhibitor of many crystallization processes, however, it is not clear what role, if any, it has in the prevention of calcium stone-formation. Although preliminary reports indicated that some stone-formers might have a decreased excretion of pyrophosphate (FLEISCH and BISAZ 1962b; RUSSELL et al. 1964), this has not been confirmed in larger series of patients (LEWIS et al. 1966; RUSSELL and HODGKINSON 1966; O'BRIEN et al. 1967) apart from one report from FLEISCH's own group (BAUMANN et al. 1977). Furthermore, it has been claimed that at normal urinary concentrations of pyrophosphate (10–50 μmol/l), its contribution towards the overall inhibitory activity of urine is very small with respect to both calcium oxalate (10–15%) (ROBERTSON et al. 1973a; MEYER and SMITH 1975b; DRACH et al. 1978) and calcium phosphate (9%) (BISAZ et al. 1978). Therefore any reduction in pyrophosphate excretion from normal would be of little consequence as regards the crystallization of calcium salts in urine. However, if pyrophosphate excretion is increased above normal, the contribution towards the overall level of inhibitory activity may be increased (ROBERTSON et al. 1976d; ROBERTSON 1985). This may be achieved by oral administration of orthophosphate (FLEISCH et al. 1964; RUSSEL et al. 1964; LEWIS et al. 1966; RUSSELL and HODGKINSON 1966; O'BRIEN et al. 1967; ROBERTSON et al. 1976d; THOMAS 1978). This increases pyrophosphate excretion through some renal mechanism which results in the rapid clearance of pyrophosphate without a change in the blood concentration (RUSSELL et al. 1976).

Many other urinary ions, many of them trace constituents, have been shown to modify the in vitro precipitation of calcium salts. For calcium phosphate, zinc, cadmium, magnesium and cobalt inhibit both the mineralization of rachitic rat cartilage and the precipitation of calcium phosphate in vitro (THOMAS et al. 1963; BIRD and THOMAS 1963; MEYER and ANGINO 1977). Other suggested inhibitors for this salt include sodium (SOBEL and HANOK 1952; MODLIN 1967b), fluoride (TAVES and NEUMAN 1964; BACHRA and FISCHER 1969; JETHI and WADKINS 1971; MEYER and NANCOLLAS 1972), tin (MEYER and NANCOLLAS 1972; MEYER and ANGINO 1977), copper and aluminium (MEYER and ANGINO 1977), citrate (SMITH et al. 1973a; SUTOR et al. 1978; BISAZ et al. 1978; BRECEVIC and FÜREDI-MILHOFER 1979) and its trace metal complexes with iron, chromium and aluminium (MEYER and THOMAS 1982a), nucleoside phosphate (MEYER et al. 1974) and, more recently, phosphocitrate (HOWARD and BECKER 1976; WILLIAMS and SALLIS 1981; TEW et al. 1981) and N-sulpho-2-amino tricarbyllate (a sulphamate analogue of phosphocitrate (BROWN and SALLIS 1983)). Non-physiological ions, such as imidodiphosphate (ROBERTSON and FLEISCH 1970) and diphosphonates (FRANCIS 1969; FLEISCH et al. 1970; MEYER and NANCOLLAS 1973; OHATA and PAK 1973), are also potent inhibitors of calcium phosphate precipitation.

Many of the above-mentioned ions are also known to inhibit the crystallisation of calcium oxalate, namely, tin (EUSEBIO and ELLIOT 1967), although not in the physiological concentration range (MEYER and ANGINO 1977), and phosphocitrate (HOWARD 1976; WILLIAMS and SALLIS 1981). Of the other trace metals, vanadium and lead are said to be effective inhibitors of calcium oxalate crystal growth in physiological concentrations (EUSEBIO and ELLIOT 1967) but copper, zinc and aluminium are not (MEYER and ANGINO 1977). Some trace metal complexes with citrate have been shown to inhibit crystal growth (MEYER and THOMAS 1982b). Certain non-physiological ions are also effective inhibitors of calcium oxalate crystallization and some may be of interest from the point of view of treatment of the disorder. These include phytate (SUTOR 1969), certain synthetic dye-stuffs (SUTOR 1969), methylene blue (SUTOR 1969; ROLLINS and FINLAYSON 1973) (although others have not confirmed this (ROBERTSON et al. 1973b)), N-sulpho-2-amino tricarbyllate (BROWN and SALLIS 1983) and diphosphonates (FRASER et al. 1972; ROBERTSON et al. 1973b; PAK et al. 1975b; WILL et al. 1976; MEYER et al. 1977b).

One of the most commonly studied ions is citrate (LIGHT and ZINSSER 1961; WELSHMAN and McGEOWN 1972; SMITH et al. 1973b; MEYER and SMITH 1975b; DOREMUS et al. 1978; BAUMANN and WACKER 1979) but this appears only to be active at concentrations high enough to cause significant complexing of calcium ions (MEYER and SMITH 1975b; FELIX et al. 1977). Several reports claim that idiopathic stone-formers excrete significantly less citrate in their urine than do normal subjects (HODGKINSON 1962; ELLIOT and RIBEIRO 1972; WELSHMAN and McGEOWN 1976; SCHWILLE et al. 1979; PYLYPCHUK et al. 1979; BUTZ 1982; RUDMAN et al. 1982; NICAR et al. 1983; MENON and MAHLE 1983). Others, however, have not confirmed this difference (ROBERTSON et al. 1968, 1971, 1978; MODLIN 1969; MARSHALL and BARRY 1973; RUDMAN et al. 1980). One of the problems with citrate excretion, as with that of magnesium, is that it is dependent on age and sex; it changes with age (WELSHMAN and McGEOWN 1976; ROBERTSON (unpublished results) and is generally higher in women than in men (HODGKINSON 1962; ROBERTSON et al. 1968; ELLIOT and RIBEIRO 1972; WELSHMAN and McGEOWN 1976, SCHWILLE et al. 1979). Since several of the above studies did not take these factors (particularly the age-related changes) into account when comparing stone-formers and normals, the comparisons are often between groups whose average age is 10 or more years different (HODGKINSON 1962; WELSHMAN and McGEOWN 1976; PYLYPCHUK et al. 1979). Since a difference of 10 years reduces urinary citrate by about 0.4 mmol/day, this alone accounts for a large proportion of the supposed differences between patients and normals in these studies. When normals and stone-formers are matched for age and sex, the apparent difference between them is almost completely lost (ROBERTSON et al. 1968).

Other factors which may cause a reduction in urinary citrate (and must therefore be taken into account in any comparison between stone-formers and normals) are renal tubular acidosis (FOURMAN and ROBINSON 1953; ROBERTSON et al. 1968), renal failure (HODGKINSON 1962), primary hyperoxaluria (ROBERTSON et al. 1968), bowel disease (ELLIOT and SOLES 1974; SMITH et al. 1979; RUDMAN et al. 1980) and, to some extent, urinary tract infection (CONWAY et al. 1949; HODGKINSON 1962; ROBERTSON et al. 1968). If the stone-formers are not well screened to remove patients with these abnormalities, the data of the stone-formers may be biased towards low values.

Since only a small fraction of total urinary inhibitory activity towards calcium oxalate appears to be due to small ions such as magnesium, pyrophosphate and citrate (ROBERTSON et al. 1973a, b; MEYER and SMITH 1975b), attention has again been drawn to the effectiveness of certain urinary polyelectrolytes as inhibitors of the crystallization of this salt in urine (CRAWFORD et al. 1968; ROBERTSON et al. 1973a, b, 1976a; GILL et al. 1977; ITO and COE 1977; FELIX et al. 1977; GARDNER and DOREMUS 1978; DOREMUS et al. 1978; NAKAGAWA et al. 1978, 1981; SALLIS and LUMLEY 1979; BOWYER et al. 1979; SCHRIER et al. 1979, 1981; COE et al. 1980; SCURR et al. 1981; ROBERTSON et al. 1981d; RYALL et al. 1981b). These macromolecular inhibitors have been variously claimed to be glycosaminoglycans (ROBERTSON et al. 1973a, b, 1976a, 1981b; GARDNER and DOREMUS 1978; SALLIS and LUMLEY 1979; BOWYER et al. 1979; SCURR et al. 1981; RYALL et al. 1981b; RESNICK et al. 1982; GJALDBAEK 1982), acidic peptides (ITO and COE 1977), glycoproteins (GILL et al. 1977; NAKAGAWA et al. 1981, 1983) and RNA-like material (SCHRIER et al. 1979, 1981). More recently, non-polymerized Tamm-Horsfall mucoprotein has also been shown to be an inhibitor of the crystallization of this salt (SCURR et al. 1981; ROBERTSON et al. 1981d, 1984).

Studies on the effect of macromolecular inhibitors on the crystallization of calcium phosphate have shown that although they may inhibit the aggregation of pre-formed crystals of the salt (HANSEN et al. 1976), quantitatively they only account for a small percentage of the overall inhibition of the precipitation of this salt (BAUMANN et al. 1977; BISAZ et al. 1978; SUTOR et al. 1979).

When comparisons have been made between idiopathic stone-formers and normals, some workers claim that the patients have less net inhibitory activity than do normals in their urine towards the crystallization of both calcium oxalate (DENT and SUTOR 1971; ROBERTSON and PEACOCK 1972; TEOTIA and TEOTIA 1975; ROBERTSON et al. 1976c; LIGABUE et al. 1979; COE et al. 1980; TISELIUS and FORNANDER 1981) and calcium phosphate (BAUMANN et al. 1977). Others, however, have not been able to show any such difference between the two groups (ROSE 1975; PYLYPCHUK et al. 1979; BAUMANN and WACKER 1979).

One problem arising from the comparison of urinary inhibitor measurements from different centres is that each group of workers tends to use a different method for assessing "inhibitory activity" in urine. Furthermore, some have concentrated on factors affecting the crystallization of calcium oxalate, while others have studied inhibitors of calcium phosphate crystallization. Another problem is that there is no concensus in the literature about the definition of "inhibitory activity" or of "inhibitors of crystallization". Some workers have used these terms to refer to ions (or fractions of urine) which reduce the *rate of nucleation* (homogeneous or, more usually, heterogeneous) of new crystals of calcium salts; others refer to inhibitors as factor which reduce the *rate of crystal growth* of added or newly formed seed crystals of the salt concerned; and others still describe them as inhibitors of the *growth and aggregation* (or agglomeration) of added or newly formed crystals.

A further problem in the definition of an inhibitor is deciding on whether it acts as a complexor of calcium, oxalate or phosphate (thereby reducing the rate of some crystallization process by reducing the supersaturation pressure on the system) or whether it functions primarily as a "crystal poison" at concentrations below those at which significant complexation occurs. Some inhibitors, such as citrate, may even operate through both mechanisms (MEYER and SMITH 1975b). In future, studies on inhibitory activity should state clearly which particular stage in the crystallization is being retarded and which salt is being studied (RANDOLPH and DRACH 1981b).

However, even when the use of the term "inhibitor" is properly defined, there is the problem of how to treat and store urine between the time of voiding and the time of measurement of inhibitory activity. The main concern must be to ensure the survival of any labile inhibitors during the collection and storage period. The main causes of loss of activity are infection of the urine and precipitation on cooling and standing of one or more of the stone-forming salts which may adsorb inhibitors thereby reducing the concentration in the urine supernatant. Usually the first problem can be avoided by using either freshly voided urine, deep-frozen urine or urine collected and stored with some preservative added, provided the latter has no effect on any of the inhibitors. If, however, urine does become infected with (say) a urea-splitting organism, this may alter the balance between the inhibitors and promoters in urine since pyrophosphate and citrate may be destroyed. Urinary pH is increased thereby increasing the risk of precipitation of phosphatic salts which may adsorb the very inhibitors in which one is interested.

The problem of precipitation of stone-forming salts and adsorption of inhibitors, however, is more difficult to overcome since the measures taken to prevent the crystallization of one salt (or to dissolve any crystals which do precipitate) may initiate the precipitation of another. For example, acidification of urine to dissolve any phosphatic deposits will cause uric acid to precipitate out and conversely alkalinization to dissolve uric acid crystals will initiate calcium phosphate precipitation.

At first sight, the answer to these problems is to use freshly voided urine, diluted to between 1% and 5% in (say) saline to re-dissolve any crystals present and at the same time re-solubilize any inhibitors (or promoters) bound to the crystal surfaces. There are, however, possible objections to using diluted urine (FLEISCH 1978; ROBERTSON 1985). There are also objections to using freshly voided samples of urine, since the inhibitor level in any one sample may not be typical for that individual. It is known, for example, that there are diurnal variations in the excretion of the glycosaminoglycan inhibitors (ROBERTSON 1976b), magnesium and citrate (ROBERTSON 1969c; MARSHALL et al. 1972b) and this probably applies to pyrophosphate as well since its excretion rate is strongly related to that of orthophosphate (RUSSELL et al. 1976) which is known to have a diurnal rhythm (ROBERTSON 1969c). To compare individuals correctly, urine samples would have to be collected over a standard period of time at a set point during the day.

To overcome the problem of diurnal fluctuations, one alternative is to collect a 24-hour sample of urine (assuming that infection can be prevented by deep-freezing or by adding a preservative). Provided that precautions are taken to re-dissolve any crystals which form during the collection period, it might be possible to measure the inhibitory effect of various extracts of the 24-hour sample *at the same concentration* as in the whole urine.

The main problem, however, in assessing inhibitory activity in urine concerns the choice of a suitable test system which will measure the effect of the inhibitor under study only on the *rate processes occurring at the crystal-solution interface* and not some secondary effect on the rate of crystallization such as a reduction in urinary supersaturation owing to the complexation of one of the crystallizing species. Ideally, the test should be carried out in whole urine (FLEISCH 1978; FLEISCH et al. 1984) but, under these conditions, the rate of crystallization will also be influenced by the level of supersaturation and the oxalate/calcium or calcium/phosphate ratio of the urine (ROBERTSON and PEACOCK 1980). These latter factors must be fixed since at any given initial level of supersaturation, the *amount* of crystalline material forming before equilibrium is reached is dependent on these ratios (ROBERTSON et al. 1981 c, d). There is a further problem if the voided urine has already exceeded the formation product of either calcium oxalate or calcium phosphate since it will have crystals of one of these salts present in it. These cannot be re-dissolved without drastically reducing the saturation of the urine. There is therefore an immediate impasse. Prior removal of any such crystals to provide a clear supernatant is also undesirable since, firstly, this may remove inhibitors (and/or promoters) adsorbed on the surface of the crystals and, secondly, will leave behind a saturation level which is unknown and bears no relationship to that of the original urine. Even if this saturation level were known precisely (by taking into account all the possible complexing of calcium, oxalate and phosphate ions), some standard activity product with a fixed oxalate/calcium or calcium/phosphate ratio would have to be established in the urine before measuring the inhibitory activity. Urinary pH too would have to be fixed as both the calcium phosphate saturation level (ROBERTSON and NORDIN 1969, 1976) and the activities of certain of the known inhibitors in urine, particularly pyrophosphate (FELIX et al. 1977), are strongly dependent on hydrogen ion activity. To achieve this set of conditions, carefully calculated amounts of calcium, oxalate and buffered phosphate would have to be added to the urine. In theory, this would be possible, but in practice it would be extremely difficult to carry out. Some attempts have been made to measure the inhibitory activity of whole urine with respect to both calcium phosphate (BISAZ et al. 1978) and calcium oxalate (BAUMANN and WACKER 1980) but there are criticisms with both procedures. Clearly it is not going to be simple to measure inhibitory activity satisfactorily in whole urine.

The alternative to working with whole (or nearly whole) urine is to add an aliquot or an extract of urine to a standard metastable inorganic solution. This may consist either of a simple calcium oxalate or calcium phosphate solution in buffered saline (ROBERTSON et al. 1973b; MEYER and SMITH 1975a, b; LIGABUE et al. 1979) or of a more complex "artificial urine" containing many of the ions at the concentrations found in urine (BARKER et al. 1974; ROSE 1975; MILLER et al. 1977; GARDNER and DOREMUS 1978; DOREMUS et al. 1978; BURNS and FINLAYSON 1980). The concentrations used by some of these workers, however, are much higher than normal (for review see BURNS and FINLAYSON 1980). Indeed, some authors (including BURNS and FINLAYSON themselves) have merely adopted the average 24-hour excretion of the various ions (DIEM and LENTNER 1970) and have assumed that these are excreted in 1 litre of urine. It seems unlikely that this volume can be considered as average for a 24-hour sample from a normal individual, the true mean figure lying between 1.4 and 1.7 litres. Indeed the "artificial urine" recommended by BURNS and FINLAYSON exceeds the upper limit of metastability for calcium oxalate and crystals of the salt form spontaneously. Since this should be preferably avoided, it would seem reasonable to increase the volume of the "artificial urine" from 1 litre to 1.4 litres or more, thereby bringing the saturation level within the metastable region.

Using a standard metastable solution of calcium oxalate of this type, with a known initial level of supersaturation and oxalate/calcium ratio, the crystal growth and/or aggregation of calcium oxalate on to seed crystals of that salt may be followed until the supersaturation eventually becomes depleted and an equilibrium of "quasiequilibrium state" is attained (ROBERTSON et al. 1973b; MEYER and SMITH 1975a). Addition of between 1% and 5% (v/v) of urine to the metastable solution is usually sufficient to modify the rate of crystal growth and/or aggregation (ROBERTSON et al. 1973b; MEYER and SMITH 1975b; LIGABUE et al. 1979). This addition is usually insufficient, however, to perturb significantly the saturation of the metastable solution and any reduction in the rate of growth and/or aggregation can be attributed solely to the influence of inhibitors in the urine. The main argument against the use of diluted urine is that theoretically some inhibitor(s) or promoter(s), which may be active in whole urine, may be diluted out and therefore underestimated or missed altogether (FLEISCH 1978).

A modification to this system is one in which the level of supersaturation is kept constant throughout the study. This "constant composition" technique avoids the problems associated with the depletion of ions and possible change of crystal phase (KOUTSOUKOS et al. 1980a; SHEEHAN and NANCOLLAS 1980). The effect of inhibitors can be tested very quickly using such a system (i.e. within 30 minutes).

Another improvement to the seeded growth system is to add various urinary extracts of amounts of known inhibitors to the metastable growth solution *in the concentrations in which they are found in whole urine.* Even this measure may be criticised, however, on the grounds that the level of metastable supersaturation of calcium oxalate generally used (log relative supersaturation value of 0.75 on the scale of ROBERTSON et al. (1976c)) is not as high as the mean value found in the urine of recurrent stone-formers (log relative supersaturation of 1.15), although it is almost the same as that in normal urine (log relative supersaturation of 0.82). Furthermore, the time of incubation (usually 3 to 4 hours) is considered too long in comparison with normal urinary transit times. Some of these objections may be overcome by using a test system in which the initial supersaturation exceeds the formation product of calcium oxalate (thereby allowing crystals to form spontaneously) and by incubation over a shorter time period. The initial level of supersaturation (log relative supersaturation of 1.17) (ROBERTSON et al. 1981 d) is set close to that of recurrent calcium oxalate stone-formers (ROBERTSON et al. 1976c) and is similar to that employed in the test system of GARDNER and DOREMUS (1978) (log relative supersaturation of 1.18). By adding various urinary extracts or amounts of known inhibitors in the concentrations found in whole urine, the effects on the rates of nucleation, crystal growth and aggregation can be measured separately (ROBERTSON et al. 1973b; RYALL et al. 1981 a, b, c).

More recently, a variation on this technique has been reported which also employs a high initial level of calcium oxalate supersaturation but which maintains a high level by continuously supplying calcium and oxalate solutions to the crystallization vessel at a steady rate (RANDOLPH and LARSON 1971; FINLAYSON 1972; MILLER et al. 1977; NYVLT 1978; ROBERTSON et al. 1984). This dynamic system is termed "mixed suspension mixed product removal" (MSMPR) and is based on the continuous crystallizer principle described in Section II. 2(e). It has been argued that by maintaining a high level of supersaturation, the MSMPR system reproduces more closely the situation occurring in the kidney (FINLAYSON 1972).

After the initial surge of nucleation in the MSMPR system a steady state is reached at which the rate of production of calcium oxalate crystals is constant and a "pseudo-equilibrium" state of saturation is attained. Analysis of the crystal size distributions at various times allows both nucleation and growth rates to be measured but the system suffers from the disadvantage that for the theory to be followed rigorously, the degree of aggregation occurring during the crystallization process should be nil. Whereas this may be an ideal system from the chemical engineer's viewpoint, it may be less satisfactory for the stone researcher, since aggregation is the most rapid process by which particle size may be increased and as such may be the most important factor in the initiation of stone-formation. In practice, however, most MSMPR systems do generate a small amount of aggregation. This may only amount to as little as 1 to 2% by weight of the total crystalline product and may be negligible as far as the chemical engineer is concerned, but from the stone researcher's standpoint this would be more than adequate to increase the risk of stone initiation. The MSMPR system has already been used to study the effects of various inhibitors and promoters on the nucleation and growth rates of calcium oxalate (MILLER et al. 1977; DRACH et al. 1978, 1980; RODGERS and GARSIDE 1981; RANDOLPH and DRACH 1981; RANDOLPH et al. 1981) and aggregation may be taken into account (ROBERTSON et al. 1984).

The choice of which inhibitory process to measure and which system to use depends on the model of stone-formation being tested. Those workers who feel that the critical step in the initiation of a stone is nucleation (either heterogeneous or homogeneous) will choose a test system which basically measures effects on the nucleation rate of crystals (for example, the MSMPR system).

Those who believe in the "free particle theory" of stone-formation (Section II.5(b)), see the critical stage as one involving the growth rates of crystals or particles as they pass down the renal tubules and will use a system which primarily measures crystal growth or some combination of growth and aggregation. Of the various possibilities, the last is by far the most potent means of rapidly increasing particle size such that a critical particle may be produced within the transit time of urine through the urinary system, for, unless crystal growth is extremely fast, individual crystals will be expelled from the urinary system before they are large enough to become trapped. Proponents of the "fixed particle theory" (Section II.5(c)) may also be interested in factors which influence growth rates, although rapid growth may not be so important in this situation, since once the nucleus is "fixed" at some site in the urinary tract the time necessary for growth into a stone nucleus will be less critical than that for the "free particle theory".

b) Inhibitors of Nucleation

As mentioned earlier, classically there are two types of nucleation – homogeneous and heterogeneous. The question arises as to what effect inhibitors have on these two processes. The answer, unfortunately, is clouded by the lack of agreement among stone researchers on whether or not homogeneous nucleation of calcium salts ever actually occurs in urine. ROBERTSON (1973) reviewing the published data on the spontaneous precipitation of calcium phosphate, concluded that the then known inhibitors of calcium phosphate precipitation mainly acted on the heterogeneous nucleation of that salt at supersaturation levels up to the empirical formation product. They had little or no effect on nucleation beyond this point, an observation recently confirmed by BAUMANN and WACKER (1980). In his papers, however, PAK disagrees with this conclusion and claims to show that the empirical formation products of both calcium phosphate and calcium oxalate are increased by a variety of inhibitors including pyrophosphate (PAK 1972), a diphosphonate (OHATA and PAK 1973; PAK et al. 1975b), heparin and chondroitin sulphate (PAK et al. 1979). However, PAK's value for the empirical formation product of calcium (which he measures after a 3-hour incubation) is lower than that of MARSHALL and ROBERTSON (1976) (measured after a 10-minute incubation) and only approaches the latter value in the presence of inhibitors such as pyrophosphate and diphosphonates (OHATA and PAK 1973). Furthermore, the apparent increase in the formation product of calcium oxalate in the presence of inhibitors reported by PAK et al. (1975b) must also be suspect since the point of precipitation, although measured after only 15 to 20 minutes incubation, was detected "by eye". Since, however, the inhibitors concerned are known to retard both the crystal growth and aggregation of calcium oxalate, it is likely that the initial microcrystals of calcium oxalate which form after nucleation would not grow sufficiently to become visible to the naked eye within the 15 minutes of the experiment. For this, a higher level of supersaturation would be necessary even although nucleation may have already occurred at the normal formation product. This is evident from more recent studies which show that the 10-minute formation product, as detected by a light-scattering technique (a more sensitive method than that relying on the human eye) is, in fact, independent of the concentration of inhibitor added (ROBERTSON, unpublished results). The rate of increase of light-scattering after initiation of crystallization, on the other hand, is considerably retarded in the presence of inhibitors, indicating that the rate of crystal growth is reduced.

Studies comparing the inhibitors of nucleation in the urine of stone-formers and normals have produced conflicting results. According to ROBERTSON et al. (1972a, b), there is no difference in the empirical formation product (as determined in whole urine by a light-scattering technique) between stone-formers and normals. Nor is this level of spontaneous precipitation in urine different from that in simple inorganic solutions. PAK, however, using his formation product ratio (FPR) (defined as the ratio of the activity product at which a precipitate forms in 3 hours divided by the activity product in the supernatant solution after "equilibrium" is reached), claims that urine from stone-formers precipitates at a lower level of supersaturation than does normal urine (PAK and GALOSY 1980). This suggests either that there is some heterogeneous nucleating agent present in stone-forming, but not in normal, urine or that there is some inhibitor present in normal urine which is absent from or deficient in stone-forming urine. The problem with the determination of FPR, however, is that it may not be measuring only inhibitory activity since it is also some function of supersaturation and the calcium/oxalate (or calcium/phosphate) ratio. Moreover, the measurement of FPR requires the prior removal of any crystals present in the urine on voiding or which precipitate before the FPR is measured. This would predictably reduce the concentrations of any inhibitors present by adsorption on the precipitates removed. Another complication of PAK's method is his use of an empirically derived "apparent solubility product" in the denominator of the expression for FPR. In the presence of inhibitors, this "apparent solubility product" is often higher than the true thermodynamic solubility product (as determined in simple aqueous solution) and is undoubtedly influenced by the presence of inhibitors (FINLAYSON 1978; ROBERTSON 1981). Thus the FPR represents the ratio of two variables which are both to some degree affected by the presence of inhibitors.

The most likely explanation for the apparent difference between PAK's observations and those of ROBERTSON is that the 10-minute empirical formation product measured by the latter approximates to that of homogeneous nucleation, and as such is probably independent of inhibitors, whereas the 3-hour value determined by PAK represents heterogeneous nucleation and is almost certainly influenced by trace inhibitors (ROBERTSON 1973). In this context, FLEISCH's data on long-term (1-day or 3-day) formation products probably also represent the effect of inhibitors on heterogeneous nucleation (FLEISCH and BISAZ 1962a, b, 1964) since the maximum value of the formation product achieved is equal to the 10-minute formation product found by ROBERTSON (1973) for spontaneous (homogeneous) nucleation. Assuming that the 10-minute formation product of ROBERTSON are near approximations to homogeneous nucleation, then it would appear that no inhibitors have yet been found to increase this upper limit of metastability apart from those which reduce the level of supersaturation by complexing with one or other of the precipitating ions.

Assuming that both PAK's and FLEISCH's techniques for the measurement of the formation product of calcium phosphate and calcium oxalate are measuring heterogeneous nucleation, then their subsequent data show that urine from stone-formers inhibits heterogeneous nucleation less than does normal urine (PAK and HOLT 1976; BAUMANN et al. 1977; PAK and GALOSY 1980). BAUMANN et al. (1977) attribute this mainly to an increase in calcium phosphate nucleation caused by a decrease in pyrophosphate excretion, and PAK and GALOSY (1980) attribute it to increases in both the nucleation of brushite and calcium oxalate in stone-formers. Several inhibitors are now known to affect heterogeneous nucleation (Tables 2 and 3). These may act either by complexing or by blocking active growth sites on potential heterogeneous nuclei.

c) Inhibitors of Crystal Growth

Most of the system developed for measuring inhibitory activity are based on measuring the growth of seed crystals of calcium oxalate or hydroxyapatite added to the corresponding metastable solutions of these salts. The findings are summarised in Tables 2 and 3.

Inhibitors of crystal growth fall into three main categories. Firstly, there are those which act by complexing one of the ions constituting the growing salt, for example, citrate (MEYER and SMITH 1975b; BAUMANN and WACKER 1979; BRECEVIC and FÜREDI-MILHOFER 1979), magnesium (ROBERTSON et al. 1973b; MEYER and SMITH 1975b; FELIX et al. 1977), phosphate and sulphate (ROBERTSON 1969a; FINLAYSON 1977a) and chondroitin 4-sulphate (CRAWFORD et al. 1968). Secondly, there are those which act in trace concentrations as true crystal poisons by adsorption to active growth sites on the seed crystal surface (NANCOLLAS 1976). Examples of these are pyrophosphate (FLEISCH and BISAZ 1962a, b, 1964; ROBERTSON et al. 1973b; NANCOLLAS and GARDNER 1974; MEYER and SMITH 1975b; GARDNER and DOREMUS 1978; WERNESS et al. 1979), phosphocitrate (WILLIAMS and SALLIS 1981), diphosphonates (FRANCIS 1969; FLEISCH et al. 1970; FRASER et al. 1972; MEYER and NANCOLLAS 1973; OHATA and PAK 1973; ROBERTSON et al. 1973b; PAK et al. 1975b; MEYER et al. 1977b), imidodiphosphate (ROBERTSON and FLEISCH 1970), acidic peptides (ITO and COE 1977; NAKAGAWA et al. 1978, 1981), nucleoside phosphates (MEYER et al. 1974), fluoride (MEYER and NANCOLLAS 1972), RNA (ITO and COE 1977; ITO and SHIMAZAKI 1978; SCHRIER et al. 1979,1981; SCURR et al. 1981) and certain trace metals (MEYER and ANGINO 1977). Thirdly, there are those substances, usually of high molecular weight, which, if present in high enough concentration, inhibit the crystal growth of calcium salts (GILL et al. 1977; GJALDBAEK and ROBERTSON 1980). These include certain glycosaminoglycans (CRAWFORD et al. 1968), an acidic glycoprotein (NAKAGAWA et al. 1983) and non-polymerized Tamm-Horsfall mucoprotein (ROBERTSON et al. 1981d, 1984; SCURR et al. 1981).

Table 2. Inhibitors of calcium phosphate crystallization

Inhibitor	Strength and mechanism of inhibition of process of			
	Homogeneous nucleation	Heterogeneous nucleation	Seeded crystal growth	Crystal aggregation
Magnesium	Moderate (complexation)	Moderate (complexation)	Moderate (complexation and adsorption)	Weak
Citrate	Moderate (complexation)	Moderate (complexation)	Moderate (complexation and adsorption)	Moderate (charge repulsion)
Fluoride	–	–	Moderate (lattice incorporation)	–
Phosphate	Weak (complexation)	Weak (complexation)	Weak (complexation and adsorption (?))	Very weak (charge repulsion)
Sulphate	Weak (complexation)	Weak (complexation)	Weak (complexation and adsorption (?))	Very weak (charge repulsion)
Trace metals	–	–	Weak to moderate (Ca, Zn, Sn & Al)	Weak (charge repulsion)
Pyrophosphate	No effect	Very strong (adsorption)	Very strong (adsorption)	Very strong (charge repulsion)
Phosphocitrate	–	Strong (adsorption)	Strong (adsorption)	–
Nucleotides	–	Strong (adsorption)	Strong (adsorption)	–
Chondroitin-4-sulphate	–	Weak (complexation and adsorption)	Weak (adsorption)	Moderate (charge repulsion)
Urinary macromolecules	–	–	–	Moderate (charge repulsion)
Uromucoid (or Tamm-Horsfall mucoprotein)	–	–	–	–
Urine	Strong (complexation)	Strong (complexation and adsorption)	Strong (complexation and adsorption)	Strong (charge repulsion)
Imidodiphosphate	–	Strong (adsorption)	Strong (adsorption)	–
Diphosphonates	No effect	Very strong (adsorption)	Very strong (adsorption)	Very strong (charge repulsion)
Heparin	No effect	–	Weak (adsorption)	Strong (charge repulsion)
Matrix substance A	–	–	Weak promoter (?)	–

Table 3. Inhibitors of calcium oxalate crystallization

Inhibitor	Strength and mechanism of inhibition of the process of			
	Homogeneous nucleation	Heterogeneous nucleation	Seeded crystal growth	Crystal aggregation
Magnesium	Moderate (complexation)	Moderate (complexation)	Moderate (complexation and adsorption (?))	No effect
Citrate	Moderate (complexation)	Moderate (complexation)	Moderate (complexation and adsorption)	Weak (charge repulsion)
Phosphate	Weak (complexation)	Weak (complexation)	Weak (complexation)	–
Sulphate	Weak (complexation)	Weak (complexation)	Weak (complexation)	–
Trace metals	–	–	Moderate (Sn, V, Pb); no effect (Cu, Zn, Al)	–
Pyrophosphate	No effect	Strong (adsorption)	Strong (adsorption)	Strong (charge repulsion)
Phosphocitrate	–	–	Moderate to strong (adsorption)	Strong (charge repulsion)
Chondroitin-4-sulphate	No effect	Weak (complexation and adsorption)	Weak (complexation and adsorption)	Very strong (charge repulsion)
Urinary macromolecules	No effect	Promote nucleation (?)	Weak (complexation and adsorption)	Strong (charge repulsion)
Uromucoid (Tamm-Horsfall mucoprotein)	No effect	Promotes nucleation (?)	Weak (complexation and adsorption)	Moderate (charge repulsion)
RNA	–	–	Strong (adsorption)	Strong (charge repulsion)
Glycoproteins	–	–	Strong (adsorption)	–
Matrix substance A	–	–	No effect	–

Urine	Strong (complexation)	Strong (complexation and adsorption)	Strong (complexation and adsorption)	Strong (charge repulsion)
Diphosphonates	No effect	Strong (adsorption)	Strong (adsorption)	Strong (charge repulsion)
Heparin	No effect	Moderate (complexation and adsorption)	Weak to moderate (complexation and adsorption)	Very strong (charge repulsion)
Alginates	–	–	–	Strong (charge repulsion)
Methylene blue	–	No effect	Weak (adsorption)	No effect

Some studies on urine have shown that stone-formers have less inhibitory activity towards the crystal growth of calcium oxalate than normals (DENT and SUTOR 1971; TEOTIA and TEOTIA 1975; LIGABUE et al. 1979; COE et al. 1980) although others have failed to show this (ROSE 1975; BAUMANN and WACKER 1979).

d) Inhibitors of Aggregation

As mentioned earlier, the most effective means of increasing particle size within a short space of time is crystal aggregation. According to the "free-particle theory" of stone-formation, the combination of aggregation and crystal growth are likely to play a major role in determining the risk of stones forming in a given individual. Consequently, any factor which inhibits the aggregation phase will be of importance in reducing the risk of stones.

In recent years evidence for a number of such inhibitors of aggregation in urine have been identified. These include, for inhibition of calcium phosphate aggregation, citrate (HANSEN et al. 1976), pyrophosphate (ROBERTSON 1973; HANSEN et al. 1976; BISAZ et al. 1976), chondroitin-4-sulphate and heparin (HANSEN et al. 1976; BISAZ et al. 1976) and to a lesser extent magnesium and trace metals (HANSEN et al. 1976). Inhibitors of calcium oxalate aggregation include citrate (FELIX et al. 1977), pyrophosphate (ROBERTSON et al. 1973b; FLEISCH and MONOD 1973; FELIX et al. 1977; RYALL et al. 1981b), phosphocitrate (ROBERTSON and SALLIS unpublished results), chondroitin-4-sulphate (ROBERTSON et al. 1973b, 1976a; BOWYER et al. 1979; SALLIS and LUMLEY 1979; RYALL et al. 1981b), alcian blue precipitable material (ROBERTSON et al. 1976a), RNA and non-polymerized Tamm-Horsfall mucoprotein (SCURR et al. 1981; ROBERTSON et al. 1984).

The most likely mechanism by which these inhibitors function is by adsorption to the crystal surface, establishment of a large negative charge on the surface and mutual repulsion of other similary-coated crystals. Studies on both the adsorption of these ions to crystal surfaces (JUNG et al. 1973; LEAL and FINLAYSON 1977; WAGNER and FINLAYSON 1978) and on the zeta potential produced (CURRERI et al. 1979; ROBERTSON et al. 1984) (Fig. 9) support this mechanism.

Studies on the inhibitory activity of urine towards aggregation have shown that the urine of stone-formers has less such activity than urine from normal subjects (ROBERTSON and PEACOCK 1972; ROBERTSON et al. 1976c; KOIDE et al. 1981). Both groups attribute this difference to a reduction in the amount of macromolecular inhibitor but one claims that it is primarily due to a reduction in alcian blue precipitable material, namely, glycosaminoglycans, non-polymerized Tamm-Horsfall mucoprotein and RNA (ROBERTSON et al. 1976c, 1978, 1981d, 1984), whereas the other suggests that the reduction is in the protein fraction of urine (KOIDE et al. 1981). The latter group states that it is not in the "RNA-like fraction" of urine as suggested by SCHRIER et al. (1979, 1981).

e) Modifiers of Inhibitory Activity

A number of urinary factors are now known to modify the effects of certain inhibitors in urine. The commonest of these is urinary pH which affects the inhibitory activity of pyrophosphate (WILL et al. 1976; FELIX et al. 1977; SCHRIER et al. 1979; ROBERTSON (unpublished results)), diphosphonates (MEYER et al. 1977 b) and probably citrate (WAGNER and FINLAYSON 1978).

It has been suggested that the inhibitory activity of the glycosaminoglycans may be influenced by the presence of high concentrations of urates (ROBERTSON 1976 b, ROBERTSON et al. 1976 a; PAK et al. 1979; ROBERTSON and PAK (unpublished results)), although others have not found this (McCULLOCH et al. 1981). One possible explanation for this effect is that hyperuricosuria leads to an increase in the saturation of urine with sodium acid urate (ROBERTSON et al. 1976 a, b; PAK et al. 1977 b, 1978, 1980 a, b) which, in turn, may lead to the formation of colloidal sodium or ammonium acid urate (PORTER 1963, 1966; ROBERTSON et al. 1976 a; PAK et al 1978) or calcium urate (ROBERTSON and PAK (unpublished results)). Since urates are known to adsorb proteoglycans (KATZ and SCHUBERT 1970), proteins (KOZIN and McCARTY 1977) and glycosaminoglycans (KATZ 1973; ROBERTSON et al. 1976 a; FINLAYSON and DUBOIS 1978; PAK et al. 1979), this effectively reduces the concentration of macromolecular inhibitor available to inhibit the crystallization of calcium oxalate. It follows that the mechanism by which hyperuricosuria appears to increase the risk of calcium oxalate stone-formation (COE and RAISEN 1973; COE and KAVALICH 1974; ROBERTSON et al. 1978) may involve urate acting, not as a heterogeneous nucleator as originally suggested by COE et al. (1975) and by PAK and ARNOLD (1975), but by interfering with the glycosaminoglycan inhibitors of calcium oxalate crystal growth and aggregation ROBERTSON et al. 1976 a). This hypothesis is supported by later data (PAK et al. 1979, 1980 a, b; FELLSTRÖM et al. 1982) which show that sodium acid urate attenuated the inhibitory effect of glycosaminoglycans on the crystallization of calcium oxalate. Polymerized Tamm-Horsfall mucoprotein may also interfere with the inhibitors (ROBERTSON 1985).

f) Naturally Occurring Inhibitors

It is clear from the above sections that there is a considerable number of inhibitors of crystallization in urine. There is also considerable controversy about which are the most important. Tables 2 and 3 summarise the current state of knowledge in this field.

g) Synthetic Inhibitors

During the various studies on inhibitors a number of synthetic material have been identified which are good inhibitors of the crystallization of one or both calcium salts. The interest in these derives from their possible therapeutic applications. The list includes a number of dye-stuffs (SUTOR 1969) including methylene blue (ROLLINS and FINLAYSON 1973; DRACH et al. 1978) (although others have not confirmed this except in very high concentrations (WELSHMAN and McGEOWN 1972; ROBERTSON et al. 1973b)), various diphosphonates (FRANCIS 1969; FLEISCH et al. 1970; ROBERTSON et al. 1973b; OHATA and PAK 1973; MEYER and NANCOLLAS 1973; PAK et al. 1975; FELIX et al. 1977; MEYER et al. 1977b; DOREMUS et al. 1978), heparin (CRAWFORD et al. 1978; ROBERTSON et al. 1973b; FELIX et al. 1977; GARDNER and DOREMUS 1978; BOWYER et al. 1979; WERNESS et al. 1979), polyphosphates (NANCOLLAS and GARDNER 1974; TOMAZIC and NANCOLLAS 1980a) and certain polyacidic peptides (GARTI et al. 1980).

Some of these synthetic inhibitors have been tried in vivo with varying degrees of success. Methylene blue, although originally claimed to be beneficial in reducing stone recurrence (BOYCE et al. 1967), has not been confirmed as a good inhibitor of calcium oxalate crystallization in vitro (ROBERTSON et al. 1973b) except in high concentrations (SUTOR 1969; WELSHMAN and McGEOWN 1972; ROLLINS and FINLAYSON 1973). Diphosphonates, although found to have some beneficial effect on urinary inhibitory activity (ROBERTSON et al. 1974) also increase urinary oxalate (ROBERTSON et al. 1974; BAUMANN et al. 1978). The net result in many instances is to increase the overall risk of calcium oxalate stones (ROBERTSON et al. 1980b). They may, however, be more beneficial in the treatment of calcium phosphate stones (FRASER et al. 1972; BAUMAN et al. 1978).

5. Unified Theories

a) General Principles

It is clear from the foregoing sections that stone disease is a multifactorial disorder of some complexity. In recent years, however, attempts have been made to integrate certain features of the various theories into composite models of stone-formation. In essence, this involves combining the factors which influence the thermodynamic and kinetic aspects of crystallization in order to define a measure of the risk of forming stones in a given individual. There are two main groups of such theories; firstly, the "free particle" theories and secondly, the "fixed particle" theory, the phrases having been originally coined by FINLAYSON (1977b).

b) "Free-Particle" Theories of Stone-Formation

The concept of free particle stone disease was first advanced by VERMEULEN and his colleagues (VERMEULEN et al. 1967; VERMEULEN and LYON 1968) when they reported that diets containing small amounts of a lithogenic substance (in this instance, oxamide) only caused stones in rats if they had initially been fed a large "trigger" dose of the same substance. In the papillae of these animals crystals of oxamide were found growing in the collecting tubules and ducts of Bellini. The particles grew fast enough to become trapped in the ducts by virtue of their size and identifiable stones of oxamide were formed. Rats fed only the low dose of oxamide did not have crystals and rats fed only the trigger dose had initial crystalluria which eventually cleared. Neither of the latter groups formed stones. Thus the concept developed that stone-formation might be an episodic process, occurring after a period of excessive urinary supersaturation (during which the urinary system fails to rid itself of the stone nuclei produced) followed by a period of metastable supersaturation during which the initial embryos grow into papillary stones (VERMEULEN et al. 1967).

Studies on crystalluria of the various stone salts and acids has shown that, indeed, periods of abnormal crystalluria may trigger off stone-formation both in animals (VERMEULEN et al. 1966) and in man (DENT and SENIOR 1955; SENGBUSCH and TIMMERMANN 1957; ROBERTSON et al. 1969; ETTINGER and KOLB 1971; CIFUENTES DELATTE et al. 1973; VALYASEVI and DHANAMITTA 1974; ELLIOT and RABINOWITZ 1976; SMITH 1976; BERG et al. 1976; WERNESS et al. 1981). In the case of calcium oxalate stone-formation, for example, patients with recurrent stones pass more calcium oxalate crystals in their urine than do normal subjects and their crystals are generally larger and more aggregated (SENGBUSCH and TIMMERMANN 1957; ROBERTSON et al. 1969; ROBERTSON and PEACOCK 1972; WERNESS et al. 1981; BRANDES et al. 1981). These abnormal crystals and aggregates (which may be up to 300 μm in diameter) have also been shown to exist in calyceal urine and are therefore likely to have started forming in the collecting ducts whose maximum diameter is 200 μm at the ducts of Bellini. There is, therefore, considerable risk that the largest of these particles might become trapped in the papillary region or become lodged in one of the lower calyces of the kidney. Alternatively, blockage may come about by a "log-jamming" mechanism in a urinary stream overcrowded with crystals. Indeed, it has been reported that the passage of large crystals and aggregates (gravel) of calcium oxalate in the urine is often accompanied by attacks of renal colic (ROBERTSON et al. 1969) and the passage of stones (SENGBUSCH and TIMMERMANN 1957; VALYASEVI and DHANAMITTA 1974). Furthermore, the severity of the disorder in a given individual, as defined by his number of stone episodes per year, is related to the percentage of large crystals and aggregates of calcium oxalate excreted in his urine (Fig. 11) (ROBERTSON et al. 1981 d).

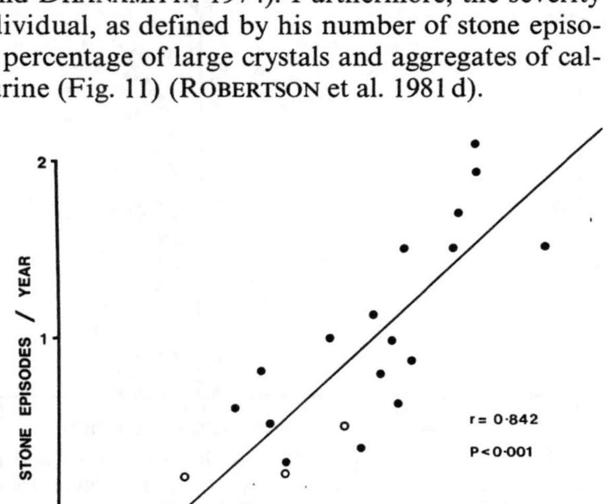

Fig. 11. The relationship between the severity of stone-formation (as defined by the stone episode rate) in calcium oxalate stone-formers and the proportion of large calcium oxalate crystals and aggregates in their urine: (●) untreated patients; (○) patients on orthophosphate treatment

In recent years attempts have been made to account biochemically for abnormal crystalluria by combining various factors which influence the nucleation, crystal growth and aggregation of free particles in the urinary stream. In essence this involves measuring, firstly, urinary saturation with the various stone salts and acids, secondly, any inhibitors of crystal nucleation, growth or aggregation and, thirdly, any promoters of crystallization. The majority of the methods apply to calcium stone-formation, although it would be a simple exercise to extend these models to cover cystine, uric acid and infected stone-formation.

α) Saturation-Inhibition Index (SII)

In the first of these, which applies to CaOx stone-formation, urine saturation with calcium oxalate and the inhibitory activity towards crystal growth and aggregation are combined into a "saturation-inhibition index" of stone-formation (Robertson et al. 1976c). This model was developed from the observation (Robertson 1976b) that calcium oxalate stone-formation is due to an imbalance between the degree of supersaturation (which was higher in recurrent, idiopathic stone-formers than normals (Robertson et al. 1971)) and the level of protective inhibitory activity (which was lower in stone-formers than normals (Robertson and Peacock 1972; Robertson et al. 1976c; Coe et al. 1980). This is seen in Fig. 12, which shows the relationship between inhibitory activity and saturation with CaOx in two groups of recurrent stone-formers and normals. Clearly, the best separation between the groups is defined, not by either variable alone, but by a line relating the two variables. The line of best separation is calculated using discriminant analysis when the distance of each individual from the discriminant line is calculated and replotted, the overlap between

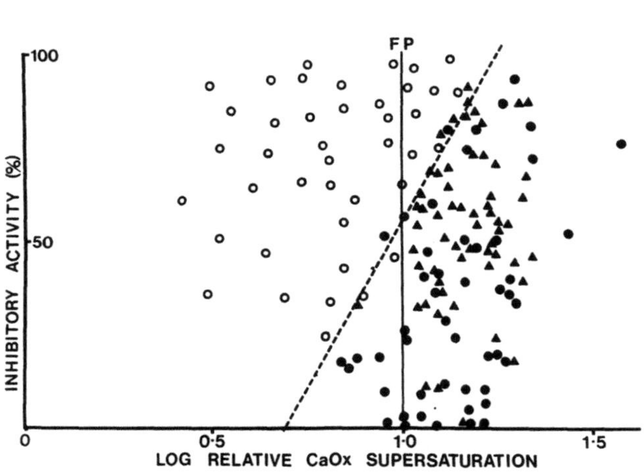

Fig. 12. The relationship between inhibitory activity and urine saturation with calcium oxalate in the urines of normal controls (○), "pure" CaOx stone-formers (●), and "mixed" CaOx/CaP stone-formers (▲). The discriminant line of best separation between the stone-formers and controls is shown by the dotted line (- - - - -)

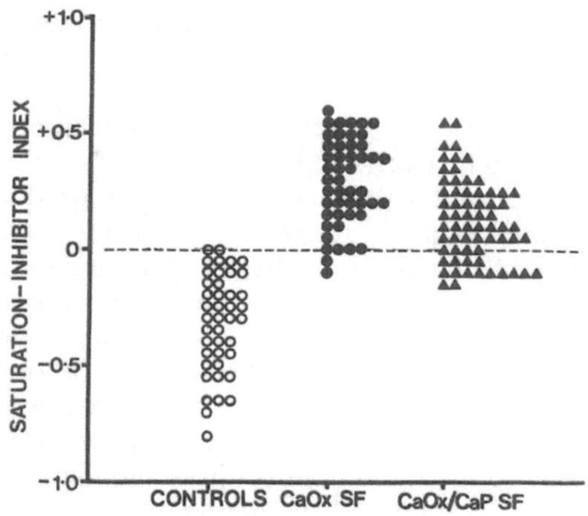

Fig. 13. The saturation-inhibition index in the urines of normal controls (○), "pure" CaOx stone-formers (●) and "mixed" CaOx/CaP stone-formers (▲) in relation to the discriminant line (- - - - -)

the three populations is markedly reduced (Fig. 13). Points to the right of the discriminant line in Fig. 12 are defined as having positive values, and points to the left as having negative values. This value has been termed the "saturation-inhibition index" (SII). It appears to be a quantitative indicator of the risk of forming calcium oxalate-containing stones since both the passage of large crystals and the severity of the disorder correlate with the mean SII of the individual patient (ROBERTSON 1976b).

The main disadvantages with the SII model is that it requires some 13 biochemical measurements in urine to obtain a single SII value. Furthermore, it does not necessarily apply to stone-formation in which calcium phosphate is the major constituent.

β) Crystal Growth Factor (CGF)

The second model does overcome this last criticism in that it incorporates saturation and inhibition measurements on both calcium oxalate and calcium phosphate (SMITH 1976). The composite measure of the risk of calcium stone-formation is termed the "crystal growth factor" and is given by the expression:

$$\mathrm{CGF} = \frac{\text{Supersaturation of CaOx}}{\text{Inhibition of CaOx growth}} + \frac{\text{Supersaturation of brushite}}{\text{Inhibition of hydroxyapatite growth}}.$$

From data published by SMITH and his colleagues, it is clear that idiopathic calcium stone-formers and stone-formers with enteric or congenital hyperoxaluria have abnormal CGF values (SMITH 1976; SMITH et al. 1980a, b). The main disadvantage of this technique is again the large number of laboratory estimations necessary to evaluate the risk.

It should be noted that in the determination of both the SII and the CGF, the measurement of inhibitory activity represents the net effect of inhibitors and promoters of crystallization in urine. In both instances, the dominant factor appears to be the protective effect of the inhibitors.

γ) Urinary Formation Product Ratio-Activity Product Ratio (FPR-APR) Discriminant Score

More recently another method has been described which combines the formation product ratio and activity product ratio measurements on both calcium oxalate and calcium phosphate to produce a discriminant score which is claimed to give a quantitative measure of the propensity for spontaneous nucleation of calcium stone disease (PAK and GALOSY 1980). Since, as discussed earlier, the FPR-APR discriminant incorporate factors which are a function of saturation, inhibitory activity and heterogeneous nucleating activity, then it probably represents another expression of the balance between the agonistic and protective factors, which influence the risk of the disorder.

The FPR-APR score also discriminates well between various groups of stone-formers and their controls and there is a relationship between the severity of the disorder and the degree of abnormality of the score (PAK and GALOSY 1980). However, in the latter instance, the FPR-APR score in terms of calcium oxalate appears to be a better indicator of the risk of stones than the combined calcium oxalate and brushite scores.

One again a large number of laboratory estimations (about 20) are necessary to evaluate the overall score and the technique would appear to be unwieldy for large numbers of samples.

δ) Risk factor model

In order to reduce the amount of analytical work necessary for the determination of an overall measure of the risk of calcium stones, an alternative approach has been proposed by ROBERTSON and his colleagues (ROBERTSON et al. 1978, 1981 a). This has the advantage of requiring only 6 measurements in each urine sample and does not depend directly on any particular physical chemical model of stone-formation. As it happens, however, each of the 6 urinary risk factors can be ascribed a possible chemical role in the stone-forming process.

To understand the risk factor model of calcium stone-formation it is helpful to look first of all at cystine stone-formation. As will be shown later, the formation of cystine stones has a simple physical chemical explanation and depends solely on the abnormally high excretion of cystine found in the urines of those affected by the disorder. Indeed, urinary cystine is so much higher in cystine stone-formers than in normals that there is no overlap at all between the frequency distribution of urinary cystine in the two groups (CRAWHALL et al. 1969). In calcium stone disease, on the other hand, there is no such clear-cut separation between stone-formers and normals in terms of any individual urinary constituent or even of combinations of these such as saturation levels and inhibitory activities (ROBERTSON et al. 1978). It follows that there is unlikely to be a single cause of calcium stone-formation and it must therefore be due to a combination of factors, each one of which contributes towards the overall risk of the disorder. Out of all the urinary factors measured over many years in Leeds, only six had mean values which were significantly different between age- and sex-matched groups of stone-formers and normal controls (ROBERTSON et al. 1978, 1981 a). In this approach, it was assumed that only those factors whose mean values were significantly different between the two groups, are the main risk factors for the disorder. The six risk factors so far identified using this criterion are urinary volume and pH and the excretions of calcium, oxalate, uric acid and the alcian blue precipitable macromolecular inhibitors (mainly glycosaminoglycans and glycoproteins) of calcium oxalate crystal growth and aggregation. In the case of each risk factor, there is a considerable overlap between the frequency distribution of values in the two populations (Fig. 14 a, b).

It is possible to make use of the overlapping distributions to quantitate the contribution of each risk factor to the overall probability of forming stones. The method is shown in Fig. 15 for the case of urinary calcium. The top half of the diagram shows the smoothed frequency distributions for urinary calcium excretion in stone formers and normals. The mean values of the two populations are significantly different (5.95 mmol/day in normals and 8.00 mmol/day in recurrent stone-formers; $P < 0.001$) but there is a large degree of overlap between the distributions. The lower half of Fig. 15 shows the ratio (α) of the (frequency of stone-formers) divided by the (frequency of normals) which provides a measure of the relative "odds" of being a stone-former rather than a normal at each

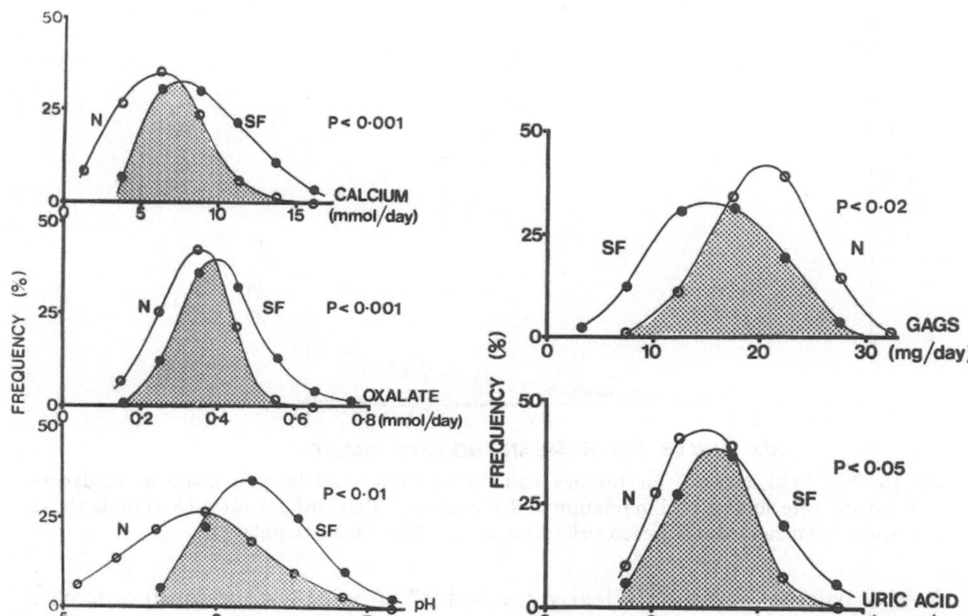

a b

Fig. 14 a, b. Frequency distributions of **a** the 24-h urinary excretions of calcium and oxalate and urinary pH and **b** the 24-h urinary excretions of polyanionic inhibitiors (mainly GAGS) and uric acid in normal subjects (○) and recurrent stone formers (●). The shaded areas define the regions of overlap between the two populations

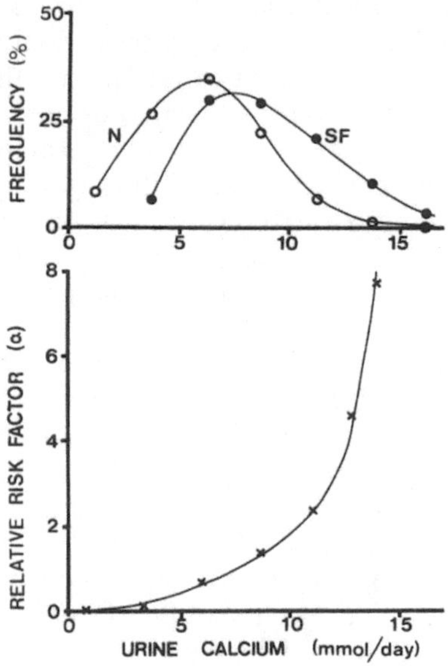

Fig. 15. A diagram showing the derivation of the relative risk (α_{Ca})
Top: Frequency distributions of 24-h urinary calcium in male normals (○) and in male recurrent stone-formers (●).
Bottom: The ratio (α_{Ca}) of the frequency of stone-formers/frequency of normals at various levels of calcium excretion

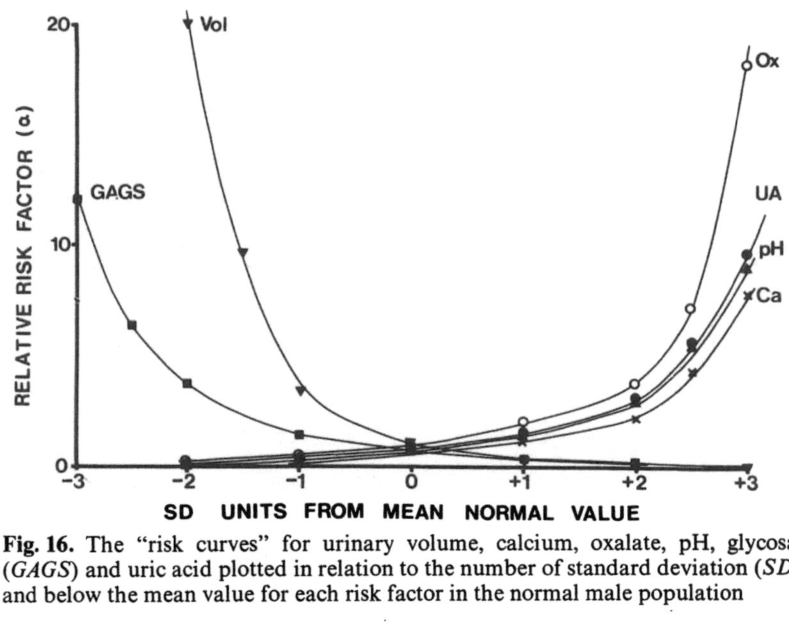

Fig. 16. The "risk curves" for urinary volume, calcium, oxalate, pH, glycosaminoglycans (*GAGS*) and uric acid plotted in relation to the number of standard deviation (*SD*) units above and below the mean value for each risk factor in the normal male population

level of calcium excretion. Clearly, the "odds" of being a stone-former increase as urinary calcium increases, the risk rising sharply above an excretion of 9 to 10 mmol/day. The relationship between α_{Ca} and urinary calcium is called the "risk curve" for calcium.

Similarly, risk curves for urinary volume, pH, oxalate, uric acid and the polyanionic macromolecular inhibitors (GAGS) may be derived from the corresponding frequency distributions of these factors in stone-formers and normals. Figure 16 shows the relative risk attributable to each risk factor plotted in relation to the number of standard deviations (SD) about the mean value (O) for each constituent in the normal population. From Fig. 16 it is possible to compare the relative importance of each constituent as a risk factor in the genesis of calcium-containing stones. Clearly, by themselves a decrease in urine volume or an increase in urinary oxalate are the most critical factors in increasing the risk of stones whereas hypercalciuria per se is much less important than has been previously considered.

It can be shown from a simple multiplicative model for combining odds that the overall relative probability of forming stones (P_{SF}) is given by the equation:

$$P_{SF} = (\alpha_{Vol}\alpha_{Ca}\alpha_{Ox}\alpha_{pH}\alpha_{GAGS}\alpha_{UA})/(1 + \alpha_{Vol}\alpha_{Ca}\alpha_{Ox}\alpha_{pH}\alpha_{GAGS}\alpha_{UA})$$

where α_{Vol} etc. are the relative risks for each of the six urinary risk factors. By measuring each of these factors in a 24-hour urine sample from a given individual on a free diet, it is therefore possible to derive a measure of his risk of forming calcium-containing stones.

As will be shown in the section on calcium stone-formation P_{SF} generally discriminates well between calcium stone-formers and normal subjects and also correlates with the severity of the disorder (ROBERTSON et al. 1978, 1981a). Furthermore, the determination of P_{SF} requires only 4 biochemical estimations plus urinary volume and pH on each urine sample and is useful for testing the possible efficacy of a treatment for the disorder. The technique of risk factor analysis has also been applied to uric acid stone-formation (BAMBACH et al. 1981).

Based on the concept of stone-formation being a multifactorial disorder resulting from the combination of a number of urinary constituents, a general risk factor model may be constructed to describe the disorder (Fig. 17). This defines

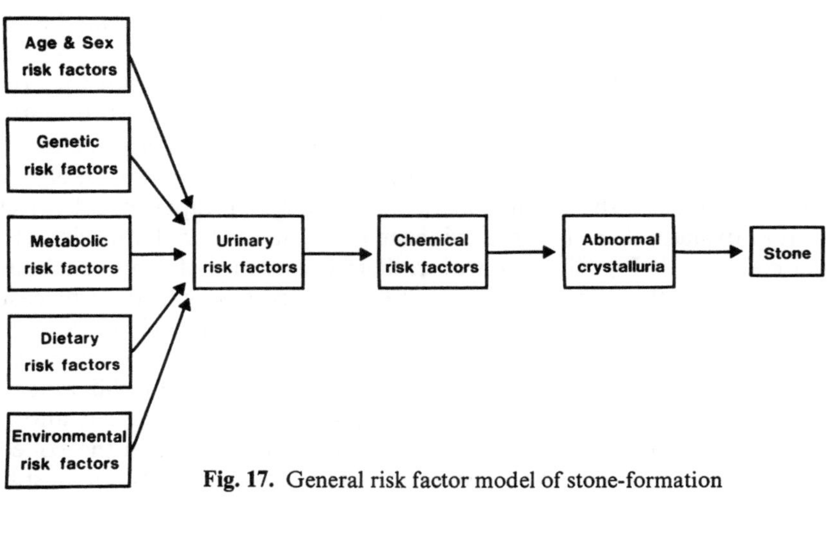

Fig. 17. General risk factor model of stone-formation

the first prerequisite of stones as being a period of abnormal crystalluria when, for some reason, large crystals and/or aggregates of one of the stone-forming salts are produced in the urine. In turn, the risk of forming large crystals depends on a set of "chemical risk factors", including urine saturation, the concentration of inhibitors of crystallization and, perhaps, also the concentration of nucleating material. These chemical risk factors are controlled by a number of "urinary risk factors" which are basically the concentrations of ions which constitute the stone-forming salts and the concentrations of the various inhibitors and anti-inhibitors in urine. Beyond the urinary risk factors, however, are a multitude of "pre-urinary risk factors" including the metabolic state of the patient, the disease state, genetic factors, hormonal imbalance, environmental factors and dietary composition and intake.

c)"Fixed Particle" Theory of Stone-Formation

In spite of the reasonable success of the four preceding approaches to the problem of discriminating biochemically between patients who have had stones and those who have not, some workers have expressed doubt about the probability of the "free particle" mechanism of stone-formation which is implicit in most of the purely chemical models (FINLAYSON 1977b; FINLAYSON and REID 1978). These authors have attempted to calculate the expectation of stone-formation being initiated by a "free particle"mechanism in the renal tubules, in the renal pelvis and in the bladder. On the basis of certain assumptions concerning urine flow rate, the dimensions of collecting ducts, urinary composition and calcium oxalate crystal growth rates, it appears that the probability of a crystal growing to a sufficient size (within the transit time of urine through the urinary collecting system) to be trapped is extremely low. Similar calculations indicate that initiation of stone-formation by a "free-particle" mechanism in the renal pelvis is also unlikely but that in the bladder it is quite feasible. FINLAYSON concludes that upper urinary tract stone disease can only be initiated if the urinary crystals become attached in some way to the renal epithelium. This he terms the "fixed particle" theory.

According to FINLAYSON, there is much evidence to support the "fixed particle" theory of stone-formation. In particular, there are reports of particles being attached to tubular epithelium, such as in intranephronic calculosis (OLIVER et al. 1966) and in primary hyperoxaluria (MORGENROTH et al. 1968). More recent studies have shown that in rats given large intraperitoneal injections of sodium oxalate, there is some evidence of crystal-cell wall adhesion (DYKSTRA and HACKETT 1979). Since, however, there is evidence of some renal damage in rats treated in this way (KHAN et al. 1981a, b), some doubt must be cast on this being a representative model of idiopathic stone-formation in man.

A major problem with FINLAYSON's calculations on the probability of "free particle" stone-formation concerns the assumptions made in his model regarding urine and particle flow. For example, he does not include any allowance for Stokes drag and the effect of gravity on crystals moving in the collecting tubules. At any point in time a proportion of the collecting tubules must be draining uphill against the force of gravity. If the urine contains growing crystals of only 1 to 2 μm in diameter it can be shown that some of these may become stationary in the urine flow (ROBERTSON, unpublished results). If held for only 5 to 10 minutes, and if the saturation-inhibitor relationship in the urine is abnormal, then the crystals may grow sufficiently to fall back in the collecting tubule. Unless the collecting tubule is inverted or urine flow increases, the retained crystals may continue to grow and aggregate, since now other smaller crystals may be impinging on them, and eventually reach a critical size which prevents the particle being excreted. A stone would then be initiated.

Another possible objection to the model of FINLAYSON (1977b) is that it assumes that urinary flow is laminar. This implies firstly, that there is no significant turbulence which would allow crystals to make contact, thereby reducing the probability of aggregation. Secondly, the model implies that there are no vortices where retention of particles may be long enough to allow them to reach a critical size above which they cannot be easily passed out in the urine. A recent study by SCHULZ and SCHNEIDER (1981) has shown, however, that there are a number of such possible sites in the urinary system where the local flow is reduced relative to the main urinary stream. The region of highest expectation of such risk sites is the pyelocalyceal system. Together the above modifications to FINLAYSON's original model suggest that the initiation of stones by a "free particle" mechanism may not be as improbable as first suggested.

III. Types of Stone Disease

Urinary stone disease can be classified into five main types in terms of pathogenesis and clinical features. The most common is calcium stone disease which can be further subdivided into a number of diseases each with a set of distinct clinical features and causes. Infected stone disease is the second most common type and arises directly from bacterial infection within the urinary tract. Uric acid stone disease and cystine stone disease occur less frequently accounting between them for about 5 to 6% of all stone patients and lastly there are a few such as xanthine stone disease which only occur very rarely.

This classification corresponds, in general, with the chemical composition of the stones formed and reflects, to a large extent, the urinary abnormalities responsible for the stones. Sometimes, however, the stone may be of mixed composition, often indicating a combination of these disease types. Infection of the urinary tract, for example, can complicate any of the non-infected types of stone disease and, as a result, the stone will contain calcium phosphate and magnesium ammonium phosphate in addition to the main stone component. Mixed stones of calcium oxalate and uric acid, or calcium phosphate and cystine (or xanthine) are sometimes encountered. Calcium stones can themselves be considered as "mixed stones" since "pure" calcium oxalate and "pure" calcium phosphate form only in diseases such as hereditary hyperoxaluria and renal tubular acidosis. However, it is common practice to consider calcium stone disease as a single type although this probably overemphasises the role of calcium in its pathogenesis at the expense of oxalate.

In each type of stone disease a number of urinary factors are involved. Some, such as urine volume and pH, are common to more than one type because of their major role in determining solubility. Others, such as cystine excretion in cystine stone disease, are unique. Abnormalities in these urinary factors which put the patient at risk of forming stones are always due to a derangement in metabolism which may be due to disease, to environment or to diet. Proper management of patients with stone disease, therefore, rests on an accurate diagnosis of the type of stone disease present, on the elucidation of the urinary factors increasing the risk of forming a particular type of stone, and on understanding the pathogenesis responsible for the urinary abnormalities.

1. Cystine Stone Disease

a) Introduction

Urinary stone formation is the sole manifestation of the disease cystinuria. Indeed the discovery of cystine in bladder stones (WOLLASTON 1810; BERZELIUS 1833) as its name implies, initiated the studies which culminated in showing that cystine stone-formation resulted from an inherited metabolic disorder of amino acid transport (THIER and SEGAL 1978). It is now generally agreed that cystinuria involves not only the amino cystine but also lysine, arginine and ornithine (Fig. 18) (YEH et al. 1951; STEIN 1951) and that the transport defect is present both in the renal tubule (DENT et al. 1954; ARNOW and WESTALL 1958) and in the gut epithelium (MILNE et al. 1961). Cystinuria is distinct from the inherited disease, cystinosis, in which there is an accumulation of cystine within cells and it is only part of a generalised aminoaciduria due to tubular damage

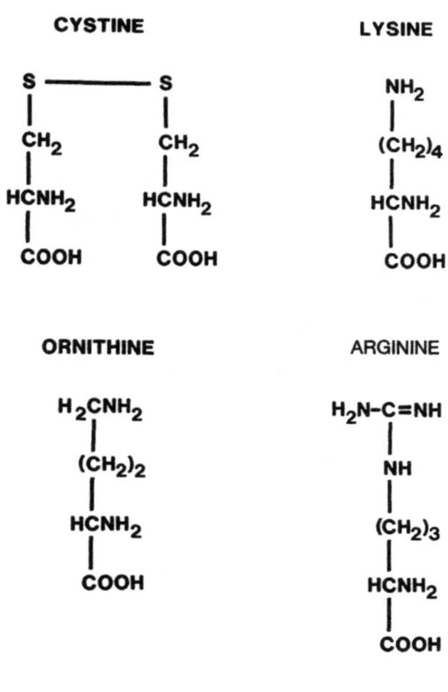

Fig. 18. The chemical structures of the amino acids whose tubular reabsorption is decreased in cystinuria

with no specific increase in urinary cystine excretion (SCHNEIDER et al. 1978. Patients with cystinosis present in childhood with various manifestations of tubular disfunction and renal impairment but do not form cystine stones.

b) Urinary Risk Factors

α) Cystine

Biochemistry. Cystine, cysteine and methionine are the main sources of sulphur in humans. Methionine is an essential amino acid although about 90% of it can be replaced by cystine and cysteine (ROSE and WIXOM 1955). The major fraction of the ingested sulphur-containing amino acids, however, is catabolised in the liver – the nitrogen appearing in urine as urea and the sulphur as sulphate. The trans-sulphuration pathway (Fig. 19) is the main disposal route for methionine and converts the sulphur of methionine through cysteine, cystine and finally to sulphates which are excreted in the urine. Intracellularly, cyst(e)ine exists mainly as cysteine (the free thiol) (CRAWHALL and SEGAL 1967). The sulphur-containing amino acids are used in the formation and repair of tissue proteins and for the production of vital hormones and polypeptides (MUDD and LEVY 1978).

Physiology. Over 99% of the filtered amino acid load in the kidney is reabsorbed in the proximal tubule (SILBERNAGL 1976). Hyperaminoaciduria arises, either because of a rise in the plasma amino acid concentration with a subsequent increased urinary excretion or because of a defect in tubular re-

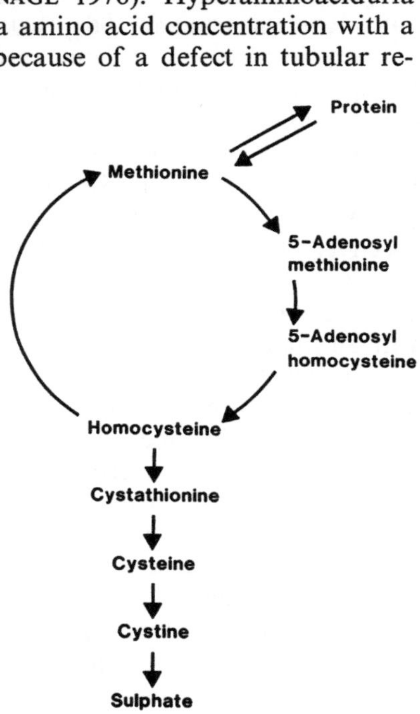

Fig. 19. The trans-sulphuration pathway

absorption giving rise to increased urinary excretion in the presence of normal or low plasma concentrations. In cystinuria the latter occurs (DENT et al. 1954; ARNOW and WESTALL 1958). To account for the decreased tubular reabsorption of cysteine, arginine, lysine and ornithine, it has been postulated that they share the same transport system in the renal tubule as a result of their common dibasic amino acid structure (Fig. 18) (DENT and ROSE 1951). To a large extent this is true since infusion of one amino acid both in normal subjects and in cystinuric patients affects the reabsorption of the other three (ROBSON and ROSE 1957; LESTER and CUSWORTH 1973). This simple hypothesis, however, may not be the total explanation for the aminoaciduria. It has been shown in the rat kidney cortex, for example, that lysine and cystine do not share the same transport system (SEGAL et al. 1967) and cystinuria without dibasic aminoaciduria (BRODEHL et al. 1967) and dibasic aminoaciduria without cystinuria (OYANAGI et al. 1970) do occur. Although increased excretion of cystine, ornithine, lysine and arginine are the main urinary amino acid abnormalities, other have been reported including glycine (FRIMPTER et al. 1962), methionine (KING and WAINER 1967), cystathionine (FRIMPTER 1969) and homocysteine-cysteine disulphide (FRIMPTER 1961).

In addition to the transport defect in the renal tubule cystinurics have the same abnormality in the gut epithelium. The initial clue to the gut abnormalities was that urinary diamines and heterocyclic amines, which result from the bacterial breakdown of lysine, arginine and ornithine, are excreted in excessive amounts in cystinuric patients (MILNE et al. 1961). Failure of the plasma cystine concentration to rise after oral loading with cystine confirmed that the defect in the gut epithelium was similar to that in the renal tubule (LONDON and FOLEY 1965; ROSENBERG et al. 1965; SILK et al. 1974) and in vitro examination of the amino acid transport in jejunal mucosal biopsies confirmed that the failure in transport involved all the dibasic amino acids (MCCARTHY et al. 1964; THIER et al. 1964).

The prevalence of cystinuria depends on the population studied. In the United Kingdom and in Sweden it has been estimated to be about 1 in 20,000 (CRAWHALL et al. 1969) and 1 in 100,000 (BOSTRÖM and HAMBRAEUS 1964) respectively. On the other hand, it has been estimated to be as high as 1 in 2500 in certain Jewish groups (WEINBERGER et al. 1974). In populations where cystinuria has been screened for in babies the prevalence is approximately 1 in 7000 with an equal distribution between both sexes (LEVY 1973).

The genetic abnormality is inherited as a recessive trait. Homozygous subjects excrete more than 1 mmol of cystine per g of creatinine and their excretion of lysine, ornithine and arginine is almost always increased. In subjects heterozygous for the trait the excretion of the dibasic amino acids may be normal or increased although never as great as that seen in the homozygous subject (CRAWHALL et al. 1969).

Taking into account the renal and intestinal abnormalities and the plasma response after ingesting a cystine load, homozygous cystinuria subjects can be classified into three types (ROSENBERG et al. 1966b): in heterozygous members of the families of Type 1 there is no abnormality in the urinary excretion of the dibasic amino acids; in the heterozygous members of the families of Type 2 and

Type 3 increased amounts of the dibasic amino acids are excreted in the urine but Type 2 excretes higher amounts than Type 3. It appears, therefore, that multiple genetic factors affect the amount of the amino acids excreted in the urine and the final phenotypic expression (ROSENBERG et al. 1966a).

c) Stone Disease

The main urinary risk factor for cystine stone-formation is the concentration of cystine in the urine. Stone-formation, the sole clinical manifestation of cystinuria, is only seen in subjects homozygous for the disease (CRAWHALL et al. 1969). Although urinary pH and volume affect the solubility of cystine in urine (DENT and SENIOR 1955), the range of these two variables is such that they play only a minor role in stone-formation. However, the increased morbidity and prevalence of stones in males, the variable recurrence rate, and the wide age range of presentation (THIER and SEGAL 1978) may be partly explained by minor urinary risk factors such as urinary pH and volume.

Stone-formation usually presents by the second or third decade of life (ROSENBERG and SCRIVER 1974). The stones are radio-opaque due to their high sulphur content (SHAW and SUTOR 1972) and may occur in any part of the urinary tract. In the pelvis of the kidney they often grow to large size and may even assume a staghorn shape similar to that of infected stones. Like all other forms of recurrent stone disease they can give rise to secondary infection and impaired renal function. The stones have a yellow beeswax appearance and microscopically are composed of characteristic hexagonal crystals. Occasionally crystals of other urinary salts may be present, particularly if the patient has been treated with large doses of alkali which increases the risk of calcium phosphate precipitation in the urine.

The diagnosis is made by establishing the presence of an increased excretion of cystine, the formation of cystine stones and the passage of characteristic crystals in the urine. The cyanide-nitroprusside test is a simple test for screening for increased cystine concentration in urine and can be used to analyse for cystine in stones (HODGKINSON 1971). It is sound clinical practice to screen every patient with stone disease for cystinuria and every stone passed should be analysed for the presence of cystine. Urinary screening of relatives of cystinurics will yield a number of patients at risk of developing stone.

d) Stone Formation

The chemical cause of cystine stone-formation is fairly simple to understand. Cystine is normally excreted in urine in low concentrations within the range 10–100 μmol/l. In cystinuria this is increased to 20–600 μmol/l in the heterozygous patients and to 1400–4200 μmol/l in the homozygotes (as calculated from the data of CRAWHALL et al. 1969). Since the limit of solubility of cystine in physiological saline within the pH range 5–7 at 37° is about 1250 μmol/l, urine from normal subjects and heterozygous cystinurics is well undersaturated

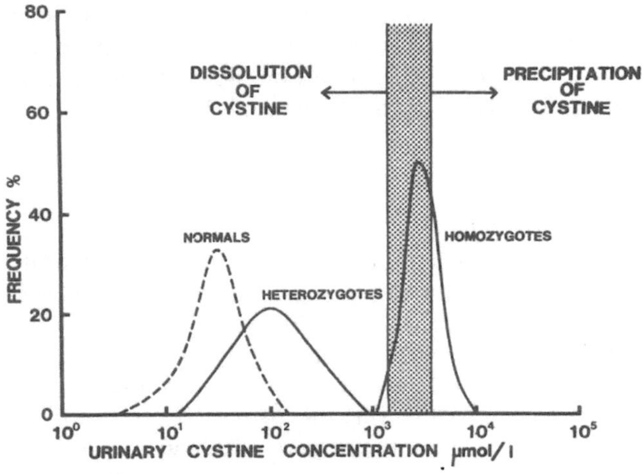

Fig. 20. Frequency distributions of urinary cystine concentration in normal subjects, heterozygous cystinurics and homozygous cystinurics in relation to the limiting concentrations of cystine below which the acid dissolves and above which it precipitates spontaneously

with cystine (Fig. 20) (ROBERTSON and PEACOCK 1981) and both groups are free of stone symptoms (CRAWHALL et al. 1969). Urine from homozygous cystinurics, on the other hand, is excessively supersaturated with cystine (Fig. 20). This accounts for the frequent crystalluria (ETTINGER and KOLB 1971; DAHLBERG et al. 1977; VAN DEN BERG et al. 1980) and stone-formation in this group since most of the urines exceed the upper limit of solubility of cystine (ROBERTSON and PEACOCK 1981).

Chemically, cystine exists in an undissociated form (H_2Cys) under acid conditions. It is this form which is insoluble in urine. As urinary pH is increased, the acid dissociates to from the more soluble cystinate ion (Cys^{2-}) according to the equilibrium: $H_2Cys \rightleftarrows 2H^+ + Cys^{2-}$. Since the pK_a values of cystine are about 8.2 and 9.1, essentially all the cystine is present in the relatively insoluble H_2Cys form at normal urinary pH levels. The true activity product may be calculated from the expression:

$$K_{Cys} = \{H^+\}^2 \{Cys^{2-}\}$$

where $\{H^+\}$ and $\{Cys^{2-}\}$ are the activities of the hydrogen ion and the fully dissociated cystine ion respectively (MARSHALL and ROBERTSON 1976). This more accurate measure of cystine saturation (NORDIN et al. 1979) supports the simpler assessment of the risk of cystine stones made from Fig. 20.

In the general model of stone-formation (Fig. 17), the criterion of excessive supersaturation leading to spontaneous crystalluria is satisfied. There is no evidence that inhibitors or promoters play a role in the formation of such stones. This form of the disorder is therefore the simplest to explain in chemical terms. The risk factor model of cystine stone-formation is summarised in Fig. 21.

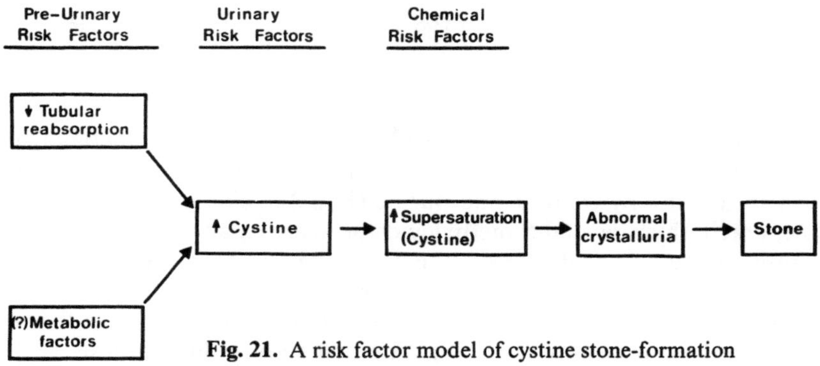

Fig. 21. A risk factor model of cystine stone-formation

2. Uric Acid Stone Disease

a) Introduction

The association of urinary stone disease with gout has been recognised for centuries. In the seventeenth century SYDENHAM (1683), one of the first physicians to recognise gout as an entity, suffered from both conditions and clearly recognised their close association. These clinical observations on the association between gout and stones were confirmed when uric acid was isolated first from urinary stones in 1776 (SCHEELE 1776) and later in tophi of patients with gout (WOLLASTON 1797; PEARSON 1798). More recently it has been established in a large number of patients that over 20% with primary gout and over 40% with secondary gout have uric acid stone disease (YÜ and GUTMAN 1967).

Geographically there are wide variations in the prevalence of uric acid stone disease in the general population and values between 5 and 33% have been reported (ATSMON et al. 1963; WYNGAARDEN and KELLEY 1976). Uric acid stone disease is also closely associated with small bowel disease (CLARKE and MCKENZIE 1969) particularly if it results in a permanent ileostomy (DAREN et al. 1962; BENNETT and JEPSON 1966). In a number of patients, with uric acid stones, however, no underlying disease nor hyperuricosuric state is present and such patients are classified as having idiopathic uric acid stone disease. It is clear, therefore, that increased uric acid excretion is not the only urinary risk factor for stone-formation. Both decreased urinary pH and volume induce oversaturation of urine with acid even in subjects with a normal uric acid excretion (PEACOCK and ROBERTSON 1980). Inhibitors of uric acid crystallization may also be involved but their role in uric acid stone-formation has not been clearly established (SPERLING et al. 1965).

b) Urinary Risk Factors

α) Uric Acid

Biochemistry. Uric acid is an end-product of purine metabolism which plays a fundamental role in nucleic acid production. The two common bases of nucleic acid are pyrimidine and purine (Fig. 22). The pyrimidine bases – cytosine, uracil, thymine and 5-methylcytosine – are catabolised to β-alanine and to β-aminoisobutyric acid whereas the purine bases adenine and guanine (Fig. 22) are catabolised to uric acid which is excreted in the urine.

Studies using labelled substrates have defined the origins of the individual atoms in the purine ring (Fig. 22). The first step in the synthesis of the purine ring is the formation of phosphoribosylamine, from phosphoribosylpyrophosphate and the amido nitrogen of glutamine which reacts with glycine to form glycinamide ribonucleotide. This compund acquires a carbon atom from formate, in the form of the formyl derivative of tetrahydrofolic acid, and after reacting with a second molecule of glutamine undergoes ring closure to give aminoimidazole ribonucleotide. The latter compound accepts carbon dioxide from bicarbonate reacts with aspartic acid and forms aminoimidazole carboxamide ribonucleotide. Ring closure occurs by accepting a further carbon atom from formate to form inosine-5-monophosphate, the latter readily converts to adenosine monophosphate or guanosine monophosphate. It is probable that the reaction of pyrophosphoribosly pyrophosphate with glutamine to form phosphoribosyl-l-amine is the rate determining reaction for the entire sequence of purine nucleotide production. The enzyme catalysing this reaction, amidophosphoribosyltransferase, catalyses the reaction irreversibly and can be inhibited by purine nucleotide end-products.

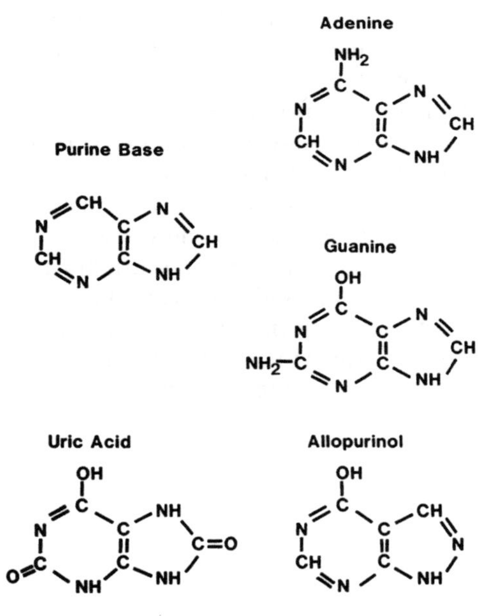

Fig. 22. The chemical structures of various purine-based molecules

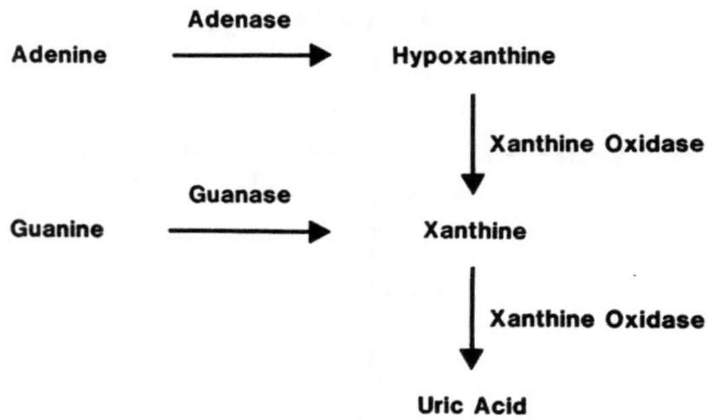

Fig. 23. The main steps in the catabolism of adenine and guanine to uric acid

Both adenine and guanine are catabolysed to uric acid (Fig. 23). Adenine is deaminated by adenase to yield hypoxanthine and guanine by guanase to xanthine. Further oxidation is brought about by the liver enzyme, xanthine oxidase, to yield uric acid which is excreted in the urine. Humans are unable to oxidise uric acid to allantoin- the major end product of purine metabolism in most mammals – because they, like the anthropoid apes, lack the enzyme uricase responsible for this final oxidation step.

Not all of the purines are oxidised completely to uric acid. Salvage pathways exist allowing the purine bases or their ribonucleotides to be re-used in the synthesis of ribonucleotides. These bases are condensed with phosphoribosylpyrophosphate with the acid of the enzyme phosphoribosyltransferase. There are two main enzymes, one acting on adenine (APRT) and the other on hypoxanthine and guanine (HGPRT).

Purine biosynthesis can be inhibited by several compounts, including allopurinol, an analogue of hypoxanthine, which competes for the phosphoribosylpyrophosphate in the phosphoribosyltransferase reactions (Fox et al. 1970). Allopurinol and its metabolic product oxypurinol also directly inhibit xanthine oxidase (Fig. 22) (Feigelson et al. 1957; Elion 1966). Maximum depression of uric acid production occurs within a few days after starting treatment and is constant thereafter (Yü and Gutman 1964).

Physiology. The main metabolic pathways of uric acid in man are illustrated in Fig. 24. The diet supplies only small amounts of uric acid, the main dietary source being the purines in food. Dietary purines are readily absorbed and taken into the purine body pool which is largely concerned with the production of nucleoproteins. Purine catabolism releases uric acid into a 'pool' of about 7 mmol, about half of which is turned over daily, with two thirds of the excretion appearing in the urine and one third passing into the gut where it is largely degraded by bacterial action (Benedict et al. 1949; Scott et al. 1969; Rieselbach et al. 1970). A small amount, about 5%, of uric acid is bound to plasma proteins (Postlethwaite et al. 1974; Kovarsky et al. 1976) and is not filtered by the kidney. The remainder is freely available for filtration yielding a clearance of uric acid in normal subjects of about 5.8 ml/min (Snaith and Scott 1971). It is now generally considered that the renal tubule reabsorbs uric acid proximally and distally and secretes it between these two sites (Steele and

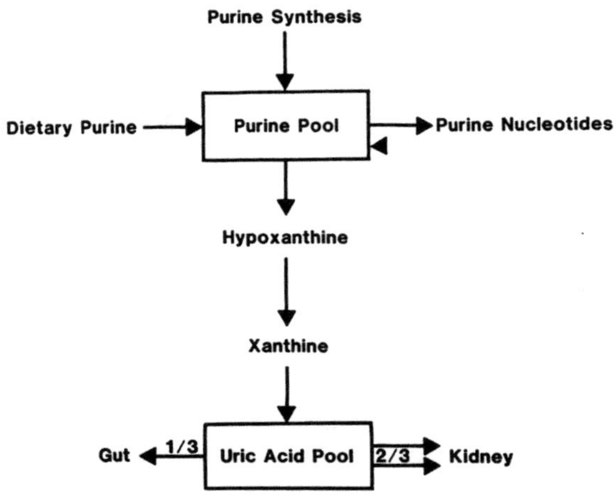

Fig. 24. The main metabolic sources of uric acid in man

BONER 1973; DIAMOND and PAOLINO 1973). The tubular reabsorption and secretion of uric acid are affected by certain drugs and vary with the age and sex of the subjects. As glomerular filtration falls in renal disease, plasma urate rises despite a concomitant fall in tubular reabsorption.

Diseases leading to increased urinary uric acid are associated with uric acid stone formation (Table 4). The hyperuricosuria may be due to increased intake or production of purine in which case there is a rise in plasma uric acid concentration and the greater the hyperuricaemia, the higher prevalence of stone disease (YÜ and GUTMAN 1967). On the other hand, where hyperuricaemia is due to changes in renal handling of uric acid, as in treatment with thiazides, there is only a marginal increase in the risk of uric acid stone-formation since urinary uric acid excretion remains normal in about half of patients treated and increases slightly in the remainder (PAK et al. 1978). Hyperuricaemia, therefore, may alert the investigator to the fact that there is an abnormality in uric acid metabolism but it is the hyperuricosuria which increases the risk of forming stones.

Table 4. Causes of hyperuricosuria

Primary gout
Increased purine intake
Glycogen storage disease – Glucose-6-phosphatase deficiency
Increased phosphoribosyl pyrophosphate synthetase activity
Hypoxanthine-guanine phosphoribosyltransferase deficiency (Lesch-Nyhan syndrome)
Neoplastic disease
Secondary polycythaemia
Anaemia and haemoglobinopathy
Psoriasis
Cystinuria

β) *Hydrogen Ion*

Biochemistry. Urinary pH is a complex function of the body's response to its dietary acid/base intake and to the metabolic needs of maintaining a constant plasma pH. Plasma hydrogen ion concentration is kept within fairly strict limits of between pH 7.35 and 7.45. This is achieved by chemical buffers in intra- and extracellular fluid and by regulation of carbon dioxide excretion by the lung and hydrogen ion excretion by the kidney. Extracellularly the main chemical buffer is bicarbonate, with protein and inorganic phosphate having a minor role. Within the cell, haemoglobin, other intracellular proteins, and organic phosphate complexes are of greater importance.

Physiology. The normal diet supplies about 50 mEq of acid per day. In diets composed largely of vegetables there may be little acid produced and conversely diets mainly composed of foods from animal sources, particularly proteins and fats, may yield a net acid production several times normal. The hydrogen ion of strong acids produced from protein and fat metabolism, namely sulphuric and phosphoric acid, are neutralised by the anions of the buffer salts to form undissociated weaks acids. The hydroxyl ions, formed by the oxidation of salts of inorganic acids, are buffered by the hydrogen ions dissociated from the body's weak buffer acids. The carbon dioxide produced by the action of acids with bicarbonate is excreted by the lung. The excretion of the fixed acids (i.e. non-volatile) is achieved by the kidney which is also the major organ concerned with the conservation of bicarbonate.

The kidney regulates acid excretion by three mechanisms: by regulating the tubular reabsorption of bicarbonate, by excreting acid salts and by its ability to produce ammonia. It is now generally accepted that bicarbonate reabsorption is accomplished by the renal tubule cell exchanging secreted hydrogen ion for sodium (Pitts 1968). This mechanism is largely dependent on an efficient sodium pump and on carbonic anhydrase production which catalyses the hydration of carbon dioxide to carbonic acid. The hydrogen from the carbonic acid is then available for secretion into the tubular fluid and the bicarbonate to return to the interstitial fluid (Fig. 25). Most of the bicarbonate is reabsorbed in the

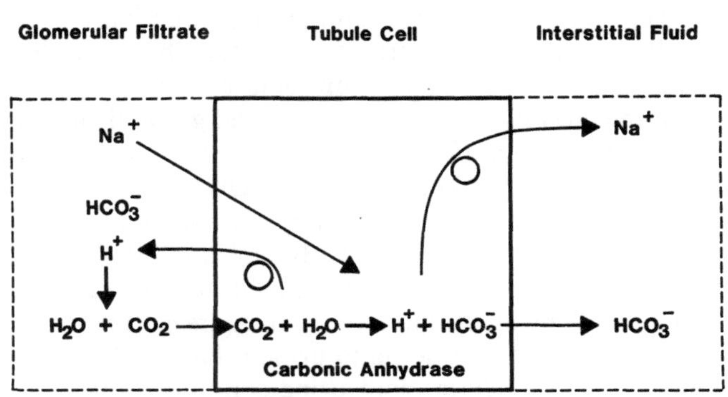

Fig. 25. Regulation of bicarbonate resorption by the renal tubule

proximal tubule when the plasma bicarbonate concentration is 25 mEq/l or less. Above this value a maximum reabsorptive capacity is quickly attained. However, this is not a true tubular reabsorptive capacity maximum in terms of mmol/minute since it is independent of glomerular filtration rate. The same phenomenon occurs with chloride and it is probable that this mechanism reflects the reabsorption characteristics of sodium to which both are closely linked in the proximal tubule (PITTS and LOTSPEICH 1946). The ability of the kidney to reabsorb bicarbonate is influenced by several factors. The first is the activity of carbonic anhydrase in the tubule, which can be altered by carbonic anhydrate inhibitors such as acetazolamide (RECTOR et al. 1960). Plasma carbon dioxide tension also plays a role: a high plasma CO_2 tension increases the capacity to reabsorb bicarbonate whereas a low tension decreases the capacity (BRAZEAU and GILMAN 1953; RELMAN et al. 1953; RECTOR et al. 1960). Plasma potassium also alters bicarbonate reabsorption: hypokalaemia increases reabsorption whereas hyperkalaemia decreases it (FULLER et al. 1955; RECTOR et al. 1964). High plasma concentrations of mineral corticoids increase bicarbonate reabsorption probably by their action on potassium (GIEBISCH et al. 1955).

In the process of buffering strong acids bicarbonate is lost. The deficit is made good by regeneration of bicarbonate in the kidney. Buffer salts of the strong acids within the tubular fluid are transformed into the acid salts or into free acids. Thus disodium hydrogen phosphate is converted to sodium dihydrogen phosphate and sodium hydroxide. The amount of acid fixed in the urine in these forms is referred to as the titratable acids i.e. the amount of acid required to neutralize the urine (PITTS 1950). Other important urinary buffers apart from phosphate are creatinine and β-hydroxybutyrate. The rate at which titratable acid is produced is determined by the rate of excretion of the buffer (for example, disodium hydrogenphosphate), by its pK and the degree of acidaemia itself.

The kidney also secretes hydrogen ion by its ability to synthesize ammonia which diffuses rapidly into the tubular urine. There it acts as a base, accepts a hydrogen ion and forms the ammonium ion which can be excreted as a salt of strong acids, thus further conserving sodium bicarbonate (ORLOFF and BERLINER 1956). The reserves for ammonia production are greater than that for titratable acid and, in acidosis, ammonia production can be increased by severalfold. Precursors are delivered from arterial blood to the kidney and it has been shown that over 70% of the ammonia produced by the kidney is from plasma glutamine, although alanine, glycine and glutamic acid account for a small proportion of this total (VAN SLYKE et al. 1943). Most of the remainder is derived from preformed arterial ammonia (OWEN et al. 1960; PITTS 1968). The excretion of ammonia is controlled by the hydrogen ion content of the body. On a normal diet which supplies 50 – 100 mEq of fixed acid the ammonia excretion is between 30 and 50 mEq/day. In acidosis, this can be increased by a factor of 10 and, in alkalosis, ammonia may disappear from the urine altogether.

The transfer of ammonia to urine is largely determined by the hydrogen ion content of urine. Under acid urine conditions the ammonia diffuses from the cell down a gradient created by its "capture" in the urine as the ammonium ion.

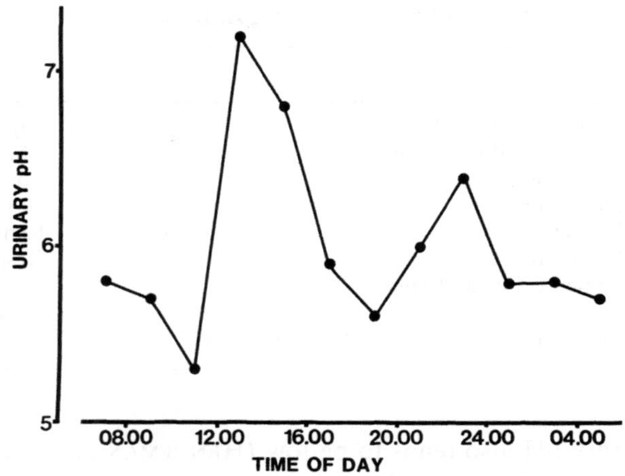

Fig. 26. The diurnal variation in urinary pH

If the urine is suddenly alkalinised the ammonium diffuses back into the blood with no immediate change in the ammonia production by the renal cell (OWEN et al. 1960). Under any particular state of acid-base balance ammonia production is controlled in an unknown way by the plasma hydrogen ion concentration. At the same time, however, ammonia excretion in the urine is determined by the urinary pH. In the urine of acidotic patients there is more ammonia at a particular pH than in the urine at the same pH of a non-acidotic subject. The control of ammonia production by hydrogen ion concentration remains unclear.

There is a diurnal variation in urinary pH such that with the onset of sleep there is a small but gradual decrease in urinary pH. Throughout the 24 hours, however, the urinary pH fluctuates widely from near 5 up to 7 (Fig. 26). These changes are mainly due to food intake and its subsequent digestion which involves the transfer of large amounts of acid and alkali to and from the extracellular space and gastrointestinal tract. During the early part of digestion there is loss of acid into the stomach and the production of alkaline urine but as the food passes down into the small intestine these changes are reversed and eventually compensated. Exercise, particularly if it is severe or prolonged, produces an acid urine and starvation with excessive metabolism of fats and proteins has the same effect.

The overall urinary pH is dependent on the composition of the diet. The higher the protein and fat content of the diet the lower will be the urinary pH. Conversely, diets composed mainly of vegetable matter give rise to alkaline urine. The pH value of 24-hour urinary collections in normal subjects has a wide range but is normally distributed (ROBERTSON et al. 1978).

A persistently low urinary pH is found in most conditions causing acidosis (Table 5). Increased acid ingestion (ammonium chloride), excessive loss of stomach secretions (pyloric stenosis or gastric fistula), diabetes, starvation, renal failure, respiratory acidosis and uretero-colic anastomosis are among some of the many causes of a persistently low urinary pH. In patients with gout the uri-

Table 5. Causes of chronic urinary pH changes

Low pH	High pH
High protein/fat diet	High vegetable diet
Chronic acid ingestion	Chronic alkali ingestion
Loss of stomach secretions	Loss of small bowel secretions
Starvation	Hypokalaemia
Diabetes	Renal tubular acidosis
Renal failure	Respiratory alkalosis
Ureterocolic anastomosis	Urinary infection
Gout	Acetazolamide
Idiopathic defect in ammonia production	

nary pH also tends to be low (HENNEMAN et al. 1962; BARZEL et al. 1964; METCALFE-GIBSON et al. 1965; YU and GUTMAN 1967) and oral alkali gives a subnormal rise in urinary pH. This abnormality has been attributed by some to a low ammonia excretion for a given pH (HENNEMAN et al. 1962; GUTMAN and YU 1965) and by others to increased values of titratable acidity (BARZEL et al. 1964; METCALFE-GIBSON et al. 1965; RAPOPORT et al. 1967). It is probable that both mechanisms are involved since dietary intake determines whether a change is observed in ammonia or in titratable acidity (FALLS 1972). A familial form of uric acid stone disease has been described (ATSMON et al. 1963) in which the urinary pH is low suggesting that genetic factors may influence urinary pH – although through what mechanism is not clear.

A persistently high urinary pH is caused by alkalosis. This occurs after excessive alkali ingestion (sodium bicarbonate), after excessive loss of small bowel secretions (ileostomy or pancreatic fistula), in hypokalaemia, in respiratory alkalosis, and after drugs which inhibit carbonic anhydrase activity such as acetazolamide.

In some patients a high urinary pH is due to congenital defects in the reabsorption of bicarbonate or in the ability of the tubule to achieve a normal hydrogen ion gradient between the tubule cell and the urine. Less severe defects may be acquired through diseases such as the Fanconi syndrome and infection which result in tubular damage. The failure to excrete acid or leak bicarbonate results in a low blood pH and these conditions are usually referred to as renal tubular acidosis (Table 5).

γ) Water Excretion

Physiology. The concentration of a stone-forming salt or acid in the urine is due not only to the amount excreted but also to the volume of urine in which it is excreted. The volume of urine produced, therefore, may be one of the risk factors involved in any type of stone disease. The osmolality of the extracellular fluid is regulated through water excretion. The volume of the extracellular fluid, on the other hand, is regulated by excretion of both water and sodium. Both salt appetite and thirst are integral parts of these control mechanisms. The

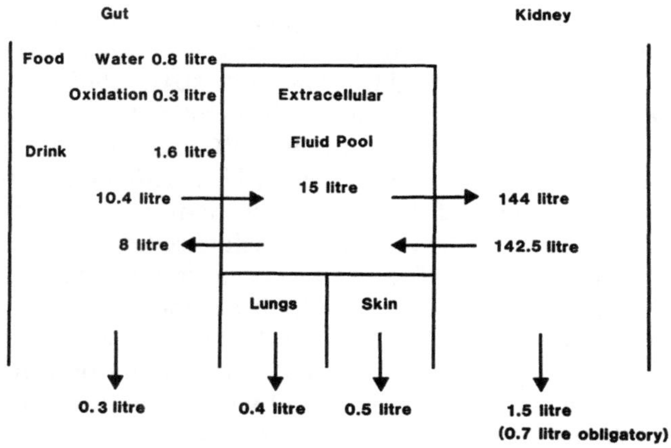

Fig. 27. Daily fluid balance in a normal adult

volume of urine in health has a diurnal variation, being lower during sleep. It varies widely from hour to hour depending on the volume of fluid ingested, the amount of fluid lost by routes other than the kidney and by the type of food consumed. Figure 27 illustrates the normal throughput of fluid in the body. About 500 ml of urine is the minimum amount which must be passed daily to allow the kidneys to eliminate the end-products of normal protein metabolism. This is often referred to as the obligatory urine output. If salt or protein intake is greater than normal then this obligatory loss has to be increased. About 100 g of water is lost daily in the faeces although over 8 litres per day is secreted into the gastrointestinal tract and in certain bowel diseases fluid loss from the bowel can be very high. Water is continuously lost through the skin by evaporation as insensible perspiration and in a normal environment amounts to about 500 ml/day. In hot environments, either due to geographical or occupational factors, sweating can increase the loss of water many times this value. Water is also lost through the expired air which is saturated with water vapour. Excessive exercise, particularly in a dry atmosphere can increase the water loss by respiration from 300 ml/day to several times this value. Shortage of water gives rise to thirst and conservation of water is achieved in the kidney by the posterior pituitary anti-diuretic hormone.

Environmental temperature is probably the commonest cause of low urinary volumes. In certain parts of the world, near the Equator, it may be virtually impossible under normal circumstances to maintain a normal urinary volume in the face of such excessive losses from the skin and from respiration. Loss of fluid through the bowel is another common cause of reduced urinary volume. Nowadays, ileostomy patients are particularly at risk but any gastrointestinal fistula which is freely draining can deplete body fluid rapidly.

c) Stone Disease

Uric acid stone usually accounts for less than 10% of patients with urinary stone disease (Boyce et al. 1956; Herring 1962; Prien 1963) although there are wide geographical variations reaching as high as 40% in some South American countries (MATOUSCHEK and HUBER 1981). Uric acid stone must not be confused with stones composed of ammonium hydrogen urate/calcium oxalate which are characteristic of endemic bladder stone (LONSDALE 1968a; SUTOR 1976; THALUT et al. 1976), a disease with a quite different pathogenesis (VALYASEVI et al. 1967; VALYASEVI and DHANAMITTA 1981; BROCKIS et al. 1981) from that of upper urinary tract uric acid stone disease. Uric acid stones are more common in men than in women and their prevalence is increased at both extremes of life with elderly males having the highest incidence (PEACOCK et al. 1979a).

These stones are friable, have a characteristic cinnamon appearance and are composed of a mixture of anhydrous and dihydrate uric acid crystals (LONSDALE and MASON 1966; SHIRLEY 1966; HESSE et al. 1975). They are radiolucent on radiography. The stones may form in any part of the urinary tract. In the kidney they tend to be small and visible only when lodged in the ureter blocking the excretion of dye given for pyelography. In the bladder, they may grow to a large size. They occasionally appear as small mixed stones with calcium oxalate or in larger stones with calcium phosphate and magnesium ammonium phosphate. The diagnosis of uric acid stone can often be suspected when urinary flow can be shown to be obstructed on intravenous pyelography by a non-radio-opaque stone and the presence of gout or an ileostomy make the diagnosis of uric acid stone very probable. But, as in other stone types, diagnosis must be established by screening all stone-forming patients after their first episode of stone, by stone and urine analysis for uric acid.

The frequency of uric acid stone-formation is increased in all conditions causing a raised uric acid excretion (Table 4). A diet rich in purines is an increasing cause of such stones in many industrialised countries because of their higher dietary intake of animal protein and, pari passu, purine intake (ROBERTSON et al. 1980a, 1981b). The high purine intake increases urinary uric acid and the high protein intake decreases urinary pH, both of which increase the risk of uric acid stone-formation. In countries such as Australia where a high meat intake is common and where the ambient temperature is high (BATESON 1973) (and therefore the urinary volume low), the prevalence of uric acid stone is relatively high (LAVAN et al. 1971). This partly accounts for the wide geographical variations in uric acid stone prevalence.

The majority of patients with idiopathic uric acid stone are accounted for by some combination of these urinary risk factors. Of those with secondary uric acid stones, gout is probably the commonest disease associated with uric acid stones and as discussed this is not only due to an increased urinary excretion of uric acid but also to a defect in urinary acidification in some patients. Patients with bowel disease, particularly if it has resulted in an ileostomy, are at particular risk of forming uric acid stones (CLARKE and MCKENZIE 1969; BAMBACH et al. 1981). The main urinary factors leading to stone-formation in this condition are the low urine volume and low urine pH due to loss of water and bicarbonate through the ileostomy. The prevalence of stone is less in patients with bowel disease where colonic function has been retained although these patients run an increased risk of calcium oxalate stones.

Familial stone disease is probably due to a hereditary defect in urine acidification.

d) Stone-Formation

Since uric acid has a dissociation constant (pK_a) of 5.46, at urinary pH values below 5 most of the uric acid is in the undissociated form of the acid (HU) according to the equilibrium: $HU \rightleftarrows H^+ + U^-$. It is the undissociated form of the acid which is insoluble in acid urine. Under these conditions urine is nearly always oversaturated with uric acid to such an extent that crystalluria is likely to be persistent. As urinary pH increases, uric acid dissociates to give the relatively soluble urate ion (U^-). The concentration of HU then falls to levels at which spontaneous crystalluria does not occur. At pH levels above 6.5, urine is nearly always undersaturated with uric acid and any pre-existing crystals of the acid would be expected to dissolve. The true uric acid activity product (K_{UA}) may be calculated from the expression:

$$K_{UA} = \{H^+\}\{U^-\}$$

where $\{U^-\}$ is the activity of the free urate ion.

Studies have shown that most normal urines are undersaturated with uric acid (Sperling and De Vries 1964; Nordin et al. 1979). In contrast, patients with idiopathic uric acid stones have significantly higher uric acid saturation levels than normal, most values being close to or exceeding the level of spontaneous crystalluria (Fig. 28) (Nordin et al. 1979). Ileostomy patients also have a high level of uric acid saturation (Bambach et al. 1981). In terms of our risk factor model, both groups have abnormal P_{SF} values (Fig. 29). Crystalluria is a common finding in the majority of uric acid stone-formers (Clarke and McKenzie 1969; Cifuentes Delatte et al. 1973). In most idiopathic patients, the high uric acid saturation levels result from the passage of a relatively acid urine (mean 24-hour urinary pH of the group is 5.32) and in ileostomy patients from the combination of an acid urine (mean 24-hour pH of 5.24) and a low urine volume (0.99 litre/day). In our general model of stone-formation (Fig.

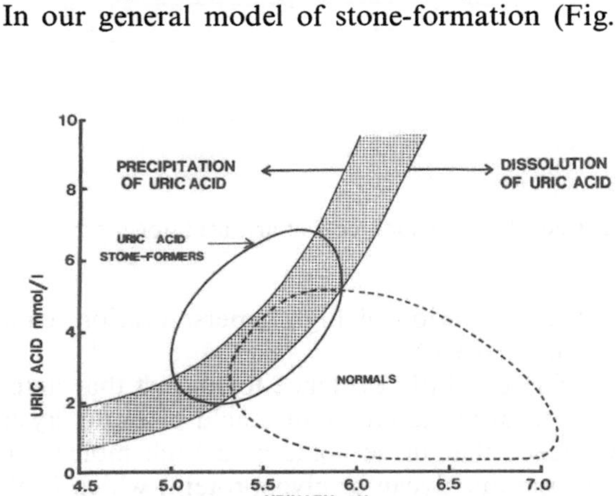

Fig. 28. Cluster diagrams of urinary uric acid concentration plotted against urinary pH in normal subjects and in patients with uric acid stones. The data are shown in relation to the upper and lower limits of solubility of uric acid in urine

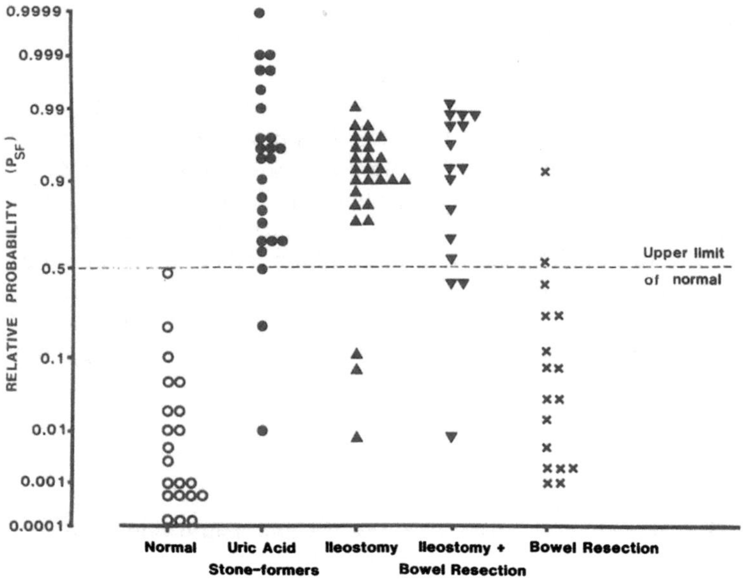

Fig. 29. The relative probability of forming uric acid stones (P_{SF}) in normal subjects, in uric acid stone-formers and in various groups of patients

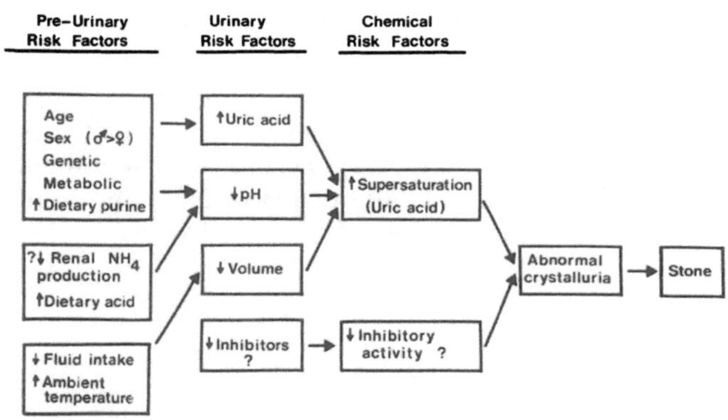

Fig. 30. A risk factor model of uric acid stone-formation

17), the criterion of high supersaturation leading to periods of crystalluria is again satisfied.

There is little evidence to suggest that heterogeneous nucleators are necessary to promote either uric acid or urate crystalluria. However, there is some evidence that urine contains a high molecular weight compound (possibly a glycosaminoglycan or glycoprotein) which is able to reduce the rate of crystallisation of both uric acid and urates from urine (SPERLING et al. 1965; PORTER 1966). One possibility is that the inhibitor stabilises uric acid or urate in the colloidal state by adsorption to the surface of colloidal-sized particles of urate as they start to crystallize out, thereby allowing the precipitating urate to be passed harmlessly in the urine in the form of colloidal particles. Interestingly, it has been reported that proteoglycans can inhibit the crystallization of sodium acid urate (KATZ and SCHUBERT 1970). Low molecular weight inhibitors, however, such as pyrophosphate, have no modifying effect on the crystallization of uric acid (FLEISCH et al. 1967). The risk factor model of uric acid stone-formation, based on the general model shown in Fig. 17, is summarised in Fig. 30. In addition to the urinary risk factors are a number of "pre-urinary risk factors" which include abnormal purine metabolism, ammonia production, purine ingestion and environmental factors.

3. Infected Stone Disease

a) Introduction

The association between urinary stone disease and urinary infection has been clearly recognised by clinicians for centuries (ADAMS 1939). By 1803 it was appreciated that it was ammonia produced by certain infections which was in part responsible for the formation of these stones (BUTT 1956) and by the early part of this century the biochemical relationship between urinary infection and stone-formation was being actively investigated (BROWN 1901; JOLY 1929; HELLSTRÖM 1938). In 1925 it was suggested that the enzyme urease, produced by the infecting organisms, catabolized urea thereby creating the abnormal urine chemistry from which stones were likely to form (HAGAR and MAGRATH 1925). Since then this hypothesis has become increasingly accepted, that only organisms possessing the enzyme, urease, produce an alkaline urine with a high ammonia concentration in which mixed stones of magnesium ammonium phosphate and calcium phosphate are likely to form.

b) Urinary Risk Factors

In most industrialised societies infected stone disease accounts for between 20–30% of all stone-formers (HELLSTRÖM 1938; PRIEN and PRIEN 1968; HODGKINSON et al. 1969; WESTBURY 1974; NORDIN et al. 1979). The main urinary risk factors responsible for the formation of magnesium ammonium phosphate/calcium phosphate stones are bacterial infection within the urinary tract and the excretion of urinary mucoproteins (PEACOCK and ROBERTSON 1979).

α) Infection

Urinary tract infection is a common disease which is often asymptomatic (covert bacteriuria). In the United Kingdom it accounts for up to 6% of all consultations in general practice and is three times more common in women that men. Children and the elderly, particularly males, are also frequently affected (Fig. 31). In

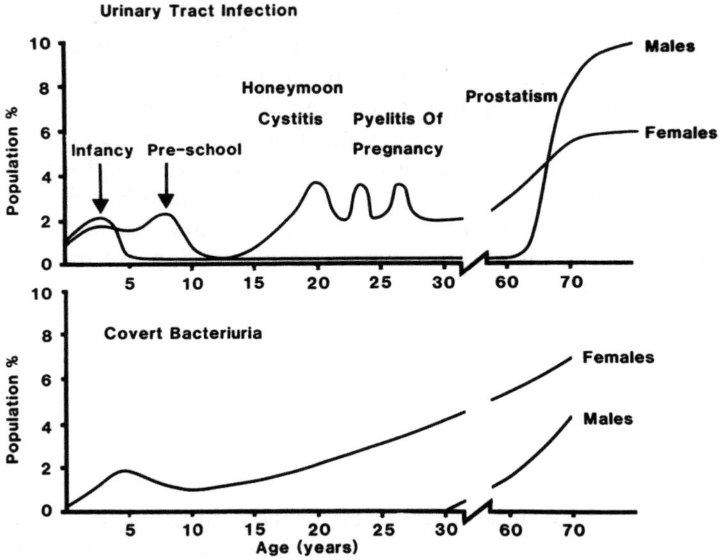

Fig. 31. Prevalence of urinary tract infection and covert bacteriuria according to age (Taken from BROWN 1980, with the permission of the author and publisher)

children, the main predisposing factors are congenital abnormalities of the urinary tract, particularly those causing obstruction such as ureteric reflux, urethral valve or ectopia vesicae. In women, sexual activity and pregnancy are important. In the elderly, particularly males in whom there is a high prevalence of bladder neck obstruction from prostate disease, poor bladder function is frequently complicated by infection. In any patient, however, who has had surgery or frequent instrumentation to the urinary tract, infection is a common sequela (COX 1974).

Not all urinary tract infections, however, lead to stone-formation since only a number of the commonly infecting organisms produce urease (Table 6) and even in these not all colonies which are isolated are capable of doing so

Table 6. The relative prevalence of organisms causing urinary tract infection (BRUMFITT 1972) and their ability to produce urease (COWAN and STEELE 1965)

Organisms causing urinary tract infection	% Patients with infection		Ability to produce urease	
	In hospital	At home	Frequently	Occasionally
Escherichia	59	90	0	0
Proteus	16	5	+	0
Klebsiella	9	2	0	+
Streptococcus	7	0	0	0
Staphylococcus	5	3	+	0
Pseudomonas	3	0	0	+
Others	1	0	–	–

(COWAN and STEELE 1965). Proteus infections are probably the commonest offenders but stone-formation does not necessarily develop (HALLETT et al. 1976). However, the recurrent nature of urinary tract infection particularly with antibiotic-resistant organisms, its increased frequency in diseases such as diabetes, steroid and antimitotic drug treatment often leads to uncommon organisms, which are capable of producing urease, infecting the urinary tract.

Ureolysis. Urease was one of the first enzymes to be crystallized (SUMMER 1926). It is present in bacteria and in plants but not in vertebrates. In man, urease is present in the gastrointestinal tract but is bacterial in origin (DELLUVA et al. 1968). Urease hydrolyses urea, probably with ammonium carbamate as an intermediate, to ammonium carbonate which undergoes spontaneous hydrolysis to ammonia and carbon dioxide (WANG and TARR 1955). Other systems are capable of catalysing urea to ammonia and carbon dioxide but they are probably of no clinical significance.

Urease inhibitors. One of the most potent groups of compounds which inhibit urease are the hydroxamic acids (KOBASHI et al. 1962), the structure of which are shown in Fig. 32. Studies on structural activity indicate that the aliphatic hydroxymates are more potent inhibitors than the aromatic and that toxicity increases as the carbon chain lengthens (KUMAKI et al. 1972; KOBASHI et al. 1975).

Fig. 32. The chemical structures of hydroxamic acid and urea

Hydroxamic acid

Urea

Both hydroxyurea and acetylhydroxamic acid have been used in patients with infected stone disease to inhibit bacterial urease (SMITH 1978; GRIFFITH et al. 1978). In these studies it has been shown that urinary pH and ammonia concentration can be effectively reduced by both agents and in some patients long-term treatment with acetylhydroxamic acid has resulted in partial dissolution of stones (GRIFFITH et al. 1979). Both compounds, however, have toxic side effects since they are potent inhibitors of DNA synthesis; the haemopoietic system is frequently involved with leukopenia, haemolytic anaemia and aplastic anaemia sometimes occurring (SMITH 1978; GRIFFITH et al. 1978).

Matrix proteins. The percentage of matrix in infected stones is usually much higher than in the other stone types. It is probable that matrix protein accumulates in the stone by non-specific absorption of proteins normally present in urine and is, therefore, invariably a mixture of serum proteins and mucoproteins (BOYCE 1968). Immunological studies on stone matrix have shown the presence of albumin, α_1- and α_2-globulins and occasionally γ-globulins. Tamm-Horsfall mucoprotein and uromucoid are also present. It is clear that there is preferential uptake of some urinary proteins to form matrix since their concentrations are higher in the matrix than in the corresponding urine. So it still remains a possibility that these proteins may play a role in promoting stone-formation and growth. In some patients with infected stone disease, particularly those with low urinary calcium concentrations due to renal failure, the stone may be almost completely composed of matrix protein; the so-called matrix stone. The increased excretion of protein and mucoprotein in infected stone disease probably represents a response of the renal cells to inflammation and there are no data to suggest that bacterial production of protein itself plays any part.

c) Stone Disease

The patient with infected stones usually gives a history of urinary tract disease. In the child, this is usually due to a congenital abnormality resulting in obstruction of urinary flow. Urethral valve syndrome, ureteric reflux, ectopia vesicae and neurogenic bladder secondary to spina bifida, are often the cause. In the young adult, traumatic quadriplegia, neurological disease or a prolonged period of immobilization following an accident are the commonest causes. In the elderly, prostatic enlargement, urethral structure and bladder dysfunction are frequently present. In all age groups, however, and particularly in women, there may be no history of renal disease and only an uneventful history of occasional dysuria and frequency. Women usually date the appearance of symptoms, when they are present, to marriage or their first pregnancy. The stone, however, in many patients is first discovered on radiographs taken for investigation of a suspected urinary tract abnormality, for investigation of recurrent urinary infection, for haematuria or, indeed, during investigation of completely unrelated conditions. The stones are rarely passed spontaneously since they tend to grow rapidly in situ often to a large size and may fill the pelvis and calyces where they assume a staghorn appearance. Radiographs of the urinary tract are, therefore, of particular importance in this type of stone disease for the diagnosis of the stone type and for establishing the presence of anatomical abnormalities.

The stone is usually composed of a mixture of magnesium ammonium phosphate and calcium phosphate. Matrix protein is often conspicuous, in contrast to the other types of stone, and gives this type of stone a variable density on radiographs. Infected stones may form secondary to any of the other types of stone disease, particularly if it has been recurrent and has resulted in frequent surgery and instrumentation of the urinary tract.

Renal failure is a frequent result of infected stone disease. Unlike most other types of stone disease the onset of and increase in renal failure does not noticeably decrease the rate of stone growth or recurrence of infected stones. The renal failure is due to the combined effects of the anatomical abnormality, the destruction of renal tissue by infection and obstruction by the stone. In severe renal failure urinary calcium and magnesium become so low that their salts fail to precipitate and a matrix stone results.

The diagnosis of infected stone disease is usually straightforward in patients with anatomical abnormalities of the urinary tract or haematuria and clinical evidence of recurrent urinary infection. In patients with more silent forms of the disease, a past history of dysuria, frequency, urgency and nocturia, particularly in relation to pregnancy, should be sought. Frequent cultures and white cell and bacterial counts on urine collected asceptically may be required before a diagnosis of infection can be established, but even when these are negative, it may be possible to diagnose chronic pyelonephritis radiographically. The stones are usually large, obstructing the urinary tract and almost always have to be removed surgically. Stone analysis and histological examination of renal tissue biopsied at operation establishes the diagnosis. The presence of chronic renal failure usually indicates that the type of stone present is infected. The measurement of urinary pH and ammonia may be helpful but are often normal once the infection is eradicated with antibiotics.

d) Stone-Formation

As mentioned above, infection-induced stones usually consist of a mixture of magnesium ammonium phosphate (MAP) and calcium phosphate (CaP). MAP is relatively soluble in urine within the normal pH range of 5–7, but becomes increasingly insoluble under more alkaline conditions owing to the formation of the insoluble PO_4^{3-} ion. Normal urine is well undersaturated with MAP (ELLIOT et al. 1959; ROBERTSON et al. 1968). Only in patients with urinary infections involving urea-splitting organisms, which produce a high ammonium ion concentration, does urine become sufficiently alkaline to cause MAP to precipitate (ROBERTSON et al. 1968; GRIFFITH et al. 1976; NORDIN et al. 1979). This is depicted in the form of cluster diagrams in Fig. 33 in which the two main urinary risk factors for infected stone-formation, namely, pH and ammonium ion

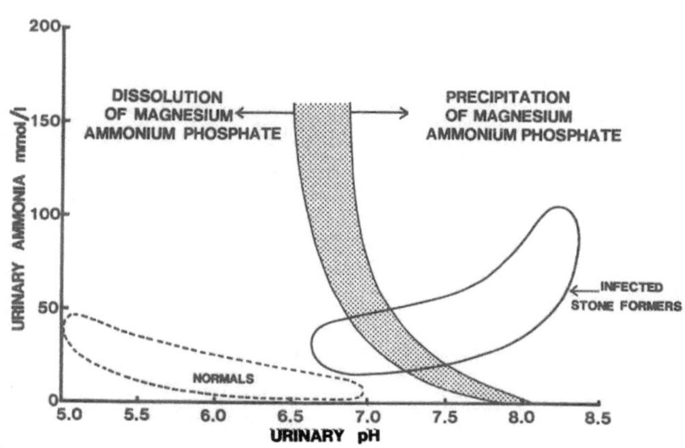

Fig. 33. Cluster diagrams of values of urinary ammonia concentration plotted against urinary pH in normal subjects and in stone-formers with a urinary tract infection involving a urea splitting-organism. The data are shown in relation to the upper and lower limits of solubility of magnesium ammonium phosphate in urine

concentration, are plotted against each other in infected stone-formers and normals. The clusters are shown in relation to the formation and solubility levels of MAP under average urinary conditions. This simple assessment of the risk of MAP crystalluria and stone-formation is in agreement with the more accurate activity product analysis (NORDIN et al. 1979). The true MAP activity product (K_{MAP}) may be calculated from the expression:

$$K_{MAP} = \{Mg^{2+}\} \{NH_4^+\} \{PO_4^{3-}\}$$

where { } contain the activities of the free ion concentrations of Mg^{2+}, NH_4^+ and PO_4^{3-}.

Although phosphatic stones arise in many patients from persistent oversaturation of urine with MAP, very few stones consist solely of this salt. The main constituent of infection stones is calcium phosphate (CaP) (HODGKINSON et al. 1969). Indeed CaP crystalluria is likely to be more common than MAP crystalluria in these patients (GRIFFITH et al. 1976), since the saturation levels with CaP more often exceed the level of spontaneous precipitation than do those of MAP (NORDIN et al. 1979). This may be seen in Fig. 34 which shows cluster diagrams in terms of the three main urinary risk factors for CaP precipitation, namely, calcium and phosphate (combined into a simple concentration product) and pH. Clearly infected stone-formers are at considerable risk of persistent CaP crystalluria. These data are consistent with the activity products of CaP (K_{CaP}) expressed in terms of octocalcium phosphate and calculated from the expression:

$$K_{CaP} = \{Ca^{2+}\}^4 \{H^+\} \{PO_4^{3-}\}^3$$

where { } contain the activities of the free ion concentrations of Ca^{2+}, H^+ and PO_4^{3-}.

A small number of patients with urinary tract infections form calculi consisting only of a "jelly-like" matrix which contains little or no mineral. Usually

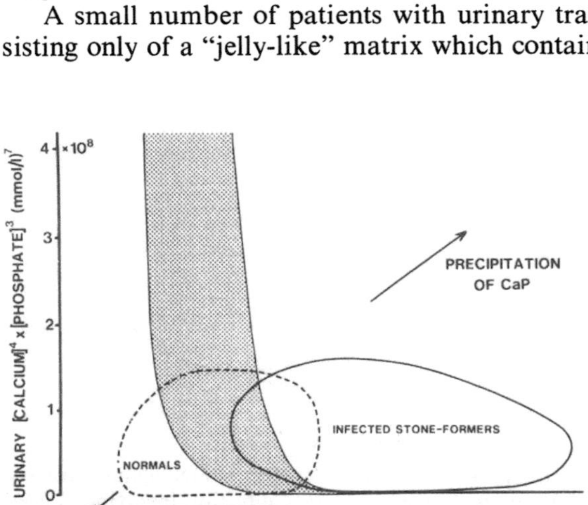

Fig. 34. Cluster diagrams of values of urinary [*calcium*]^4 × [*phosphate*]^3 concentration product against urinary pH in normal subjects and in stone-formers with a urinary tract infection involving a urea-splitting organism. The data are shown in relation to the upper and lower limits of solubility of calcium phosphate in urine

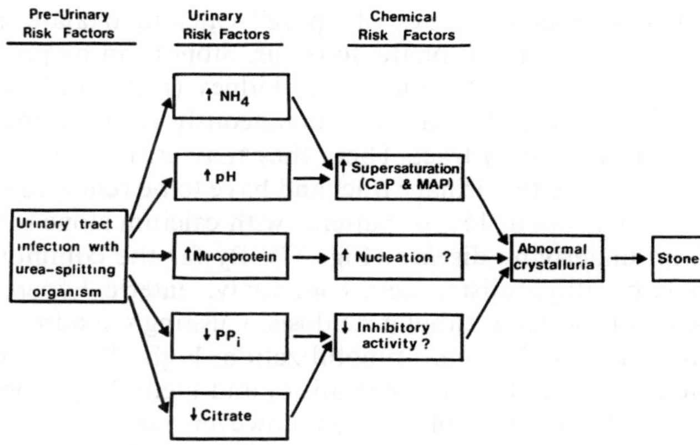

Fig. 35. A risk factor model of infected stone-formation

this occurs in urines with very low calcium levels some of which may be as low as 1 to 1.2 mmol/day (BOYCE and KING 1959; ALLEN and SPENCE 1966). Under these conditions the saturation of urine is too low to allow spontaneous precipitation of CaP. Whether this matrix material, mainly a mucoprotein, actually promotes mineral deposition under more saturated conditions is not yet clear but remains a possible additional risk factor (FINLAYSON et al. 1961; WICKHAM 1976).

As far as inhibitors of crystallization are concerned, there is no evidence that urine contains any inhibitor of the crystallization of MAP. Pyrophosphate, however, is a potent inhibitor of the crystallization of calcium salts, particularly CaP (FLEISCH and BISAZ 1962a, b). Since urinary pyrophosphate levels may be reduced in patients with urinary tract infections, this may allow crystals of CaP to grow and aggregate more readily than in normal urine. Moreover, the excretion of citrate, another inhibitor of CaP crystallization (SMITH et al. 1973a; BISAZ et al. 1978) is also slightly reduced in some patients with urinary tract infections (ROBERTSON et al. 1968) and this will contribute to the risk of large crystals and aggregates of CaP forming in urine.

In the general model of stone-formation (Fig. 17), the criterion of abnormal urine biochemistry leading to spontaneous crystalluria is again satisfied. The detailed risk factor model of infected stone-formation is summarised in Fig. 35.

4. Calcium Stone Disease

a) Introduction

Calcium stones are the commonest type of stone formed in the urinary tract (PRIEN and FRONDEL 1947; HERRING 1962; HODGKINSON et al. 1969; HESSE and SCHNEIDER 1976; PEACOCK et al. 1979a, b). They are composed of a mixture of calcium oxalate and calcium phosphate with calcium oxalate predominating but a number of stones of "pure" calcium oxalate and, less commonly, of "pure" calcium phosphate do occur. Stones can be present throughout the urinary tract but most occur in the kidney (Fig. 36). The majority of stones are small enough to be passed spontaneously in the urine, but a number remain within the urinary tract. There they may enlarge or become lodged in the narrower sites of the urinary tract and have to be removed surgically (Fig. 36).

In only about 15% of patients with calcium stone is the condition secondary to an underlying disease (Fig. 37). By far the commonest of these is primary hyperparathyroidism. Less commonly, enteric hyperoxaluria, hereditary hyperoxaluria, renal tubular acidosis, Cushing's syndrome, steroid treatment, vitamin D intoxication, immobilization, high alkali and calcium ingestion (for the treatment of peptic ulceration) and medullary sponge kidney may be present. In the majority of patients, however, none of these diseases is present and the stone disease is referred to as "idiopathic" or primary.

The prevalence of calcium stone disease is rising in most industrialised countries (ANDERSEN 1969, 1973; BLACKLOCK 1976, 1979). The rise mainly reflects the increasing incidence of idiopathic disease in the adult male (ROBERT-

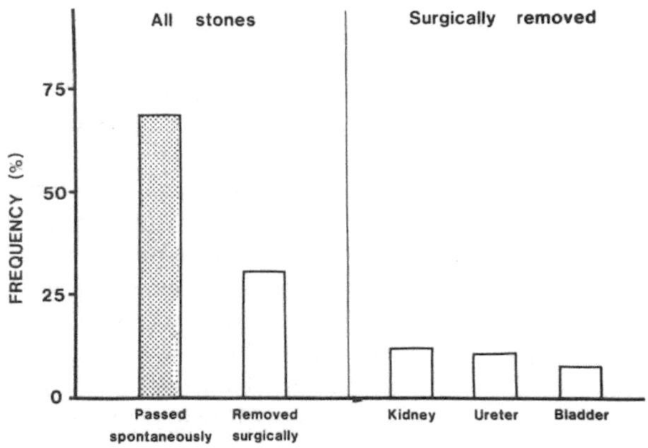

Fig. 36. The relative frequency of stones passed spontaneously and removed surgically and the site from which the stones were removed

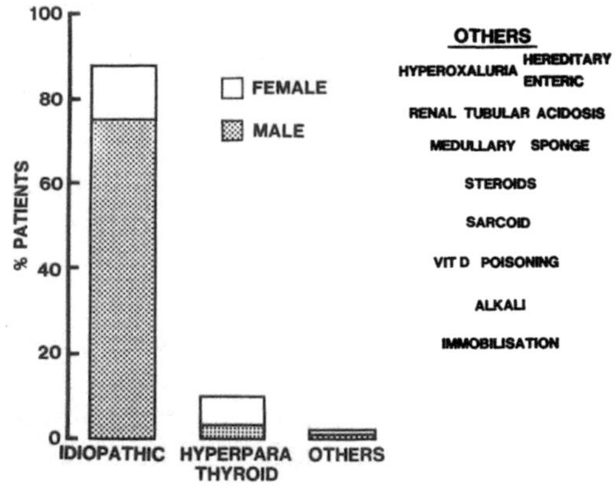

Fig. 37. Relative frequency of different types of calcium stone-formation

SON and PEACOCK 1982; ROBERTSON et al. 1983) and is probably related to increasing standards of living. Increasing affluence could affect the prevalence of calcium stone disease in many ways but a change in dietary habits is probably one of the most important. Several dietary factors have been considered including animal protein (ROBERTSON et al. 1979a, b, 1981b), refined carbohydrate (BLACKLOCK 1976; RAO et al. 1982) and dietary fibre (BLACKLOCK 1979). In our view, dietary animal protein plays a major role since differences in intake of this constituent of the diet reflect, both nationally and internationally, the temporal, geographical and social class changes in stone prevalence rates. (ROBERTSON et al. 1979a, b, 1980a, 1981b, 1983).

b) Urinary Risk Factors

As mentioned earlier, the main urinary factors responsible for calcium stone disease are volume, calcium, oxalate, pH, uric acid, GAGS. In addition, a number of urinary factors such as magnesium, citrate and pyrophosphate excretion may also be involved in a few specific cases. Calcium stone-formation is invariably due to an interaction of several of these urinary abnormalities. Where it is secondary to an underlying disease, particular urinary risk factors are affected. However, not all patients with the underlying disease develop stones, indicating that the effect of the disease on the urinary risk factors can be modified. In primary stone disease, the abnormalities in urine tend to be less pronounced but more are involved (ROBERTSON et al. 1978, 1980a, 1981a), although these data have not been confirmed by RYALL and MARSHALL (1983).

α) *Calcium*

Biochemistry and Physiology. FLOCKS (1939, 1940) was the first to point out that in a proportion of patients with calcium stone the daily urinary calcium excretion was above the normal range. He suggested that the increased urinary calcium might be the result of an abnormal sensitivity to vitamin D although he failed to confirm the hypothesis (FLOCKS 1940). Subsequent workers established that these patients had normal plasma calcium concentrations and were unlikely, therefore, to have primary hyperparathyroidism. Nor could they define an underlying disease such as sarcoidosis, hyperthyroidism, Cushing's syndrome, malignant tumor, or osteoporosis to account for the increased urinary calcium and they therefore classified the hypercalciuria as being "idiopathic" (ALBRIGHT et al. 1953; HENNEMAN et al. 1958), thus confirming FLOCK's original concept that those patients constituted a new syndrome of unknown aetiology. A number of these patients also had hypophosphataemia, an increased calcium absorption, and a higher urinary calcium than normal subjects on a low calcium intake. It was suggested, therefore, that this hypercalciuria represented a defect in the tubular reabsorption of calcium. HENNEMAN et al. (1958) suggested that this was an acquired defect due to urinary tract infection. Others, however, proposed that it was a primary defect and that the increased calcium absorption represented a compensatory response to the loss of calcium in the urine (MELICK and HENNEMAN 1958; JACKSON and DANCASTER 1959; EDWARDS and HODGKINSON 1965). On the other hand, the relationship between urinary and dietary calcium in idiopathic hypercalciuria is steeper than normal and at a theoretical zero calcium intake there is no difference in the urinary calcium between normal and hypercalciuric subjects (PEACOCK et al. 1967). Furthermore, no defect in tubular reabsorption of calcium was found in studies of renal calcium clearance in patients with idiopathic hypercalciuria (PEACOCK and NORDIN 1968).

At about the same time it became clear that hypercalciuria occurred not only in calcium stone-formers but also in normal subjects and that the condition lacked a clear definition to separate it from other types of increased urinary calcium. If it was defined on a 24-hour urinary excretion, the dietary intake of calcium had to be considered (PEACOCK et al. 1967) and if it was defined on the urinary excretion in the fasting state (i.e. the relationship between urinary and plasma calcium), the subject had to be fasted so that the previously absorbed dietary intake had been cleared from the plasma (PEACOCK et al. 1968). Measurements of calcium absorption, using either stable calcium (PEACOCK et al. 1968) or radiocalcium (CANIGGIA et al. 1965; NORDIN et al. 1972), were introduced in an attempt to quantitate the degree of absorption. This lead to formulation of criteria for various types of hypercalciuria (CANIGGIA et al. 1965; PEACOCK and NORDIN 1969; NORDIN et al. 1972; PAK et al. 1974) according to the organ responsible for the increased urine calcium, namely the gut, the bone or the kidney.

With the development of immunoassays to measure plasma parathyroid hormone and plasma and urinary cyclic AMP, it became possible to test whether the hypercalciuria was primarily an absorption problem, or whether the kidney and bone were involved. In absorptive hypercalciuria, the levels of parathyroid hormone (PTH) and cyclic AMP should be within the normal range, or indeed suppressed, whereas in renal hypercalciuria plasma PTH should be high-normal or elevated since the compensation in absorption should act through a fall in plasma calcium causing secondary hyperparathyroidism. Some workers reported that renal hypercalciuria based on raised PTH plasma levels occurred in over 70% of patients with idiopathic hypercalciuria, and the resulting secondary hyperparathyroidism probably accounted for the observed hypophosphataemia (COE et al. 1973). Others, however, found that it occurred in only about 20% of idiopathic hypercalciuric patients (PAK et al. 1975a; PAK and GALOSY 1979). The nature of the defect in tubular calcium reabsorption as defined by these workers has not yet been defined and remains elusive. On the other hand, many centres studying calcium stone disease have found renal hypercalciuria to be uncommon and consider that the main defect is a primary increase in calcium absorption (PEACOCK et al. 1976a, b; SMITH et al. 1973b; BORDIER et al. 1976; BROADUS et al. 1978). More recently it has been shown that plasma $1,25(OH)_2$ vitamin D, the main vitamin D metabolite controlling calcium absorption, is increased in idiopathic hypercalciuria (SHEN et al. 1977; PEACOCK et al. 1981b). The cause of the increased plasma $1,25(OH)_2$ vitamin D has been considered to be hypophosphataemia although this is not universally agreed (KAPLAN et al. 1977; GRAY et al. 1977; CALDAS et al. 1978).

The hypophosphataemia of patients with idiopathic calcium stone disease has also been the centre of much investigation (HENNEMAN et al. 1958; COE et al. 1973; PEACOCK et al. 1976a, b; SHEN et al. 1977; GRAY et al. 1977). Most workers agree that it is largely due to a decrease in tubular reabsorption of phosphate but the mechanism remains obscure and its role in controlling calcium absorption controversial (GRAY et al. 1977; PEACOCK and ROBERTSON 1978). It is difficult at the present time to fit the various abnormalities which have been described in patients with idiopathic calcium stone into one cause. On the other hand, they may be considered as pre-urinary risk factors for stone disease and if stone-formers are selected from the outer limits of the normal distribution then these "abnormalities" will have a higher frequency in the stone-forming population (NORDIN et al. 1976).

In most industrialised countries the intake of calcium in the diet varies from 15 to 35 mmol/day. About two-thirds of the dietary calcium is taken in the form of milk products, which also have a high phosphate content. Changes in calcium intake are, therefore, usually associated with corresponding changes in phosphate. In some countries, however, supplementation of the diet with calcium is practised. In the United Kingdom, for example, calcium carbonate was added to flour for many years.

Many dietary factors are known to affect the availability of calcium for absorption by the intestine. Phytic acid, phosphate, oxalic acid and fats can be shown to decrease calcium absorption whereas proteins and sugars increase it. The importance, however, of these digestive factors in determining the absolute amount of calcium absorbed remains unclear (IRVING 1973; WILKINSON 1976). In an adult in calcium balance there is a net absorption of calcium – mainly from the duodenum and jejunum – of about 6 mmol/day (Fig. 38). The other major input of calcium to the extracellular pool is from bone resorption. However, in the steady state, an amount equal to resorption leaves the ECF pool for bone mineralisation and the net contribution from bone over a 24-hour period tends to zero. Since the kidney, under normal circumstances, is the main route of calcium excretion, the major part of the absorbed calcium eventually appears

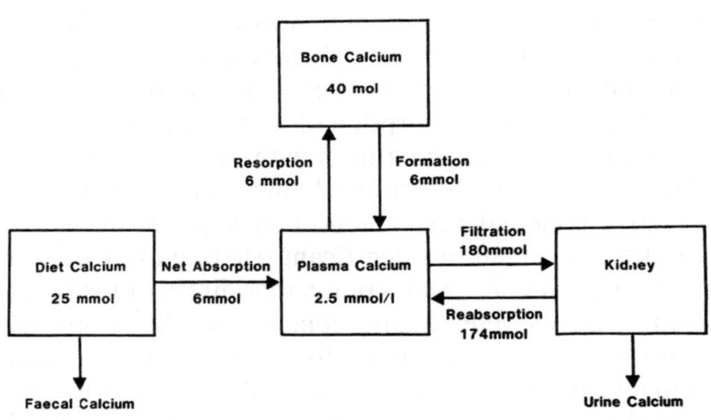

Fig. 38. Schema of calcium metabolism in a normal adult in balance on an average intake of calcium

in the urine. The urinary calcium in an adult in balance closely approximates, therefore, the amount of calcium absorbed in any 24-hour period. There appear to be two main mechanisms responsible for calcium absorption in humans. The first, located mainly in the upper part of the small intestine, is an active transport system and is largely regulated by plasma 1,25$(OH)_2$ vitamin D (Haussler et al. 1977). The second occurs in the small intestine and is due to a diffusion process (Wilkinson 1976).

Hypercalciuria can, therefore, be classified into five types depending on the source of calcium (Nordin et al. 1972; Pak et al. 1974) (Fig. 39). Dietary hypercalciuria, resulting from an increased intake of calcium, probably accounts for the higher urinary calcium in men than women (Bulusu et al. 1970; Nordin et al. 1972). It does not explain, however, the major part of the hypercalciuria of calcium stone-forming patients since their dietary calcium intake is normal (Nordin et al. 1972). Increased availability of calcium from a normal calcium intake is a theoretical cause of hypercalciuria but in practice is extremely difficult to diagnose. It may be suspected in patients on a normal cal-

Dietary

Digestive

Absorptive

Skeletal

Renal

Fig. 39. Classification of hypercalciuria

cium intake who have a normal active calcium absorption but nevertheless have hypercalciuria. It is not known whether or not this occurs in stone-forming patients but several dietary factors may act in this way (Boyce et al. 1958a; Smith et al. 1973b; Peacock et al. 1976a, b). Absorptive hypercalciuria is due to increased active absorption of dietary calcium. This is the commonest type of hypercalciuria seen in patients with calcium stone disease (Nordin et al. 1972; Pak et al. 1974). Resorptive hypercalciuria from bone occurs when there is negative bone balance. The normal response to a primary increase in bone resorption is a small but significant rise in plasma calcium which reduces plasma 1,25$(OH)_2$ vitamin D secretion either directly or through suppression of PTH secretion. Only severe negative bone balance, therefore, manifests itself by hypercalciuria and even in the major forms of osteoporosis with negative bone balance, urinary calcium is rarely increased above the normal range. Tubular hypercalciuria due to a decreased reabsorption of calcium implies that the subject must be in negative calcium balance which must be compensated for by secondary hyperparathyroidism acting on the skeleton and on calcium absorption.

In patients with renal stone disease hypercalciuria is approximately defined by the urinary calcium excretion over a 24-hour period on a normal diet. Using this criterion, hypercalciuria is commonly found in about 30% of patients with calcium stone disease as compared to normals (BULUSU et al. 1970). It must be remembered, however, that urinary calcium excretion in normal subjects is not normally distributed but is skewed towards higher values (ROBERTSON and MORGAN 1972). It is common practice to take the upper end of the normal range as two standard deviations above the normal mean. This, however, defines almost 5% of normal subjects having hypercalciuria. Since urinary calcium is greater in men than women, the sexes should be considered separately unless the urinary calcium is expressed as a calcium/creatinine ratio which brings the two populations together (BULUSU et al. 1970). Because of the wide geographical variations in urinary calcium (NORDIN et al. 1967), in any given study the stone-formers should only be related to the normal population from which they are drawn.

β) Oxalate

Introduction. The history of oxalic acid has many interesting facets (HODGKINSON 1977). Oxalate is widely distributed in both the animal and plant kingdom either as the acid or, more commonly, as its potassium or calcium salts. BERGMAN (1776) was the first to show that it was a constituent of urinary stones. Thereafter, it was found that oxalate was a normal urinary constituent and that calcium oxalate crystalluria occurred both in patients with urinary stone disease and in normal subjects (PROUT 1821; DONNÉ 1839; BIRD 1853). Towards the end of last century it became clear that only a proportion of ingested oxalate appeared in urine (DUNLOP 1896) and that ingestion of large amounts was toxic and could result in death. Primary hyperoxaluria, a congenital defect in oxalate metabolism which often presents with renal stones, was first described in 1925 (LE POUTRE 1925) and by 1964 the findings in over a hundred patients with this disease were reviewed (HOCKADAY et al. 1964). The recognition that hyperoxaluria was a feature of patients with small bowel disease and was an important factor in the renal stone-formation of these patients was made in 1970 (HOFMANN et al. 1970). More recently mild hyperoxaluria in patients with calcium stone-formation particularly of the idiopathic type has been stressed (THOMAS et al. 1972; ROBERTSON and PEACOCK 1980; WALLACE et al. 1981; BAGGIO et al. 1983).

Throughout this period the methodology for measuring oxalic acid in biological fluids has developed but the techniques remain difficult, especially for measuring plasma oxalic acid at its normal circulating concentrations (HODGKINSON 1977; ROSE et al. 1979; ROBERTSON and RUTHERFORD 1980). There are, therefore, still a number of areas of uncertainty in the biochemistry and physiology of oxalate metabolism in humans, particularly with respect to the absorption and renal handling of oxalate.

Biochemistry. Oxalic acid is an end-product of metabolism in humans – over 90% of carbon-labelled oxalate given intravenously is recovered unchanged

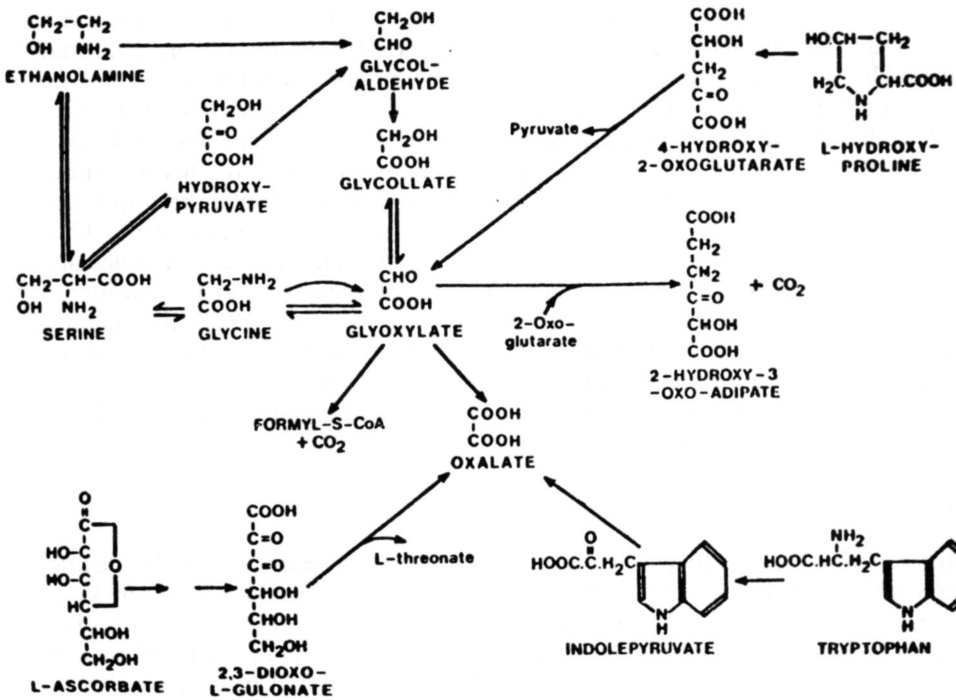

Fig. 40. Metabolic pathways involved in the synthesis of oxalic acid in animals and in man (Taken from HODGKINSON (1977) with the permission of the author and publishers)

in the urine within 48 hours with no label appearing in the expired CO_2 (ELDER and WYNGAARDEN 1960; HODGKINSON and WILKINSON 1974). The major pathways of oxalic acid production – the ascorbic acid pathway and the glyoxylic acid pathway – are shown in Fig. 40. Between 17 and 40% of urinary oxalate is derived from ascorbic acid (ATKINS et al. 1964; BAKER et al. 1966). It is probable that this pathway is normally working at a maximum since ingestion of small amounts of ascorbic acid does not increase urinary oxalate further (LAMBDEN and CHRISTOWSKI 1954; TAKENOUCHI et al. 1966). When the diet is supplemented with doses of ascorbic acid over 4 g/day the rise in urinary oxalate is slightly greater (BRIGGS et al. 1973) but at intakes over 9 g there is a marked increase in oxalate excretion (LAMBDEN and CHRYSTOWSKI 1954; SCHMIDT et al. 1981). It may be necessary to repeat some of these studies in the light of the observation that ascorbic acid may be converted to oxalate during many of the oxalate methods in common usage. The enzymatic control of this pathway has still to be established.

A similar amount of urinary oxalate is derived from the glyoxylic acid pathway. At least three enzymes are involved in this reaction, none of which is specific for the precursor. These are xanthine oxidase (GIBBS and WATTS 1966), glycollic acid oxidase (RICHARDSON and TOLBERT 1961) (both flavoproteins) and lactic dehydrogenase (BANNER and ROSALKI 1967; SAWAKI et al. 1967). The main precursors of glyoxylate are glycine (CRAWHALL et al. 1959; DEAN et al. 1968), glycollic acid (HOCKADAY et al. 1964) and 4-hydroxy-2-oxoglutarate (DEKKER and MAITRA 1962). The latter is a product of hydroxyproline metabolism although not the only important one. Quantitatively, glycine seems to be the major precursor although the glyoxylate pathway may be only a minor route for glycine metabolism. Tryptophan ingestion has been shown to increase urinary oxalate (GERSHOFF and PRIEN 1960) which may explain the increase in urinary oxalate on a high intake of animal protein (ZAREMBSKI and HODGKINSON 1969; ROBERTSON et al. 1979a).

In congenital hyperoxaluria two biochemical types can be recognised (Fig. 40). In Type I (glycollic aciduria), the commonest type, there is a deficiency of the 2-oxoglutarate:glyoxylate carboligase enzyme. Glyoxylate accumulates and results in hyperoxaluria, glycollic aciduria and glyoxylic aciduria (KOCH et al. 1967). In Type II (L-glyceric aciduria) there is a deficiency of D-glyceric dehydrogenase (WILLIAMS and SMITH 1968a, b) which gives rise to hyperoxaluria and L-glyceric aciduria with decreased urinary excretion of glycollate and glyoxylate.

Physiology. The high content of oxalate in plants has been known for centuries; one plant specimen goes under the name 'oxalis'. The Sorrel plant is one of the best known oxalate-containing plants and salts of sorrel (potassium hydrogen oxalate) are widely used in the home and in industry. About 70–170 mg of oxalate is ingested in the diet per day in the form of vegetables or plant beverages (ZAREMBSKI and HODGKINSON 1962; ANDERSON et al. 1971) (Fig. 41). In the British diet, tea is normally the largest single source of oxalate, although chocolate and coffee can also be important (FINCH et al. 1981). However, there is wide seasonal and geographical variation in dietary oxalate (ROBERTSON et al. 1977) due to the variable oxalate content of vegetables (HODGKINSON 1977).

Only a small fraction of the dietary oxalate is absorbed. Between 2–8% of orally administered oxalate is excreted in the urine (DUNLOP 1896; ARCHER et al. 1957; ZAREMBSKI and HODGKINSON 1969; CHADWICK et al. 1973). Oxalate

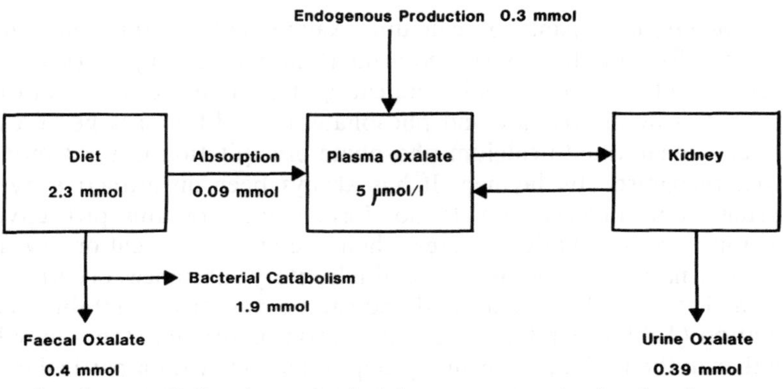

Fig. 41. Schema of oxalate metabolism in a normal adult on an average intake of oxalate

is absorbed throughout the gastrointestinal tract; quantitatively the colon seems to be an important site of absorption. There is little oxalate secreted by the gut back into the bowel lumen (ELDER and WYNGAARDEN 1960; HODGKINSON and WILKINSON 1974). Bacteria in the colon catabolise oxalate and only about a third of the dietary oxalate is excreted in the faeces (BARBAR and GALLIMORE 1940). The absorption of oxalate is not dependent on an active process. The most important factors, therefore, which govern oxalate absorption are the amount of oxalate ingested and the digestive factors making oxalate available for transport across the bowel wall. Of the latter, the amount of calcium in the diet seems to be the most important. A high intake of calcium reduces oxalate absorption and a low calcium intake enhances oxalate absorption (MARSHALL et al. 1972a). Steatorrhoea, which reduces the free calcium in the bowel, also enhances oxalate absorption.

The plasma concentration of oxalate is probably about 2 – 5 μmol/l (HODGKINSON 1977; ROSE et al. 1979) although there is still considerable controversy about the exact figure mainly because of the difficulty of measuring plasma oxalate (HODGKINSON 1977). Most biological membranes appear to be freely permeable to oxalate and it is found in most tissues of the body. The half-life of radioactive oxalate injected intravenously is almost 2 hours and the pool size ranges from 0.03 to 0.12 mmol. The rate of endogenous synthesis has been estimated to be between 0.4 and 0.8 mmol/day (ELDER and WYNGAARDEN 1960; HODGKINSON and WILKINSON 1974) which is close to the daily excretion of oxalate in normal subjects.

Oxalate is probably secreted by the proximal tubule and it has been estimated that the oxalate/creatinine clearance in the dog is 1.28 (CATTELL et al. 1962) and in man 1.6 (WILLIAMS et al. 1971). Urinary oxalate excretion varies normally between 0.2 and 0.55 mmol/day. This is mainly due to variations in dietary intake and digestion. In disease of the small bowel urinary oxalate may increase to several times the normal range (enteric hyperoxaluria). The highest urinary excretion of oxalate is found in primary hyperoxaluria.

γ) *Inhibitors*

Introduction. Crystals of calcium oxalate and calcium phosphate are frequently found in freshly voided urine from normal subjects (DYER and NORDIN 1967; ROBERTSON et al. 1969) indicating that the urine is oversaturated with respect to calcium oxalate and phosphate. Indeed the passage of a cloudy urine after a meal, due to calcium phosphate precipitation is a common observation well recognised by laymen. It has always been an attractive hypothesis that urine from subjects who do not form stones contains protective substances against stone-formation whereas their excretion is absent or low from patients with urinary stone disease. Several inhibitory substances occurring naturally in urine have now been identified and can be classified as inhibitors of stone-formation (Tables 2 and 3). The risk of forming urinary stones may be increased either in the individual or in a group of patients with a particular disease, by a decrease in excretion of one or more of these natural inhibitors.

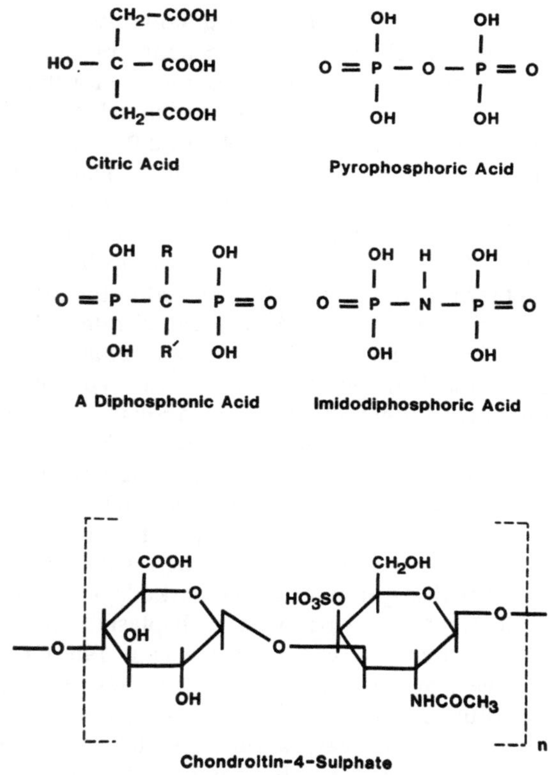

Fig. 42. The chemical structures of various inhibitors of crystallization of calcium salts

Citrate. It has been estimated that approximately 50% of the inhibitory activity of urine to calcium phosphate precipitation is due to urinary citrate (FLEISCH 1978). Changes in citrate excretion potentially therefore could have marked effects on calcium phosphate precipitation. The range of citrate excretion in normal subjects is 0.6 to 5.7 mmol per day and the plasma concentration is 0.12–0.21 mmol/l.

Citric acid is a simple organic acid (Fig. 42) which plays a fundamental role in intermediate metabolism (KREBS and JOHNSON 1937; LOWENSTEIN 1969). About 90% of the citrate in the body is located in bone where it accounts for nearly 1% of its net weight (DICKENS 1941; MARTIN et al. 1958). The gastrointestinal tract is the other major source of citrate production (MARTENSSON 1940). The main organs responsible for citrate utilisation are the kidney (MARTENSSON 1940; ELLIOT and FREEMAN 1956; SIMPSON 1963), and the liver (GORDON and CRAIGE 1960; HENNEMAN and SHOEMAKER 1961). Blood citrate concentration in the steady state is regulated largely by the production and release of citrate from bone and intestine and by its uptake by liver and kidney. Only a small part of an ingested citrate load appears in the urine (KUYPER and MATILL 1933), the major part being metabolised. Since plasma citrate does not remain raised for more than a few days following nephrectomy, the blood level is mainly controlled by the production rate of citrate in bone and the intestine and there is a feedback control mechanism on production through the plasma concentration. The mechanism responsible for the high specificity of the kidney for citrate uptake is not clear. A similar selective uptake occurs with α-ketoglutarate (SELLECK and COHEN 1965) and it has been postulated that both share a common membrane transport mechanism. Within the kidney, plasma citrate enters the tubular cell from the peritubular plasma and its rate of uptake is proportional to the plasma concentration of citrate (HERNDON and FREEMAN 1958). Some of the filtered citrate is taken up by the tubular cell by reabsorption but whether this fraction is metabolised in the same way as that entering from plasma is not known. In acidosis lower citrate utilisation is found (CRAWFORD et al. 1959; EVANS et al. 1957; GROLLMAN et al. 1961; GORDON 1963; SIMPSON 1964; KOOK and LOTSPEICH 1968). Several hypotheses have been put forward for the role of the kidney in citrate metabolism. The first is to utilise the citrate released by bone resorption thus allowing the ECF ionized calcium pool to remain high. Secondly, it may enhance calcium and sodium reabsorption (WALSER 1961; VISHWAKARMA and MILLER 1963). Thirdly, on oxidation it may provide hydrogen ion for secretion as titratable acid.

The infusion of sodium citrate results both in an increased rate of excretion and of reabsorption. There is marked splay in the titration curve and no T_m can be demonstrated since very high plasma citrate levels cannot be achieved because of the toxicity (GROLLMAN et al. 1961). Citrate excretion is also said to be increased by oestrogens, by the administration of calcium salts and by alkaline potassium citrate (BUTZ 1982; SAKHAEE et al. 1983; NICAR et al. 1984).

Citrate acid plays a fundamental role in energy production from carbohydrate and lipid metabolism as part of the tricarboxylic acid pathway (KREBS and JOHNSON 1937; LOWENSTEIN 1969). The large stores of citrate in bone are probably accounted for by the low rate of citrate metabolism in bone (VAES and NICHOLS 1961). The direct relationship between bone resorption and citrate accumulation which is accentuated by bone-resorbing agents has been considered by some to be strong evidence that bone citrate is intimately involved in the resorption of bone (REYNOLDS 1972).

Glycosaminoglycans. The glycosaminoglycans (or acid mucopolysaccharides) are a group of related heteropolysaccharides widely distributed throughout the body in connective tissue where they play a fundamental role in the structure and integrity of this basic tissue. The characteristic disaccharide repeating unit is an N-acylated hexosamine. The commonest forms are hyaluronic acid, chondroitin sulphate, dermatan sulphate, keratin sulphate and heparin. One of the striking properties of these compounds is that they are large polyvalent anions and it is probably this property which makes them important in urine as inhibitors of stone-formation. The factors controlling the synthesis and metabolism of the compounds are poorly understood. There are a group of hereditary clinical disorders, the mucopolysaccharide storage diseases (McKUSICK et al. 1978) in which various enzyme deficiencies have been described. One of the features is excessive excretion of mucopolysaccharides in the urine.

The glycosaminoglycans occurring naturally in urine have been shown to influence the aggregation and growth of calcium oxalate crystals (CRAWFORD et al. 1968; ROBERTSON et al. 1973b). Urinary excretion usually amounts to 12–15 mg of GAGS/day in normal subjects. A major fraction of this material is probably produced by the renal tubules themselves but inflammation and damage to the kidney can also increase their excretion. Their excretion tends to be higher through the day than at night and is higher in males than females (ROBERTSON et al. 1976a). The factors controlling the excretion of these substances have not been clearly defined.

Pyrophosphate. Since the initial experiments (FLEISCH and NEUMAN 1961) showing that pyrophosphate inhibited the precipitation of calcium phosphate, there has been continued interest in this ion as a regulator of calcification in bone and as a natural urinary inhibitor of calcium stone-formation (FLEISCH 1978). In these respects it is analogous to citrate with a possible major role in bone metabolism and only a coincidental role in urine as an inhibitor of stone-formation. About 34 μmol of pyrophosphate are excreted in the urine daily in normal men (RUSSELL and HODGKINSON 1966), with less in women, at a plasma concentration of 3.5 μmol/l (RUSSELL et al. 1971).

Pyrophosphate is produced intracellularly by a larger number of reactions, the most typical involving the removal of pyrophosphate from a nucleotide triphosphate (KORNBERG 1962). The pyrophosphate produced from these reactions is hydrolysed within the cell to orthophosphate by intracellular pyrophosphatases. This renders most of these reactions irreversible and as such represents a fundamental metabolic step in the synthesis of nucleotide and peptide bonds and in fatty acid activation. Injected radio-labelled pyrophosphate has a rapid half-life of only a few minutes (FLEISCH and BISAZ 1962a; JUNG et al. 1970). The major route of removal is by hydrolysis, less than 5% being excreted in the urine. In congenital absence of alkaline phosphate, hypophosphatasia, the urinary excretion of pyrophosphate is greatly increased (RUSSELL 1965). It is probable that little pyrophosphate is absorbed from the diet although ingestion of orthophosphate increases the urinary excretion of pyrophosphate (FLEISCH et al. 1964; RUSSELL et al. 1964). The relationship between urinary pyrophosphate and urinary orthophosphate is probably due to a renal effect of orthophosphate and it is present in normal subjects and in subjects on a low and high phosphorus intake (RUSSELL and FLEISCH 1969; RUSSELL et al. 1976). The success of orthophosphate in preventing renal stone disease is in part probably due to its action to increase urinary pyrophosphate (SMITH et al. 1973b; PEACOCK et al. 1981c).

Because pyrophosphate itself is rapidly hydrolysed it has not been used therapeutically. However, synthetic analogues (diphosphonates) in which the P-O-P bond (Fig. 42) is replaced by a P-C-P bond have been found to be more stable and to possess many of the properties of pyrophosphate. They have marked effects on both calcium phosphate and oxalate crystal growth and aggregation in vitro (see Section II.4(g)). Some of these compounds have been used to treat urinary stone disease and although they are excreted in urine in low concentration because of poor absorption and a high affinity for bone they do effect calcium crystallization (FRASER et al. 1972; ROBERTSON et al. 1974, 1980b; OHATA and PAK 1973, 1974).

Magnesium. Magnesium oxalate is more soluble than calcium oxalate and the high excretion of magnesium in the urine reduces the concentration of oxalate available for calcium oxalate precipitation (ROBERTSON 1969a; MEYER and SMITH 1975b; FINLAYSON 1977a). In addition to this action, however, magnesium has also been considered by some to be an inhibitor of calcium stone-formation by its action on the crystallization of calcium salts (MUKAI and HOWARD 1963; DESMARS and TAWASHI 1973).

Magnesium is present in most foods of plant and animal origin since it is the major intracellular divalent cation of all tissues. It is present in the porphyrin complex of chlorophyll and more than two-thirds of the daily magnesium intake is contributed by cereals and vegetables (DAVIDSON and PASSMORE 1969). Substantial amounts can also be taken in with water since in some areas the water may naturally be high in magnesium, a litre of water sometimes supplying over a third of the daily magnesium intake (SCHROEDER et al. 1969). The availability of magnesium for absorption is influenced by digestive factors which release intracellular magnesium from food, solubilizing it within the gastrointestinal tract (WILKINSON 1976). Approximately 40% of dietary magnesium is absorbed (HEATON and PYRAH 1963; KING and STANBURY 1970) and the relationship between net absorption and dietary intake is linear over a wide range of dietary intakes (WILKINSON 1976). Magnesium absorption occurs throughout the gastrointestinal tract. Following a dose of labelled magnesium, peak magnesium absorption occurs 4 to 6 hours later with a steady rate of absorption occurring up to about 8 hours (AIKAWA et al. 1958; GRAHAM et al. 1960). The small intestine, therefore, is the major site of magnesium absorption, although the colon is capable of transporting magnesium under certain situations. Certainly magnesium deficiency occurs in patients with small bowel resection (FLETCHER et al. 1960; NIELSEN and THAYSEN 1971).

Many factors have been shown to alter magnesium absorption. There is an interrelationship between magnesium and calcium absorption such that increasing one reduces the absorption of the other. This reciprocal relationship can be explained by assuming that part of their absorptive processes are linked and that competitive inhibition occurs. The same end result can occur through digestive factors, however, since any substance chelating one cation will also be competing for chelation with the other. In man, in diseases which affect calcium absorption, there tends to be a direct relationship between calcium and magnesium, probably reflecting specific effects of vitamin D and parathyroid hormone on the transport of these two cations (WILKINSON 1976).

Under normal situations the urinary excretion of magnesium equals the amount absorbed and about 90–95% of the filtered magnesium is reabsorbed by the tubule. In situations of increased magnesium intake a rise in plasma magnesium results in an increased excretion of magnesium. In situations of decreased magnesium, urinary magnesium falls to extremely low levels and only if this low level is continued does the plasma magnesium then begin to fall (SHILS 1964). Unlike calcium, there is no hormonal control mechanism to maintain the

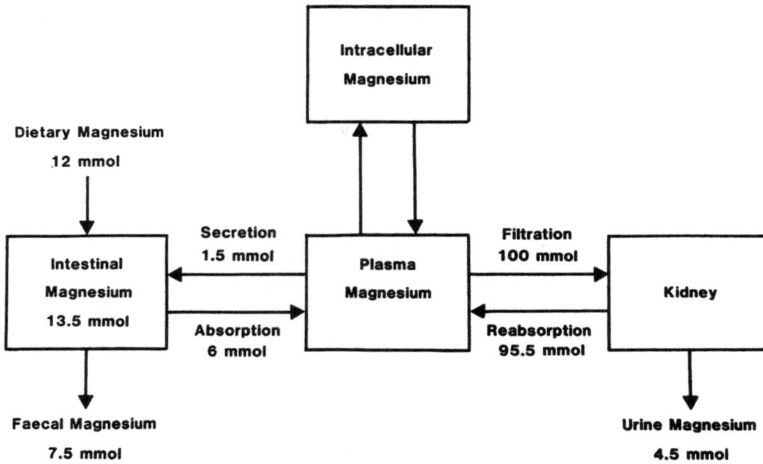

Fig. 43. Schema of magnesium metabolism in a normal adult in balance on an average intake of magnesium

plasma magnesium within a narrow range and, although the plasma magnesium in normal subjects is remarkably constant, wide changes in plasma magnesium occur in diseases affecting magnesium intake and absorption or renal function (Fig. 43).

δ) Other Urinary Risk Factors

The other factors influencing calcium stone-formation are volume, pH, uric acid and possibly phosphate. The control of urine volume has been discussed above (see Section III.2(b) (*γ*)). In calcium stone-formation, changes in urine volume have two main effects which tend to act in opposite directions.

A decrease in urine volume causes an increase in the saturation level of the calcium salts. This promotes precipitation and crystal formation. On the other hand, the concentrations of urinary inhibitors are increased and crystal growth and aggregation will be retarded. The overall effect tends to follow that on saturation since a low urine volume (< 1 litre/day) is generally associated with a high risk of stones and a high urine volume is associated with a low risk. However, there appears to be no further beneficial effect on the risk of stones above urine volumes of 2.5 to 3 litres per day (Robertson et al. 1980a, 1981a).

Uric acid has also been discussed above (see Section III.2(b) (*α*)). Its importance in calcium stone-formation is probably through its inhibitory action on the GAG inhibitors. In urines with a high uric acid concentration, the GAG inhibitors appear to be less active in preventing stone-formation (see Section II.4(e)). This relationship could possibly also be altered by fluid volume since it is not clear over what range of uric acid concentrations the attenuating effect on the GAG inhibitors remains linear.

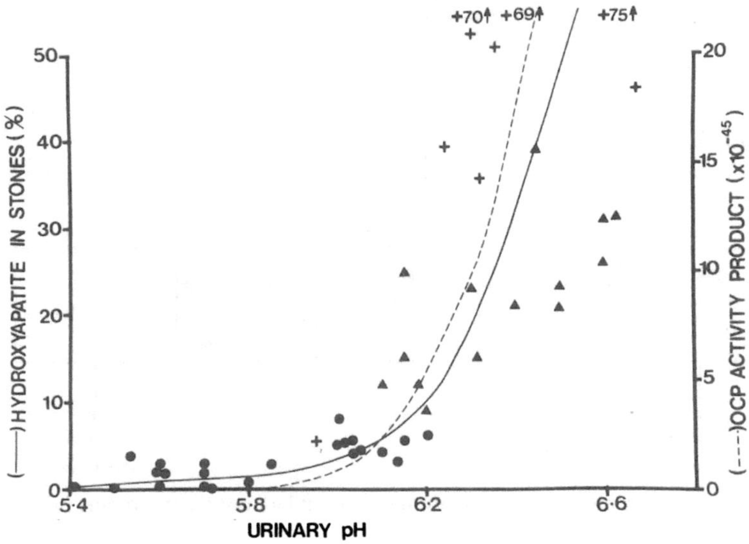

Fig. 44. The proportion of hydroxyapatite (——) in the urinary calculi of "pure" CaOx stone-formers (●), "mixed" CaOx/CaP stone-formers (▲) and hyperparathyroid stone-formers (+) in relation to their average 24-hour urinary pH. Also shown is the corresponding relationship between the saturation of urine with octocalcium phosphate (OCP) (- - - - -) and urinary pH

Control of urine pH has been discussed above (see Section III.2(b) (β)). It is an important risk factor for the precipitation of calcium phosphate. Above a urine pH of 6.2, calcium phosphate will precipitate out over a wide range of urinary phosphate; in persistently acid urines, on the other hand, calcium phosphate will not precipitate out even in the presence of a high phosphate concentration. The amount of calcium phosphate in the stone is largely determined by the prevailing pH of the urine during the time of stone-formation (Fig. 44).

It follows, from the above argument, that urinary phosphate itself is not an important risk factor for calcium stones (ROBERTSON et al. 1978). The urinary excretion of phosphate is for the most part determined by the dietary intake of phosphorus. Approximately 60% of dietary phosphorus is absorbed and appears in the urine. There is, however, an important relationship between phosphorus intake and pyrophosphate excretion, as mentioned earlier. The higher the intake of phosphorus, the greater is the excretion of pyrophosphate (FLEISCH et al. 1964; RUSSELL et al. 1964).

c) Stone Disease

α) Idiopathic calcium stone disease

Idiopathic stone disease accounts for about 80% of all patients with calcium stones (NORDIN et al. 1979; COE 1980; PEACOCK and ROBERTSON 1980). It is at least two to three times more common in men than women (WILLIAMS 1963,

1969). Most patients first present between the ages of 30 and 40 and it is uncommon in children and people over the age of 65 (COE 1980). The effect of age and sex on stone occurrence is reflected by their effect on the urinary risk factors. Children have a high excretion of GAG inhibitors which prevent stone-formation despite high concentrations of calcium oxalate due to low fluid volume (ROBERTSON et al. 1978, 1980a, 1981a). In the elderly, calcium excretion and, probably, oxalate excretion, are lower than in the young adult (BULUSU et al. 1970). Women have lower excretions of both calcium and oxalate than men of comparable age (ROBERTSON et al. 1978). The recurrence rate of stones between and within individuals is high. Some patients may only have one or two episodes of stone throughout their lives whereas others may have that number every year (WILLIAMS 1963, 1969; BLACKLOCK 1969). The mean recurrence time is approximately 5 years (WILLIAMS 1963, 1969; BLACKLOCK 1969; COE 1977). The disease affects both kidneys equally (HARRISON et al. 1945; MATES and KRICEK 1955; AHLGEN and LORSTAD 1965) although unilateral involvement is more common than bilateral (BLACKLOCK 1969). Several studies have indicated that renal stone disease is more common in the siblings and parents of stone-formers than is expected from the prevalence of the disease in the general population (McGEOWN 1960; PRIDGEN et al. 1968; LJUNGHALL 1979). However, not all studies have shown this and, furthermore, there is little doubt that environmental factors, such as diet, could account for a major proportion of the familial tendency to stone-formation (WHITE et al. 1969). There are wide geographical and racial variations in the prevalence of urinary stone disease and although this could be accounted for by variations in stone-formation other than calcium stone, it is probably that these variations reflect different prevalence rates mainly in calcium stone disease (ANDERSEN 1969, 1973; BLACKLOCK 1969, 1976; SIERAKOWSKI et al. 1978; ROBERTSON et al. 1979c, 1980a). Calcium stone disease is more common in people in the higher social classes, reflecting the effect of income and diet on the prevalence rate (WHITE et al. 1969; SUTOR 1976; ROBERTSON et al. 1979c, 1980a). Several dietary factors have been implicated (including calcium, refined carbohydrate, fibre, purine and animal protein); of these, a high intake of animal protein (coupled with purine) is probably the major factor (COE et al. 1976; ROBERTSON et al. 1979c, 1980a).

The diagnosis of calcium stone disease is made on stone analysis of a stone passed spontaneously or removed surgically (PEACOCK and ROBERTSON 1980). Idiopathic calcium stone disease is diagnosed by excluding the other types of calcium stone disease which can all be diagnosed on positive criteria. Although there are no specific criteria for establishing the diagnosis of idiopathic disease it does have, however, a number of biochemical abnormalities. These only occur in a proportion of patients and in the individual may not be consistently present. From the studies reported from various centres it is difficult to be sure exactly what proportion of the idiopathic population have these abnormalities – particularly in the plasma. Some studies include male and female patients together without consideration of the effect of age and sex on normal ranges. A further problem in any series of idiopathic stone patients studied is how much selection has occurred since many of these patients are referred for further study and the exclusion of calcium stone formers with an underlying disease, particularly primary hyperparathyroidism, has not always been meticulous. Nevertheless, it is clear that a number of biochemical abnormalities are present. The urinary excretions of calcium (FLOCKS 1939; HODGKINSON and PYRAH 1958; ROBERTSON et al. 1968, 1978), oxalate (ROBERTSON et al. 1969, 1978; HODGKINSON 1974) and uric acid (COE and KAVALICH 1974; ROBERTSON et al. 1978) are increased in about 30% of patients. The glycosaminoglycan inhibitors are reduced (ROBERTSON et al. 1978) and urinary pH tends to be high, particularly in those patients with the highest amounts of calcium phosphate in the stone (MARSHALL et al. 1972b; ROBERTSON et al. 1978). It has been reported that the urinary excretions of magnesium (SUTTON and WATSON 1968; HODGKINSON 1974, 1978), pyrophosphate (FLEISCH and BISAZ 1962b; BAUMANN et al. 1977) and citrate (HODGKINSON 1962; WELSHMAN and MCGEOWN 1976; SCHWILLE et al. 1979) are also reduced but these have not been universal findings (LEWIS et al. 1966; RUSSELL and HODGKINSON 1966; O'BRIEN et al. 1967; ROBERTSON et al. 1968, 1971, 1978, 1984; JOHANSSON et al. 1980b; RUDMAN et al. 1980).

A low plasma phosphate concentration with a decreased tubular reabsorption of phosphate occurs in about 30% of patients (ALBRIGHT et al. 1953; PEACOCK et al. 1976a, b). Plasma 1,25-dihydroxyvitamin D concentration is increased or is in the high-normal range in a proportion of patients (SHEN et al. 1977; PEACOCK et al. 1981b). Plasma parathyroid hormone concentration is in the normal range (PAK et al. 1974; PEACOCK et al. 1976a, b) although some workers have reported an increase in a proportion of their patients (COE et al. 1973). The significance of these raised plasma parathyroid hormone concentrations still remains unclear since only some immunoassays show up this abnormality. Apart from these abnormalities, plasma biochemistry, in particular plasma calcium, both totel and ionized, is normal.

In addition to these biochemical abnormalities, hyperabsorption of calcium is present in many of these patients, which in general correlates with the raised concentration of plasma $1,25(OH)_2$ vitamin D. A few of these may also have a raised fasting urinary calcium and have been defined as having tubular hypercalciuria. This often occurs in women and there remains some doubt whether these patients may or may not have a mild form of primary hyperparathyroidism.

It is difficult, at the present time, to bring these various abnormalities into a unified hypothesis of cause and effect which leads to a disease resulting in renal stones. Two possible explanations are possible. The first is that idiopathic stone disease is made up of several conditions which at present are grouped together thus explaining the variety and non-uniformity of the biochemical abnormalities observed. The second, which is more likely, is that patients with idiopathic calcium stone disease have been selected from the normal population to form stones by their risk factors (both urinary and metabolic). They tend to lie at the extremes of the normal ranges for those variables and it is the overall combination of these (sometimes) small abnormalities which increases their risk of stones.

β) Primary Hyperparathyroid Stone Disease

Calcium stone-formation secondary to an underlying disease is most commonly due to primary hyperparathyroidism (Fig. 37) which accounts for between 5 and 10% of the calcium stone-forming population (HELLSTRÖM and IVEMARK 1962; McGEOWN 1963; WILLIAMS 1969; YENDT 1970; LAVAN et al. 1971; BROADUS 1980). Since primary hyperparathyroidism is more common (MULLER 1969) and idiopathic calcium stone disease less common (NORDIN et al. 1979) in women than men, then the chance of a female calcium stone-former being a case of hyperparathyroidism is much higher than it is in a male calcium stone-former (PEACOCK 1978).

The prevalence of primary hyperparathyroidism in the population is between 0.1 and 1 in 1000 (BOONSTRA and JACKSON 1971). In about 30–60% of patients, the disorder first presents with renal stone disease (KEATING 1961; PYRAH et al. 1966; COPE 1966; LLOYD 1968; PURNELL et al. 1971; BROADUS 1980); the exact percentage is to a large extent dependent on the population from which the primary hyperparathyroid patients are drawn. In centres specially interested in renal stone disease, often with an interest in hyperparathyroidism, the percentage may be high. In centres where routine plasma calcium is measured in all hospital patients or in biochemical screening programmes of the normal population, a large number of primary hyperparathyroid patients present with hypercalcaemia which is usually completely asymptomatic (TASHIMA 1970). Once patients with asymptomatic hyperparathyroidism have been screened from any population the incidence of the disease decreases since asymptomatic hyperparathyroidism can remain so for a considerable time without progressing (PURNELL et al. 1971; BROADUS 1980).

The stone recurrence rate in primary hyperparathyroidism is similar to that of idiopathic calcium stone disease and there is a wide variation between and within individuals. The age of onset, however, is different from that of idiopathic stone disease, coming on at a later age (PYRAH et al. 1966). This is largely influenced by the number of women who become hyperparathyroid after the menopause.

The composition of the stone passed in patients with primary hyperparathyroidism tends to have a higher content of phosphate than oxalate (HODGKINSON et al. 1969; HODGKINSON and MARSHALL 1975). Indeed some patients may pass almost pure calcium phosphate stones and in this respect are similar to patients with renal tubular acidosis. Both kidneys are involved and occasionally there is associated nephrocalcinosis. This may take one of two forms. In the first, multiple small stones form within the collecting ducts. They have a similar appearance radiographically to the deposits in medullary sponge kidney. In the second, there is true nephrocalcinosis consisting of calcium salts deposited in the cortex and the medulla. These may or may not be associated with urinary stone-formation.

The urinary abnormalities present in idiopathic stone disease are also present in hyperparathyroid stone disease (PEACOCK et al. 1976a; ROBERTSON et al. 1980a, 1981a). Hypercalciuria and a high urinary pH are, however, the most consistent findings (PEACOCK et al. 1976a). Plasma calcium is elevated in all patients. Normocalcaemic primary hyperparathyroidism has been described but this diagnosis is difficult to sustain unless there is concomitant vitamin D deficiency or renal failure (both of which tend to reduce the risk of forming stones) to account for the normal plasma calcium. Patients with mild forms of the disease, however, are common and in these the plasma calcium concentrations may move in and out of the high normal range. These patients are difficult to distinguish from patients with idiopathic stone disease and a slightly raised parathyroid hormone concentration. Plasma parathyroid hormone concentration, like plasma calcium, should be elevated in all patients. However, the plasma level of parathyroid hormone is dependent on the assay used and some assays actually measure plasma parathyroid hormone concentrations in the normal range in a proportion of hyperparathyroid patients particularly in the milder forms of the disease. Urinary cyclic AMP is usually raised and may be helpful, although in the milder forms of the disease there is a large overlap with normal values (DREZNER et al. 1976; BABKA et al. 1976; BROADUS et al. 1977). Plasma phosphate is reduced due to decreased tubular reabsorption of phosphate. The tubular reabsorption of calcium is increased. Plasma $1{,}25(OH)_2$ vitamin D concentrations are elevated or in the high-normal range and correlate with hyperabsorption of calcium (KAPLAN et al. 1977). Plasma alkaline phosphatase and hydroxyproline excretion due to increased bone turnover may be elevated but in many patients with stone disease they are both commonly within the normal range. This is not the case in patients with hyperparathyroidism and clinical bone disease. These patients, however, are at less risk of forming urinary stones since the bone disease is accelerated by a relative malabsorption of calcium due to low plasma $1{,}25(OH)_2$ vitamin D levels (PEACOCK 1978).

γ) Hyperoxaluric Stone Disease

In idopathic calcium stone disease, mild hyperoxaluria occurs in a proportion of patients, the urinary oxalate excretion lying just above the normal range (ROBERTSON and PEACOCK 1980). On the other hand, in hyperoxaluric stone disease, the urinary excretion of oxalate is at least three times that of normal subjects (SHEPARD et al. 1960; HOCKADAY et al. 1964; HOFMANN et al. 1970). There are two main forms of this condition. In hereditary hyperoxaluria, the abnormalities lie in oxalate metabolism. It is often also referred to as primary or congenital hyperoxaluria. The second form is an acquired condition, probably due to increased absorption of oxalate from the gastrointestinal tract and generally referred to as enteric hyperoxaluria.

Other forms of hyperoxaluria occur but are extremely uncommon (SMITH 1980). Dietary hyperoxaluria is due to an excessive intake of foods high in oxalate content. It can also be due to a high intake of oxalate precursors such as ethylene glycol or ascorbic acid. The former has been taken as a poison and the latter for the non-specific treatment of several diseases. Since 40% of endogenous oxalate is derived from the ascorbic acid pathway a high ascorbic acid intake is potentially dangerous. However, it requires a massive increase in ascorbic acid ingestion to increase urinary oxalate appreciably (LAMBDEN and CHRYSTOWSKI 1954; SCHMIDT et al. 1981). Zylotal (THOMAS et al. 1976) given as an intravenous source of calories, anaesthesia with methoxyflurane (FRASCINO et al. 1970), and experimental pyridoxine deficiency (FABER et al. 1963) can induce increased excretion of urinary oxalate from endogenous production. Pyridoxine deficiency itself is unusual in humans and is unlikely ever to be a cause of hyperoxaluria. It is interesting, however, that some patients with congenital hyperoxaluria reduce their urine oxalate excretion when pyridoxine is given in massive doses (GERSHOFF 1964; SMITH and WILLIAMS 1967; GIBBS and WATTS 1970; WILL and BIJVOET 1979). There is also a recent report of 2 cases of idiopathic calcium stone disease with hyperoxaluria whose urinary oxalate fell on treatment with pyridoxine (HARRISON et al. 1981). Infection with *aspergillus* tends to cause local deposition of calcium oxalate; this is presumably due to the ability of this organism to manufacture and excrete high amounts of oxalate (NIME and HUTCHINS 1973).

Hereditary Hyperoxaluria. Hereditary hyperoxaluria Type I (and probably Type 2) appear to be inherited as an autosomal recessive character with equal frequency in both sexes and there is often a history of consanguinity in the family (HOCKADAY et al. 1964; WILLIAMS and SMITH 1968b). However, it has been suggested that there is some genetic heterogeneity in its inheritance pattern (SHEPARD et al. 1960). The two types of hereditary hyperoxaluria may be differentiated by measuring the urinary excretions of glyoxylic and glyceric acids (HODGKINSON 1977; SMITH 1980).

Hereditary hyperoxaluria is uncommon and usually accounts for less than 1% of all calcium stone-formers. The majority of patients develop symptoms before the age of five and present with renal colic or haematuria. Some children may present with renal failure and delayed growth. Patients, however, tend to be referred to special Stone Centres and in 1964 over a hundred patients from several countries could be reviewed (HOCKADAY et al. 1964). The condition should always be suspected in children presenting with urinary stone disease, particularly if siblings are affected. The diagnosis is established by determining the urinary excretion of oxalate which is consistently raised. Plasma oxalate is usually high enough to be measured even by the poor methods which are at present available. Plasma biochemistry usually also shows the effects of renal failure. Indeed, the prognosis is poor because of the early onset of renal failure due to a high stone recurrence rate and the deposition of calcium oxalate in the tissues, particularly the kidney.

Enteric Hyperoxaluria. This condition is defined by an increased urinary oxalate due to altered bowel function and not to an abnormally high intake of oxalate, nor, as far as is known, to altered oxalate metabolism. Urinary oxalate excretion may be increased from just above the normal range to as high as the urinary oxalate excretion found in patients with hereditary hyperoxaluria. The association between disease of the bowel and urinary stone-formation was clearly recognised (LINDAHL and BARGEN 1941; DEREN et al. 1962; MARATKA and NEDBAL 1964; BENNETT and JEPSON 1966; GELZAYD et al. 1968) before it was appreciated that many of these patients had hyperoxaluria (SMITH et al. 1970; ADMIRAND et al. 1971; DOWLING et al. 1971). Hyperoxaluria occurs in a number of bowel diseases, the common factors probably being malabsorption and steatorrhoea in the presence of a normally functioning colon.

Surgical bypass of the small bowel for morbid obesity frequently gives rise to hyperoxaluria and calcium oxalate stone disease (DICKSTEIN and FRAME 1973; O'LEARY et al. 1974). It is also a common sequela of small bowel resection usually for inflammatory diseases such as Crohn's disease or small bowel infarction (GREGORY et al. 1977; BAMBACH et al. 1981). It can also be present, although less commonly, in coeliac disease and in the bacterial overgrowth of blind-loop syndrome.

The increase in urinary oxalate is now generally considered to be due to increased oxalate absorption from the colon (EARNEST et al. 1974; DOBBINS and BINDER 1977). Various hypotheses have been put forward to explain the increased absorption of oxalate. Malabsorption of bile acids and their subsequent increased concentration in the colon may increase the permeability of the colon to oxalate (SMITH and HOFMANN 1974; CHADWICK et al. 1977). The glycine in glycocholic acid could also act as a precursor for bacterial production of oxalate which is subsequently absorbed (HOFMANN et al. 1970; DOWLING et al. 1971; HOFMANN and POLEY 1972; SMITH and HOFMANN 1974). Another factor which may increase the absorption of oxalate is the increased availability of oxalate after removal of calcium by fatty acid-binding in the intestine since calcium oxalate is not readily absorbed by the bowel (EARNEST et al. 1974).

Although hyperoxaluria is usually the main urinary risk factor for the formation of stones, a decreased urine volume is often an important contributory factor (BAMBACH et al. 1981). A reduced urinary citrate excretion, induced by acidaemia, may also play a minor role in those patients acidaemic from persistent loss of bowel secretions. Hypomagnesaemia may also be present in a number of patients and promote stone formation by a reduction of inhibitory power in the urine (SMITH et al. 1979).

It should be remembered that uric acid stone-formation, particularly in patients with ileostomies, is also a common complication and it cannot be assumed that all stones passed by patients with bowel disease are necessarily composed of calcium oxalate (CLARKE and MCKENZIE 1969; BAMBACH et al. 1981). The overall occurrence of stone disease in patients with bowel disease is between 10 and 30% (BAMBACH et al. 1981).

It is probable, however, that patients with enteric hyperoxaluria would have a very high incidence of stone disease if calcium metabolism were normal. In patients with bowel disease, urinary excretion of calcium is low because of calcium malabsorption and an increased prevalence of vitamin D-deficient osteomalacia (PEACOCK et al. 1981 a). Severe hypocalciuria is often a striking abnormality in these patients and despite the high oxalate excretion frequently prevents the urine from being oversaturated with calcium oxalate (BAMBACH et al. 1981; PEACOCK et al. 1981 a). When these patients are treated with vitamin D for osteomalacia, urinary calcium eventually rises and the risk of forming calcium oxalate stones is greatly increased (PEACOCK et al. 1981 a).

The diagnosis of calcium oxalate stone disease due to enteric hyperoxaluria is made on the history of bowel disease or surgery, and the excessive excretion of urinary oxalate. Tests for malabsorption are usually performed. The hyperabsorption of oxalate can be demonstrated by measuring urinary oxalate on a high and low oxalate diet or after a standard load of oxalate (CHADWICK et al. 1973; EARNEST et al. 1974; GREGORY et al. 1977; BARILLA et al. 1978). In some patients the history of bowel disease, particularly resection of the bowel, may have been carried out in childhood and forgotten; a detailed history is, therefore, always important. Plasma biochemistry is usually unhelpful apart from showing up other biochemical features of malabsorption such as osteomalacia.

δ) *Renal Tubular Acidosis Stone Disease*

The formation of calcium phosphate stones in patients with renal tubular acidosis is common; indeed, urinary stone is often the presenting feature of the condition. Renal tubular acidosis can occur as a primary condition or secondary to renal disease. In the primary form there are no underlying diseases which give rise to the tubular defect in acidification and the symptoms, signs and biochemical abnormalities are all attributable to a failure of urinary acidification. Females are more often affected than males and the disease presents from childhood onwards. In childhood, there is a variant of the disease which usually affects boys and which, uncommonly, produces urinary stones. This form of the disorder regresses with treatment. It is sometimes referred to as 'infantile renal tubular acidosis' as opposed to 'adult' but is probably best referred to as 'transient renal tubular acidosis' (HUTH et al. 1960; LIGHTWOOD and BUTLER 1963). In the persistent or adult type of primary tubular acidosis the majority of the patients are female and nephrocalcinosis and urinary stone disease affects over 70% of patients (SELDIN and WILSON 1978). Nephrocalcinosis occurs more frequently than urinary stone itself (PYRAH and HODGKINSON 1960) and the renal calcification tends to be dense and have a medullary distribution particularly affecting the calyces. The radiological findings are similar to those seen in nephrocalcinosis due to primary hyperparathyroidism and in medullary sponge kidney. In both of these latter disorders further diagnostic difficulties may arise since occasionally renal tubular acidosis may occur secondary to both these conditions. Calcification of the kidneys, the passage of urinary stones, attacks of renal colic and haematuria may be the first presentation of the disease. Urinary tract infection is a frequent complication and may be the first indication that tubular acidosis and stone disease are present. Some of these patients may produce infected stones rather than calcium stones and may be difficult to distinguish from urinary tract infection with secondary impairment of renal function. In the latter, however, nephrocalcinosis is rare. Electrolyte abnormalities particularly hypokalaemia are also common and patients may present with severe muscle weakness, chronic acidaemia, anorexia and lethargy. Occasionally osteomalacia or rickets may be the presenting features.

Renal tubular acidosis can be due to failure of bicarbonate reabsorption (Type 1) or to a failure of achieving a normal pH gradient between blood and urine (Type 2). In the former the response to bicarbonate treatment is slow since much of it leaks into the urine whereas in the latter the response is rapid and the urine pH is uniformly high irrespective of the degree of systemic acidosis. The majority of cases of primary renal tubular acidosis are sporadic with a negative family history (PIEL 1957). In some patients, however, there is a clear family history suggesting that an autosomal dominant type of inheritance is responsible (SCHREINER et al. 1953; RANDALL 1967).

In secondary renal tubular acidosis a number of identifiable diseases is present which have in common the ability to cause injury to the renal tubule. These include: disproteinaemic disease (MORRIS and FUDENBERG 1967), vitamin D intoxication (FERRIS et al. 1961), hyperthyroidism (HUTH et al. 1959), metal poisoning with such as cadmium (KAZANTZIS et al. 1963) and mercury (MacGREGOR and RAYNER 1964), treatment with out-dated tetracyclines (FRIMPTER et al. 1963) or amphotericin B (McCURDY et al. 1968), Sjögren's syndrome (TALAL et al. 1968), Wilson's disease (MORGAN et al. 1962), Lowe's syndrome (SCHOEN 1959), galactosaemia (BICKEL and THURSBY-PEKHAM 1954), hereditary fructose intolerance (MORRIS 1968), chronic urinary tract infection (ALBRIGHT and REIFENSTEIN 1948; COCHRAN et al. 1968), medullary sponge kidney (MORRIS 1969) and primary hyperparathyroidism (FOURMAN et al. 1960). These conditions usually give rise to Type 1 tubular acidosis with nephrocalcinosis being less common than in Type 2 but stone disease is equally common (SELDIN and WILSON 1978).

Diagnosis is easily established in those patients with acidaemia who have a persistently high urinary pH. In the patients without acidaemia the diagnosis can be established by measuring the urinary pH after an oral acid load (WRONG and DAVIES 1959). In these occult cases where there is a failure to establish a pH-gradient, a bicarbonate infusion to determine the maximum tubular reabsorption capacity is necessary. Either hyper- or hypokalaemia may be present although the effects of renal failure may overshadow the biochemical picture in some patients.

In most centres dealing with renal stone disease, renal tubular acidosis is encountered only occasionally. In some, however, a high percentage of patients who appear to be idiopathic calcium stone-formers have been reported to show a failure in urinary acidification after a standard acid load (BACKMAN et al. 1980). Patients with idopathic calcium stone disease and predominantly calcium phosphate stones tend to have a higher 24-hour urine pH (WRONG and DAVIES 1959) and calcium phosphate saturation levels in their urine (MARSHALL et al. 1972b). However, no defect in acidification has been found in this group (personal observation).

ε) *Medullary Sponge Kidney Stone Disease*

Medullary sponge kidney usually accounts for less than 1% of all stone-formers and about 3 to 4% of recurrent stone-formers (MAYALL 1970; LAVAN et al. 1971; BACKMAN et al. 1981) although in one series a mild form of the disorder (tubular ectasia) is reported in 13% of calcium stone-formers (YENDT et al. 1981). It is diagnosed essentially by radiology (LENARDUZZI 1939; CACHI and RICCI 1949). This shows, on intravenous urography, that there are multiple small cysts up to about 5 mm in diameter representing dilatations in the collecting ducts (LINDWALL 1959; LALLI 1969). These may be present in a single pyramid or all may be affected. This may lead to enlargement of the papillae. Some cysts appear to be unconnected with the urinary excretory system (EKSTRÖM et al. 1959; HARRISON and ROSE 1979). The radiological appearance must be distinguished, however, from that of medullary calcinosis due to hyperparathyroidism and that of renal tubular acidosis. Tuberculosis of the kidney can also occasionally have a similar appearance.

Histologically, dilated collecting ducts can be found in continuity with the tubules and/or the renal pelvis. Spotty calcification may be seen, often bulging into the calyces. In the majority of patients, small calcium stones occur within the areas of dilatation. Urinary tract infection is a fairly common complication (HARRISON and ROSE 1979). Patients usually present with renal colic, passage of urinary stones, haematuria or pyelonephritis (HARRISON and ROSE 1979), but the prevalence of the disease is uncertain since patients without urinary stone or infection may never present for investigation. The disease is thought by some (KUIPER 1971), but not others (EKSTRÖM et al. 1959; MORRIS et al. 1965; BUTLER et al. 1973; HARRISON and ROSE 1979) to be familial although the mode of inheritance is not clear. Renal tubular acidosis of the secondary type is sometimes present (MORRIS 1969).

The prognosis of medullary sponge kidney is good and renal failure is not a direct consequence of the disease. This contrasts with medullary cystic disease which has a much more serious prognosis.

It has been reported recently that ectasia of the collecting ducts is common in patients with idiopathic calcium stone disease (YENDT et al. 1981). It is unlikely, however, that the changes described by these workers would be accepted as constituting medullary sponge kidney by most investigators and histological evidence corresponding to these changes has not been produced.

The formation of urinary stones in this condition is poorly understood but it probably represents a local problem related to urine flow and water reabsorption which results in a high concentration of calcium stone-forming salts within these cysts. There are no distinguishing biochemical abnormalities either in urine or blood to help with the diagnosis which is still primarily based on the radiological features seen on intravenous pyelography, although some workers have reported a tendency to hypercalciuria (EKSTRÖM et al. 1959; FELTS et al. 1964; STEYN and LOGIE 1964; HARRISON and ROSE 1979; BACKMAN et al. 1981).

Φ) Uncommon Forms of Calcium Stone-Formation

Several other diseases are associated with calcium stone formation. In all of these there has been no thorough examination of the urinary risk factors involved. Usually urinary volume, pH and calcium have been measured but there are few data on the excretion of uric acid, inhibitors or oxalate.

Cushing's Disease and Steroid Treatment. There is a high prevalence of calcium stone disease in patients with Cushing's disease or Cushing's syndrome (WANG and ROBBINS 1956; SCHOLZ et al. 1957; ROSS et al. 1966). On the other hand, steroid treatment, which is considerably more common than Cushing's disease, seems to give rise to calcium stone-formation much less often. In part, this may be due to the fact that patients treated with steroids are often suffering from serious debilitating diseases which by themselves may reduce the urinary risk factors responsible for calcium stone-formation.

In Cushing's disease it is not clear what factors in the urine are responsible for stone-formation. Urinary calcium is not excessively high in spite of the fact that the patient often develops osteoporosis from negative calcium balance. The hypokalaemic alkalosis probably gives rise to a persistently alkaline urine which increases the risk of calcium phosphate stone-formation. The origin of the stones may be partly explained by the observation that patients with Cushing's syndrome often have microscopic renal calcification (SHORTLAND and CRANE 1969).

Immobilization. During immobilization a negative skeletal balance occurs and calcium appears in the urine in excessive amounts for a variable period (DEITRICK et al. 1948; SMITH et al. 1969). In some patients, the hypercalciuria may be quite marked and there is an increased risk of calcium stone (PYRAH and FOWWEATHER 1938; PULVERTAFT 1939; SMITH et al. 1969). In many of these patients, however, for example in paraplegics and in patients with multiple injury, catheterisation of the bladder is frequently necessary. Recurrent urinary tract infection is common in such patients and infected stone disease is a common complication (ELLIOT and TODD 1961). The high urinary pH and hypercalciuria promote calcium phosphate precipitation which may overlay the magnesium ammonium phosphate stone (SMITH et al. 1969). Interestingly, the incidence of stones in immobilized patients fell markedly after the general introduction of antibiotic therapy in the mid-1940s, suggesting that urinary infection must have been the major cause of stones in this condition. Nevertheless, a few idiopathic stone formers do give a history of immobilization prior to symptoms of stone disease and it is likely that non-infected quiescent stone-formation may have developed during the immobilization period.

Vitamin D Intoxication. Vitamin D, its hydroxylated metabolites, and synthetic analogues given in quantities in excess of requirements, give rise to hyperabsorption of calcium from the intestine and to increased bone resorption (WILKINSON 1976). Hypercalciuria results in the absence of hypercalcaemia and the risk of calcium stone-formation is increased (TAYLOR 1972). Nephrocalcinosis is also a frequent complication of vitamin D excess (ANDERSON 1976) and frequently leads to renal failure (ANNING et al. 1948). On the other hand, in hypoparathyroid patients treated with vitamin D, urinary calcium is frequently in the hypercalciuric range yet calcium stone-formation is uncommon.

Sarcoidosis. Recurrent calcium stone disease, particularly with the production of small stones which are spontaneously passed in the urine, is present in some patients with sarcoidosis (LONGCOPE and FREIMAN 1952; SCHOLZ and KEATING 1956; ANDERSON and GRAHAM 1960). The stones found in patients with sarcoidosis are usually composed of calcium oxalate with or without an admixture of calcium phosphate. Hypercalciuria and mild hypercalcaemia are common (HARRELL and FISHER 1939; LE BACQ et al. 1970). Medullary calcinosis, particularly in the papillae, also occurs and these patients must be distinguished from patients with medullary sponge kidney, vitamin D intoxication and primary hyperparathyroidism. In occasional patients sarcoidosis and primary hyperparathyroidism may co-exist and it may be extremely difficult to be sure which condition is responsible for the urinary stone disease and the biochemical abnormalities.

Milk-alkali Syndrome. The increased ingestion of milk and alkali, with which peptic ulceration used to be treated, occasionally gives rise to calcium stone disease (DUFAULT and TOBIAS 1954; SCHOLZ and KEATING 1955; PYRAH 1979; ORWOLL 1982). The increase in urine calcium and pH are probably the main urinary risk factors responsible. Management of patients with peptic ulceration, however, has changed such that the milk-alkali regimen is now uncommon. There has been a concomitant decrease in the occurrence of calcium stone in patients with peptic ulceration. A small number of patients with idiopathic stone may give a history of high alkali ingestion for dyspepsia.

d) Stone-Formation

Calcium oxalate and calcium phosphate are the most insoluble of the stone-forming salts under the ionic conditions present in urine, which probably accounts for them being the most common constituents of urinary stones (HODGKINSON et al. 1969). Most evidence, however, points to calcium oxalate crystalluria as being the primary cause of this type of stone; the amount of CaP in the stone being largely determined by the prevailing pH of urine. The more alkaline the urine, the more CaP is present in the stone (Fig. 44).

The urinary factors leading to calcium stone-formation are more complex than those responsible for the other types of stone and appear to be largely dependent on the balance between the factors influencing the saturation of urine and those affecting the inhibitory activity (Section II.5(b)). As mentioned earlier, the urinary concentrations of calcium and oxalate along with urinary pH primarily determine the saturation of urine with calcium oxalate (CaOx) and calcium phosphate (CaP). The true activity product for CaOx (K_{CaOx}), which requires about 12 biochemical estimations in every urine sample may be calculated from the expression:

$$K_{CaOx} = \{Ca^{2+}\} \{C_2O_4^{2-}\}$$

where $\{Ca^{2+}\}$ and $\{C_2O_4^{2-}\}$ are the activities of the free ion concentrations of calcium and oxalate. That for CaP may be calculated as described in Section II.2(c).

When the urinary concentrations of these ions are translated into saturation levels of calcium oxalate and calcium phosphate, there is a progressive rise in the mean saturation values from normals through single stone-formers to recurrent stone-formers. In particular, the recurrent groups are frequently exposed to the risk of calcium oxalate crystalluria (ROBERTSON 1976b). Thus the first prerequisite of stone-formation i.e. that of excessive supersaturation leading to spontaneous crystalluria is satisfied.

The second important factor in calcium stone-formation is the role played by the inhibitor(s) of crystallization. In recent years, it has been shown that male, idiopathic calcium oxalate stone-formers, in fact, tend to have reduced levels of inhibitory activity in their urine with respect to the crystallization of calcium salts in vitro (THOMAS and HOWARD 1959; ROBERTSON and PEACOCK 1972; ROBERTSON et al. 1976c; BAUMANN et al. 1977; COE et al. 1980), although others have failed to confirm these observations (ROSE 1975). In about 50% of these patients, the reduction of inhibitory activity can be attributed to a lower than normal concentration of the polyanionic inhibitors (mainly glycosaminoglycans) mentioned earlier (ROBERTSON et al. 1976a). In the remainder, however, the reduction in inhibitory activity is associated with an apparently normal concentration of glycosaminoglycans in the urine. In these patients, most of whom have a tendency to hyperuricosuria in addition to their high calcium and oxalate excretions, the *effective* concentration of glycosaminoglycans is reduced by adsorption to the surface of colloidal particles of urate (ROBERTSON et al. 1976a). A similar phenomenon has been reported in the urines of Dalmatian dogs which excrete large amounts of "uric acid" in their urine in the form of colloidal urate. This is stabilised by adsorption of high molecular weight polyanions (PORTER 1966). This reduction in "free" glycosaminoglycans in the urine of hyperuricosuric calcium oxalate stone-formers makes less available to inhibit the growth and aggregation of the load of calcium oxalate crystal excreted by these patients and so a reduced level of inhibitory activity is measured in their urine (ROBERTSON et al. 1976a). This colloidal urate may be looked on as an "anti-inhibitor" of calcium oxalate crystallization and may explain the reported association between hyperuricosuria and calcium oxalate stone-formation (COE and KAVALICH 1974). It may also explain the mechanism by which allopurinol (a xanthine oxidase inhibitor which reduces uric acid excretion) apparently reduces the incidence of calcium oxalate stones in hyperuricosuric stone-formers (COE and KAVALICH 1974). The level of inhibitory activity towards growth and aggregation appears, therefore, to be determined by the balance between the urinary concentration of polyanionic macromolecules (mainaly glycosaminoglycans) which increase inhibitory activity and that of colloidal urate which decreases it (ROBERTSON et al. 1976a; PAK et al. 1979). These five urinary risk factors, together with a low urine volume, between them appear to determine the chemical risk of forming calcium-containing stones (ROBERTSON et al. 1978, 1981a).

Using the risk factor model of calcium stone-formation discussed earlier (Section II.5(b) (δ), it is possible to calculate the overall biochemical probability of forming calcium-containing stones from the combination of the six urinary risk factors. Figure 45 shows the relative probability of forming stones,

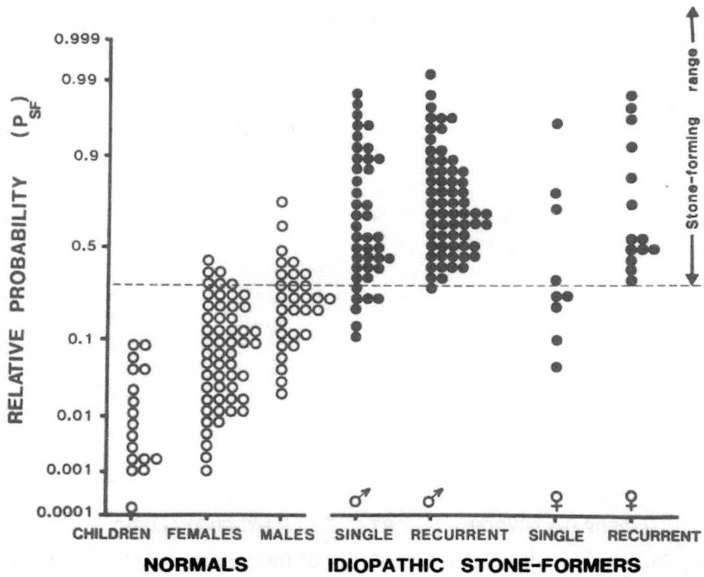

Fig. 45. The overall relative probability of forming calcium-containing stones (P_{SF}) in normal children and adults and in single and recurrent idiopathic calcium stone-formers

calculated in this way, in groups of normal subjects and idiopathic calcium stone-formers. In the normals the P_{SF} values range between 0.0001 and 0.55, the lowest values being in children and the highest in men. The P_{SF} values in women lie in an intermediate position. It is interesting that the relative magnitude of the values reflects the pattern of incidence of idiopathic calcium stones in these three sections of the population.

The underlying reasons for this order of overall risk of stones is that men have higher excretions of calcium, oxalate and uric acid than women and children. The latter actually have about the same urinary *concentrations* of calcium oxalate and uric acid as adults but are greatly protected from stones by having very high concentrations of protective GAG inhibitors.

Single stone-formers have P_{SF} values overlapping with normals and recurrent stone-formers. Presumably, some of these patients will eventually become recurrent stone-formers (since about 50–70% of all first-time stone-formers pass another stone in the following 10 years (WILLIAMS 1963)) and some will form no further stones during their lifetime. It will be interesting to see whether or not the single stone-formers with the highest P_{SF} values join the recurrent group and whether or not the patients with the lowest values form no more stones.

Figure 46 shows that the values of P_{SF} in various groups of patients who are at risk of forming calcium-containing stones secondary to some identifiable genetic or metabolic abnormality. In most of these individuals there is an increased risk of stones. The hyperparathyroid group is sub-divided into patients

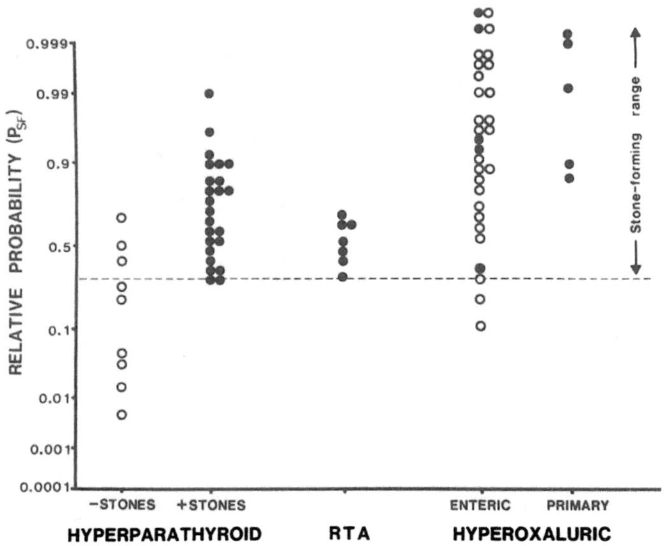

Fig. 46. The overall relative probability of forming stones (P_{SF}) in various groups of patients at risk of forming secondary calcium stones (○ = patients who have not yet formed stones: ● = patients who have formed stones)

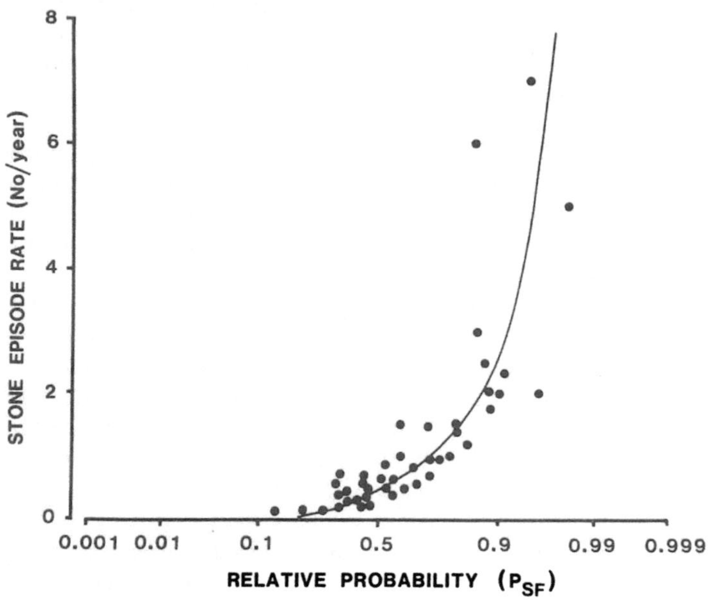

Fig. 47. The stone episode rate in recurrent calcium stone-formers in relation to their calculated relative probability of forming stones (P_{SF})

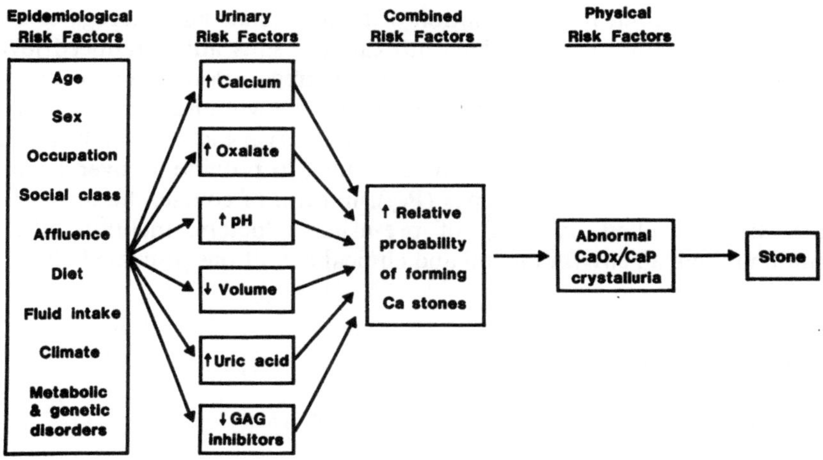

Fig. 48. A risk factor model of calcium stone-formation

with and without stone disease. Those with stones have significantly higher P_{SF} values, mainly due to their hypercalciuria and increased urinary pH, than the patients who have not formed stones. In this latter group the lower P_{SF} values are also due to a higher excretion of GAG inhibitors. This is possibly derived from increased bone resorption since many of this group have bone disease. In the patients with renal tubular acidosis (RTA) the main risk factor is the increase in urinary pH, although a small number are hypercalciuric as well. In the hyperoxaluric group, the high excretion of oxalate is the critical factor. These are sub-divided into the patients with the congenital form of the disorder and those with so-called enteric hyperoxaluria secondary to small bowel surgery.

Figure 47 shows that amongst the recurrent stone-formers the severity of the disease (as defined by the stone episode rate of each patient) is proportional to individual's P_{SF} value (ROBERTSON et al. 1978). Above P_{SF} values of 0.6, the relationship rises steeply such that patients with P_{SF} values greater than 0.98 would be expected to form multiple stones each year.

Thus the risk factor approach to the study of calcium stone-formation appears to be a useful tool for assessing the relative probability of forming stones in the various clinical conditions which predispose towards stone disease. It also explains the influence of most of the epidemiological factors said to be of importance in increasing the risk of stones such as age, sex, occupation, social class, climate, season and, most important of all, dietary and fluid intake, each of which has been shown to influence adversely one or more of the six urinary risk factors (ROBERTSON et al. 1980a, 1981a).

A model of stone-formation based on the risk factor concept is outlined in Fig. 48 which is an expansion of the general model in Fig. 17. According to this model the first pre-requisite of stones is a period of abnormal crystalluria, usually of calcium oxalate, during which a particle is formed which is large enough to become trapped at some narrow portion of the urinary tract. The chemical factors which control the formation of large crystals and aggregates are an excessive supersaturation of urine with calcium salts and a reduced level of inhibitory activity against the growth and aggregation of large crystals of these salts. These are basically determined by urinary volume, pH, calcium, oxalate, GAGS and uric acid which are the same six risk factors which may be combined, independently of the chemical model, to provide an overall measure of the probability of forming stones (P_{SF}). In turn, of course, the urinary risk factors are controlled by a set of pre-urinary factors, including the various epidemiological, environmental and clinical conditions discussed above.

5. Uncommon Stones

a) Introduction

There are a number of uncommon forms of urinary stone disease which result from some rare metabolic disorder, from the administration of some drug with which the patient is being treated for some other condition or from the obsessive intake of some unusual type of diet. In all these instances, the stone forms because of the relative insolubility of some excretory product in the urine, whether it derives naturally from the processes of metabolism or iatrogenically from drug administration.

α) Xanthine Stones

An increased urinary excretion of xanthine, because of its limited solubility in urine, may lead to the formation of xanthine stones. The great rarity of these calculi is shown by the fact that xanthine was found in only 4 out of 10,000 calculi analysed by HERRING (1962) in 1 out of 17,000 calculi analysed by HESSE and SCHNEIDER (1976).

There are two conditions which give rise to an increased excretion of xanthine. The first of these is a rare hereditary disease of purine metabolism, probably autosomal recessive in character, which is characterised by a deficiency of xanthine oxidase activity (DENT and PHILPOT 1954; DICKINSON and SMELLIE 1959; WATTS et al. 1964). This leads to an increase in plasma and urinary xanthine and hypoxanthine and a corresponding fall in plasma and urinary uric acid (WATTS 1976). Stone disease usually affects males and can occur in children and adults (WYNGAARDEN 1978). Not all patients with xanthine stones have xanthine oxidase deficiency and there are other conditions which may give rise to increased excretion of urinary xanthine, such as treatment with allopurinol. Xanthine stone-formation in this situation is rare, however, except in patients with very high uric acid production rates such as in the Lesch-Nyhan syndrome (GREENE et al. 1969) or in neoplastic disease (BAND et al. 1970).

β) Silica Stones

Urinary calculi containing silica are not uncommon in grazing animals (KELLER 1963). In man, however, they are very rare and are found almost exclusively in patients who have been taking magnesium trisilicate antacids over a prolonged period (LAGERGREN 1962). When acid reacts with a silicate, part of the silica so-formed is precipitated as a gel and part remains in solution in the form of a colloid. The breakdown products in the digestive tract include various silicic acids which are soluble and can therefore be absorbed and excreted in the urine. Thus the urinary excretion of silica is higher after administration of magnesium trisilicate than before (PAGE et al. 1941). Recurrence is usually prevented by discontinuing the drugs.

γ) 2,8-Dihydroxyadenine Stones

In a rare inborn error of metabolism there is a defect in the adenine salvage enzyme, adenine phosphoribosyltransferase. This leads to a build up of 2,8-dihydroxyadenine in the tissues with a subsequent increase in its urinary concentration. The stones usually present in childhood and may be easily confused with uric acid stones because of their similar chemical reactions (SIMMONDS et al. 1976, 1981).

References

Achilles W, Cumme GA, Scheffel M (1976) Investigation of complex-chemical equilibria in urinary systems with respect to calcium oxalate formation. In: Fleisch H, Robertson WG, Smith LH, Vahlensieck W (eds) Urolithiasis research. Plenum, New York, p 229–232

Achilles W, Scheidt B, Hoppe H, Cumme GA (1977) Eine Ionenaustauschmethode zur Bestimmung freier Metallionenkonzentration, geeignet zur Anwendung in biologischen Flüssigkeiten. Acta Biol Med Germ 36:17–28

Adams F (1939) The genuine works of Hippocrates, Williams & Wilkins, Baltimore

Adamthwaite DN (1983) Urinary particulate activity in urinary calculus disease. Br J Urol 55:95–99

Admirand WH, Earnest DL, Williams HE (1971) Hyperoxaluria and bone disease. Trans Assoc Am Physcians 84:307–312

Ahlgen SA, Lorstadt M (1965) An epidemiological investigation of 1429 roentgenologically verified cases. Acta Chir Scand 130:344–353

Aikawa JK, Rhoades EL, Gordon GS (1958) Urinary and faecal excretion of orally administered Mg^{28}. Proc Soc Exp Biol (Med) 98:29–31

Albright F, Reifenstein EC (1948) Parathyroid glands and metabolic bone disease. Williams & Wilkins, Baltimore

Albright F, Henneman P, Benedict PH, Forbes AP (1953) Idiopathic hypercalciuria. Proc R Soc Med 46:1077–1081

Allen TD, Spence HM (1966) Matrix stones. J Urol 95:284–290

Alonso J, Somacarrera E (1973) Scanning microscopy in renal lithiasis. In: Cifuentes Delatte L, Rapado A, Hodgkinson A (eds) Urinary calculi. Karger, Basel, p 256–263

Andersen DA (1969) Historical and geographical differences in the pattern of incidence of urinary considered in relation to possible aetiological factors. In: Hodgkinson A, Nordin BEC (eds) Proceedings of the renal stone research symposium, Churchill, London. p 7–31

Andersen DA (1973) Environmental factors in the aetiology of urolithiasis. In: Cifuentes Delatte L, Rapado A, Hodgkinson A (eds) Urinary calculi, Karger, Basel, p 130–144
Anderson AJ, Lepper MH, Winzler RJ (1960) The fractionation of urine colloids on anion-exchange cellulose. Biochem J 77:581–591
Anderson CK (1969) Renal histological changes in stone-formers and non-stone-formers. In: Hodgkinson A, Nordin BEC (eds) Proceedings of the renal stone research symposium. Churchill. London, p 113–136
Anderson CK (1974) Partial nephrectomy – a pathological evaluation. Proc R Soc Med 67:459–464
Anderson CK (1976) Pathology of nephrocalcinosis and stone-formation In: Williams DI, Chisholm GD (eds) Scientific foundations of urology, vol I. Heinemann, London, p 282–289
Anderson CK (1979) The anatomical aetiology of renal lithiasis. In: Wickham JEA (ed) Urinary calculous disease. Churchill Livingstone, Edinburgh, p 40–68
Anderson GS, Graham AG (1960) Renal sarcoidosis and nephrolithiasis. Soc Med J 5:392–396
Anderson L, McDonald JR (1946) The origin, frequency and significance of microscopic calculi in the kidney. Surg Gynecol Obstet 82:275–282
Anderson W, Hollings JG, Bond PS (1971) The composition of tea infusions examined in relation to the association between mortality and water hardness. J Hyg (Lond) 69:1–15
Anning ST, Dawson J, Dolby DE, Ingram JT (1948) Toxic effects of calciferol. Quart J Med 37:79–96
Archer HE, Dormer AE, Scowen EF, Watts RWE (1957) Studies on the urinary excretion of oxalate by normal subjects. Clin Sci 16:405–411
Arnow VK, Westall RG (1958) Amino acid clearances in cystinuria. J Physiol (Lond) 142:141–146
Atkins GL, Dean BM, Griffin WJ, Watts RWE (1964) Quantitative aspects of ascorbic acid metabolism in Man. J Biol Chem 239:2975–2980
Atsmon A, De Vries A, Frank M (1963) Uric acid lithiasis. Elsevier, Amsterdam
Babka JC, Bower RH, Sode J (1976) Nephrogenous cyclic AMP levels in primary hyperparathyroidism. Arch Intern Med 136:1140–1144
Bach D, Hesse A, Strenge A, Vahlensieck W (1981) Magnesium excretion in urine on condition of individual as well as standard diet in healthy controls and calcium oxalate stone-formers. In: Smith LH, Robertson WG, Finlayson B (eds) Urolithiasis – clinical and basic research. Plenum, New York, p 45–49
Bachra BN, Fischer HRA (1969) The effect of some inhibitors on the nucleation and crystal growth of apatite. Calcif Tissue Res 3:348–357
Backman U, Danielson BG, Johansson G, Ljunghall S, Wikström B (1980) Incidence and clinical importance of renal tubular defects in recurrent renal stone-formers. Nephron 25:96–101
Backman U, Danielson BG, Fellström B, Johansson G, Ljunghall S, Wikström B (1981) Clinical and laboratory findings in patients with medullary sponge kidney. In: Smith LH, Robertson WG, Finlayson B (eds) Urolithiasis – clinical and basic research. Plenum, New York, p 113–120
Baggio B, Gambaro G, Favaro S, Borsatti A (1983) Prevalence of hyperoxaluria in idiopathic calcium oxalate kidney stone disease. Nephron 35:11–14
Baker EM, Saari JC, Tolbert BM (1966) Ascorbic acid metabolism in man. Am J Clin Nutr 19:371–378
Bambach CP, Robertson WG, Peacock M, Hill GL (1981) Effect of intestinal surgery on the risk of urinary stone-formation. Gut 22:257–263
Band PR, Silverberg DS, Henderson JF, Ulan RA, Wensel RH, Banerjee TK, Little AS (1970). Xanthine nephropathy in a patient with lymphosarcoma treated with allopurinol. N Engl J Med 283:354–357
Banner MR, Rosalki SB (1967) Glyoxylate as a substrate for lactate dehydrogenase. Nature 213:726–727
Barbar HH, Gallimore EJ (1940) The metabolism of oxalic acid in the animal body. Biochem J 34:144–148

Barilla DE, Notz C, Kennedy D, Pak CYC (1978) Renal oxalate excretion following oral oxalate loads in patients with ileal disease and with renal and absorptive hypercalciurias. Am J Med 64:579–585

Barker LM, Pallante SL, Eisenberg H, Joule JA, Becker GL, Howard JE (1974) Simple synthetic and natural urines have equivalent anticalcifying properties. Invest Urol 12:79–81

Barzel US, Sperling O, Frank M, De Vries A (1964) Renal ammonium excretion and urinary pH in idiopathic uric acid lithiasis. J Urol 92:1–5

Bateson EM (1973) Renal tract calculi and climate. Med J Aust 2:111–113

Baumann JM, Wacker M (1979) Experience with the measurement of inhibitory activity of urine and crystallisation inhibitors by different techniques. Urol Res 7:183–188

Baumann JM, Wacker M (1980) The direct measurement of inhibitory capacity to crystal growth of calcium oxalate on undiluted urine and in other inhibitor containing solutions. Urol Res 8:171–175

Baumann JM, Bisaz S, Felix R, Fleisch H, Ganz U, Russell RGG (1977) The role of inhibitors and other factors in the pathogenesis of recurrent calcium-containing renal stones. Clin Sci Molec Med 53:141–148

Baumann JM, Bisaz S, Fleisch H, Wacker M (1978) Biochemical and clinical effects of ethane-1-hydroxy-1,1-diphosphonate in calcium nephrolithiasis. Clin Sci Molec Med 54:509–516

Beck CW, Mulvaney WP (1966) Apatitic urinary calculi from early American Indians. JAMA 195:168–169

Benedict JD, Forsham PH, Stetten D (1949) The metabolism of uric acid in the normal and gouty human studied with the aid of isotopic uric acid. J Biol Chem 181:183–193

Bennett AH, Colodny AH (1973) Urinary tract calculi in children. J Urol 109:318–320

Bennett RC, Jepson RP (1966) Uric acid stone formation following ileostomy. Aust NZ J Surg 36:153–158

Berg W, Schneider H-J, Hesse A (1976) Crystal optical findings on calcium oxalate of uric concretions. In: Fleisch H, Robertson WG, Smith LH, Vahlensieck W (eds) Urolithiasis research. Plenum, New York, p 241–247

Bergmann TO (1776) Observations nonullae de calculis urinaris XVII. Opuscula Physica et Chemie (Upsala) 1

Bernshtam J, Pinto B (1976) Epitaxy mechanism of urinary mucoprotein. In: Fleisch H, Robertson WG, Smith LH, Vahlensieck W (eds) Urolithiasis research. Plenum, New York, p 249–251

Berzelius JJ (1833) Calculus urinaires. Traité Chem 7:424

Bichler K-H, Kirchner C, Ideler V (1976) Uromucoid excretion of normal individuals and stone-formers. Br J Urol 47:733–738

Bickel H, Thursby-Pelham DC (1954) Hyperaminociduria in Lignac-Fanconi disease, in galactosaemia and in an obscure syndrome. Arch Dis Child 29:224–231

Bird ED, Thomas WC (1963) Effect of various metals on mineralisation in vitro. Proc Soc Exp Biol Med 112:640–643

Bird G (1853) Urinary deposits, their diagnosis, pathology and therapeutical indications. John Churchill, London, p 207–249

Bisaz S, Felix R, Hansen NM, Fleisch H (1976) Disaggregation of hydroxyapatite crystals. Biochim Biophys Acta 451:560–566

Bisaz S, Felix R, Neuman WF, Fleisch H (1978) Quantitative determination of inhibitors of calcium phosphate precipitation in whole urine. Min Electrolyte Metab 1:74–83

Blacklock NJ (1969) The pattern of urolithiasis in the Royal Navy. In: Hodgkinson A, Nordin BEC (eds) Proceedings of the renal stone research symposium, Churchill, London, p 33–47

Blacklock NJ (1976) Epidemiology of urolithiasis. In: Williams DI, Chisholm GD, (eds) Scientific foundations of urology, vol 1. Heinemann, London, p 235–243

Blacklock NJ (1979) Epidemiology of renal lithiasis. In: Wickham JEA (ed) Urinary calculous disease. Churchill Livingstone, Edinburgh, p 21–39

Blomen LJMJ, Bijvoet OLM, Will EJ, Van der Linden H (1979) Kristallwachstum und Harnsteinerkrankung: die Wachstumskonstante. Fortschr Urol Nephrol 14:210–218

Bommer J, Ritz E, Tschöpe W, Waldherr R, Gebhardt M (1979) Urinary matrix calculi consisting of microfibrillar protein in patients on maintenance haemodialysis. Kidney Int 16:722–728

Boonstra CA, Jackson CE (1971) Serum calcium survey for hyperparathyroidism. Am J Clin Path 55:523–526

Bordier PJ, Berbir NN, Queille ML, Kahn MF, DeSèze S (1976) Phosphate metabolism, hyperparathyroidism and skeletal remodeling in idiopathic hypercalciuria. In: Phosphate metabolism, kidney and bone. Nouvelle Imprimirie Fournie, Toulouse, p 79–91

Boskey AL, Posner AS (1974) Magnesium stabilization of amorphous calcium phosphate: a kinetic study. Mat Res Bull 9:907–916

Boström H, Hambraeus L (1964) Cystinuria in Sweden. VII. Clinical, histopathological and medico-social aspects of the disease. Acta Med Scand [Suppl 411] 175:1–128

Bowyer RC, Brockis JG, McCulloch RK (1979) Glycosaminoglycans as inhibitors of calcium oxalate crystal growth and aggregation. Clin Chim Acta 95:23–28

Boyce WH (1968) Organic matrix of human urinary concretions. Am J Med 45:673–683

Boyce WH (1969a) Organic matrix of native human urinary concretions. In: Hodgkinson A, Nordin BEC (eds) Proceedings of the renal stone research symposium. Churchill, London, p 93–104

Boyce WH (1969b) Macromolecular components of kidney calculi in urine. In: Hodgkinson A, Nordin BEC (eds) Proceedings of the renal stone research symposium. Churchill, London, p 181–189

Boyce WH (1973) Ultrastructure of human renal calculi. In: Cifuentes Delatte L, Rapado A, Hodgkinson A (eds) Urinary calculi. Karger, Basel, p 247–255

Boyce WH, Garvey FK (1956) The amount and nature of the organic matrix of urinary calculi. A review. J Urol 76:213–227

Boyce WH, King JS (1959) Crystal-matrix interrelations in calculi. J Urol 81:351–365

Boyce WH, King JS (1963) Present concepts concerning the origin of matrix and stones. Ann NY Acad Sci 104:563–578

Boyce WH, Sulkin NM (1956) Biocolloids of urine in health and in calculous disease. III. The mucoprotein matrix of urinary calculi. J Clin Invest 35:1067–1079

Boyce WH, Garvey FK, Norfleet CM (1954a) Proteins and other biocolloids of urine in health and in calculous disease. I. Electrophoretic studies at pH 4.5 and 8.6 of those components soluble in molar sodium chloride. J Clin Invest 33:1287–1297

Boyce WH, Garvey FK, Norfleet CM (1954b) Ion-binding properties of electrophoretically homogeneous mucoproteins of urine in normal subjects and in patients with calculous disease. J Urol 72:1019–1031

Boyce WH, Garvey FK, Norfleet CM (1954c) The turbidity of urine in the normal and in patients with urinary calculi. Exp Med Surg 12:450–459

Boyce WH, Garvey FK, Norfleet CM (1955) The metal chelate compounds of urine. Am J Med 19:87–95

Boyce WH, Garvey FK, Strawcutter HE (1956) Incidence of urinary calculi among patients in general hospital 1948–1952. JAMA 161:1437–1442

Boyce WH, Garvey FK, Goven CE (1958a) Abnormalities of calcium metabolism in patients with "idiopathic" urinary calculi. Effect of oral administration of sodium phytate. JAMA 166:1577–1583

Boyce WH, Poole CS, Meschan I, King JS (1958b) Organic matrix of urinary calculi. Acta Radiol [Diagn] (Stockh) 50:543–560

Boyce WH, King JS, Fielden ML (1962) Total nondialyzable solids in human urine. XIII. Immunological detection of a component peculiar to renal calculous matrix and to urine of calculous patients. J Clin Invest 41:1180–1189

Boyce WH, McKinney WM, Long TT, Drach GW (1967) Oral administration of methylene blue to patients with renal calculi. J Urol 97:783–789

Boyce WH, Willard J, Prater TF (1973) Intra-nephronic calculosis in surgical biopsies of human kidney in urinary calculi. In: Cifuentes Delatte L, Rapado A, Hodgkinson A (eds) Urinary calculi. Karger, Basel, p 339–346

Brandes L, Oreopoulos DG, Husdan H, Crassweller P (1981) Study of crystals in patients with kidney stones. In: Smith LH, Robertson WG, Finlayson B (eds) Urolithiasis – clinical and basic research. Plenum, New York, p 23–27

Brazeau P, Gilman A (1953) Effect of plasma CO_2 tension on renal tubular reabsorption of bicarbonate. Am J Physiol 175:33–38

Brecevic L, Füredi-Milhofer H (1979) Precipitation of calcium phosphates from electrolyte solutions. V. The influence of citrate ions. Calcif Tissue Int 28:131 – 136
Briggs MH, Garcia-Webb P, Davies P (1973) Urinary oxalate and vitamin C supplements. Lancet II:201
Broadus AE (1980) Nephrolithiasis in primary hyperparathyroidism. In: Coe FL (ed) Nephrolithiasis. Churchill Livingstone, New York, p 58 – 85
Broadus AE, Mahaffey JE, Bartter FC, Neer RM (1977) Nephrogenous cyclic adenosine monophosphate as a parathyroid function test. J Clin Invest 60:771 – 783
Broadus AE, Dominguez M, Barter FC (1978) Pathophysiological studies in idiopathic hypercalciuria: use of an oral calcium tolerance test to characterise distinctive hypercalciuria subgroups. J Clin Endocrinol Metab 47:751 – 760
Brockis JG, Bowyer RC, McCulloch RK, Taylor TA, Wisniewski ZS (1981) Physiopathology of endemic bladder stones. In: Brockis JG, Finlayson B (eds) Urinary calculus. PSG Publishing Co. Littleton, Mass, p 225 – 236
Brodehl J, Gellissen K, Kowalewski S (1967) Isolated cystinuria (without lysine-ornithine-argininuria) in a family with hypocalcaemic tetany. Klin Wochenschr 45:38 – 40
Brown CB (1980) Urinary tract infections. Medicine (Baltimore) 26:1341 – 1346
Brown MR, Sallis JD (1983) The synthesis and characterization of N-sulfo-2-amino tricarbyllate: an analog of phosphocitrate and inhibitor of calcification. Analyt Biochem 132:115 – 123
Brown TR (1901) On the relationship between the variety of microorganisms and the composition of stone in calculous pyelonephritis. JAMA 36:1395 – 1397
Brown WE, Chow LC (1981) Thermodynamics of apatite crystal growth and dissolution. J Crystal Growth 53:31 – 41
Brumfitt W (1972) Bacteriological aspects of renal disease. In: Black D (ed) Renal disease, 3rd ed. Blackwell Scientific Publications, Oxford, p 367 – 397
Bruwer A (1979) Primary renal calculi: Anderson-Carr-Randall progression. Am J Roentgenol 132:751 – 758
Bulusu L, Hodgkinson A, Nordin BEC, Peacock M (1970) Urinary excretion of calcium and creatinine in relation to age and body weight in normal subjects and patients with renal calculus. Clin Sci 38:601 – 612
Burch PRJ, Dawson JB (1969) Aetiological implications of the sex- and age-distributions of renal lithiasis. In: Hodgkinson A, Nordin BEC (eds) Proceedings of the renal stone research symposium. Churchill, London, p 71 – 84
Burns JR, Finlayson B (1980) A proposal for a standard reference artificial urine in in vitro urolithiasis experiments. Invest Urol 18:167 – 169
Butler MR, Devine HF, O'Flynn JD (1973) Medullary sponge kidney: review of the literature and presentation of 33 cases. J Irish Med Assoc 66:5 – 13
Butt AJ (1952) Role of protective urinary colloids in prevention of renal lithiasis. J Urol 67:450 – 459
Butt AJ (1956) Etiologic factors in renal lithiasis. Thomas, Springfield, Illinois
Butz M (1982) Oxalatsteinprophylaxe durch Alkali-Therapie. Urologe [Ausg A] 21:142 – 146
Cacchi R, Ricci V (1949) Sur une rare maladie kystique multiple des pyramides rénales, Le "rein en éponge". J Urol (Paris) 55:497 – 519
Caldas AE, Gray RW, Lemon J (1978) The simultaneous measurement of vitamin D metabolites in plasma studies in healthy adults and patients with calcium nephrolithiasis. J Lab Clin Med 91:840 – 849
Caniggia A, Gennari C, Cesari L (1965) Intestinal absorption of ^{45}Ca in stone forming patients. Br Med J 1:427 – 429
Carr JA (1953) The pathology of urinary calculi: radial striation. Br J Urol 25:26 – 32
Carr JA (1956) The pathology of urinary calculi: sedimentation. Br J Urol 28:240 – 242
Carr RJ (1954) A new theory on the formation of renal calculi. Br J Urol 26:105 – 117
Carr RJ (1969) Aetiology of renal calculi: micro-radiographic studies. In: Hodgkinson A, Nordin BEC (eds) Proceedings of the renal stone research symposium. Churchill, London, p 123 – 132
Cattell WR, Spencer AG, Taylor GW, Watts RWE (1962) The mechanism of the renal excretion of oxalate in the dog. Clin Sci 22:43 – 51

Chadwick VS, Modha K, Dowling RH (1973) Mechanism for hyperoxaluria in patients with ileal dysfunction. N Engl J Med 289:172–176
Chadwick VS, Philips SF, Hofmann AF (1977) Measurement of intestinal permeability using low molecular weight polyethylene glycols (PEG 400). Gastroenterology 73:247–251
Chow F-HC, Hamar DW, Udall RH (1968) Studies on urolithiasis. XI. Interaction of urine polyelectrolytes and inorganic ions. Invest Urol 5:557–567
Churchill DN, Maloney CM, Nolan R, Gault MH, Winsor G (1980) Pediatric urolithiasis in the 1970s. J Urol 123:237–238
Cifuentes Delatte L, Rapado A, Abehsera A, Traba ML, Cortes M (1973). Uric acid lithiasis and gout. In: Cifuentes Delatte L, Rapado A, Hodgkinson A (eds) Urinary calculi, Karger, Basel, p 115–118
Clarke AM, McKenzie RG (1969) Ileostomy and the risk of uric acid stones. Lancet II:395–397
Cochran M, Peacock M, Smith DA, Nordin BEC (1968) Renal tubular acidosis of pyelonephritis with renal stone disease. Br Med J 32:721–729
Coe FL (1977) Treated and untreated recurrent calcium nephrolithiasis in patients with idiopathic hypercalciuria, hyperuricosuria or no metabolic disorder. Ann Intern Med 87:404–410
Coe FL (1978) Nephrolithiasis. Year Book Medical Publishers, Chicago
Coe FL (1980) Hyperuricosuric calcium oxalate nephrolithiasis. In: Coe FL (ed) Nephrolithiasis. Churchill Livingstone, New York, p 116–135
Coe FL, Kavalich AG (1974) Hypercalciuria and hyperuricosuria in patients with calcium nephrolithiasis. N Engl J Med 291:1344–1350
Coe FL, Raisen L (1973) Allopurinol treatment of uric acid disorders in calcium-stone formers. Lancet I:129–131
Coe FL, Canterbury JM, Firpo JJ, Reiss E (1973) Evidence for secondary hyperparathyroidism in idiopathic hypercalciuria. J Clin Invest 52:134–142
Coe FL, Lawton RL, Goldstein RB, Tembe V (1975) Sodium urate accelerates precipitation of calcium oxalate in vitro. Proc Soc Exp Biol Med 149:926–929
Coe FL, Moran E, Kavalich AG (1976) The contribution of dietary purine over-consumption to hyperuricosuria in calcium oxalate stone-formers. J Chronic Dis 29:793–800
Coe FL, Margolis HC, Deutsch LH, Strauss AL (1980) Urinary macromolecular crystal growth inhibitors in calcium nephrolithiasis. Miner Electrolyte Metab 3:268–275
Conways NS, Maitland AIL, Rennie JB (1949) The urinary citrate excretion in patients with renal calculi. Br J Urol 21:30–38
Cooke SAR (1970) The site of calcification in the human renal papilla. Br J Surg 57:890–896
Cooke SAR (1971) The distribution of calcium in the human kidney. Br J Urol 43:130–139
Cooke SAR (1973) Calcium concentration within the nephron and calcium stone-formation. In: Cifuentes Delatte L, Rapado A, Hodgkinson A (eds) Urinary calculi. Karger, Basel, p 333–338
Cope O (1966) The story of hyperparathyroidism at the Massachusetts General Hospital. N Engl J Med 274:1174–1182
Cornelius CE, Mia AS, Rosenfeld S (1965) Ruminant urolithiasis. VII. Studies on the origin of Tamm-Horsfall urinary mucoprotein and its presence in urine calculous matrix. Invest Urol 2:453–457
Cowan ST, Steele KJ (1965) Manual for the identification of medical bacteria. Cambridge University Press, London
Cox CE (1974) Urinary tract infection and renal lithiasis. Urol Clin North Am 1:279–297
Crawford JE, Crematy EP, Alexander AE (1968) The effect of natural and synthetic polyelectrolytes on the crystallisation of calcium oxalate. Aust J Chem 21:1067–1072
Crawford MA, Milne MD, Scribner BH (1959) The effect of changes in acid-base balance on urinary citrate in the rat. J Physiol (Lond) 149:413–423
Crawhall JC, Segal S (1967) The intracellular ratio of cysteine and cystine in various tissues. Biochem J 105:891–896
Crawhall JC, Scowen EF, Watts RWE (1959) Conversion of glycine to oxalate in primary hyperoxaluria. Lancet II:806–809
Crawhall JC, Purkiss P, Watts RWE, Young EP (1969) The excretion of amino acids by cystinuric patients and their relatives. Ann Hum Genet 33:149–169

Curreri P, Onada GY, Finlayson B (1979) An electrophoretic study of calcium oxalate monohydrate. J Colloid Interface Sci 69:170–182
Dahlberg PJ, Van Den Berg CJ, Kurtz SB, Wilson DM, Smith LH (1977) Clinical features and management of cystinuria. Mayo Clin Proc 52:533–542
Danielson BG, Backman U, Fellström B, Johansson G, Ljunghall S, Wikström B (1979) Prophylactischer Einsatz von Thiaziden, Magnesium und Zellulosephosphate. Fortschr Urol Nephrol 14:391–397
Davidson S, Passmore R (1969) Human nutrition and dietetics. Livingstone, Edinburgh
Dean BM, Watts RWE, Westwick WJ (1968) The conversion of [1^{13}C] glycine and [2^{13}C] glycine to [^{13}C] oxalate in primary hyperoxaluria:evidence for the existence of more than one metabolic pathway from glycine to oxalate in man. Clin Sci 35:325–335
Debye P, Hückel E (1923) Zur theorie der elektrolyte. I. Gefrierpunktserniedrigung und verwandte Erscheinungen. Physik Z 24:185–206
Deitrick JE, Whedon GD, Shorr E (1948) Effect of immobilisation upon various metabolic and physiologic functions of normal men. Am J Med 4:3–36
Dekker EE, Maitra U (1962) Conversion of γ-hydroxyglutamate to glyoxylate and alanine, purification and properties of the enzyme system. J Biol Chem 237:2218–2227
Delluva AM, Markley K, Davies RE (1968) The absence of gastric urease in germ free animals. Biochim Biophys Acta 151:646–650
Dent CE, Philpot GR (1954) Xanthinuria an inborn error (or deviation) of metabolism. Lancet I:182–185
Dent CE, Rose GA (1951) Amino acid metabolism in cystinuria. Q J Med 20:205–230
Dent CE, Senior B (1955) Studies on the treatment of cystinuria. Br J Urol 27:317–332
Dent CE, Sutor DJ (1971) Presence or absence of inhibitor of calcium oxalate crystal growth in urine of normals and of stone-formers. Lancet II:775–778
Dent CE, Senior B, Walshe JM (1954) The pathogenesis of cystinuria. II. Polarographic studies of the metabolism of sulphur-containing amino acids. J Clin Invest 33:1216–1226
Deren JJ, Porush JG, Levitt MF, Khilnani MT (1962) Nephrolithiasis as a complication of ulcerative colitis and regional enteritis. Ann Intern Med 56:843–853
Desmars JF, Tawashi R (1973) Dissolution and growth of calcium oxalate monohydrate. I. Effect of magnesium and pH. Biochim Biophys Acta 313:256–267
Desnos ME (1914) In: Pousson A, Désnos E (eds) Encyclopédie Françaisе d'Urologie. Octane Doin et Fils, Paris, p 1–294
Diamond HS, Paolino JS (1973) Evidence for a post-secretory reabsorptive site for uric acid in Man. J Clin Invest 52:1491–1499
Dickens F (1941) Citric acid content of animal tissues with reference to its occurrence in bone and tumour. Biochem J 35:1011–1023
Dickinson CJ, Smellie JM (1959) Xanthinuria. Br Med J 2:1217–1221
Dickstein JW, Frame B (1973) Urinary tract calculi after intestinal shunt operations for the treatment of obesity. Surg Gynaecol Obstet 136:257–260
Diem K, Lentner C (1970) Documenta Geigy – Scientific Tables, 7th ed. Geigy, Basel
Dobbins JW, Binder HJ (1977) Importance of the colon in enteric hyperoxaluria. N Engl J Med 296:298–301
Donné MA (1839) Sur la formation de cristaux d'oxalate de chaux dans l'urine determinée par l'usage de l'oseille. Comptes Rendus Hebdomadaires des Seances de l'Academie des Sciences (Paris) 8:805–806
Doremus RH, Teich S, Silvis PX (1978) Crystallization of calcium oxalate from synthetic urine. Invest Urol 15:469–472
Dowling RH, Rose GA, Sutor DJ (1971) Hyperoxaluria and renal calculi in ileal disease. Lancet I:1103–1106
Drach GW, Boyce WH (1972) Nephrocalculosis as a source for renal stone nuclei, observations on humans and squirrel monkeys and on hyperparathyroidism in the squirrel monkey. J Urol 107:897–904
Drach GW, Randolph AD, Miller JD (1978) Inhibition of calcium oxalate dihydrate crystallization by chemical modifiers: I. Pyrophosphate and methylene blue. J Urol 119:99–103
Drach GW, Thorson S, Randolph A (1980) Effects of urinary organic macromolecules on crystallization of calcium oxalate: enhancement of nucleation. J Urol 123:519–523

Drach GW, Kraljevich Z, Randolph AD (1982a) Effects of high molecular weight urinary macromolecules on crystallization of calcium oxalate dihydrate. J Urol 127:805–810
Drach GW, Sarig S, Randolph AD, Thorson S (1982b) The paradox of inhibition and enhancement of the formation of urinary stones. Urol Res 10:165–168
Drezner MK, Neelon FA, Curtis HB, Lebovitz HL (1976) Renal cyclic adenosine monophosphate: an accurate index of parathyroid function. Metabolism 25:1103–1112
Dufault FX, Tobias GJ (1954) Potentially reversible renal failure following excessive calcium and alkali intake in peptic ulcer therapy. Am J Med 16:231–236
Dulce HJ (1958a) Einflüsse von hydrophilen Kolloiden auf Oxalatfällungen und ihre Beziehungen zum Dispersionsgrad des Calciumoxalats. Z Physiol Chem 311:185–190
Dulce H-J (1958b) Einflüsse von Kristalloiden des Harnes auf Oxalatfällungen. Z Physiol Chem 311:191–196
Dulce H-J (1958c) Einflüsse von Kristalloiden und hydrophilen Kolloiden auf Oxalatfällungen mit normalen Harn. Z Physiol Chem 311:197–200
Dunlop JC (1896) The excretion of oxalic acid in urine and its bearing on the pathological condition known as oxaluria. J Pathol Bact 3:389–429
Dyer R, Nordin BEC (1967) Urinary crystals and their relation to stone formation. Nature 215:751–752
Dykstra MJ, Hackett RL (1979) Ultrastructural events in early calcium oxalate crystal formation in rats. Kidney Int 15:640–650
Eanes ED, Posner AS (1968) Intermediate phases in the basic solution preparation of alkaline earth phosphate. Calcif Tissue Res 2:38–48
Earnest DL, Johnston G, Williams HE, Admirand WH (1974) Hyperoxaluria in patients with ileal resection: an abnormality in dietary oxalate absorption. Gastroenterology 66:1114–1122
Edwards NA, Hodgkinson A (1965) Metabolic studies in patients with idiopathic hypercalciuria. Clin Sci 29:147–157
Ekström T, Engfeldt B, Lagergren C, Lindwall N (1959) Medullary sponge kidney: a roentgenologic, clinical and histopathologic and biophysical study. Almquist & Wiksell, Stockholm
Elder TD, Wyngaarden JB (1960) The biosynthesis and turnover of oxalate in normal and hyperoxaluric subjects. J Clin Invest 39:1337–1344
Elion GB (1966) Enzymatic and metabolic studies with allopurinol. Ann Rheum Dis 25:608–614
Elliot JR, Freeman S (1956) Parathyroid function and the plasma citric acid and calcium response to nephrectomy. Endocrinology 59:181–189
Elliot JS (1973) Optical analysis of urinary calculi: the value of low power dissection. In: Cifuentes Delatte L, Rapado A, Hodgkinson A (eds) Urinary calculi. Karger, Basel, p 216–219
Elliot JS, Rabinowitz IN (1976) Crystal habit, structure and incidence in the urine of a hospital population. In: Fleisch H, Robertson WG, Smith LH, Vahlensieck W (eds) Urolithiasis research. Plenum, New York, p 257–260
Elliot JS, Ribeiro ME (1972) The urinary excretion of citric, hippuric, and lactic acid in normal adults and in patients with calcium oxalate urinary calculus disease. Invest Urol 10:102–106
Elliot JS, Sharp RF, Lewis L (1959) The solubility of struvite in urine. J Urol 81:366–368
Elliot JS, Soles WP (1974) Excretion of calcium and citric acid in patients with small bowel disease. J Urol 111:810–812
Elliot JS, Todd HE (1961) Calculous disease in patients with poliomyelitis. J Urol 86:484–488
Erwin DT, Roberts JA, Sledge G, Bennett DJ, Finlayson B (1976) Estimating urine supersaturation, a comparison of the results of two methods evaluating changes induced by drinking milk. In: Fleisch H, Robertson WG, Smith LH, Vahlensieck W (eds) Urolithiasis research. Plenum, New York, p 261–264
Ettinger B, Kolb FO (1971) Factors involved in crystal formation in cystinuria. In vivo and in vitro crystallization dynamics and a simple quantitative colorimetric assay for cystine. J Urol 106:106–110
Eusebio E, Elliot JS (1967) Effect of trace metals on the crystallization of calcium oxalate. Invest Urol 4:431–435

Evans BM, MacIntyre I, McPherson CR, Milne MD (1957) Alkalosis and sodium and potassium depletion with special reference to organic acid excretion. Clin Sci 16:53–65

Evans JR, Robertson WG, Morgan DB, Fleisch H (1980) Effects of pyrophosphate and diphosphonates on the dissolution of hydroxyapatites using a flow system. Calcif Tissue Int 31:153–159

Faber SR, Feitler WW, Bleiler RE, Ohlson NA, Hodges RE (1963) The effects of an induced pyridoxine and pantothenic acid deficiency on excretion of oxalic and xanthurenic acids in the urine. Am J Clin Nutr 12:406–412

Falls WF (1972) Comparison of urinary acidification and ammonium excretion in normal and gouty patients. Metabolism 21:433–445

Feagin FF, Walker AA, Pigman W (1969) Evaluation of the calcifying characteristics of biological fluids and inhibitors of calcification. Calcif Tissue Res 4:231–244

Feigelson P, Davidson JD, Robins RK (1957) Pyrazolo pyrimidines as inhibitors and substrates of xanthine oxidase. J Biol Chem 226:993–1000

Felix R, Monod A, Broge L, Hansen NM, Fleisch H (1977) Aggregation of calcium oxalate crystals: effect of urine and various inhibitors. Urol Res 5:21–28

Fellström B, Backman U, Danielson BG, Holmgren K, Ljunghall S, Wikström B (1982) Inhibitory activity of human urine on calcium oxalate crystal growth: effects of sodium urate and uric acid. Clin Sci 62:509–514

Felts JH, Headley RN, Whitley JE, Yount EH (1964) Medullary sponge kidney. Clinical appraisal. JAMA 188:233–236

Ferris T, Kashgarian M, Levitin H, Braudt I, Epstein FH (1961) Renal tubular acidosis and renal potassium wasting acquired as a result of hypercalcaemic nephropathy. N Engl J Med 265:924–928

Fetner CD, Barilla DE, Townsend J, Pak CYC (1978) Effects of magnesium oxide on the crystallization of calcium salts in urine in patients with recurrent nephrolithiasis. J Urol 120:399–401

Fidalgo B, Chordi A (1964) Urinary α_2-mucoprotein in patients with renal lithiasis. Lancet II:235

Finch AM, Kasidas GP, Rose GA (1981) Urine composition in normal subjects after oral ingestion of oxalate-rich foods. Clin Sci 60:411–418

Finlayson B (1972) The concept of a continuous crystallizer. Invest Urol 9:258–263

Finlayson B (1974) Renal lithiasis in review. Urol Clin North Am 1:181–212

Finlayson B (1977a) Calcium stones: some physical and clinical aspects. In: David DS (ed) Calcium metabolism in renal failure and nephrolithiasis. Wiley, New York, p 337–382

Finlayson B (1977b) Where and how does urinary stone disease start? An essay on the expectation of free – and fixed-particle urinary stone disease. In: Van Reen R (ed) Idiopathic urinary bladder stone disease. DHEW, Washington, p 7–31

Finlayson B (1978) Physico-chemical aspects of urolithiasis. Kidney Int 13:344–360

Finlayson B, Du Bois L (1978) Adsorption of heparin on sodium acid urate. Clin Chim Acta 84:203–206

Finlayson B, Miller GH (1969) Urine ion equilibria. Invest Urol 6:428–440

Finlayson B, Reid F (1978) The expectation of free and fixed particles in urinary stone disease. Invest Urol 15:442–448

Finlayson B, Vermeulen CW, Stewart EJ (1961) Stone matrix and mucoprotein from urine. J Urol 86:355–363

Fleisch H (1978) Inhibitors and promoters of stone formation. Kidney Int 13:361–371

Fleisch H, Bisaz S (1962a) Isolation from urine of pyrophosphate, a calcification inhibitor. Am J Physiol 203:671–675

Fleisch H, Bisaz S (1962b) Mechanism of calcification: inhibitory role of pyrophosphate. Nature 195:911

Fleisch H, Bisaz S (1964) The inhibitory effect of pyrophosphate on calcium oxalate precipitation and its relation to urolithiasis. Experientia 20:276–277

Fleisch H, Monod A (1973) A new technique for measuring aggregation of calcium oxalate crystals in vitro: effect of urine, magnesium, pyrophosphate and diphosphonates. In: Cifuentes Delatte L, Rapado A, Hodgkinson A (eds) Urinary calculi. Karger, Basel, p 53–56

Fleisch H, Neuman WF (1961) Mechanisms of calcification: role of collagen, polyphosphates and phosphatase. Am J Physiol 200:1296–1300

Fleisch H, Bisaz S, Care AD (1964) Effect of orthophosphate on urinary pyrophosphate excretion and the prevention of urolithiasis. Lancet I:1065–1067

Fleisch H, Russell RGG, Straumann F (1966) Effect of pyrophosphate on hydroxyapatite and its implications in calcium homeostasis. Nature 212:901–903

Fleisch H, Bisaz S, Russell RGG (1967) Influence of pyrophosphate on the crystallisation of uric acid and magnesium ammonium phosphate and its implications in phosphate therapy for urolithiasis. Urol Int 22:483–491

Fleisch H, Russell RGG, Bisaz S, Termine JD, Posner AS (1968) Influence of pyrophosphate on the transformation of amorphous to crystalline calcium phosphate. Calcif Tissue Res 2:49–59

Fleisch H, Russell RGG, Bisaz S, Mühlbauer RC, Williams DA (1970) The inhibitory effect of phosphonates on the formation of calcium phosphate crystals in vitro and on aortic and kidney calcification in vivo. Eur J Clin Invest 1:12–18

Fleisch H (1985) Round table on the comparison of models for the study of inhibitory activity in urine. In: Schwille PO, Smith LH, Robertson WG, Vahlensieck W (eds) Urolithiasis and related clinical research. Plenum, New York, p 903–908

Fletcher RF, Henley AA, Sammons HG, Squire JR (1960) A case magnesium deficiency following massive intestinal resection. Lancet I:522–525

Flocks RH (1939) Calcium and phosphorus excretion in the urine of patients with renal or ureteral calculi. JAMA 113:1466–1471

Flocks RH (1940) Calcium urolithiasis: The role of calcium metabolism in the pathogenesis and treatment of calcium urolithiasis. J Urol 43:214–233

Fourman P, Robinson JR (1953) Diminished urinary excretion of citrate during deficiencies of potassium in Man. Lancet II:656–657

Fourman P, McConkey B, Smith JWG (1960) Defects of water reabsorption and of hydrogen-ion excretion by the renal tubules in hyperparathyroidism. Lancet I:619–623

Fox IH, Wyngaarden JB, Kelley WN (1970) Depletion of erythrocyte phosphoribosyl pyrophosphate in man, a newly observed effect of allopurinol. N Engl J Med 283:1177–1182

Foye WH, Hong HS, Kim CM, Prien EL (1976) Degree of sulfation in mucopolysaccharide sulfates in normal and stone-forming urines. Invest Urol 14:33–37

Francis MD (1969) The inhibition of calcium hydroxyapatite crystal growth by polyphosphonates and polyphosphates. Calcif Tissue Res 3:151–162

Frascino JA, Venamee P, Rosen PP (1970) Renal oxalosis and azotemia after methoxyflurane anesthesia. N Engl J Med 283:676–679

Fraser D, Russell RGG, Pohler O, Robertson WG, Fleisch H (1972) The influence of disodium ethane-1-hydroxy-1,1-diphosphonate (EHDP) on the development of experimentally induced urinary stones in rats. Clin Sci 42:197–207

Frimpter GW (1961) The disulfide of L-cysteine and L-homocysteine in urine of patients with cystinuria. J Biol Chem 236:PC51–PC53

Frimpter GW (1969) Cystathioninuria in a patient with cystinuria. Am J Med 46:832–836

Frimpter GW, Horwith M, Furth E, Fellows RE, Thompson DD (1962) Inulin and endogenous amino acid renal clearances in cystinuria: evidence for tubular secretion. J Clin Invest 41:281–288

Frimpter GW, Timpanelli AE, Eisenmenger WJ, Stein HS, Ehrlich LI (1963) Reversible "Fanconi syndrome" caused by degraded tetracycline. JAMA 184:111–113

Fuller GR, MacLeod MB, Pitts RF (1955) Influence of administration of potassium salts on the renal reabsorption of bicarbonate. Am J Physiol 182:111–118

Füredi-Milhofer H, Skrtic D, Markovic M, Komunjer L (1981) Crystal growth and aggregation of calcium oxalate in high ionic strength solutions. In: Smith LH, Robertson WG, Finlayson B (eds) Urolithiasis – clinical and basic research. Plenum, New York, p 401–409

Gale RO, Cornelius CE, Bishop JA (1966) Fractionation of urinary biocolloids in children and adults by gel filtration. Invest Urol 4:33–38

Gardner GL (1975) Nucleation and crystal growth of calcium oxalate trihydrate. J Crystal Growth 30:158–168

Gardner GL (1976) Kinetics of the dehydration of calcium oxalate trihydrate crystals in aqueous solution. J Colloid Interface Sci 54:298–310

Gardner GL (1978) The effect of pyrophosphate and phosphonate anions on the crystal growth kinetics of calcium oxalate hydrates. J Phys Chem 82:864–870
Gardner GL, Doremus RH (1978) Crystal growth inhibitors in human urine. Effect on calcium oxalate kinetics. Invest Urol 15:478–485
Garti N, Sarig S, Tibika F (1980) Retardation of calcium oxalate formation by polyacidic peptides. Invest Urol 18:149–150
Gelzayd EA, Breuer RI, Kirsner JB (1968) Nephrolithiasis in inflammatory bowel disease. Am J Dig Dis 13:1027–1034
Gershoff SN (1964) Vitamin B_6 and oxalate metabolism. Vitamins Hormones 22:581–589
Gershoff SN, Prien EL (1960) Excretion of urinary metabolites in calcium oxalate lithiasis. Effect of tryptophan and vitamin B_6 administration. Am J Clin Nutr 8:812–816
Ghazali S, Barratt TM, Williams DI (1973) Childhood urolithiasis in Britain. Arch Dis Child 48:291–295
Gibbs DA, Watts RWE (1966) An investigation of the possible role of xanthine oxidase in the oxidation of glyoxylate to oxalate. Clin Sci 31:285–297
Gibbs DA, Watts RWE (1970) The action of pyridoxine in primary hyperoxaluria. Clin Sci 38:277–286
Giebisch G, MacLeod MB, Pitts RF (1955) Effect of adrenal steroids on renal tubular reabsorption of bicarbonate. Am J Physiol 183:377–386
Gill WB, Roma MJ (1976) Determinants of supersaturation levels and crystallization rates of calcium oxalate from urines of normal humans and stone-formers: effects of non-dialyzable materials. J Surg Res 21:45–49
Gill WB, Silvert MA, Roma MJ (1974) Supersaturation levels and crystallization rates of calcium oxalate from urines of normal humans and stone-formers determined by a ^{14}C-oxalate technique. Invest Urol 12:203–209
Gill WB, Karesch JW, Garsin L, Roma MJ (1977) Inhibitory effect of urinary macromolecular on the crystallisation of calcium oxalate. Invest Urol 15:95–99
Gjaldbaek JC (1982) Inhibition of chondroitin sulphate and heparin on the growth and agglomeration of calcium oxalate monohydrate crystals in vitro. Clin Chim Acta 120:363–365
Gjaldbaek JC, Robertson WG (1980) Does urine from stone-formers contain macromolecules which promote the crystal growth rate of calcium oxalate crystals in vitro? Clin Chim Acta 108:75–80
Glimcher MJ, Krane SM (1964) The identification of serine phosphate in enamel proteins. Biochim Biophys Acta 90:477–483
Goldberg V (1934) Über die Verträglichkeit des chondroitinschwefelsauren Natriums und dessen Ausscheidung in die Harnwege. Z Urol Chir 39:308–313
Gordon EE (1963) Effect of acute metabolic acidosis and alkalosis on acetate and citrate metabolism in the rat. J Clin Invest 42:137–142
Gordon EE, Craige A (1960) Effect of intravenous glucose on splanchnic and peripheral metabolism of endogenous pyruvate and citrate in patients with cirrhosis and in subjects without liver disease. J Lab Clin Med 55:841–848
Graham LA, Caesar JJ, Burgen ASV (1960) Gastrointestinal absorption and excretion of Mg^{28} in man. Metabolism 9:646–659
Gray RW, Wilz DR, Caldos AE, Lemann J (1977) The importance of phosphate in regulating plasma $1,25(OH)_2$ vitamin D levels in humans. Studies in healthy subjects in calcium-stone formers and patients with primary hyperparathyroidism. J Clin Endocrinol Metab 45:299–306
Greene ML, Fuyimoto WY, Seegmiller JE (1969) Urinary xanthine stones – a rare complication of allopurinol therapy. N Engl J Med 283:354–357
Gregory JG, Park KY, Schoenberg HW (1977) Oxalate stone disease after intestinal resection. J Urol 117:631–634
Griffith DP, Musher DM, Itin C (1976) Urease. The primary cause of infection induced urinary stones. Invest Urol 13:346–350
Griffith DP, Gibson JR, Clinton CW, Musher DM (1978) Acetohydroxamic acid: clinical studies of a urease inhibitor in patients with staghorn renal calculi. J Urol 119:9–15
Griffith DP, Moskowitz PA, Carlton CE (1979) Adjunctive chemotherapy of infection-induced staghorn calculi. J Urol 121:711–715

Grollman AP, Harrison HC, Harrison HE (1961) The renal excretion of citrate. J Clin Invest 40:1270–1296
Gutman AB, Yü TF (1965) Urinary ammonium excretion in primary gout. J Clin Invest 44:1474–1481
Hagar BH, Magrath TB (1925) The etiology of incrusted cystitis with alkaline urine. JAMA 85:1352–1355
Haggitt RC, Pitcock JA (1971) Renal medullary calcification: a light and electron microscopic study. J Urol 106:342–347
Hallett RJ, Pead L, Maskell R (1976) Urinary infection in boys. Lancet II:1107–1110
Hallson PC, Rose GA (1979) Uromucoids and urinary stone formation. Lancet I:1000–1002
Hallson PC, Rose GA, Samuell CT (1981) The role of uromucoids in urinary stone formation. In: Brockis JG, Finlayson B (eds) Urinary calculus. PSG Publishing Co. Littleton, Mass, p 285–295
Hallson PC, Rose GA, Sulaiman S (1982a) Magnesium reduces calcium oxalate crystal formation in human whole urine. Clin Sci 62:17–19
Hallson PC, Rose GA, Sulaiman S (1982b) Urate does not influence the formation of calcium oxalate crystals in whole human urine at pH 5.3. Clin Sci 62:421–425
Hammersten G (1929) On calcium oxalate and its solubility in the presence of inorganic salts with special reference to the occurrence of oxaluria. C R Lab Carlsberg 17:1–85
Hansen NM, Felix R, Bisaz S, Fleisch H (1976) Aggregation of hydroxyapatite crystals. Biochim Biophys Acta 451:549–559
Harrell GT, Fisher S (1939) Blood chemical changes in Boeck's sarcoid with particular reference to protein, calcium and phosphatase values. J Clin Invest 18:687–693
Harrison AR, Rose GA (1979) Medullary sponge kidney. Urol Res 7:197–207
Harrison AR, Kasidas GP, Rose GA (1981) Hyperoxaluria and recurrent stone-formation apparently cured by short courses of pyridoxine. Br Med J 282:2097–2098
Harrison JH, Botsford TW, Pierce FR (1945) Management of urinary lithiasis in army general hospital. J Urol 53:282–294
Hartung R, Leskovar P, Kratzer M (1980) Mechanisms of the influence of uric acid on the precipitation of Ca-oxalate crystals out of metastable solution (urine). Croat Chim Acta 53:381–388
Haugen H, Åkesson I, Enger E, Meberg A (1978) Uromucoid in normal urine. Scand J Clin Lab Invest 38:49–51
Haugen H, Åkesson I, Strømme SB, Refsum HA (1980) Excretion of casts and uromucoid in urine after prolonged heavy exercise. Scand J Clin Lab Invest 40:545–549
Hauschka PV, Lian JB, Gallop PM (1975) Direct identification of the calcium-binding amino acid. γ-carboxyglutamic acid, in mineralized tissue.
Haussler MR, McCain TA (1977) Basic and clinical concepts related to vitmain D metabolism and action. N Engl J Med 297:974–983
Hautmann R, Osswald H (1983) Concentration profiles of calcium and oxalate in urine, tubular fluid and renal tissue – some theoretical considerations. J Urol 129:433–436
Hautmann R, Lehmann A, Komor S (1980) Calcium and oxalate concentrations in human renal tissue: the key to the pathogenesis of stone-formation? J Urol 123:317–319
Heaton FW, Pyrah LN (1963) Magnesium metabolism in patients with parathyroid disorders. Clin Sci 25:475–485
Hellström J (1938) The significance of staphylococci in the development and treatment of renal and ureteral stones. Br J Urol 10:348–372
Hellström J, Ivemark BI (1962) Primary hyperparathyroidism, clinical and structural findings in 138 cases. Acta Chir Scand [Suppl] 294:1–113
Henneman DH, Shoemaker WC (1961) Effect of glucagon and epinephrenic on regional metabolism of glucose, pyruvate lactate and citrate on normal conscious dogs. Endocrinology 68:889–898
Henneman PH, Benedict PH, Forbes AP, Dudley HR (1958) Idiopathic hypercalciuria. N Engl J Med 259:802–808
Henneman PH, Wallach S, Dempsey EF (1962) The metabolic defect responsible for uric acid stone formation. J Clin Invest 41:537–542
Hering F, Burschardt WG, Pyhel N, Lutzeyer W (1981) The relation between relative supersaturation and crystal aggregation in urine – an SEM study and a computerized calculation

of the ion equilibrium. In: Smith LH, Robertson WG, Finlayson B (eds) Urolithiasis – clinical and basic research. Plenum, New York, p 441–445
Herndon RF, Freeman S (1958) Renal citric acid utilization in the dog. Am J Physiol 192:369–372
Herring LC (1962) Observations on the analysis of ten thousand urinary calculi. J Urol 88:545–562
Hesse A, Schneider H-J (1976) Results of the standardization and centralization of stone analysis in the German Democratic Republic. In: Fleisch H, Robertson WG, Smith LH, Vahlensieck W (eds) Urolithiasis research. Plenum, New York, p 295–298
Hesse A, Schneider H-J, Berg W, Hienzsch E (1975) Uric acid dehydrate as urinary calculus component. Invest Urol 12:405–409
Hockaday TDR, Clayton JE, Frederick EW, Smith LH (1964) Primary hyperoxaluria. Medicine (Baltimore) 43:315–345
Hodgkinson A (1962) Citric acid excretion in normal adults and in patients with renal calculus. Clin Sci 23:203–212
Hodgkinson A (1971) A combined qualitative and quantitative procedure for the chemical analysis of urinary calculi. J Clin Pathol 24:147–151
Hodgkinson A (1974) Relations between oxalic acid, calcium, magnesium and creatinine excretion in normal men and male patients with calcium oxalate kidney stones. Clin Sci Molec Med 46:357–367
Hodgkinson A (1977) Oxalic acid in biology and medicine. Academic Press, London
Hodgkinson A (1978) Evidence of increased oxalate absorption in patients with calcium-containing renal stones. Clin Sci Molec Med 54:291–294
Hodgkinson A (1980) Solubility of calcium oxalate in human urine, simulated urine, and water. Invest Urol 18:123–126
Hodgkinson A, Marshall RW (1972) Stone composition, urine saturation and treatment of patients with calcium-containing renal stones. In: Hioco D (ed) Rein et calcium. Sandoz Editions, Paris, p 319–339
Hodgkinson A, Marshall RW (1975) Changes in the composition of urinary tract stones. Invest Urol 13:131–135
Hodgkinson A, Pyrah LN (1958) The urinary excretion of calcium and inorganic phosphate in 344 patients with calcium stone of renal origin. Br J Surg 46:10–18
Hodgkinson A, Wilkinson R (1974) Plasma oxalate concentration and the renal excretion of oxalate in man. Clin Sci Molec Med 46:61–73
Hodgkinson A, Peacock M, Nicholson M (1969) Quantitative analysis of calcium-containing urinary calculi. Invest Urol 6:549–561
Hofmann AF, Poley JR (1972) Role of bile acid malabsorption in pathogenesis of diarrhoea and steatorrhea in patients with ileal resection. I. Response to cholestyramine or replacement of dietary long chain triglyceride by medium chain triglyceride. Gastroenterology 62:918–934
Hofmann AF, Thomas PJ, Smith LH, McCall JT (1970) Pathogenesis of secondary hyperoxaluria in patients with ileal resection and diarrhoea. Gastroenterology 58:960
Howard JE (1962) Urinary stone. Can Med Assoc J 86:1001–1007
Howard JE (1976) Studies on urinary stone formation: a saga of clinical investigation. Johns Hopkins Med J 139:239–252
Howard JE, Becker G (1976) Phosphate-citrate interactions as a source of anticalcifying activity in simple synthetic urines. In: Finlayson B, Thomas WC (eds) Colloquium on renal lithiasis. University Presses of Florida, Gainesville, p 119–126
Howard JE, Thomas WC (1958) Some observations on rachitic rat cartilage of probable significance in the etiology of renal calculi. Trans Am Clin Climatol Assoc 70:94–102
Howard JE, Thomas WC, Mukai T, Johnston RA, Pascoe BJ (1962) The calcification of cartilage by urine, and a suggestion for therapy in patients with certain kinds of calculi. Trans Assoc Am Physicians 75:301–306
Howard JE, Thomas WC, Barker LM, Smith LH, Wadkins CL (1967) The recognition and isolation from urine and serum of a peptide inhibitor to calcification. Johns Hopkins Med J 120:119–136
Hunt LD, King JS (1963) Ionic calcium in the urine of stone-formers. Invest Urol 1:83–86

Huth EJ, Maycock RL, Kerr RM (1959) Hyperthyroidism associated with renal tubular acidosis. Am J Med 26:818–826
Huth EJ, Webster GD, Elkington JR (1960) The renal excretion of hydrogen ion in renal tubular acidosis. III. An attempt to detect latent cases in a family: comments on nosology, genetics and etiology of the primary disease. Am J Med 29:586–598
Irving JT (1973) Calcium and phosphorus metabolism. Academic Press, New York
Ismail SI, Tawashi R (1980) Effect of organic matrix on the dissolution of uric acid stones. Eur Urol 6:237–240
Ito H, Coe FL (1977) Acidic peptide and polyribonucleotide crystal growth inhibitors in human urine. Am J Physiol 233:F455–F463
Ito H, Shimazaki J (1978) High molecular weight substances which inhibit calcium oxalate crystal growth. Jpn J Urol 69:1342–1348
Jackson WPU, Dancaster C (1959) A consideration of the hypercalciuria in sarcoidosis, idiopathic hypercalciuria and that produced by vitamin D. A new suggestion regarding calcium metabolism. J Clin Endocrinol Metab 19:658–680
Jacobson AL, Singhal PC, Mandin H, Hyne JB (1979a) Urinary ionic calcium and binding sites in normocalciuric idiopathic calcium urolithiasis. Invest Urol 17:218–222
Jacobson AL, Singhal PC, Mandin H, Hyne JB (1979b) Variability of ionized calcium with pH or normal urine. Biochem Med 22:383–386
Jacobson AL, Singhal PC, Mandin H, Hyne JB (1983) New methods to determine the date of saturation of urine and to discriminate between the urine of control subjects and stone-formers. Clin Biochem 16:79–86
Jaques LW, Riesco BF, Weltner W (1980) NMR spectroscopy and calcium binding of sialic acids: N-glycolylneuraminic acid and periodate-oxidized N-acetylneuraminic acid. Carbohyd Res 83:21–32
Jethi RK, Wadkins CL (1971) Studies of the mechanism of biological calcification: II. Evidence for a multi-step mechanism of calcification by tendon matrix. Calcif Tissue Res 7:277–289
Johansson G, Backman U, Danielson BG, Fellström B, Ljunghall S, Wikström B (1980a) Biochemical and clinical effects of the prophylactic treatment of renal calcium stones with magnesium hydroxide. J Urol 124:770–774
Johansson G, Backman U, Danielson BG, Ljunghall S, Wikström B (1980b) Magnesium metabolism in renal stone disease. Invest Urol 18:93–96
Johansson G, Backman U, Danielson BG, Fellström B, Ljunghall S, Wikström B (1981) Prophylactic treatment with magnesium hydroxide in renal stone disease. In: Smith LH, Robertson WG, Finlayson B (eds) Urolithiasis – clinical and basic research. Plenum, New York, p 267–273
Johnson RG (1959) The solubility of magnesium ammonium phosphate hexahydrate at 38 °C, with considerations pertaining to the urine and the formation of urinary calculi. J Urol 81:681–690
Joly SS (1929) Stone and calculous disease of the urinary organs. CV Moshy, St. Louis
Joost J, Silbernagl S, Jarosch E (1981a) Excretion of the Ca-binding amino acid, γ-carboxyglutamic acid, in stone formers. In: Smith LH, Robertson WG, Finlayson B (eds) Urolithiasis – clinical and basic research. Plenum, New York, p 81–88
Joost J, Jarosch E, Egger G, Hohlbrugger G (1981b) γ-Carboxyglutamic acid in recurrent calcium stone-formers. In: Brockis JG, Finlayson B (eds) Urinary calculus. PSG Publishing Co, Littleton, Mass, p 129–138
Jung A, Russell RGG, Bisaz S, Morgan DB, Fleisch H (1970) Fate of intravenously injected pyrophosphate – ^{32}P in dogs. Am J Physiol 218:1757–1764
Jung A, Bisaz S, Fleisch H (1973) The binding of pyrophosphate and two diphosphonates by hydroxyapatite crystals. Calcif Tissue Res 11:269–280
Kaplan RA, Haussler MR, Deftos LJ, Bone H, Pak CYC (1977) The role of 1α,25-dihydroxyvitamin D in the metabolism of intestinal hyperabsorption of calcium in primary hyperparathyroidism and absorptive hypercalciuria. J Clin Invest 59:756–760
Katz WA (1973) Effect of glycosaminoglycans on urate precipitation in gout. Clin Res 21:973
Katz WA, Schubert M (1970) The interaction of monosodium urate with connective tissue components. J Clin Invest 49:1783–1789

Kazantzis G, Flynn FV, Spowage JS, Trott DG (1963) Renal tubular malfunction and pulmonary emphysema in cadmium pigment workers. Q J Med 32:165–192
Keating FR (1961) Diagnosis of primary hyperparathyroidism. JAMA 178:547–555
Keeler RF (1963) Silicon metabolism and silica-protein matrix interrelationship in bovine urolithiasis. Ann NY Acad Sci 104:592–611
Keutel HJ, King JS (1964) Further studies of matrix substance A. Invest Urol 2:115–122
Keutel HJ, King JS, Boyce WH (1964) Further studies of uromucoid in normal and stone urine. Urol Int 17:324–341
Khan SR, Finlayson B, Hackett RL (1979) Histology study of the early events in oxalate induced intranephronic calculosis. Invest Urol 17:199–202
Khan SR, Finlayson B, Hackett RL (1981 a) Rat renal papillary structure in oxalate-induced microlithiasis. A scanning electron microscope study. In: Smith LH, Robertson WG, Finlayson B (eds) Urolithiasis – clinical and basic research. Plenum, New York, p 517–521
Khan SR, Finlayson B, Hackett RL (1981 b) The ultrastructure of rat renal tubules in experimental calcium oxalate nephrolithiasis. In: Smith LH, Robertson WG, Finlayson B (eds) Urolithiasis – clinical and basic research. Plenum, New York, p 523–525
Khan SR, Finlayson B, Hackett RL (1983) Agar-embedded urinary stones: a technique useful for studying microscopic architecture. J Urol 130:992–995
Kimura Y, Kisaki N, Ise K (1976) The role of the matrix substance in formation of urinary stones. Urol Int 31:355–367
King JS (1967) Etiologic factors involved in urolithiasis: a review of recent research. J Urol 97:583–591
King JS, Boyce WH (1957) Amino acid and carbohydrate composition of the mucoprotein matrix in various calculi. Proc Soc Exp Biol Med 95:183–187
King JS, Boyce WH (1963 a) Immunological studies on serum and urinary proteins in urolith matrix in man. Ann NY Acad Sci 104:579–591
King JS, Boyce WH (1963 b) Invitro production of simulated renal calculi. J Urol 89:546–551
King JS, Wainer A (1967) Cystinuria with hyperuricemia and methioninuria: biochemical study of a case. Am J Med 43:125–130
King RG, Stanbury SW (1970) Magnesium metabolism in primary hyperparathyroidism. Clin Sci 39:281–303
Kitamura T, Pak CYC (1982) Tamm and Horsfall glycoprotein does not promote spontaneous precipitation and crystal growth of calcium oxalate in vitro. J Urol 127:1024–1026
Kitamura T, Zerwekh JE, Pak CYC (1982) Partial biochemical and physiochemical characterization of organic macromolecules in urine from patients with renal stones and control subjects. Kidney Int 21:379–386
Kjølhede KT, Lassen HK (1942) The significance of Randall papillary lesions in the causation of renal calculi. J Urol 47:45–57
Kobashi K, Hase J, Uehara K (1962) Specific inhibition of urease by hydroxamic acids. Biochim Biophys Acta 65:380–383
Kobashi K, Takebe S, Terashima N, Hase J (1975) Inhibition of urease activity by hydroxamic acid derivatives of amino-acids. J Biochem (Tokyo) 77:837–843
Koch J, Stokstad ELR, Williams HE, Smith LH Jr (1967) Deficiency of 2-oxo-glutarate: glyoxylate carboligase activity in primary hyperoxaluria. Proc Natl Acad Sci USA 57:1123–1129
Koide T, Takemoto M, Itatani H, Takaha M, Sonoda T (1981) Urinary macromolecular substances as natural inhibitors of calcium oxalate crystal aggregation. Invest Urol 18:382–386
Kook YJ, Lotspeich WD (1968) Citrate excretion during intrarenal arterial precursor infusion in the alkalotic dog. Am J Physiol 215:282–288
Kornberg A (1962) On the metabolic significance of phosphorolytic and pyrophosphorolytic reactions. In: Kasha M, Pullman D (eds) Horizons in biochemistry. Academic Press, New York, p 251–264
Koutsoukos PG, Nancollas GH (1981) Crystal growth of calcium phosphate – epitaxial considerations. J Crystal Growth 53:10–19
Koutsoukos PG, Amjad Z, Tomson MB, Nancollas GH (1980 a) Crystallisation of calcium phosphates. A constant composition study. J Am Chem Soc 102:1553–1557

Koutsoukos PG, Lam-Erwin CY, Nancollas GH (1980b) Epitaxial considerations in urinary stone formation. I. The urate-oxalate-phosphate system. Invest Urol 18:178–184
Koutsoukos PG, Sheehan ME, Nancollas GH (1981) Epitaxial considerations in urinary stone-formation: II. The oxalate-phosphate system. Invest Urol 18:358–363
Kovarsky J, Holmes E, Kelley WN (1976) Absence of significant urate binding to human serum proteins. Clin Res 24:21
Kozin F, McCarty DJ (1977) Protein binding to monosodium urate monohydrate, calcium pyrophosphate dihydrate and silicon dioxide crystals. I. Physical characteristics. J Lab Clin Med 89:1314–1325
Krebs HA, Johnson WA (1937) The role of citric acid in intermediate metabolism in animal tissues. Enzymologia 4:148–156
Kuiper JJ (1971) Medullary sponge kidney in three generations. NY State J Med 71:2665–2669
Kumaki K, Tomioka S, Kobashi K, Hase H (1972) Structure activity correlations between hydroxamic acids and their inhibitory powers on urease activity. I. A quantitative approach to the effect of hydrophobic character of acyl residue. Chem Pharm Bull (Tokyo) 20:1599–1606
Kuyper AC, Matill HA (1933) Some aspects of citric acid metabolism. J Biol Chem 103:51–60
Labeeuw M, Gerbaulet C, Pozet N, Zech P, Divry P, Traeger J (1980) Uric acid, monosodium urate and ammonium urate urinary relative saturations in normo-uricosuric calcium oxalate stone formers. Eur Urol 6:241–246
Lagergren C (1956) Biophysical investigations of urinary calculi. Acta Radiol [Suppl] (Stockh) 133:1–72
Lagergren C (1962) Development of silica calculi after oral administration of magnesium trisilicate. J Urol 87:994–996
Lalli AF (1969) Medullary sponge kidney disease. Radiology 92:92–96
Lam C-Y, Nancollas GH, Ko S-J (1978) The kinetics of formation and dissolution of uric acid crystals. Invest Urol 15:473–477
Lambden MP, Chrystowski GA (1954) Urinary oxalate excretion by man following ascorbic acid ingestion. Proc Soc Exp Biol Med 85:190–192
Lanzalaco AC, Sheehan ME, White DJ, Nancollas GH (1982) The mineralization inhibitory potential of ùrines, a constant composition approach. J Urol 128:845–849
Lavan JN, Neale FC, Posen S (1971) Urinary calculi – clinical, biochemical and radiological studies in 619 patients. Med J Aust 2:1049–1061
Leal JJ, Finlayson B (1977) Absorption of naturally occurring polymers onto calcium oxalate crystal surfaces. Invest Urol 14:278–283
Lebacq E, Desmet V, Verhaegen H (1970) Renal involvement in sarcoidosis. Postgrad Med J 46:526–529
Legeros RZ, Morales P (1973) Renal stone crystals grown in gel systems. Invest Urol 11:12–20
Lenarduzzi G (1939) Reporto pielografico poco commune dilatazione delle view urinarie intrarenali. Radiol Med (Torino) 26:346–351
Lepoutre C (1925) Calculs multiples chez un enfant. Infiltration du parenchyme rénal par des dêpôts cristallins. J d'Urol Médicale et Chirurg 20:424
Leskovar P (1979) Das ionisierte Kalzium in Serum und im Harn. Bestimmungsmethoden und methodische Schwierigkeiten. Z Urol Nephrol 72:259–268
Lester FT, Cusworth DC (1973) Lysine infusion in cystinuria: theoretical renal thresholds for lysine. Clin Sci 44:99–111
Levy HL (1973) Genetic screening. In: Herns H, Hirschorn K (eds) Progress in human genetics, vol 4. Plenum Press, New York, p 1–50
Lewis AM, Thomas WC, Tomita A (1966) Pyrophosphate and the mineralizing potential of urine. Clin Sci 30:389–397
Lian JB, Prien EL, Glimcher MJ, Gallop PM (1977) The presence of protein-bound γ-carboxyglutamic acid in calcium-containing renal calculi. J Clin Invest 59:1151–1157
Lichtwitz L (1944) The formation of concretions. In: Alexander J (ed) Colloid chemistry, vol 5. Reinhold, New York, p 1063–1082
Lichtwitz L, Rosenbach O (1909) Untersuchungen über Kolloide im Urin. Z Physiol Chem 61:122–128

Ligabue A, Fini M, Robertson WG (1979) Influence of urine in vitro crystallisation rate of calcium oxalate: determination of inhibitory activity by a ^{14}C-oxalate technique. Clin Chim Acta 98:39–46

Light IS, Zinsser HH (1961) Determination of rate of formation and nucleation time of calcium oxalate in various systems. Arch Biochem Biophys 92:487–496

Light IS, Gursel, Zinsser HH (1973) Urinary ionised calcium in urolithiasis. Effect of cranberry juice. Urology 1:67–70

Lightwood R, Butler N (1963) Decline in primary infantile renal acidosis Aetiological implications. Br Med J 1:855–857

Lindahl WW, Bargen JA (1941) Nephrolithiasis complicating chronic ulcerative colitis after ileostomy. A report of six cases. J Urol 46:183–192

Lindvall N (1959) Roentgenologic diagnosis of medullary sponge kidney. Acta Radiol 51:193–206

Ljunghall S (1979) Family history of renal stones in a population study of stone-formers and healthy subjects. Br J Urol 51:249–252

Lloyd HM (1968) Primary hyperparathyroidism: an analysis of the role of the parathyroid tumor. Medicine (Baltimore) 47:53–71

London DR, Foley TH (1965) Cystine metabolism in cystinuria. Clin Sci 29:133–141

Longcope WT, Freiman DG (1952) A study of sarcoidosis based on a combined investigation of 160 cases including 30 autopsies from the Johns Hopkins Hospital and Massachusetts General Hospital. Medicine (Baltimore) 31:1–132

Lonsdale K (1968a) Human stones. Science 159:1199–1207

Lonsdale K (1968b) Epitaxy as a growth factor in urinary calculi and gallstones. Nature 217:56–58

Lonsdale K, Mason P (1966) Uric acid, uric acid dehydrate and urates in urinary calculi, ancient and modern. Science 152:1511–1512

Lowenstein JM (ed) (1969) Citric acid cycle control and compartmentation. Marcel Dekker, New York

MacGregor ME, Rayner PHW (1964) Pink disease and primary renal tubular acidosis. Lancet II:1083–1085

Malek RS, Boyce WH (1973) Intranephronic calculosis: its significance and relationship to matrix in nephrolithiasis. J Urol 109:551–555

Malek RS, Boyce WH (1977) Observations on the ultrastructure and genesis of urinary calculi. J Urol 117:336–341

Malek RS, Kelalis PP (1975) Pediatric nephrolithiasis. J Urol 113:545–551

Mandel NS, Mandel GS (1981) Epitaxis between stone-forming crystals at the atomic level. In: Smith LH, Robertson WG, Finlayson B (eds) Urolithiasis – clinical and basic research. Plenum, New York, p 469–480

Maratka Z, Neobal J (1964) Urolithiasis as a complication of the surgical treatment of ulcerative colitis. Gut 5:214–217

Markovic M, Komunjer L (1979) A new method to follow crystal growth by Coulter Counter. J Crystal Growth 46:701–705

Marshall RW, Barry H (1973) Urine saturation and the formation of calcium containing calculi: the effects of various forms of therapy. In: Cifuentes Delatte L, Rapado A, Hodgkinson A (eds) Urinary calculi. Karger, Basel, p 164–169

Marshall RW, Nancollas GH (1969) The kinetics of crystal growth of dicalcium phosphate dihydrate. J Phys Chem 73:3838–3844

Marshall RW, Robertson WG (1976) Nomograms for the estimation of the saturation of urine with calcium oxalate, calcium phosphate, magnesium ammonium phosphate, uric acid, sodium acid urate, ammonium acid urate and cystine. Clin Chim Acta 72:253–260

Marshall RW, Cochran M, Hodgkinson A (1972a) Relationship between calcium and oxalic acid intake in the diet and their excretion in the urine of normal and renal stone-forming subjects. Clin Sci 43:91–99

Marshall RW, Cochran M, Robertson WG, Hodgkinson A, Nordin BEC (1972b) The relation between urine saturation and stone composition in patients with calcium-containing renal stones. Clin Sci 43:433–441

Marshall V, White RH, Chaput de Saintonge M, Tresidder GC, Blandy JP (1975) The natural history of renal and ureteric calculi. Br J Urol 47:117–124

Martensson J (1940) On the citric acid metabolism in mammals. Acta Physiol Scand [Suppl] 11:1–96

Martin GR, Firschein HE, Mulryan BJ, Newman WF (1958) Concerning the mechanism of action of parathyroid hormone. II. Metabolic effect. J Am Chem Soc 80:6201–6204

Mates J, Krizek V (1955) Die Steinkrankheit im Lichte von 3340 beobachteten Fällen. Z Urol 48:478–487

Matouschek E, Huber R (1981) Ergebnisse einer internationalen kooperativen Studie über das Harnsteinleiden. Fortschr Urol Nephrol 17:23–32

Maxfield M (1959) Physicochemical study in salt solution of urinary mucoprotein with virus-inhibiting activity. Arch Biochem Biophys 85:382–390

Maxfield M (1960) Fractionation of the urinary mucoprotein of Tamm and Horsfall. Arch Biochem Biophys 89:281–288

Maxfield M (1963) Urinary mucopolysaccharide and calculi. Annu Rev Med 14:99–110

May P, Schindler E (1973) Methods and results of conservative treatment of uric acid stones. In: Cifuentes Delatte L, Rapado A, Hodgkinson A (eds) Urinary calculi. Karger, Basel, p 111–114

Mayall GF (1970) The incidence of medullary sponge kidney. Clin Radiol 21:171–174

McCarthy CF, Borland JL, Lynch HJ, Owen EE, Tyor MP (1964) Defective uptake of basic amino acids and L-cystine by intestinal mucosa of patients with cystinuria. J Clin Invest 43:1518–1524

McCulloch RK, Bowyer RC, Brockis JG (1981) Possible roles of urate in calcium urolithiasis. In: Brockis JG, Finlayson B (eds) Urinary calculus. PSG Publishing Co., Littleton, Mass., p 347–352

McCurdy DT, Frederic M, Elkinton JR (1968) Renal tubular acidosis due to amphotericin B. N Engl J Med 278:124–131

McDonald DF, Roth L, McFadden A (1964) In vitro calculogenesis with human urine: 1. Method and reproducibility of results. J Urol 91:676–680

McGeown MG (1960) Heredity in renal stone disease. Clin Sci 19:465–471

McGeown MG (1963) The causes of kidney stones. Irish J Med Sci 451:301–320

McKusick VA, Neufeld EF, Kelly TE (1978) The mucopolysaccharide storage diseases. In: Stanbury JB, Lsyngaarden JB, Fredrickson DS (eds) The metabolic basis of inherited disease. McGraw-Hill, London, p 1282–1307

McQueen E (1962) The nature of urinary casts. J Clin Pathol 15:367–373

McQueen E (1966) Composition of urinary casts. Lancet I:397–398

McQueen E, Engel G (1966) Factors determining the aggregation of urinary mucoprotein. J Clin Pathol 19:392–396

Meberg A, Haugen H, Åkesson I, Sande H (1979) Uromucoid (Tamm-Horsfall's mucoprotein) in amniotic fluid and in urine in children. Nephron 23:28–31

Melick RA, Henneman PH (1958) Clinical and laboratory studies of 207 consecutive patients in a kidney stone clinic. N Engl J Med 259:307–314

Melick RA, Quelch KJ, Rhodes M (1980) The demonstration of sialic acid in kidney stone matrix. Clin Sci 59:401–404

Menon M, Mahle CJ (1983) Urinary citrate excretion in patients with renal calculi. J Urol 129:1158–1160

Metcalfe-Gibson A, MacCallum FM, Morrison RBI, Wrong O (1965) Urinary excretion of hydrogen ion in patients with uric acid calculi. Clin Sci 28:325–345

Meyer AS, Finlayson B, Dubois L (1971) Direct observation of urinary stone ultra-structure. Br J Urol 43:154–164

Meyer JL (1981) Nucleation kinetics in the calcium oxalate-sodium urate monohydrate system. Invest Urol 19:197–201

Meyer JL, Angino EE (1977) The role of trace metals in calcium urolithiasis. Invest Urol 14:347–350

Meyer JL, Eanes ED (1978) A thermodynamic analysis of the secondary transition in the spontaneous precipitation of calcium phosphate. Calcif Tissue Res 25:209–216

Meyer JL, Nancollas GH (1972) Effect of stannous and fluoride ions on the rate of crystal growth of hydroxyapatite. J Dent Res 51:1443–1450

Meyer JL, Nancollas GH (1973) The influence of multidentate organic phosphonates on the crystal growth of hydroxyapatite. Calcif Tissue Res 13:295–303

Meyer JL, Smith LH (1975a) Growth of calcium oxalate crystals. I. A model for urinary stone growth. Invest Urol 13:31–35
Meyer JL, Smith LH (1975b) Growth of calcium oxalate crystals. II. Inhibition by natural urinary crystal growth inhibitors. Invest Urol 13:36–39
Meyer JL, Thomas WC (1982a) Trace metal-citric acid complexes as inhibitors of calcification and crystal growth I. J Urol 128:1372–1375
Meyer JL, Thomas WC (1982b) Trace metal-citric acid complexes as inhibitors of calcification and crystal growth II. J Urol 128:1376–1378
Meyer JL, McCall JT, Smith LH (1974) Inhibition of calcium phosphate crystallization by nucleoside phosphates. Calif Tissue Res 15:289–293
Meyer JL, Bergert JH, Smith LH (1975) Epitaxial relationships in urolithiasis: the calcium oxalate monohydrate-hydroxyapatite system. Clin Sci Molec Med 49:369–374
Meyer JL, Bergert JH, Smith LH (1976) The epitaxially induced crystal growth of calcium oxalate by crystalline uric acid. Invest Urol 14:115–119
Meyer JL, Bergert JH, Smith LH (1977a) Epitaxial relationships in urolithiasis the brushite-whewellite system. Clin Sci Molec Med 52:143–148
Meyer JL, Lee KE, Bergert JH (1977b) The inhibition of calcium oxalate crystal growth by multidentate organic phosphonates. Calcif Tissue Res 28:83–86
Miller JD, Randolph AD, Drach GW (1977) Observations upon calcium oxalate crystallization kinetics in simulated urine. J Urol 117:342–345
Milne MD, Asatoor AM, Edwards KDG, Loughridge LW (1961) The intestinal absorption defect in cystinuria. Gut 2:323–337
Modlin M (1967a) Urinary ionized calcium and renal stone. An interracial study. J Urol 97:567–572
Modlin M (1967b) The aetiology of renal stone: a new concept arising from studies on a stone-free population. Ann R Coll Surg Engl 40:155–178
Modlin M (1969) Renal calculus in the Republic of South Africa. In: Hodgkinson A, Nordin BEC (eds) Proceedings of the renal stone research symposium. Churchill, London, p 49–58
Mogg RA (1964) Matrix calculi. Proc R Soc Med 57:935–937
Moore CA, Bunce GE (1964) Reduction in frequency of renal calculus formation by oral magnesium administration. Invest Urol 2:7–13
Moreno EC, Varughese K (1981) Crystal growth of calcium apatites from dilute solutions. J Crystal Growth 53:20–30
Morgan HG, Stewart WK, Lowe KG, Stowers JM, Johnstone JH (1962) Wilson's disease and the Fanconi syndrome. Q J Med 31:361–384
Morgenroth K, Backmann R, Blaschke R (1968) Über die Formen der Calciumoxalate Ablagerungen und der menschlichen Niere bei Oxalase. Beitr Pathol Anat 136:454–463
Morris RC (1968) An experimental acidification defect in patients with hereditary fructose intolerance. I. Its resemblance to renal tubular acidosis. J Clin Invest 47:1389–1398
Morris RC (1969) Renal tubular acidosis. N Engl J Med 281:1405–1413
Morris RC, Fudenberg HH (1967) Impaired renal acidification in patients with hypergammaglobulinemia. Medicine (Baltimore) 46:57–69
Morris RC, Yamauchi H, Palubinskas AJ, Howerstine J (1965) Medullary sponge kidney. Am J Med 38:883–892
Mudd SH, Levy HL (1978) Disorders of transsulfuration. In: Stanbury JB, Wyngaarden JB, Fredrickson DS (eds) The metabolic basis of inherited disease. McGraw Hill, New York, pp 458–503
Mukai I, Howard JE (1963) Some observations on the calcification of rachitic rat cartilage by urine. Bull Johns Hopkins Hosp 112:279–290
Muller H (1969) Sex, age and hyperparathyroidism. Lancet I:449–450
Murphy BT, Pyrah LN (1962) The composition, structure, and mechanisms of the formation of urinary calculi. Br J Urol 34:129–159
Nakagawa Y, Kaiser ET, Coe FL (1978) Isolation and characterization of calcium oxalate crystal growth inhibitors from human urine. Biochim Biophys Res Commun 84:1038–1044
Nakagawa Y, Margolis HC, Yokoyama S, Kezdy FJ, Kaiser ET, Coe FL (1981) Purification and characterization of a calcium oxalate monohydrate crystal growth inhibitor from human kidney tissue culture medium. J Biol Chem 256:3936–3944

Nakagawa Y, Abram V, Kezdy FL, Kaiser ET, Coe FL (1983) Purification and characterization of the principal inhibitor of calcium oxalate monohydrate crystal growth in human urine. J Biol Chem 258:12594–12600
Nancollas GH (1976) The kinetics of crystal growth and renal stone-formation. In: Fleisch H, Robertson WG, Smith LH, Vahlensieck W (eds) Urolithiasis research. Plenum, New York, p 5–23
Nancollas GH, Gardner GL (1974) Kinetics of crystal growth of calcium oxalate monohydrate. J Crystal Growth 21:267–276
Nancollas GH, Tomazic BB (1974) Growth of calcium phosphate on hydroxyapatite crystals. Effect of supersaturation and ionic medium. J Physiol Chem 78:2218–2225
Nancollas GH, Tomazic B, Tomson M (1976) The precipitation of calcium phosphates in the presence of magnesium. Croatica Chem Acta 48:431–438
Nelsestuen GL, Suttie JW (1973) The mode of action of vitamin K. Isolation of a peptide containing the vitamin K – dependent portion of prothrombin. Proc Natl Acad Sci USA 70:3366–3370
Newcomb C (1930) Role of urinary colloids in prevention of stone formation. Indian J Med Res 18:275–281
Nicar MJ, Holt K, Pak CYC (1980) Ion binding by small molecular weight substances (1000–10,000 daltons) in urine. Invest Urol 18:162–164
Nicar MJ, Skurla C, Sakhaee K, Pak CYC (1983) Low urinary citrate excretion in nephrolithiasis. Urology 21:8–14
Nicar MJ, Peterson R, Pak CYC (1984) Use of potassium citrate as potassium supplement during thiazide therapy of calcium nephrolithiasis. J Urol 131:430–433
Nielsen JA, Thaysen EH (1971) Acute and chronic magnesium deficiency following extensive small gut resection. Scand J Gastroenterol 6:663–666
Nine FA, Hutchins GM (1973) Oxalosis caused by aspergillus injection. Johns Hopkins Med J 133:183–194
Nordin BEC (1959) The estimation of 'free' calcium in the urine and its relevance to calculus formation. Br J Urol 31:404–413
Nordin BEC, Tribedi K (1962) Ionised calcium in normal and stone-forming urine. Lancet I:409–410
Nordin BEC, Hodgkinson A, Peacock M (1967) The measurement and meaning of urinary calcium. Clin Orthop 52:392–322
Nordin BEC, Peacock M, Wilkinson R (1972) Hypercalciuria and renal stone disease. Clin Endocrinol Metab 1:169–183
Nordin BEC, Peacock M, Marshall DH (1976) Calcium excretion and hypercalciuria. In: Fleisch H, Robertson WG, Smith LH, Vahlensieck W (eds) Urolithiasis research. Plenum Press, New York, p 101–115
Nordin BEC, Hodgkinson A, Peacock M, Robertson WG (1979) Urinary tract calculi. In: Hamburger J, Crosnier J, Grunfeld JP (eds) Nephrology. Wiley, New York Paris, p 1091–1130
Nyvlt J (1978) Dynamics of steady state establishing in continuous crystallizers. Coll Czech Chem Commun 43:2531–2535
O'Brien MM, Uhlemann I, McIntosh HW (1967) Urinary pyrophosphate in normal subjects and in stone-formers. Canad Med Assoc J 96:100–103
Ohata M, Pak CYC (1973) The effect of diphosphonate on calcium phosphate crystallization in urine in vitro. Kidney Int 4:401–406
Ohata M, Pak CYC (1974) Preliminary study of the treatment of nephrolithiasis (calcium stones) with diphosphonate. Metabolism 23:1167–1173
O'Leary JP, Thomas WC, Woodward ER (1974) Urinary tract stone after small bowel surgery for morbid obesity. Am J Surg 127:142–147
Oliver J, MacDowell M, Whang R, Welt LG (1966) The renal lesions of electrolyte imbalance. IV. The intranephronic calculosis of experimental magnesium depletion. J Exp Med 124:263–278
Ord WM (1879) On the influence of colloids upon crystalline forms and cohesion with observations on the structure and mode of formation of urinary and other calculi. Stanford, London

Oreopoulos DG, Soyannwo MAO, McGeown MG (1968) Magnesium/calcium ratio in urine of patients with renal stones. Lancet II:420–422
Orloff J, Berliner RW (1956) The mechanism of the excretion of ammonia in the dog. J Clin Invest 35:223–235
Orwoll ES (1982) The milk-alkali syndrome: current concepts. Ann Intern Med 97:242–248
Owen EE, Tyor MP, Flanagan JF, Berry JN (1960) The kidney as a source of blood ammonia in patients with liver disease. The effects of acetozolamide. J Clin Invest 39:288–294
Oyanagi K, Miura R, Yamanouchi T (1970) Congenital lysinuria: a new inherited transport disorder of dibasic amino acids. J Pediatr 77:259–266
Page RC, Heffner RR, Frey A (1941) Urinary excretion of silica in humans following oral administration of magnesium trisilicate. Am J Dig Dis 8:13–15
Pak CYC (1969) Physico-chemical basis for formation of renal stones of calcium phosphate origin: calculation of the degree of saturation of urine with respect to brushite. J Clin Invest 48:1914–1922
Pak CYC (1972) Effects of cellulose phosphate and sodium phosphate on formation product and activity product of brushite in urine. Metabolism 21:447–455
Pak CYC (1978) Calcium urolithiasis: is it analogous to bone formation? Calcif Tissue Res 26:195–197
Pak CYC (1981) Potential etiology role of brushite in the formation of calcium (renal) stones. J Crystal Growth 53:202–208
Pak CYC, Arnold LH (1975) Heterogeneous nucleation of calcium oxalate by seeds of monosodium urate. Proc Soc Exp Biol Med 149:930–932
Pak CYC, Chu S (1973) A simple technique for the determination of urinary state of saturation with respect of brushite. Invest Urol II:211–221
Pak CYC, Galosy RA (1979) Fasting urinary adenosine 3′5′ monophosphate: A discriminant analysis for the identification of renal and absorption hypercalciurias. J Clin Endocrinol Metab 48:260–265
Pak CYC, Galosy RA (1980) Propensity for spontaneous nucleation of calcium oxalate. Am J Med 69:681–689
Pak CYC, Holt K (1976) Nucleation and growth of brushite and calcium oxalate in urine of stone-formers. Metabolism 25:665–673
Pak CYC, Williams HE, Ruskin B (1971) Physicochemical basis for the formation of Ca-containing renal stones. Clin Res 19:482
Pak CYC, Kaplan RA, Bone H, Townsend J, Waters O (1975a) A simple test for the diagnosis of absorptive, resorptive and renal hypercalciurias. N Engl J Med 292:497–500
Pak CYC, Ohata M, Holt K (1975b) Effect of diphosphonate on crystallization of calcium oxalate in vitro. Kidney Int 7:154–160
Pak CYC, Ohata M, Lawrence EC, Snyder W (1974) The hypercalciurias. J Clin Invest 54:387–400
Pak CYC, Hayashi Y, Arnold LH (1976) Heterogeneous nucleation with urate, calcium phosphate and calcium oxalate. Proc Soc Exp Biol Med 153:83–87
Pak CYC, Hayashi Y, Finlayson B, Chu S (1977a) Estimation of the state of saturation of brushite and calcium oxalate in urine: A comparison of three methods. J Lab Clin Med 89:891–901
Pak CYC, Waters O, Arnold L, Holt K, Cox C, Barilla D (1977b) Mechanism for calcium urolithiasis among patients with hyperuricosuria. J Clin Invest 59:426–431
Pak CYC, Tolentino R, Stewart A, Galosy RA (1978) Enhancement of renal excretion of uric acid during long-term thiazide therapy. Invest Urol 16:191–193
Pak CYC, Holt K, Zerwekh JE (1979) Attenuation by monosodium urate of the inhibitory effect of glycosaminoglycans on calcium oxalate nucleation. Invest Urol 17:138–140
Pak CYC, Barilla DE, Holt K, Brinkley L, Tolentino R, Zerwekh JE (1980a) Effect of oral purine load and allopurinol on the crystallization of calcium salts in urine of patients with hyperuricosuria calcium urolithiasis. Am J Med 65:593–599
Pak CYC, Holt K, Britton F, Peterson R, Crowther C, Ward D (1980b) Assessment of pathogenetic roles of uric acid, monopotassium urate, monoammonium urate and monosodium urate in hyperuricosuric calcium oxalate nephrolithiasis. Miner Electrolyte Metab 4:130–136

Papathanassiadis S, Swinney J (1966) Results of partial nephrectomy compared with pyelolithotomy and nephrolithotomy. Br J Urol 38:403–409
Paternain JL, Bernshtam J, Pinto B (1980) Isolation of a mucoprotein possessing mineral nucleating activity. Invest Urol 18:119–122
Peacock M (1978) The endocrine control of calcium and phosphorus metabolism and its diseases. Medicine (Baltimore) 9:407–417
Peacock M, Nordin BEC (1968) Tubular reabsorption of calcium in normal and hypercalciuric subjects. J Clin Pathol 21:353–358
Peacock M, Nordin BEC (1969) The hypercalciuria of renal stone disease. In: Hodgkinson A, Nordin BEC (eds) Proceedings of renal stone research symposium. Churchill, London, p 253–262
Peacock M, Robertson WG (1978) Metabolic factors in calcium stone disease. In: Barcelo R (ed) Proceedings of the VIIth international congress of nephrology. Karger, Basel, p 371–377
Peacock M, Robertson WG (1979) The biochemical aetiology of renal lithiasis. In: Wickham JEA (ed) Urinary calculous disease. Churchill, Livingstone, Edinburgh, p 69–95
Peacock M, Robertson WG (1980) Renal calculi. Medicine (Baltimore) 27:1372–1379
Peacock M, Hodgkinson A, Nordin BEC (1967) Importance of dietary calcium in the definition of hypercalciuria. Br Med J 3:469–471
Peacock M, Knowles F, Nordin BEC (1968) Effect of calcium administration and deprivation on serum and urine calcium in stone-forming subjects. Br Med J 2:729–731
Peacock M, Marshall RW, Robertson WG, Varnavides CK (1976a) Renal stone disease in primary hyperparathyroid and idiopathic stone-formers: diagnosis, etiology and treatment. In: Finlayson B, Thomas WC (eds) Colloquium on renal lithiasis. University Presses of Florida, Gainesville, p 339–355
Peacock M, Marshall RW, Robertson WG, Varnavides C, Nordin BEC (1976b) Hypercalciuria and recurrent renal calcium stone disease. Effect of oral phosphate in phosphate metabolism kidney and bone. Nouvelle Imprimerie Fournie Toulouse, p 63–76
Peacock M, Robertson WG, Heyburn PJ, Rutherford A (1979a) Urinary tract stone disease. In: Robinson BHB, Hawkins JB, Naik RB (eds) Proceedings of the european dialysis and transplant association, vol 16. Pitman Medical Publishing Co., p 556–565
Peacock M, Robertson WG, Marshall RW (1979b) Disorders associated with recurrent calcium-containing stones. In: Degroot LJ, Odell WD, Martini L, Potts JT, Nelson DH, Steinberger E, Winegrad AD (eds). Endocrinology vol 2. Grune & Stratton, New York, p 823–828
Peacock M, Bambach CP, Robertson WG, Aaron JE, Hill GL (1981a) Urinary stone-formation in bowel disease. In: Smith LH, Robertson WG, Finlayson B (eds) Urolithiasis – clinical and basic research. Plenum, New York, p 159–168
Peacock M, Heyburn PJ, Barnet M, Taylor GA, Brown WB, Davies AEJ (1981b) Plasma $1,25(OH)_2D$ in idiopathic and hyperparathyroid stone-formers. In: Smith LH, Robertson WG, Finlayson B (eds) Urolithiasis – clinical and basic research. Plenum, New York, p 825–829
Peacock M, Robertson WG, Heyburn PJ, Davies AEJ, Rutherford A (1981c) Phosphate treatment of idiopathic calcium stone disease. In: Smith LH, Robertson WG, Finlayson B (eds) Urolithiasis – clinical and basic research. Plenum Press, New York, p 259–265
Pearson G (1798) Experiments and observations, tending to show the composition and properties of urinary concretions. Philos Trans R Soc Lond (Biol) 88:15–39
Piel CF (1957) Disease of the nerve tubules in childhood. Pediatrics 20:337–357
Pinto B (1973) Oxalate binding by the mucoprotein components of renal stones. In: Cifuentes Delatte L, Rapado A, Hodgkinson A (eds) Urinary calculi. Karger, Basel, p 46–52
Pitts RF (1950) Acid base regulation by the kidneys. Am J Med 9:356–372
Pitts RF (1968) Renal regulation of acid-base balance. In: Pitts RF (ed) Physiology of the kidney and body fluids. Year Book Publishers Inc, Chicago, p 179–212
Pitts RF, Lotspeich WD (1946) Bicarbonate and the renal regulation of acid-base balance. Am J Physiol 147:136–154
Pollak VE, Arbel C (1969) The distribution of Tamm-Horsfall mucoprotein (uromucoid) in the human nephron. Nephron 6:667–672

Porter P (1963) Physico-chemical factors involved in urate calculus formation. II. Colloidal flocculation. Res Vet Sci 4:592–602
Porter P (1966) Colloidal properties of urates in relation to calculus formation. Res Vet Sci 7:128–137
Posey LC (1942) Urinary concretions. II. A study of the primary calculous lesions. J Urol 48:300–309
Postlethwaite AE, Gutman RA, Kelley WN (1974) Salicyclate-mediated increase in urate removal during haemodialysis. Evidence for urate binding to protein in vivo. Metabolism 23:771–777
Price PA, Otsuka AS, Poser JW, Kristaponis J, Raman N (1976) Characterization of a γ-carboxyglutamic acid-containing protein from bone. Proc Natl Acad Sci USA 73:1447–1451
Pridgen DB, Resnick M, Goodman HO, Boyce WH (1968) Inheritance of calcium containing renal stones. Lancet I:537–538
Prien EL (1949) Studies in urolithiasis: II. Relationships between pathogenesis, structure and composition of calculi. J Urol 61:821–836
Prien EL (1955) Studies in urolithiasis. III. Physicochemical principles in stone formation and prevention. J Urol 73:627–652
Prien EL (1963) Crystallographic analysis of urinary calculi: A 23-year survey study. J Urol 89:917–924
Prien EL (1975) The riddle of Randall's plaques. J Urol 11:500–507
Prien EL, Frondel C (1947) Studies in urolithiasis. I. The composition of urinary calculi. J Urol 57:949–991
Prien EL, Prien EL (1968) Composition and structure of urinary stone. Am J Med 45:654–672
Prout W (1821) An inquiry into the nature and treatment of gravel, calculus and other diseases connected with a deranged operation of the urinary organs. Baldwin, Cradock and Joy, London
Pulvertaft RG (1939) Nephrolithiasis occurring in recumbency. J Bone Joint Surg 21:559–575
Puri P, Guiney EJ, O'Donnell B (1975) Urolithiasis in Irish children. J Irish Med Assoc 68:192
Purnell DC, Smith LH, Scholz DA, Elveback LR, Arnaud CR (1971) Primary hyperparathyroidism: a prospective clinical study. Am J Med 50:670–678
Pylypchuk G, Ehrig U, Wilson DR (1979) Idiopathic calcium nephrolithiasis. 1. Differences in urine crystalloids, urine saturation with brushite and urine inhibitors of calcification between persons with and persons without recurrent kidney stone formation. Can Med Assoc J 17:658–665
Pyrah LN (1979) Renal calculus. Springer, Berlin Heidelberg New York
Pyrah LN, Fowweather FS (1938) Urinary calculi developing in recumbent patients. Br J Surg 26:98–112
Pyrah LN, Hodgkinson A (1960) Nephrocalcinosis. Br J Urol 32:361–373
Pyrah LN, Hodgkinson A, Anderson CK (1966) Primary hyperparathyroidism. Br J Surg 53:245–316
Raaflaub J (1962) Zur photometrischen Bestimmung des ionisierten calciums in biologischen Flüssigkeiten, insbesondere im Harn. Z Physiol Chem 328:198–203
Raaflaub J (1963) Komplexchemische Grundlagen der Harnsteingenese. Helv Med Acta 30:724–755
Randall A (1937) Origin and growth of renal calculi. Ann Surg 105:1009–1027
Randall A (1940) Papillary pathology as a precursor of primary renal calculus. J Urol 44:580–589
Randall RE (1967) Familial renal tubular acidosis revisited. Ann Intern Med 66:1024–1025
Randolph AD, Drach GW (1981a) Some measurements of calcium oxalate nucleation and growth rates in urine-like liquors. J Crystal Growth 53:195–201
Randolph AD, Drach GW (1981b) A proposal of standardized nomenclature in the study of crystallization in biological systems eg urolithiasis. In: Smith LH, Robertson WG, Finlayson B (eds) Urolithiasis – clinical and basic research. Plenum, New York, p 383–390
Randolph AD, Larson MA (1971) Theory of particulate processes. Academic Press, New York
Randolph AD, Kraljevich ZI, Drach GW (1981) Effect of urinary macromolecules on calcium oxalate dihydrate crystal growth and nucleation rates. In: Smith LH, Robertson WG, Finlayson B (eds) Urolithiasis – clinical and basic research. Plenum, New York p 427–436

Rao MVR, Agarwal JS, Taneja OP (1978) Studies in urolithiasis III. Electron optical investigation on the morphology of the colloidal matrix of urinary calculi. Invest Urol 15:452–455

Rao PN, Gordon C, Davies D, Blacklock NJ (1982) Are stone-formers maladapted to refined carbohydrates? Br J Urol 54:575–577

Rapoport A, Crassweller PO, Husdan H, From GLA, Zweig M, Johnson MD (1967) The renal excretion of hydrogen ion in uric acid stone formers. Metabolism 16:176–188

Rector FC, Seldin DW, Roberts AD, Smith JS (1960) The role of plasma CO_2 tension and carbonic anhydrase activity in the renal reabsorption of bicarbonate. J Clin Invest 39:1706–1721

Rector FC, Bloomer HA, Seldin DW (1964) Effect of potassium deficiency on the reabsorption of bicarbonate in the proximal convolution of the rat kidney. J Clin Invest 43:1976–1982

Relman AS, Estein B, Schwartz WB (1953) Regulation of renal bicarbonate reabsorption by plasma carbon dioxide tension. J Clin Invest 32:972–978

Resnick MI, Boyce WH (1978) Spherical calcium bodies in stone-forming urine. Invest Urol 15:449–451

Resnick MI, Boyce WH (1979a) Aetiological theories of renal lithiasis – a historical review. In: Wickham JEA (ed) Urinary calculous disease. Churchill Livingstone, Edinburgh, p 1–20

Resnick MI, Boyce WH (1979b) Low molecular weight urinary proteins and renal lithiasis. Invest Urol 16:270–273

Resnick MI, Oliver J, Drach GW (1978) Intranephronic calculosis in the squirrel monkey. Invest Urol 15:295–298

Resnick MI, Gammon CW, Sorrell MB, Boyce WH (1980) Calcium-binding proteins and renal lithiasis. Surgery 88:239–243

Resnick MI, Sorrell ME, Bailey JA, Boyce WH (1982) Inhibitory effects of urinary calcium-binding substances on calcium oxalate crystallization. J Urol 127:568–571

Reynolds JJ (1972) Skeletal tissue in culture. In: Bourne GH (ed) The biochemistry and physiology of bone. 2nd edition. Academic Press, New York, p 69–126

Richardson KE, Tolbert NE (1961) Oxidation of glyoxylic acid to oxalic acid by glyoxylic acid oxidase. J Biol Chem 236:1280–1284

Rieselbach RE, Sorensen LB, Shelp WD, Steele TH (1970) Diminished renal urate secretion per nephron as a basis for primary gout. Ann Intern Med 73:359 366

Robertson WG (1969a) Measurement of ionized calcium in biological fluids. Clin Chim Acta 24:149–157

Robertson WG (1969b) A method for measuring calcium crystalluria. Clin Chim Acta 26:105–110

Robertson WG (1969c) Physicochemical aspects of renal stone-formation. Ph.D. Thesis, University of Leeds

Robertson WG (1973) Factors affecting the precipitation of calcium phosphate in vitro. Calcif Tissue Res 11:311–322

Robertson WG (1976a) Urinary excretion. In: Nordin BEC (ed) Calcium, phosphate and magnesium metabolism. Churchill Livingstone, Edinburgh p 113–161

Robertson WG (1976b) Physical chemical aspects of calcium stone-formation in the urinary tract. In: Fleisch H, Robertson WG, Smith LH, Vahlensieck W (eds) Urolithiasis research. Plenum, New York, p 25–39

Robertson WG (1982) The solubility concept. In: Nancollas GH (ed) Biological mineralization and demineralization. Springer-Verlag, Berlin Heidelberg New York, p 5–21

Robertson WG (1985) Ionic and macromolecular modifiers of crystallization of calcium salts in urine. Fortschr Urol Nephrol (in press)

Robertson WG, Fleisch H (1970) The effect of imidodiphosphate (P-N-P) on the precipitation and dissolution of calcium phosphate in vitro. Biochim Biophys Acta 222:677–680

Robertson WG, Morgan DB (1972) The distribution of urinary calcium excretions in normal persons and stone-formers. Clin Chim Acta 37:503–508

Robertson WG, Nordin BEC (1969) Activity products in urine. In: Hodgkinson A, Nordin BEC (eds) – Proceedings of the renal stone research symposium. Churchill, London, p 221–232

Robertson WG, Nordin BEC (1976) Physico-chemical factors governing stone-formation. In: Williams DI, Chisholm GD (eds) Scientific foundations of urology, vol 1. Heinemann, London, p 254–267
Robertson WG, Peacock M (1972) Calcium oxalate crystalluria and inhibitors of crystallization in recurrent renal stone-formers. Clin Sci 43:499–506
Robertson WG,Peacock M (1980) The cause of idiopathic calcium stone disease: hypercalciuria or hyperoxaluria? Nephron 26:105–110
Robertson WG, Peacock M (1981) Risk factors in the formation of urinary stones. In: Williams DI, Chisholm GD (eds) Scientific foundations of urology, 2nd edition. Heinemann, London, p 267–278
Robertson WG, Peacock M (1982) The pattern of urinary stone disease in Leeds and in the United Kingdom in relation to animal protein intake during the period 1960–1980. Urol Int 37:394–399
Robertson WG, Rutherford A (1980) Aspects of the analysis of oxalate in urine – a review. Scand J Urol Nephrol [Suppl] 53:85–93
Robertson WG, Peacock M, Nordin BEC (1968) Activity products in stone-forming and non-stone-forming urine. Clin Sci 32:579–594
Robertson WG, Peacock M, Nordin BEC (1969) Calcium crystalluria in recurrent renal stone-formers. Lancet II:21–24
Robertson WG, Peacock M, Nordin BEC (1971) Calcium oxalate crystalluria and urine saturation in recurrent renal stone-formers. Clin Sci 40:365–374
Robertson WG, Peacock M, Nordin BEC (1972a) Measurement of activity products in urine from stone-formers and normal subjects. In: Finlayson B, Hench LL, Smith LH (eds) Urolithiasis – physical aspects. National Academy of Sciences, Washington, p 79–95
Robertson WG, Peacock M, Nordin BEC (1972b) Crystalluria. In: Finlayson B, Hench LL, Smith LH (eds) Urolithiasis – physical aspects. National Academy of Sciences, Washington, p 243–254
Robertson WG, Peacock M, Knowles F (1973a) Calcium oxalate crystalluria and inhibitors of crystallisation in recurrent renal stone-formers. In: Cifuentes Delatte L, Rapado A, Hodgkinson A (eds) Urinary calculi. Karger, Basel, p 302–306
Robertson WG, Peacock M, Nordin BEC (1973b) Inhibitors of the growth and aggregation of calcium oxalate crystals in vitro. Clin Chim Acta 43:31–37
Robertson WG, Peacock M, Marshall RW, Knowles F (1974) The effect of ethane-1-hydroxy-1,1-diphosphonate (EHDP) on calcium oxalate crystalluria in recurrent renal stone-formers. Clin Sci Molec Med 47:13–22
Robertson WG, Knowles F, Peacock M (1976a) Urinary acid mucopolysaccharide inhibitors of calcium oxalate crystallization. In: Fleisch H, Robertson WG, Smith H, Vahlensieck W (eds) Urolithiasis research. Plenum, New York, p 331–334
Robertson WG, Marshall RW, Peacock M, Knowles F (1976b) The saturation of urine in recurrent, idiopathic calcium stone-formers. In: Fleisch H, Robertson WG, Smith LH, Vahlensieck W (eds) Urolithiasis research. Plenum, New York, p 335–338
Robertson WG, Peacock M, Marshall RW, Marshall DH, Nordin BEC (1976c) Saturation-inhibitor index as a measure of the risk of calcium oxalate stone formation in the urinary tract. N Engl J Med 294:249–252
Robertson WG,, Peacock M, Marshall RW, Varnavides CK, Heyburn PJ, Nordin BEC (1976d) Effect of orthophosphate on calcium crystalluria in stone formers. In: Fleisch H, Robertson WG, Smith LH, Vahlensieck W (eds) Urolithiasis research. Plenum New York, p 339–342
Robertson WG, Hodgkinson A, Marshall DH (1977) Seasonal variations in the composition of urine from normal subjects: a longitudinal study. Clin Chim Acta 80:347–353
Robertson WG, Peacock M, Heyburn PJ, Marshall DH, Clark PB (1978) Risk factors in calcium stone disease of the urinary tract. Br J Urol 50:449–454
Robertson WG, Heyburn PJ, Peacock M, Hanes FA, Swaminathan R (1979a) The effect of high animal protein intake on the risk of calcium stone-formation in the urinary tract. Clin Sci 57:285–288
Robertson WG, Peacock M, Heyburn PJ, Hanes FA, Rutherford A, Clementson E, Swaminathan R, Clark PB (1979b) Should recurrent calcium oxalate stone-formers become vegetarians? Br J Urol 51:427–431

Robertson WG, Peacock M, Hodgkinson A (1979c) Dietary changes and the incidence of urinary calculi in the UK between 1958 and 1976. J Chronic Dis 32:469–476

Robertson WG, Peacock M, Heyburn PJ, Hanes FA (1980a) Epidemiological risk factors in calcium stone disease. Scand J Urol Nephrol [Suppl] 53:15–28

Robertson WG, Peacock M, Marshall RW (1980b) Treatment of calcium stone disease with diphosphonate (ethane-1-hydroxy-1,1-diphosphonate). In: Canniggia A (ed) Etidronate. Gentili, Pisa, p 147–165

Robertson WG, Peacock M, Heyburn PJ, Bambach CP (1981a) Risk factors in calcium stone disease. In: Brockis JG, Finlayson B (eds) Urinary calculus. PSG Publishing Co., Littleton, Mass, p 265–273

Robertson WG, Peacock M, Heyburn PJ, Hanes FA, Swaminathan R (1981b) The risk of calcium stone formation in relation to affluence and dietary animal protein. In: Brockis JG, Finlayson B (eds) Urinary calculus. PSG Publishing Co., Littleton, Mass, p 3–12

Robertson WG, Peacock M, Quimet D, Heyburn PJ, Rutherford A (1981c) The main risk factor for calcium stone disease in man: hypercalciuria or mild hyperoxaluria? In: Smith LH, Robertson WG, Finlayson B (eds) Urolithiasis – clinical and basic research. Plenum, New York, p 3–12

Robertson WG, Scurr DS, Bridge CM (1981d) Factors influencing the crystallisation of calcium oxalate in urine-critique. J Crystal Growth 53:182–194

Robertson WG, Peacock M, Baker M, Marshall DH, Pearlman B, Speed R, Sergeant V, Smith A (1983) Studies on the prevalence and epidemiology of urinary stone disease in men in Leeds. Br J Urol 55:595–598

Robertson WG, Latif AB, Scurr DS, Caswell AM, Drach GW, Randolph AD (1984) Inhibitors of calcium oxalate crystallization in urine from stone-formers and normals. In: Ryall R, Brockis JG, Marshall V, Finlayson B (eds) Urinary stone, Churchill Livingstone, Melbourne, p 167–172

Robson EB, Rose GA (1957) The effect of intravenous lysine on the renal clearances of cystine, arginine and ornithine in normal subjects, in patients with cystinuria and Fanconi syndrome and their relatives. Clin Sci 16:75–93

Rodgers A, Garside J (1981) The effect of some urinary constituents on the in vitro nucleation and growth kinetics of calcium oxalate. In: Smith LH, Robertson WG, Finlayson B (eds) Urolithiasis – clinical and basic research. Plenum, New York, p 641–650

Rollins R, Finlayson B (1973) Mechanism of prevention of calcium oxalate incrustation by methylene blue and demonstration of the concentration dependence of its action. J Urol 110:459–463

Rose GA, Sulaiman S (1982) Tamm-Horsfall mucoproteins promote calcium oxalate crystal formation in urine: quantitative studies. J Urol 127:177–179

Rose GA, Robertson WG, Watts RWE (eds) (1979) Oxalate in human biochemistry and clinical pathology. Wellcome Foundation, London

Rose MB (1975) Renal stone formation. The inhibitory effect of urine on calcium oxalate precipitation. Invest Urol 12:428–433

Rose MB, Follows OJ (1977) Partial nephrectomy for stone disease. Br J Urol 49:605–610

Rose WC, Wixom RL (1955) The amino acid requirements of man. XIII. The sparing effect of cystine on the methionine requirement. J Biol Chem 216:763–773

Rosenberg LE, Scriver CR (1974) Disorders of amino acid metabolism. In: Bondy PK, Rosenberg LE (eds) Duncan's diseases of metabolism: genetics and metabolism. Saunders, Philadelphia, p 465–653

Rosenberg LE, Durant JL, Holland JM (1965) Intestinal absorption and renal extraction of cystine and cysteine in cystinuria. N Engl J Med 273:1239–1245

Rosenberg LE, Downing S, Durant JL, Segal S (1966a) Cystinuria: biochemical evidence for three genetically distinct diseases. J Clin Invest 45:365–371

Rosenberg LE, Durant JL, Albrecht I (1966b) Genetic heterogeneity in cystinuria: evidence for allelism. Trans Assoc Am Physicians 79:284–296

Rosenow EC (1940) Renal calculi: a study of papillary calcification. J Urol 44:19–28

Ross EJ, Marshall-Jones P, Friedman M (1966) Cushing's syndrome; diagnostic criteria. Q J Med 35:149–192

Rudman D, Dedonis JL, Fountain MT, Chandler JB, Gerron GG, Fleming GA, Kutner MH (1980) Hypocitraturia in patients with gastrointestinal malabsorption. N Engl J Med 303:657–661
Rudman D, Kutner MH, Redd SC, Waters WC, Gerron GG, Bleier J (1982) Hypocitraturia in calcium nephrolithiasis. J Clin Endocrinol Metab 55:1052–1057
Rumpf H, Schubert H (1977) Adhesion forces in agglomeration processes. In: Onada G, Hench L (eds) Sciences of ceramic processing before firing. Wiley, New York, p 357–376
Russell RGG (1965) Excretion of inorganic pyrophosphate in hypophosphatasia. Lancet II:461–464
Russell RGG, Fleisch H (1969) Pyrophosphate and stone formation. In: Hodgkinson A, Nordin BEC (eds) Proceedings of the renal stone research symposium. Churchill, London, p 165–180
Russell RGG, Hodgkinson A (1966) Urinary excretion of inorganic pyrophosphate by normal subjects and patients with renal calculus. Clin Sci 31:51–62
Russell RGG, Edwards NA, Hodgkinson A (1964) Urinary pyrophosphate and urolithiasis. Lancet I:1446
Russell RGG, Bisaz S, Fleisch H (1976) The influence of orthophosphate on the renal handling of inorganic pyrophosphate in man and dog. Clin Sci Molec Med 51:435–443
Russell RGG, Bisaz S, Donath A, Morgan DB, Fleisch H (1971) Inorganic pyrophosphate in plasma in normal persons and in patients with hypophosphatasia osteogenesis imperfecta and other disorders of bone. J Clin Invest 50:961–969
Ryall RL, Marshall VR (1983) The value of the 24-hour urine analysis in the assessment of stone-formers attending a general hospital outpatient clinic. Br J Urol 55:1–5
Ryall RL, Bagley CJ, Marshall VR (1981 a) Independent assessment of the growth and aggregation of calcium oxalate crystals using the Coulter Counter. Invest Urol 18:401–405
Ryall RL, Harnett RM, Marshall VR (1981 b) The effect of urine, pyrophosphate, citrate, magnesium and glycosaminoglycans on the growth and aggregation of calcium oxalate crystals in vitro. Clin Chim Acta 112:349–356
Ryall RL, Ryall RG, Marshall VR (1981 c) Interpretation of particle growth and aggregation patterns obtained from the Coulter Counter: a simple theoretical model. Invest Urol 18:396–400
Sakhaee K, Nicar M, Hill K, Pak CYC (1983) Contrasting effects of potassium citrate and sodium citrate therapies on urine chemistries and crystallization of stone-forming salts. Kidney Int 24:348–352
Sallis JD, Lumley MF (1979) On the possible role of glycosaminoglycans as natural inhibitors of calcium oxalate stones. Invest Urol 16:296–299
Samuell CT (1979) Uromucoid excretion in normal subjects, calcium stone-formers and in patients with chronic renal failure. Urol Res 7:5–12
Sarig S, Raphael M, Ron A (1973) Calcium oxalate crystallization from inhibited solutions. Isr J Chem 11:635–643
Sawaki S, Hattori N, Morikawa N, Yamada K (1967) Oxidation and reduction of glyoxylate by lactate dehydrogenase. J Vitaminol 13:93–97
Schade H (1928) Concretions. In: Alexander J (ed) Colloid chemistry, vol 2. Chemical Catalog Co., New York, p 803–844
Scheele KW (1776) Examen chemicum calculi urinarii. Opuscula 2:73–90
Schmidt KH, Hagmaier V, Hornig DH, Vuilleumier J-P, Rutishauser G (1981) Urinary oxalate excretion after large intakes of ascorbic acid in man. Am J Clin Nutr 34:305–311
Schneider H-J, Hienzsch E (1979) Epidemiologie der Urolithiasis. In: Proceedings of XVIII congress of the international society of urology, vol 1. Joly, Paris, p 87–112
Schneider JA, Schulman JD, Seegmiller JE (1978) Cystinosis and the Fanconi syndrome. In: Stanbury JB, Wyngaarden JB, Fredrickson DS (eds) Metabolic basis of inherited diseases, McGraw-Hill, New York, p 1660–1682
Schoen EJ (1959) Lowe's syndrome: abnormalities in renal tubular function in combination with other congenital defects. Am J Med 27:781–792
Scholz DA, Keating FR (1955) Milk-alkali syndrome. Arch Intern Med 95:460–468
Scholz DA, Keating FR (1956) Renal insufficiency, renal calculi and nephrocalcinosis in sarcoidosis. Am J Med 21:75–84

Scholz DA, Sprague RG, Kernohan JW (1957) Cardiovascular and renal complication of Cushing's syndrome. N Engl J Med 256:833–837
Schreiner GE, Smith LH, Kyle LH (1953) Renal hyperchloremic acidosis. Am J Med 15:122–129
Schrier EE, Lee KE, Rubin JL, Werness PG, Smith LH (1979) Macromolecular inhibitors of calcium oxalate crystal growth and aggregation in urine. In: Rose GA, Robertson WG, Watts RWE (eds) Oxalate in human biochemistry and clinical pathology. Wellcome Foundation, London, p 22–27
Schrier EE, Rubin JL, Lee KE, Werness PG, Smith LH (1981) Characterization of the calcium oxalate crystal growth inhibitors in human urine. In: Smith LH, Robertson WG, Finlayson B (eds) Urolithiasis – clinical and basic research. Plenum, New York, p 579–588
Schroeder HA, Mason AP, Tipton IH (1969) Essential metals in man – magnesium. J Chronic Dis 21:815–841
Schulz E, Schneider H-J (1981) A new view of stone-formation under the aspect of flow dynamics. In: Smith LH, Robertson WG, Finlayson B (eds) Urolithiasis – clinical and basic research. Plenum, New York, p 533–537
Schwartz A (1967) The nucleation of calcium phosphate by organic matrices. M.Sc Thesis, Case Institute of Technology
Schwille PO, Scholz D, Paulus M, Engelhardt W, Sigel A (1979) Citrate in daily and fasting urine. Invest Urol 16:457–462
Scott JT, Holloway VP, Glass HT, Arnot RN (1969) Studies of uric acid pool size and turnover rate. Ann Rheum Dis 28:366–373
Scott R, Mathieson A, McLelland A (1980) The reduction in stone recurrence and oxalate excretion by allopurinol. In: Rose GA, Robertson WG, Watts RWE (eds) Oxalate in human biochemistry and clinical pathology. Wellcome Foundation, London, p 191–197
Scurr DS, Robertson WG (1985) Studies on the mode of action of polyanionic inhibitors of calcium oxalate crystallization in urine. In: Schwille PO, Smith LH, Robertson WG, Vahlensieck W (eds) Urolithiasis and related clinical research. Plenum, New York, p 835–838
Scurr DS, Bridge CM, Robertson WG (1981) Studies on inhibitors and promoters of the crystallization of calcium oxalate in urine and in matrix from calcium oxalate stones. In: Smith LH, Robertson WG, Finlayson B (eds) Urolithiasis – clinical and basic research. Plenum, New York, p 601–605
Segal S, Schwartzman L, Blair A, Bertoli D (1967) Dibasic amino acid transport in rat kidney slices. Biochim Biophys Acta 135:127–135
Seldin DW, Wilson JD (1978) Renal tubular acidosis. In: Stanbury JB, Wyngaarden JB, Fredrickson DS (eds) The metabolic basis of inherited disease. McGraw-Hill, New York, p 1618–1633
Selleck BA, Cohen JJ (1965) Specific localization of γ-ketoglutarate uptake to the dog kidney and liver in vitro. Am J Physiol 208:24–37
Seneca H, Lattimer J, Peer P (1964) The relationship among normal intestinal flora, kidney infections and kidney stones. J Urol 92:603–613
Sengbusch R, Timmermann A (1957) Das kristalline Calciumoxalat im menschlichen Harn und seine Beziehung zur Oxalatstein-Bildung. Urol Int 4:76–95
Shattock SG (1905) A prehistoric or predynastic Egyptian calculus. Trans Pathol Soc (London) 61:275–290
Shaw DG, Sutor DJ (1972) Cystine stone dissolution. Br J Radiol 45:664–666
Sheehan ME, Nancollas GH (1980) Calcium oxalate crystal growth. A new constant composition method for modelling urinary stone formation. Invest Urol 17:446–450
Sheinfeld J, Finlayson B, Reid F (1978) Ultrafiltration evidence of ion binding by macromolecules in urine. Invest Urol 15:462–464
Shen FH, Baylink DJ, Nielson RL, Sherrard D, Ivey JL, Haussler MR (1977) Increased serum 1,25-dihydroxyvitamin D in idiopathic hypercalciuria. J Lab Clin Med 90:955–962
Shepard TH, Lee LW, Krebs EG (1960) Primary hyperoxaluria II. Genetic studies in a family. Pediatrics 25:869–871
Shils ME (1964) Experimental human magnesium depletion. I. Clinical observations and blood chemistry alterations. Am J Clin Nutr 15:133–143
Shirley R (1966) Uric acid dihydrate: crystallography and identification. Science 152:1512–1513

Shortland JR, Crane WAL (1969) Histology and ultrastructure of renal biopsies in Cushing's syndrome. J Pathol 98:209

Sierakowski R, Finlayson B, Landes RR, Finlayson CD, Sierakowski N (1978) The frequency of urolithiasis in hospital discharge diagnosis in the United States. Invest Urol 15:438–441

Silbernagl S (1976) Renal handling of amino acids: Recent results of tubular microperfusion. Clin Nephrol 5:1–8

Silk DB, Perrett D, Stephens AD, Clark ML, Scowen EF (1974) Intestinal absorption of cystine and cysteine in normal human subjects and patients with cystinuria. Clin Sci Molec Med 47:393–397

Simmonds HA, Van Acker KJ, Cameron JS, Sneddon W (1976) The identification of 2,8-dihydroxyadenine, a new component of urinary stones. Biochem J 157:485–487

Simmonds HA, Van Acker KJ, Dillon MJ, Barratt TM, Potter CF, Sahota A, Cameron JS (1981) 2,8-dihydroxyadeniuria: or when is a uric acid stone not a uric acid stone? In: Smith LH, Robertson WG, Finlayson B (eds) Urolithiasis – clinical and basic research. Plenum, New York, p 125–130

Simpson DP (1963) Effect of nephrectomy on citrate metabolism in the rat. Am J Physiol 205:1049–1052

Simpson DP (1964) Influence of plasma bicarbonate concentration and pH on citrate excretion. Am J Physiol 204:875–882

Sinno K, Boyce WH, Resnick MI (1979) Childhood urolithiasis. J Urol 121:662–664

Sisk IR, Toenhart O (1937) Factors influencing the solubility of relatively insoluble salts in urine. J Urol 37:595–603

Smales FC (1972) A computer program for calculating the activities of calcium and orthophosphate ions in biological fluids and related synthetic solutions. Calcif Tiss Res 8:304–319

Smith LH (1976) Application of physical, chemical and metabolic factors to the management of urolithiasis. In: Fleisch H, Robertson WG, Smith LH, Vahlensieck W (eds) Urolithiasis research. Plenum, New York, p 199–211

Smith LH (1980) Enteric hyperoxaluria and other hyperoxaluric states. In: Coe FL (ed) Nephrolithiasis. Churchill Livingstone, New York, p 136–164

Smith LH, Hofmann AF (1974) Acquired hyperoxaluria, urolithiasis and intestinal disease: a new digestive disorder? Gastroenterology 66:1257–1261

Smith LH, McCall JT (1969) Chemical nature of peptide inhibitors isolated from urine. In: Hodgkinson A, Nordin BEC (eds) Proceedings of the renal stone research symposium. Churchill, London, p 153–163

Smith LH, Williams HE (1967) Treatment of primary hyperoxaluria. Mod Treatment 4:522–530

Smith LH, Hofmann AF, McCall JT, Thomas PJ (1970) Secondary hyperoxaluria in patients with ileal resection and oxalate nephrolithiasis. Clin Res 18:541

Smith LH, Meyer JL, McCall JT (1973a) Chemical nature of crystal inhibitors isolated from human urine. In: Cifuentes Delatte L, Rapado A, Hodgkinson A (eds) Urinary calculi. Karger, Basel, p 318–327

Smith LH, Thomas WC, Arnaud CD (1973b) Orthophosphate therapy in calcium renal lithiasis. In: Cifuentes Delatte L, Rapado A, Hodgkinson A (eds). Urinary calculi. Karger, Basel, p 188–197

Smith LH, Werness PG, Wilson DM (1979) Enteric hyperoxaluria: associated metabolic abnormalities that promote formation of renal calculi. In: Rose GA, Robertson WG, Watts RWE (eds) Oxalate in human biochemistry and clinical pathology. Wellcome Foundation, London, p 224–230

Smith LH, Werness PG, Van Den Berg CJ, Wilson DM (1980a) Orthophosphate treatment in calcium urolithiasis. Scand J Urol Nephrol [Suppl] 53:253–259

Smith LH, Werness PG, Wilson DM (1980b) Metabolic and clinical disturbances in patients with calcium urolithiasis. Scand J Urol Nephrol [Suppl] 53:213–220

Smith MJV (1977) Placebo versus allopurinol for renal calculi. J Urol 117:690–692

Smith MJV (1978) Hydroxyurea and infected stones. Urology 11:274–277

Smith PH, Cook JB, Robertson WG (1969) Stone-formation in paraplegia. Paraplegia 7:77–85

Snaith ML, Scott JT (1971) Uric acid clearance in patients with gout and normal subjects. Ann Rheum Dis 30:285–289

Sobel AE, Hanok A (1952) Calcification; reversible inactivation of calcification in vitro and related studies. J Biol Chem 197:669–685

Solomons CC, Neuman WF (1960) On the mechanism of calcification: the remineralization of dentin. J Biol Chem 235:2502–2506

Sophasan S, Chatasingh S, Thanphaichitr P, Dhanamitta S (1980) Tamm-Horsfall mucoprotein in urine of potential bladder stone formers. J Urol 124:522–524

Spector AR, Gray A, Prien EL (1976) Kidney stone matrix. Differences in acidic protein composition. Invest Urol 13:387–389

Spector M, Garden NM, Rous SN (1978) Ultrastructure and pathogenesis of human urinary calculi. Br J Urol 50:12–15

Sperling O, De Vries A (1964) Studies on the etiology of uric acid lithiasis, Part II. Solubility of uric acid in urine specimens from normal subjects and patients with idiopathic uric acid lithiasis. J Urol 92:331–334

Sperling O, De Vries A, Kedem O (1965) Studies on the etiology of uric acid lithiasis IV. Urinary non-dialyzable substances in idiopathic uric acid lithiasis. J Urol 94:286–292

Spitzer WM, Hillkowitz P (1924) The cause of stone in the urinary tract. J Urol 11:327–336

Steele TH, Boner G (1973) Origins of the uricosuric response. J Clin Invest 52:1368–1375

Stein WH (1951) Excretion of amino acids in cystinuria. Proc Soc Exp Biol Med 78:705–708

Stewart HH (1955) Calcification and calculus formation in the upper urinary tract. Br J Urol 27:352–366

Stewart HH (1960) The surgery of the kidney in the treatment of renal stone. Br J Urol 32:392–413

Steyn J, Logie NJ (1964) Medullary sponge kidney. Br J Urol 36:482–486

Sumner JB (1926) Isolation and crystallization of enzyme urease: preliminary paper. J Biol 69:435–441

Sutor DJ (1969) Growth studies of calcium oxalate in the presence of various ions and compounds. Br J Urol 41:171–178

Sutor DJ (1972) The nature of urinary stones. In: Finlayson B, Hench LL, Smith LH (eds) Urolithiasis – physical aspects. National Academy of Sciences Washington, p 43–60

Sutor DJ (1976) Crystallographic analysis of urinary calculi. In: Williams DI, Chisholm GD (eds) Scientific foundations of urology, vol I. Heinemann, London, p 244–254

Sutor DJ, O'Flynn JD (1973) Matrix formation in crystalline material in vivo. In: Cifuentes Delatte L, Rapado A, Hodgkinson A (eds) Urinary calculi. Karger, Basel, p 280–284

Sutor DJ, Percival JM, Doonan S (1978) Isolation and identification of some urinary inhibitors of calcium phosphate formation. Clin Chim Acta 89:273–278

Sutor DJ, Percival JM, Piper KAJ (1979) Urinary inhibitors of calcium phosphate formation: the inhibitory activity of normal and artificial urines. Br J Urol 51:1–5

Sutton RAL, Watson L (1968) Urinary magnesium and renal stones. Lancet II:636

Sydenham T (1683) Tractatus de podagra et hydrope. G. Kettilby, London

Tak H-K, Cooper SM, Wilcox WR (1980a) Studies on the nucleation of monosodium urate at 37 °C. Arthritis Rheum 23:574–580

Tak H-K, Wilcox WR, Cooper SM (1980b) Crystallisation of monosodium urate and calcium urate at 37 °C. J Colloid Interface Sci 77:195–201

Takasaki E (1971) An observation on the analysis of urinary calculi by infra red spectroscopy. Calcif Tissue Res 7:232–240

Takasaki E, Shimano E (1967) The urinary excretion of oxalic acid and magnesium in oxalate urolithiasis. Invest Urol 5:302–312

Takenouchi K, Aso K, Kawase K, Ichikawa H, Shiomi T (1966) On the metabolites of ascorbic acid especially oxalic acid, eliminated in urine following the administration of large amounts of ascorbic acid. J Vitaminol 12:49–58

Talal N, Zisman E, Schur PH (1968) Renal tubular acidosis, glomerulonephritis and immunologic factors in Sjögren's syndrome. Arthritis Rheum 11:774–786

Tamm I, Horsfall F (1950) Characterization and separation of an inhibitor of viral hemagglutination present in urine. Proc Soc Exp Biol Med 74:108–114

Tashima C (1970) Hypercalcemia found by multiple test screening. JAMA 214:149
Taves DR, Neuman WF (1964) Factors controlling calcification in vitro: flouride and magnesium. Arch Biochem Biophys 108:390–397
Taylor WH (1972) Renal calculi and self-medication with multi-vitamin preparations containing vitamin D. Clin Sci 42:515–522
Teotia M, Teotia SPS (1975) Inhibitor of calcium oxalate crystallisation in urine of normal and stone formers. Indian J Med Res 63:1209–1216
Termine JD, Peckauskas RA, Posner AS (1970) Calcium phosphate formation in vitro II. Effects of environment on amorphous-crystalline transformation. Arch Biochem Biophys 140:318–325
Tew WP, Malis CD, Lehninger AL, Walker GW, Howard JE (1981) Inhibition of PTH induced nephrocalcinosis by phosphocitrate. In: Smith LH, Robertson WG, Finlayson B (eds) Urolithiasis – clinical and basic research. Plenum, New York, p 559–568
Thalut K, Rizal A, Brockis JG, Bowyer RC, Taylor TA, Wisniewski ZS (1976) The endemic bladder stones of Indonesia – epidemiology and clinical features. Br J Urol 48:617–621
Thier SO, Segal S (1978) Cystinuria. In: Stanbury JB, Wyngaarden JB, Fredrickson DS (eds) The metabolic basis of inherited disease, McGraw-Hill, New York, p 1578–1592
Thier S, Fox M, Segal S, Rosenberg LE (1964) Cystinuria. In vitro demonstration of an intestinal transport defect. Science 143:482–484
Thomas DW, Hannett B, Chambers A, Rofe AM, Edwards JB, Edwards RG (1976) Oxalate crystal formation after carbohydrate administration. Int J Vitam Nutr Res 15:181–192
Thomas J, Dechosal J, Thomas E, Rabussier H, Girad M, Aboulker P, Desgrez P (1960) Comparative study of the serum and urinary mucoproteins in renal lithiasis. J Urol Med Chir 66:679–692
Thomas J, Melon JM, Thomas E, Steg A, Desgrez P, Aboulker P (1972) Données récentes sur l'élimination urinaire de l'acide oxalique dans la lithiase rénal oxalique. Ann Urol 6:31–33
Thomas WC (1978) Use of phosphates in patients with calcereous renal calculi. Kidney Int 13:390–396
Thomas WC, Howard JE (1959) Studies on the mineralising propensity of urine from patients with and without renal calculi. Trans Assoc Am Physicians 72:181–187
Thomas WC, Bird ED, Tomita A (1963) Some concepts concerning the genesis of urinary calculi. J Urol 90:521–526
Tiselius H-G, Fornander A-M (1981) Evaluation of a routine method for determination of calcium oxalate crystal growth inhibition in diluted urine samples. Clin Chem 27:565–568
Tiselius HG, Almgård LE, Larsson L, Sörbo B (1978) A biochemical basis for grouping of patients with urolithiasis. Eur Urol 4:241–249
Tomazic BB, Nancollas GH (1979) A study of the phase transformation of calcium oxalate trihydrate-monohydrate. Invest Urol 16:329–335
Tomazic BB, Nancollas GH (1980a) Crystal growth of calcium oxalate hydrates: a comparative kinetics study. J Colloid Interface Sci 75:149–160
Tomazic BB, Nancollas GH (1980b) The kinetics of dissolution of calcium oxalate hydrates II. The dihydrate. Invest Urol 18:97–101
Tovberg Jensen A (1941) On concrements from the urinary tract III. Acta Chir Scand 85:472–486
Travis DF, Francois CJ, Bonar LC, Glimcher MJ (1967) Comparative studies of the organic matrices of invertebrate mineralised tissue. J Ultrastruct Res 18:519–550
Trump BF, Dees JH, Kim KM, Sahaphong S (1972) Some aspects of kidney structure and function; with comments on tissue calcification, calcification in the kidney. In: Finlayson B, Hench LL, Smith LH (eds) Urolithiasis – physical aspects. National Academy of Sciences, Washington, p 1–39
Vaes GM, Nichols G (1961) Metabolic studies of bone in vitro. III. Citric acid metabolism and bone mineral solubility. Effects of parathyroid hormone and estradiol. J Biol Chem 236:3323–3329
Vahlensieck W, Bastian HP (1976) Clinical features and treatment of urinary calculi in childhood. Eur Urol 2:129–134
Valyasevi A, Dhanamitta S (1974) Studies of bladder stone disease in Thailand. XVII. Effect of exogenous source of oxalate on crystalluria. Am J Clin Nutr 27:877–882

Valyasevi A, Dhanamitta S (1981) Epidemiology and pathogenesis of bladder stone disease in Thailand. In: Brockis JG, Finlayson B (eds) Urinary calculus, PSG Publishing Co., Littleton, Mass, p 185–194

Valyasevi A, Dhanamitta S, van Reen R (1973) Studies of bladder stone disease in Thailand. XVI. Effect of 4-hydroxy-L-proline and orthophosphate supplementations on urinary composition and crystalluria. Am J Clin Nutr 26:1207–1211

Valyasevi A, Halstead SB, Dhanamitta S (1967) Studies of bladder stone disease in Thailand. VI. Urinary studies in children 2–10 years old, resident in a hypo- and hyperendemic area. Am J Clin Nutr 20:1362–1368

Van den Berg CJ, Jones JD, Wilson DM, Smith LH (1980) Glutamine therapy of cystinuria. Invest Urol 18:155–157

Van Leeuwen C (1979) On the driving force for crystallization: the growth affinity. J Crystal Growth 46:91–95

Van Slyke DD, Phillips RA, Hamilton PB, Archibold RM, Futcher PH, Hillar A (1943) Glutamine as a source of urinary ammonia. J Biol Chem 150:481–482

Veis A, Perry A (1967) The phosphoprotein of the dentin matrix. Biochemistry 6:2409–2416

Vermeulen CW, Lyon ES (1968) Mechanisms of genesis and growth of calculi. Am J Med 45:684–692

Vermeulen CW, Lyon ES, Miller GH (1958) Calcium phosphate solubility in urine as measured by a precipitation test: experimental urolithiasis XIII. J Urol 79:596–606

Vermeulen CW, Lyon ES, Gill WB (1964) Artificial urinary concretions. Invest Urol 1:370–386

Vermeulen CW, Lyon ES, Fried FA (1965) On the nature of the stone-forming process. J Urol 94:176–186

Vermeulen CW, Ellis JE, Hsu T-C (1966) Experimental observations on the pathogenesis of urinary calculi. J Urol 95:681–690

Vermeulen CW, Lyon ES, Ellis JE, Borden TA (1967) The renal papilla and calculogenesis. J Urol 97:573–582

Vermooten V (1941) The incidence and significance of the deposition of calcium plaques in the renal papilla as observed in the Caucasian and Negro (Bantu) population in South Africa. J Urol 46:193–200

Vermooten V (1972) The origin and development in the renal papilla of Randall's calcium plaques. J Urol 48:27–37

Vermooten V (1956) Randall's plaques and their relationship to the etiology of urolithiasis. In: Butt AJ (ed) Etiologic factors in renal lithiasis. CC Thomas, Springfield, Illinois, p 232–237

Vishwakarma P, Miller T (1963) Renal tubular transport of citrate: relations with calcium. Am J Physiol 205:281–285

Von Hemsbach JHM (1865) Mikrogeologie, Reimer, Berlin

Wagner M, Finlayson B (1978) The characteristics of adsorption of pyrophosphate and citrate onto whewellite. Invest Urol 15:456–458

Wallace MR, Mason K, Gray J (1981) Urine oxalate and calcium in idiopathic renal stoneformers. NZ Med J 94:87–89

Walser M (1960) Determination of free magnesium ions in body fluids. Analyt Chem 32:711–717

Walser M (1961) Calcium clearance as a function of sodium clearance in the dog. Am J Physiol 200:1099–1104

Walton AG (1963) Nucleation and the interfacial tension of sparingly soluble salts. Mikrochim Acta 3:422–430

Walton AG (1967) The formation and properties of precipitates. Interscience Publications, New York

Wang CC, Robbins LL (1956) Cushing's disease: its roentgenological findings. Radiology 67:17–24

Wang JH, Tarr DA (1955) On the mechanism of urease action. J Am Chem Soc 77:6205–6206

Watanaba T (1972) Histochemical studies on mucosubstances in urinary stones. Tohoku J Exp Med 107:345–357

Watts RWE (1976) Xanthinuria and xanthine stone-formation. In: Williams DI, Chisholm GD (eds) Scientific foundations of urology, vol 1. Heinemann, London, p 310–315

Watts RWE, Engleman K, Klinenberg JR, Seegmiller JE (1964) The enzyme defect in a case of xanthinuria. Biochem J 90:4P

Weinberger A, Sperling O, Rabinovitz M, Brosh S, Adam A, De Vries A (1974) High frequency of cystinuria among Jews of Libyan origin. Hum Hered 24:568–572

Weller RO, Nester B, Cooke SAR (1972) Calcification in the human renal papilla: an electron-microscopy study. J Pathol 107:211–216

Welshman SG, McGeown MG (1972) A quantitative investigation of the effects on the growth of calcium oxalate crystals of potential inhibitors. Br J Urol 44:677–680

Welshman SG, McGeown MG (1976) Urinary citrate excretion in stone-formers and normal controls. Br J Urol 48:7–11

Werness PG, Duckworth SC, Smith LH (1979) Calcium oxalate dihydrate crystal growth. Invest Urol 17:230–233

Werness PG, Bergert JH, Smith LH (1981) Crystalluria. J Crystal Growth 53:166–181

Westbury EJ (1974) Some observations on the quantitative analysis of over 1000 urinary calculi. Br J Urol 46:215–227

White RW, Cohen RB, Vince FP, Williams G, Blandy J, Tresidder GC (1969) Minerals in the urine of stone-formers and their spouses. In: Hodgkinson A, Nordin BEC (eds) Proceedings of the renal stone research symposium. Churchill, London, p 289–296

Wickham JEA (1976) The matrix of renal calculi. In: Williams DI, Chisholm GD (eds) Scientific foundations of urology, vol 1. Heinemann, London, p 323–329

Wikström B, Wieslander J (1981) Excretion of Tamm-Horsfall urinary glycoprotein (uromucoid) in renal calcium stone-formers. In: Smith LH, Robertson WG, Finlayson B (eds) Urolithiasis – clinical and basic research. Plenum, New York, p 685–689

Wilkinson R (1976) Absorption of calcium, phosphorus and magnesium. In: Nordin BEC (ed) Calcium, phosphate and magnesium metabolism. Churchill Livingstone, London, p 36–112

Will EJ, Bijvoet OLM (1979) Primary oxalosis: clinical and biochemical response to high-dose pyridoxine therapy. Metabolism 28:542–548

Will EJ, Bijvoet OLM, Van der Linden HB (1976) Inhibition of calcium oxalate crystal growth – a simple method of measurement and preliminary results. In: Fleisch H, Robertson WG, Smith LH, Vahlensieck W (eds) Urolithiasis research. Plenum, New York, p 367–370

Will EJ, Bijvoet OLM, Blomen LJMJ, Van der Linden H (1983) Growth kinetics of calcium oxalate monohydrate I. Method and validation. J Crystal Growth 64:297–305

Williams DI (1963) Matrix calculi. Br J Urol 35:411–415

Williams G, Sallis JD (1981) The sources of phosphocitrate and its role as an inhibitor of calcium phosphate and calcium oxalate crystallization. In: Smith LH, Robertson WG, Finlayson B (eds) Urolithiasis – clinical and basic research. Plenum, New York, p 569–577

Williams GD (1926) An ancient bladder stone. J Am Med Assoc 87:941

Williams HE, Smith LH (1968a) L-glyceric aciduria: a new genetic variant of primary hyperoxaluria. N Engl J Med 278:233–239

Williams HE, Smith LH (1968b) Disorders of oxalate metabolism. Am J Med 45:715–735

Williams HE, Johnson GA, Smith LH (1971) The renal clearance of oxalate in normal subjects and patients with primary hyperoxaluria. Clin Sci 41:213–218

Williams RE (1963) Long-term survey of 538 patients with upper urinary tract stone. Br J Urol 35:416–437

Williams RE (1969) The natural history of renal lithiasis. In: Hodgkinson A, Nordin BEC (eds) Proceedings of the renal stone research symposium. Churchill, London, p 65–70

Wollaston WH (1797) On gouty and urinary concretions. Phil Trans R Soc (London) 87:386–400

Wollaston WH (1810) On cystic oxide: a new species of urinary calculus. Phil Trans R Soc (London) 100:223–230

Wright RJ, Hodgkinson A (1972) Oxalic acid, calcium and phosphorus in the renal papilla of normal and stone-forming rats. Invest Urol 9:369–375

Wrong O, Davies HEF (1959) The excretion of acid in renal disease. Q J Med 28:259–311

Wyngaarden JB (1978) Hereditary xanthinuria. In: Stanbury JB, Wyngaarden JB, Fredrickson DS (eds) The metabolic basis of inherited diseases. McGraw Hill, New York, p 1037–1044

Wyngaarden JB, Kelley WN (1976) Gout and hyperuricaemia. Grune & Stratton, New York

Yeh HL, Frankl W, Dunn MS, Parker P, Hugher B, György P (1951) The urinary excretion of amino acids by a cystinuric subject. Am J Med Sci 214:507–512

Yendt ER (1970) Renal calculi. Can Med Ass J 102:479

Yendt ER, Connor TB, Howard JE (1955) In vitro calcification of rachitic rat cartilage in normal and pathological human sera with some observations on the pathogenesis of renal rickets. Bull Johns Hopkins Hosp 96:1–19

Yendt ER, Jarzylo S, Finnis WA, Cohanim M (1981) Medullary sponge kidney (tubular ectasia) in calcium urolithiasis. In: Smith LH, Robertson WG, Finlayson B (eds) Urolithiasis – clinical and basic research. Plenum, New York, p 105–112

Yü TF, Gutman AB (1965) Effects of allopurinol [4-hydroxypyrazolo (3,4-δ) pyrimidine] on serum and urinary uric acid in primary and secondary gout. Am J Med 37:885–898

Yü TF, Gutman AB (1967) Uric acid nephrolithiasis in gout: predisposing factors. Ann Intern Med 67:1133–1148

Zarembski PM, Hodgkinson A (1962) The oxalic acid content of English diets. Br J Nutr 16:627–634

Zarembski PM, Hodgkinson A (1969) Some factors influencing the urinary excretion of oxalic acid in man. Clin Chim Acta 25:1–10

Zechner O, Latal D (1978) Die Bedeutung der Magnesiumausscheidung im Harn von Patienten mit Harnsteinen unter besonderer Berücksichtigung der Rezidivneigung der Harnsteinbildung. Urologe [Ausg A] 17:258–260

Diagnosis of Urinary Calculi

W. VAHLENSIECK

I. History

1. Pain

Pain as a clinical manifestation of urolithiasis varies considerably from case to case, depending on site, size, surface structure and mobility of the stone. A careful history of the pain may nevertheless contain valuable diagnostic clues (DE VRIES 1961; HAHN et al. 1979; PYRAH 1979; TERHORST 1980; BERGMAN 1981; MARBERGER 1983).

a) Incidence

Stone patients most commonly present with classical ureteric colic, which either may be heralded by dragging discomfort or may come on suddenly. Such case have been described as "acute urolithiasis" if mobility or onward passage of the calculus give rise to severe pain and/or if superinfection occurs (VAHLENSIECK 1969, 1970; VAHLENSIECK and BASTIAN 1973; ACKERMANN 1981).

Such exceptionally severe pain is due to the sudden arrest of a calculus on its way through the urinary tract, being caused primarily by local irritation at the site of impaction. Appositional crystals on the surface of a fast moving calculus are capable of injuring the intima or of cutting so deeply into it as to bring the stone to a halt, the pain being according. Sideways impaction of an irregularly shaped calculus deforms the ureteric wall to such an extent as to give rise to local ischemia, socalled ureteric angina, of which pain is the chief symptom. Sudden overfilling of the balloon of a ureteric balloon catheter causes similar pain of distension, thus substantiating our concept of pain physiology for impacted ureteric calculi (SOEKELAND and MAY 1969). According to MELCHIOR (1981), stripping waves arise primarily within the smooth muscle and are only modulated by autonomic efferents. Cholinergic pain-, pH- and osmoreceptor fibres in the ureteric wall give rise to axon reflexes. True autonomic reflexes involving the ureter are mediated by the sympathetic system. Epinephrine and norepinephrine act via alpha receptors to exert a chronotropic effect on the ureteric pacemaker and to recruit latent local pacemakers in the lower ureter by altering their threshold. A corresponding inhibitory negative bathmotropic influence is exerted by beta adrenoreceptors and is more pronounced in the proximal than in the distal ureter. Extreme mechanical stimuli to the ureteric wall trigger local smooth muscle spasm with impaction of the calculus and ureteric colic. Even if this is not sufficient to cause complete ureteric occlusion, local edema will soon do so, thus fixing the stone even more firmly. Of necessity there will be proximal holdup of urine flow, a constant phenomenon according to BOYARSKI and LABAY (1972), ROSS et al. (1972) and PETERS (1978). The result is a rise in pressure within the proximal ureter and in the pelvicalyceal system, causing pain and tenderness to percussion in the renal angle. The pain is thought to be mediated by sympathetic pain fibres arising in the pelvicalyceal wall and travelling in the splanchnic nerves on the one hand and by local pressure ischemia on the other (RUTISHAUSER 1970; ROSS et al. 1972).

These reflex pathways and pain mechanisms also explain the frequently observed concomitant and subsequent clinical picture of sudden perspiration, rapid thready pulse, malaise, nausea, vomitting and abdominal distension. It is these phenomena which often make it so hard for the patient to give a precise history of the site and radiation of his pain. In cases where colic as such rapidly subsides, ileus may be the dominant clinical feature and simulate a primarily intestinal pathology.

Children and pregnant women often present with an atypical clinical picture, a fact worth bearing in mind when their histories are taken.

In the series of UNGER and THIEL (1977) only 27% of children presented with ureteric colic, whilst 6.4% had loin pain and 15.5% obscure abdominal pain. In MARBERGER's (1983) study this feature is even more pronounced, with only 6% of children having obvious colic and 25% vague abdominal pain. Of his pediatric patients with established ureteric calculi 22% had had colic and 38% nonspecific abdominal pain.

In this context it is as well to remember that infants are unable to give a history, and in them the presence of pain can only be deduced from abnormal behavior patterns such as persistent continuous screaming or agitation (VAHLENSIECK and BASTIAN 1976).

According to MARBERGER (1983) 33% of adults with renal calculi had typical colic whilst 6% had obscure abdominal pain. For ureteric calculi the figures were 87% and 8% respectively.

Occasionally, a previously silent calculus becomes symptomatic during pregnancy, presumably because the ureteric ectasia of pregnancy allows some movement. Such an event occurred 12 times (0.65%) in our own group of 1844 stone patients (GOEDDE and VAHLENSIECK 1965). During a subsequent four year period there were 5 (2.3%) pregnant women among 222 patients (BASTIAN and VAHLENSIECK 1976). Widely varying figures are given in the literature for the incidence of urolithiasis complicating pregnancy. McVANN (1964) quotes 0.03%, SOLOMON (1954) 0.04%. One series of 21,439 deliveries (KLEMPERER and OPPENHEIMER 1960) contains 10 cases (0.05%) of urinary calculus. Other figures are 0.2% (WOJEWSKI and ZAYACZKOWSKI 1971), 0.25% (PAPALOUCAS et al. 1970), 0.3% (HARRIS and DUNNIHOO 1967), 0.4% (CRABTREE 1942) and 0.8% (LATAL 1975).

During the first trimester urolithiasis is likely to present in the usual fashion, whilst an atypical picture is the rule in the second half of pregnancy.

b) Intensity and Radiation

The history may contain diagnostically important details on pain intensity and radiation pattern.

Nephrocalcinosis and fixed intrarenal stones are generally painless and are often only discovered during the investigation of an unrelated complaint or following abnormal urinalysis. The same is true of calyceal calculi and pelvicalyceal staghorns so long as they are held immobile and urine is able to flow past them unhindered. Under such circumstances stones may remain asymptomatic for extended periods and are then known as "silent" or "latent" calculi.

Patients with more mobile calyceal or intrapelvic calculi complain of dull backache (related to intimal injury) occurring particularly after prolonged physical activity and usually subsiding after a period of rest (CIBERT et al. 1972). Patients frequently connect such symptoms with spinal disorders, but any pain not definitely localized over the vertebral column or having only an inconstant relationship to movement and changes of posture should be suspected of denoting urolithiasis, especially where a previous orthopedic consultation has failed to reveal spinal pathology.

It may be equally difficult to interpret dragging pain in the renal or ureteric reference territory, sometimes radiating to the testicles or labia. Not uncommonly such pain is generated by crystals or crystal aggregates ("sand"; "gravel") causing intimal damage on their way down the urinary tract. In view of the many other possible causes, careful consideration should be given to differential diagnosis during periods of symptomatic activity. The demonstration of red blood cells and/or crystals in the urine may be of key significance, as may the presence of sterile pyuria.

Impaction of a calculus virtually always gives rise to colic. Attacks of pain may occur suddenly, but they are frequently preceded by a dull dragging ache, reaching a crescendo after 10–30 minutes and then persisting with waves of exacerbation or, alternatively, fading rapidly to disappear altogether (BRETLAND 1972; PYRAH 1979).

Pain will localize and radiate quite differently, depending on the exact site of impaction. Impaction in the neck of a calyx or in the pelviureteric junction will cause severe back or loin pain at the moment of occlusion, followed by a continuous dull ache in the same region, denoting obstruction.

Similar events follow impaction of a stone in the upper ureter, but there is usually a complaint of additional pain radiating along the course of the ureter to the groin or genitalia.

Should a calculus come to rest in the lower ureter, especially in its intramural segment, there will be urgency and frequency in addition to colic radiating to the genitalia. Such a history of pain continues to occur and remains diagnostic in early pregnancy. During the last four weeks before term symptoms may simulate uterine contractions (GOEDDE and VAHLENSIECK 1965; KREMLING 1977). Generally, however, the symptomatology of incipient or reactivated urolithiasis tends to become so vague during the second half of pregnancy that pyelonephritis of pregnancy is often wrongly diagnosed. The clinical picture is often compatible with appendicitis, pelvic inflammatory disease, tubal ectopic pregnancy and threatened abortion (RUMMEL and WALCH 1963; VAINBERG and GIMPELSON 1973; KREMLING 1977; KUNTZ and SCHUETZ 1982).

A further typical set of symptoms belongs to calculi that have entered the bladder but are prevented from escaping during micturition, e.g. by a vesical outflow obstruction. The symptoms are enhanced if further appositional growth occurs in the bladder or if the calculus has an irregular surface. The consequence is bladder pain, especially during violent movement, and pronounced frequency with urgency or even strangury. Pain may radiate into the distal urethra or glans.

Urethral passage of a calculus is accompanied by similar symptoms. Again, local impaction may occur, with more marked localization of pain and often retention of urine.

2. Changes in the Urine

a) Color

A careful inquiry about changes in urine color often yields valuable diagnostic or differential diagnostic information.

Although sequential urine testing reveals microscopic hematuria in virtually every stone patient, more extensive hemorrhage is generally required to darken the urine. Not infrequently patients will report dragging discomfort in the loin accompanied by passage of abnormally dark urine following vigorous exercise. Such a story suggests the temporary dislodgement of a renal pelvic or calyceal stone. The epithelium is lacerated and hematuria ensues.

Patients who report urine fluctuating between dark and pale frequently turn out to have a widely varying or generally inadequate fluid intake. The dark color of their urine is then merely the result of its high concentration, a conclusion further substantiated by the observation that their urine tends to have a penetrating odor.

A correctly taken history should be able to exclude hepatic pathology with urinary overspill of bile pigments as the cause of urine discoloration.

Dark brown urine also raises the possibility of hemoglobinuria or myoglobinuria, easily recognized in the presence of acute hemolysis or muscle damage. A detailed history will distinguish between the rarer forms such as paroxysmal nocturnal, cold and march hemoglobinuria.

The same is true of exogenous urine discoloration simulating hematuria. Intake of beetroot and drugs such as antipyrin, pyrazolones or pyridium should be inquired about.

Patients also occasionally report the settling out of brick red sediment if previously clear urine is allowed to stand after collection. This is a highly significant observation, since increased uric acid excretion is the cause of this brick dust sediment, amorphous uric acid tending to precipitate at pH below 5.5.

In the presence of colic with micro- or macroscopic hematuria, hemorrhagic diatheses and anticoagulant therapy assume special importance. Even though the patient may not have noticed hematuria, microscopic hematuria may suffice for the formation of coagula within the pelvicalyceal system. The passage of these clots is at times accompanied by colic simulating urolithiasis.

Long term cytotoxic administration can have similar effects. Firstly there may be a prerenal coagulation defect and secondly certain agents have a direct toxic action on the urothelium resulting in bleeding within the tract.

Bright blood in the urine usually results in an immediate presentation but is not at all typical of stone disease. Although injury to the bladder neck or urethra by a passing stone may on occasion cause initial hematuria or urethral bleeding, even the typical picture of a stone on the move or of a bladder neck calculus should not be taken at face value. Such a combination of phenomena always requires careful differential diagnosis to exclude alternative causes such as tumor in the bladder or urethra.

Macroscopic hematuria with passage of clots is quite uncommon as a manifestation of urolithiasis. In the series of MARBERGER (1983) 27% of children with kidney stones and 38% of those with ureteric calculi had macroscopic hematuria. Among adults he found macroscopic hematuria in only 12% and 18% respectively. Such hemorrhage presupposes extensive damage to the wall of the urinary tract, as is only possible when a papillary calculus is dislodged or as a result of pressure necrosis within the pelvicalyceal system due to a staghorn. In this situation painless macroscopic hematuria may be the first manifestation of a previously silent stone. Painless macroscopic hematuria may therefore also precede an episode of colic by 1 – 2 days, although the two events are more often simultaneous. In all these cases full investigation is essential since stones and tumors may coexist in the same patient.

b) Volume

There is rarely a history of a slight decrease in urine volume. Because they poorly understand the physiology of fluid retention and excretion, patients will occasionally complain of a feeling of not passing enough. As long as there is no history of dependent edema one may nevertheless assume adequate fluid excretion.

On the other hand one must take careful note of factors leading to marked dehydration, such as a chronically inadequate fluid intake or inappropriate intake of diuretics and laxatives. These habits can lead to anuria in their own right and independently of any stone problem.

Socalled reflex anuria is highly controversial and, at the very least, extremely rare. UEBELHOER (1976) suggested it could only occur where reflex effects of longstanding untreated colic cause severe damage to the contralateral kidney.

Bilateral urinary tract obstruction seems rather more likely, for example where intrarenal precipitation of uric acid leads to bilateral obstruction at the tubular level, as may occur after total starvation, during uricosuric treatment or during cytotoxic therapy without adequate fluid intake or urine alkalinization.

Acute postrenal effects arise not infrequently from a radioopaque calcific stone in one ureter and a simultaneous and easily overlooked radiolucent uric acid stone in the other.

Whenever colic is associated with acute anuria one must consider the possibility of ureteric obstruction combined with unilateral nonfunctioning or congenitally solitary kidney. Conversely the situation is easily explained where there is an unequivocal history of previous unilateral nonfunction.

Anuria is equally unproblematic where there is obvious occlusion of bladder neck or urethra, so long as the patient is able to give an appropriate typical history of pain and micturition symptoms.

Obstruction due to stone impaction may be complicated by pre-existing or iatrogenic infection. In either case suppurative pyelonephritis may result in severe toxic damage to the opposite kidney, with consequent oliguria or anuria (KARCHER 1959; RENYI-VAMOS et al. 1960; KARCHER and VAHLENSIECK 1964; HASCHEK and SCHUMANN 1971; VAHLENSIECK 1973).

c) Disorders of Micturition

Renal calculi are only complicated by micturition difficulties where these were pre-existing or if infection supervenes.

On the other hand ureteric stones commonly give rise to dysuria, particularly if they are situated in the lower third. UNGER and THIEL (1977) recorded dysuria in 4.6% of their children with urolithiasis. MARBERGER (1983) has found the same symptom in 5% of children and in 9% of adults with ureteric stones.

Bladder calculi also cause marked frequency and terminal dysuria, often with radiation to the distal urethra or glans penis. The classical story is of the urinary stream being suddenly interrupted, only to recommence spontaneously after sitting down or moving about.

Sudden cessation of micturition accompanied by intense urethral pain definitely denotes a stone lodging in the urethra.

3. Fever

It is relatively rare for stone sufferers to report attacks of high temperature. Among our own clinical material about 10% of in-patients give a history of previous treatment for inflammatory conditions of the kidneys and urinary tract. Even in cases of acute urolithiasis it is relatively unusual for patients to complain of fever and rigors accompanying their pain. On the other hand, 28% of our in-patients proved to have a urinary tract infection, the bulk of these no doubt contributed by chronic asymptomatic bacteriuria. Should the organisms involved be urease-positive there will be an alkaline urine in which true "infective calculi" are formed. The latter should be carefully distinguished from "infected calculi" which arise primarily under aseptic conditions and which are complicated by secondary urinary tract infection. In either case suitable events (hypothermia, flu-like illnesses, urinary obstruction) can trigger an exacerbation of pyelonephritis with fever and rigors. Where, however, there is no history of previous urologic disease (about 80% of all our stone patients) a history of fever, combined with pain suggestive of renal or ureteric colic, merits consideration as cholecystitis, pancreatitis, appendicitis, diverticulitis and pelvic inflammatory disease among other differential diagnoses. Pregnancy may render any distinction between the alternatives exquisitely difficult, since this condition in itself makes both pyelonephritis more likely and the clinical picture of urolithiasis less typical.

4. Predisposing Factors

a) First Attack or Recurrence

A survey carried out in collaboration with the Institute for Applied Sociology (INFAS) in Bonn – Bad Godesberg (FRG) revealed an 0.54% incidence of urolithiasis for the FRG (population 60 million) during 1979. This means that of every 100,000 persons 540 will have an episode of urolithiasis during the year (VAHLENSIECK et al. 1981, 1982). Careful epidemiologic studies are likely to reveal a similar quote for all the industrialized nations. Thus BENGTSON et al. (1980) arrived a yearly incidence of 3.7 per 1000 women in Gothenburg, Sweden.

One significant finding in our own study was the figure of 22% first attacks versus 78% recurrences. The recurrence rate is generally of the order of 40–45% (ETTINGER 1979; VAHLENSIECK et al. 1980; SCHNEIDER and BERG 1981; ZECHNER and LATAL 1981), although careful metaphylaxis is able to reduce this below 10% (YENDT 1970; VAHLENSIECK 1973, 1978, 1982; COE 1977; SCHNEIDER and BERG 1981; ZECHNER and LATAL 1981). Poor or ineffective prevention of recurrence may result in figures as high as 70% (LJUNGHALL 1978, 1985). Wherever there is a past history of a stone, suggestive symptoms should be assuned to be due to recurrence, whatever the intervening period.

In view of the steadily increasing incidence, however, the absence of a previous history does nothing to make the diagnosis less likely in anyone with appropriate symptoms. The age of the patient is of some importance, since urolithiasis is relatively uncommon in children and teenagers, who make up only 2–3% of all patients. SCHNEIDER and HIENSCH (1979) quote a urolithiasis rate of 0.5% for children. In a study of 1000 children (496 girls and 504 boys) aged 6–15 REMZI et al. (1979) recorded an incidence of 0.8% and a prevalence of 1%. Such low figures may be explained by the finding of ROBERTSON et al. (1980) that, within a normal population, the lowest probability of stone formation is to be found in children. Yet there can be no doubt that prevalence increases with age.

Analysis of prevalence figures for the FRG in 1979 showed a rise with age from 0.37% to 1.4% of the whole sample (n = 10,130). In terms of the number of individuals in each age cohort, however, the rise in prevalence was far more marked, increasing from 1.28% to 6.79%. Note that these figures are overall values for men and women and are thus somewhat lower than those given by LJUNGHALL et al. (1977), LJUNGHALL (1978) and LJUNGHALL et al. (1981), who quote a prevalence of 13.7% for men aged 49–50 (n = 2,322) and as much as 18.1% for men of 60 (n = 331).

The sex distribution in our study is also in accordance with the literature, giving an incidence ratio of 2:1 in favor of men.

The prevalence as percentage total population was more evenly distributed at 1.8% men and 2.2% women. In terms of male and female subpopulations the prevalence is also approximately equal at 4% of men (183/4620) and 4% of women (225/5510) (VAHLENSIECK et al. 1981). A limited epidemiologic study in Cumbernauld (SCOTT et al. 1981) also failed to show any difference in the prevalence for men and women. These studies may signify a changing trend, since urolithiasis would appear to be increasing more in women than in the past. The reason must lie in a shift in the way women live.

There is often a history of more frequent symptoms and of spontaneously passed stones or gravel in summertime and in autumn (ELLIOT et al. 1975; ROBERTSON et al. 1975). From analytical data on 30,000 calculi HESSE et al. (1977) demonstrated a statistically significant increase in the number of uric acid stones passed spontaneously during the summer and autumn months. They relate this phenomenon to increased uric acid production from a rise in cell turnover under the influence of sunlight. The same pattern exists for the excretion of calcium and oxalate, the values being significantly higher between May and October than between November and April, correlating with raised serum levels of 25-(OH)-D3 (ELOMAA et al. 1981).

ALKEN (1969) coined the term "summer colic" to describe episodes of pain the investigation of which frequently fails to reveal any pathology, thus presenting a diagnostic challenge. The problem may be one of extremely short periods of crystalluria. The calculus may be so small as to pass spontaneously and almost without delay or a uric acid stone may enter a silent phase, be missed on plain radiology and be completely enveloped in contrast on IVU. Unless a urine pH around 5.5 coupled to hyperuricemia gives the clue, such patients can only be advised to return at the first inkling of further symptoms. There will then at least be a chance of microscopic hematuria confirming the diagnosis.

b) Anatomic Anomalies and Coexisting Disease

The history of stone formers not uncommonly suggests the involvement of some anatomic malformation, of pre-existing renal or urinary tract disease, of environmental factors or of systemic illness acting to impair normal urodynamics and thus predisposing to stone formation.

The commonest cause of dystrophic *nephrocalcinosis*, i.e. of calcification of damaged tubular tissue in the absence of hypercalcemia, is chronic pyelonephritis, more rarely chronic glomerulonephritis or poisoning (ZOLLINGER 1966).

Our own observations suggest that profound hypotension may also lead to tubular degeneration or necrosis with stone formation. In many cases careful questioning will reveal a history of severe hypotension preceding the first stone episode, and of a subsequent rise in blood pressure to normal or elevated values (VAHLENSIECK 1979, 1982). The initial event must be decreased papillary perfusion. Tissue degeneration is then followed by calcific incrustation and results in a typical papillary calculus, hanging like a stalactite into the calyx. No doubt a similar process operates in diabetes mellitus and hypertension, via an atherosclerotic pathways in both cases. These latter factors are therefore important aspects of the history.

At least equal significance attaches to a history of systemic disease liable to result in predisposing change in kidneys or urine composition. Hypercalcemia – be it due to increased absorption from the gut (hyperparathyroidism, sarcoidosis) or to increased bone resorption (hyperparathyroidism, osteoporosis with Paget's disease, trauma and spinal injury, Cushing's disease, thyrotoxicosis, postmenopausal osteoporosis, myelomatosis and bone secondaries) – may in turn result in hypercalciuria and metastatic nephrocalcinosis. The same situation may arise in the hyperoxalemia and hyperoxaluria of primary oxalosis. It is as yet unknown whether the tissue lesion is primary or results from an excessive renal calcium or oxalate load. In any event, microdeposits of calcium oxalate or apatite are formed in specific segments of the tubule, depending on the exact etiology. "In a few cases the interstitial space is also calcified and so, rarely, is the vasculature. It is extremely uncommon for the glomeruli to contain any precipitate." (ZOLLINGER 1966).

Careful note must also be taken of any history of *intestinal disease* or of disease affecting intestinal function. Chief among these are chronic constipation, recurrent diarrheal illnesses, Crohn's disease, ulcerative colitis, sprue and saccharose – isomaltose intolerance. Rarer conditions include diabetic enteropathy, cirrhosis, pancreatitis and radiation enteritis. Such surgical procedures as choledochojejunostomy, ileostomy, extensive small bowel resection, jejunoileal bypass or conditions such as the blind loop syndrome may have similar effects. Malabsorption of bile acids and fatty acids will, depending on degree, result in hyperoxaluria. Water, sodium and potassium malabsorption will further so alter urine composition as to increase the risk of uric acid stone formation. Bicarbonate malabsorption tends to acidify the urine and decrease citrate excretion. Citrate is, however, not the only crystallization inhibitor to be excreted in reduced amounts, since reduced protein absorption will also reduce the excretion of magnesium and pyrophosphate (ANDERSSON 1979; BICHLER et al. 1979; FUSS et al. 1979; SCHOLZ et al. 1979; SMITH et al. 1979; BACKMANN et al. 1985; DOBBINS 1985).

Attempts should be made to detect a family history of urolithiasis in combination with hyperuricemia or gout. According to the 1980 report of the German Society for Nutrition, hyperuricemia may be considered to occur in 5–9% of the population. The chief cause seems to be overweight due to overeating, a significant point, since the Society's report also identified overweight in 30–50% of the population. A family history of gout and overweight therefore suggests either an inherited defect of renal uric acid excretion in the presence of liberal purine intake or a congenital enzyme defect leading to increased uric acid formation (ZOELLNER 1980). On the other hand the incidence quoted for nephrolithiasis in the presence of gout varies widely (GOEBEL 1980; HARTUNG 1981). YŰ (1978) related it unequivocally to the quantity of uric acid excreted, finding nephrolithiasis in 24% of patients with a daily excretion of 400 mg and in 49% of those excreting 1000 – 1600 mg uric acid per day. Note, however, that patients with gout are prone not only to uric acid but also to calcium oxalate calculi. GUTMANN and YŰ (1968) found 12% of their gouty stone formers to have calcium oxalate stones, the mechanism probably being uric acid blockade of inhibitor substances normally preventing calcium oxalate precipitation (ROBERTSON et al. 1976) or uric acid functioning as nucleator.

The possibility must also be kept in mind of secondary hyperuricemia resulting from increased uric acid formation. The purine is endogenous, arising from *raised cell turnover* in conditions such as polycythemia rubra vera, myelofibrosis with myeloid metaplasia, acute leukemias and chronic myeloid leukemia, as well as during remissions of certain anemias, especially pernicious anemia and the hemolytic group. A similar situation arises during periods of tumor tissue breakdown, usually in the wake of chemotherapy or irradiation (ZOELLNER 1980).

Lack of exercise and *bedrest* may induce a catabolic state involving urine alkalinization and, in severe cases, increased skeletal turnover leading to hypercalciuria. FUSS et al. (1979) found a significant history of bedrest in over 20% of their patients.

Inquiry must also be made into the patient's occupation. FUSS et al. (1979) found 3.6% of their patients to have an occupational exposure to *dehydration*, usually resulting from extremes of heat and low relative humidity, but not infrequently involving lack of drinking facilities.

Patients who take sauna baths may lose considerable amounts of fluid and must be asked what steps they take to replace this loss. They should be encouraged to measure losses on the weighing scales.

Any previous or current history of *anatomical abnormality* or of *renal* and *urinary tract disease* liable to interfere with normal urodynamics should be carefully noted.

Patients are quite often aware that they have a medullary sponge kidney, polycystic kidneys, pelvic ectopic kidney or congenital urinary tract stenoses. Recurrent urinary tract infection and relapsing prostatitis may suggest vesicoureteric reflux and subvesical outflow obstruction respectively.

Functional urodynamic disturbances, such as occur during longterm bedrest, in neurological conditions and in pregnancy should also be born in mind.

We have found about 70% of our patients with "idiopathic" stones to have often subtile urodynamic abnormalities and consider this to be next to urine composition in importance as an influence on the further evolution of primary free particles and on the transformation of primary fixed particles into secondary free particles. Any abnormality of urodynamics will allow particles, especially larger ones, to settle under gravity in areas of stagnation at the bottom of the ascending limb, where they will grow in persistently supersaturated urine. The same is true of stones retained within renal calyces, in the renal pelvis or in the ureter, bladder or urethra.

c) Drugs

A careful history must always be taken of medication and self-medication, of the drugs involved and of the dosage and duration. Certain preparations are urolithogenic in their own right or may perpetuate previous stone disease (DANDON and REVEILLAND 1985).

Analgesic abuse, e.g. with phenacetin, aspirin or aminophenazone (amidopyrin) immediately comes to mind. Apart from pure preparations, these substances are also common components of proprietary mixtures, often in combination with caffeine, codeine or barbiturates. Abuse of this kind is on the increase and is therefore a point never to be omitted from the history (MICHIELSEN 1972; HASCHEK and SCHMIDT 1975).

It is also worth remembering that tablet abuse is seldom restricted to one agent. NANRA (1980) noted that patients with analgesic nephropathy frequently exhibit polytoxicomania involving analgesics, psychotropic agents, purgatives, alcohol and nicotine in varying combinations.

Analgesic nephropathy is characterised by fibrosis of Bowman's capsule with scanty glomeruli, interstitial fibrosis and tubular atrophy with thickening of the basement membrane (LABERKE 1982a). Papillary necrosis can be expected to occur in about 25% of these patients (LABERKE 1982b). Depending on the duration of drug abuse, on the extent of papillary necrosis and on the severity of other factors operating to promote local calcification, radioopaque papillary encrustation and frank papillary calculi will then develop (MURPHY 1968). Thus BLACKMAN et al. (1967) found a history of analgesic abuse in 17% of a consecutive series of stone sufferers.

Patients should be asked about *vitamin D* intake, since overdosage can lead to abnormally increased calcium absorption from the gut, with consequent hypercalciuria. In severe cases calcium may be deposited in the kidneys and calculi can then occur (MICHIELSEN et al. 1972; BRONNER et al. 1976; DE LUCA 1976; SUTTON et al. 1976; PETERLIK 1979).

Continuous intake of *diphenylhydantoin* may result in vitamin D deficiency with secondary hyperparathyroidism and urolithiasis.

Long term *dihydrotachysterol* (AT10) therapy can lead to hypercalcemia, nephrocalcinosis and urolithiasis (MICHIELSEN 1972).

Any history of long term absorbable *alkali* (e.g. bicarbonate) intake is important and is common in patients with peptic ulcers. In combination with a milk diet such medication may result in the so-called milk alkali syndrome with azotemia, hypercalcemia, nephrocalcinosis and urolithiasis (HERMAN and GOLDBERG 1960). Urine alkalinization plays a key role in this condition.

If a patient has been taking *calcium preparations* a high dosage for prolonged periods hypercalciuria and urolithiasis may easily ensue. Young people in accelerated growth phases are frequently prescribed such preparations "to strengthen the skeleton", as are elderly persons with osteoporosis.

PAS-calcium therapy for tuberculosis holds similar dangers.

The use of *purgatives* is another important point in the history. Chronic purgation can lead to significant dehydration with increased urine concentration. Saturation products for lithogens may be exceeded and crystals precipitated, quite apart from the effects on oxalic acid absorption and hyperoxaluria of chronic intestinal mucosal embarassment.

Controversy surrounds high dose *vitamin C* intake. COSTELLO (1979) gave healthy subjects 8 g pure ascorbic acid daily for ten days and failed to observe any increase in oxalate excretion either during or after the conclusion of medication. If 8 g Redoxon were given there was still no effect during medication, but increased oxaluria 7 days after stopping it. He explained this effect by the concept that Redoxon contains, in addition to pure ascorbic acid, ingredients which reduce oxalate clearance. The retained oxalic acid would then be excreted once medication had ceased. SCHMIDT et al. (1981) found that healthy individuals taking 10 g ascorbic acid a day excreted between 53.8±9.4 and 87±9.3 mg oxalate in 24 hours. In 1981 these workers were able to confirm that high dose vitamin C intake leads to a moderate elevation of urinary oxalate excretion. After administration of 28.4 mMol ascorbic acid mean oxalate excretion rose to 131% of the control value (0.32 to 0.42 mMol). If the dose of ascorbic acid was increased to 56.8 mMol, oxalate excretion rose by as much as 176% (from 0.37 to 0.65 mMol). In 1982 SCHMIDT et al. recorded daily oxalate outputs of 80–100 mg for an ascorbic acid intake of 5 times 1–2 g or a single dose of 5 g daily. Since ROBERTSON et al. (1981) had already pointed out that a slight increase in oxalic acid excretion, i.e. mild hyperoxaluria, would suffice to significantly elevate the risk of stone formation, it must be clear that a history of recurrent high dose vitamin C intake represents an important diagnostic factor in anyone with typical symptoms (PENDSE et al. 1985).

The observation by LUX and MAY (1982) that a daily ascorbic acid dose of 3–5 g raises urinary pH to the region of 7.3 is also of some importance for the relative risk of stone formation.

During the course of TUR of the prostate, systemic infusion of *glycine* solution may occur, resulting in a fall in plasma sodium and osmolarity. This is followed by substantial hyperoxaluria, taking about two weeks to subside. If urine dilution is inadequate during this period stones may form (FITZPATRICK et al. 1979).

Whether or not *methoxyfluorane* anesthesia alone can provoke postoperative hyperoxaluria is as yet unanswered (SILVERBERG et al. 1971). Certainly KUZUKU (1970) has reported on a number of patients who developed a postoperative rise in BUN and serum creatinine in the wake of a methoxyfluorane anesthetic. Three of these patients died and at autopsy their renal tubules were found to be stuffed full of calcium oxalate crystals. It was, however, stressed in the original report that these patients had received pre- and postoperative tetracyclines. One cannot therefore say with certainty whether the anesthetic was responsible alone or in combination with the latter.

Uricosuric agents are also of great importance, since they both increase the risk of uric acid lithiasis and provide possible heterologous nuclei or block inhibitors of calcium oxalate stone formation. One should therefore ask patients whether or not they have ever been treated in this fashion for gout or hyperuricemia, and if so whether additional measures were taken to reduce the risk of stone formation by urine dilution and/or neutralization.

The history of infants suspected of urolithiasis should be carefully sifted through for evidence of previous *furosemide* therapy. In a series of premature infants treated with furosemide (2–4 mg/kg) for the cardiac failure of patent ductus arteriosus or of severe chronic lung disease HUFNAGLE et al. (1982) observed the onset of renal parenchymal calcification and kidney stone formation, starting 12–14 days after the onset of treatment. Kinetic studies showed that such infants receiving furosemide excreted 10–20 times the amount of calcium excreted by control infants, despite persistently normal serum calcium and phosphate levels. Calcification, consisting of small or large flecks, was mainly seen in the interstitial areas of the renal papillae, although free collecting system calculi and staghorn calculi were also noted. The composition of these calculi was primarily calcium oxalate or calcium phosphate.

It is worth mentioning in this connection that 15–17.5% of patients with gout have calcific calculi (YŰ 1978). Pronounced hypercalciuria during *probenecid* therapy has been demonstrated by WEINBERGER et al. (1982), presumably the reason why this uricosuric agent results not only in uric acid lithiasis but also in the formation of mixed calculi.

Parenteral administration of *amino acids* also lowers serum uric acid levels and consequently causes hyperuricosuria (ZOELLNER 1980).

Estrogens are also not without effect on serum uric acid and urinary uric acid excretion. These parameters have lower values in women of childbearing age than in men, and this has been regarded as explaining the lower incidence or urolithiasis among these women. Contraceptive hormones unequivocally reduce urinary calcium and phosphate excretion, an effect also seen during the treatment of postmenopausal osteoporosis with estrones or combined estrogen/progesterone preparations (TSCHOEPE et al. 1982). Men being treated with estrogens for prostatic carcinoma also exhibit both a corresponding fall in serum uric acid and a rise in its urinary excretion.

Since uric acid is more likely to precipitate the lower the urine pH, patients must be asked about *preparations likely to acidify the urine.* Chief among these are "Acidol-Pepsin", ammonium chloride, mixtures containing it such as "Extin" and lastly methionine.

Xanthine stone formation has occasionally been reported in hyperuricosuric patients receiving *allopurinol* therapy. Nevertheless, allopurinol has not emerged as likely to bring this about, except in patients with complete congenital hypoxanthine guanine phosphoribosyltransferase deficiency (LESCH-NYHAN syndrome) or with abnormal bone marrow turnover (lymphosarcome, Burkitt's lymphoma).

Patients with a history of gastrointestinal disease should be asked about *silicate* ingestion. Substances such as magnesium trisilicate are quite capable of causing stones (JOEKES et al. 1973; CIFUENTES DELATTE et al. 1978; MEDINA et al. 1978, 1981; BERG et al. 1983).

Poorly soluble *sulfonamides* are nowadays hardly ever used, so that acute renal failure due to intrarenal obstruction by sulfonamide crystals at low pH virtually never occurs.

Hypertensives may have been taking *triamterene.* ETTINGER et al. (1981) noted elderly patients to be particularly susceptible to the lithogenic effects of this drug, developing urolithiasis after only a few months exposure. One third of the calculi involved were of pure or almost pure triamterene. If the drug acts as a stone promoter is an open question (SOERGEL et al. 1985).

Finally, the importance of anticoagulants and cytotoxic agents should not be overlooked. Urinary tract bleeding may lead to clot colic simulating the clinical picture of urolithiasis.

d) Individual Dietary History

According to SCHOLZ et al. (1981) and FELLSTROEM et al. (1985) there is nothing in the dietary protein, fat or carbohydrate intake of stone sufferers to distinguish them from healthy subjects. One can only conclude that a normal dietary load is sufficient to activate a genetic predisposition resulting in lithogenesis or that the coincidence of a whole series of etiologic factors is required to initiate stone disease.

For this reason the dietary history of each individual patient assumes a special importance. Idiosyncrasies of individual diet and fluid intake must be assessed in the light of their possible involvement in stone formation.

Dietary documentation would be most accurately achieved by weighing in and recording all liquids and foodstuffs before they are consumed. Such a laborious approach may indeed be justified in patients with stubbornly recurrent disease, but in routine cases a careful interviewer of a cooperative patient will arrive at adequate results (WIRTHS 1974) and uncover valuable diagnostic data for future treatment and recurrence prevention.

One common finding is that first episodes are frequently preceded by periods of inadequate *fluid* intake. FUSS et al. (1979) report that 35% of their stone patients had been taking less than one liter a day prior to developing stones. Our own data on 23 healthy subjects is that twelve women had a daily intake of 993 ± 323 ml and that the 11 men took 1665 ± 665 ml (STRENGE 1982).

Both male and female stone formers had a higher fluid intake than did healthy controls, a phenomenon perhaps explained by prior medical advice aimed at preventing recurrence. As the data from the control subjects show, low fluid intake must be a frequent cause of stone formation.

What fluids people drink may also have a powerful effect on urine pH and on urinary lithogen excretion:

Regular intake of mineral water may either acidify or alkalinize the urine, depending on the brand of water. The same question arises in connection with citrus fruit (orange, lemon and grapefruit) or their juices. They all alkalinize the urine and, according to the German Society for Nutrition (1980), their consumption has risen sharply. Blackcurrants or blackcurrant juice are urine acidifiers (VAHLENSIECK 1979).

In our study of the dietary history of 72 stone formers we paid particularly careful attention to the nature and daily volume of fluid intake.

76% of our patients stated they drank *coffee* every day and 21% were daily *tea* drinkers. Geographical variations in dietary habits may be important here, e.g. a high tea intake in the UK (ZAREMBSKI and HODGKINSON 1962). According to our Institute of Economic Research (ifo) the average intakes of coffee and black tea in the FRG in 1981 were 198 litre and 50 litre respectively per head of the population. In almost every case one has therefore to consider whether such a tea or coffee intake could sufficiently raise the basic metabolic rate as to increase uric acid production and excretion. The further question of increased oxaluria arises in the case of tea.

On the other hand, urinary excretion is influenced by the amount of daily tea and coffee intake. 71% of our coffee drinkers took a maximum of 700 ml per day and we do not consider 4 cups of coffee a day to constitute a significant risk. The situation is, however, different for those subjects whose coffee intake ranged from 750 to over 1000 ml a day (29%). They may well carry an increased risk of stone formation.

A similar situation appertains to the 21% of our group who were regular tea drinkers. 47% of this subgroup drank up to 300 ml, 27% up to 750 ml and 26% drank 900 ml or more. Certainly for this latter group tea drinking should be looked at quite carefully as a potential risk factor, in terms both of oxaluria and of hyperuricosuria.

Alcohol consumption also warrants special consideration, since de novo synthesis of purines will result in increased uric acid excretion.

In Germany alcohol consumption has risen steadily from 3.27 litre per head of the population in 1950 to 12.67 litre in 1980 (German Society for nutrition 1980; ZIEGLER 1981). In this sense alcohol could nowadays be considered the principal drug of addiction.

Any dietary history must take account of inherent reluctance on the part of patients to admit to the true quantity of alcohol they consume. 38 (52.8%) of our 72 calcium oxalate stone formers drank alcohol every day. According to Institute for Economic Research (ifo) the average German citizen drank 147 litre of beer in 1981.

Of our 31 daily beer drinkers (43% of stone formers) 55% drank up to 700 ml, 29% exactly 1000 ml and the remainder (16%) 1000 – 2000 ml a day.

High alcohol intake leads to increased lactatemia, which in turn reduces renal uric acid elimination and hyperuricemia. There then follows secondary hyperuricosuria.

In fact the increase in alcohol consumption we have seen in Germany correlates better with the rising incidence and prevalence of urolithiasis than do, for example, increases in animal protein or calcium intake (VAHLENSIECK 1982).

The work both of ZECHNER (1981) and of ZECHNER and SCHEIBER (1981) show that rising alcohol consumption correlates both with increasing urinary uric acid levels and with the frequency with which stones contain uric acid. In addition, raised urinary uric acid levels may result both in heterogenous nucleation and in blockade of calcium oxalate precipitation inhibitors (ROBERTSON et al. 1976).

According to a report by the German Society for Nutrition, daily calcium intake in the FRG lies between 1000 and 1200 mg, as against a physiologic range of 700 – 800 mg. In a subject with such a high calcium intake the additional daily consumption of 1 – 2 litre of high calcium *mineral water* would certainly present a risk of causing hypercalciuria or of exacerbating it where already present. On the other hand the hardness of drinking water does not constitute a significant factor in the incidence of urolithiasis (SIERAKOWSKI et al. 1979; CHURCHILL et al. 1981; SCHUSTER et al. 1982; ILIEVSKI and ILIEVSKA 1985; VAHLENSIECK 1985). According to the Institute of Economic Research (ifo) per capita consumption of mineral waters in the FRG was 43 liters during the same period.

61% of stone patients in our study stated that they drank mineral water every day. Of this group 45% gave a daily intake of up to 400 ml, 39% of up to 700 ml and the remainder (16%) drank 1000 – 1400 ml. In any given case, however, the calcium content of the water concerned must be taken into account. We surveyed 100 different brands of water and found calcium levels varying from 5 to 900 mg/l. In the data of FUSS et al. (1979) 24% of patients were drinking waters with a calcium concentration in the range 100 – 500 mg/l.

Attention should also be focused on the daily consumption of *dairy produce*, since the quantity of calcium involved may be of major significance for the stone former. According to the German Society for Nutrition (DGE 1980) 41% of dietary calcium is of dairy origin. Data from the Institute for Economic Research (ifo) gives a per capita milk intake of 93 liters for the FRG in 1981.

Many of our patients had already heard about the hazards of milk as a source of calcium. This would explain why only 19% of stone formers drank milk every day. 54% of this minority drank not more than 200 ml and 46% drank 300 – 500 ml daily. There has been a steady decline in milk consumption but a simultaneous rise in cheese sales. In 63 of our stone patients dairy products alone accounted for a daily calcium intake of 551 ± 336 mg for the 25 women and 402 ± 331 mg for the 38 men (STRENGE 1982). In the light of the recommendations already mentioned for total daily calcium intake, it would seem that some stone patients are satisfying their total daily calcium needs from dairy sources alone. Any further dietary calcium would therefore represent an overload and could lead to hypercalciuria, a particular concern where milk or other dairy foods are consumed at intervals throughout the day (KALES and PHANG 1971). ZECHNER et al. (1981) have indeed noted a greater recurrence rate among patients with a marked preference for dairy produce.

Patients must be specifically asked about excessive indulgence in *purine* rich foods such as fish and meat, including offal. In 1980 the German Society for Nutrition noted a slight shortfall of protein intake among young people against the recommended level of 0.9 g/kg body weight. By contrast the recommendations were widely exceeded in all adults, both men and women, and 60% of the protein was of animal origin.

Excess dietary protein results in increased intestinal calcium absorption and hypercalciuria, with a rise in urinary oxalic acid and uric acid excretion (ANDERSEN 1973; COE et al. 1976; ROBERTSON et al. 1976; ZOELLNER 1976; KIM and LINKSWEILER 1979; ROBERTSON et al. 1979, 1981; SIMMONDS et al. 1981; FELLSTROEM et al. 1982; ARORA et al. 1985; LEMANN 1985; ROBERTSON 1985).

Under steady state conditions the ingestion of 150 g liver leads to an increase in uric acid excretion within 2 hours. The subsequent 24 h urinary uric acid of 3.67 ± 0.97 mMol is 31% above the control level (2.8 ± 0.77 mMol). 24 hours later the level was still elevated at 3.36 ± 0.69 mMol. On the test day calcium excretion remained at the control value of 4.38±2.26 mMol, but rose the day after the liver load to 5.12±2.29 mMol. Oxalate excretion was unchanged (HESSE et al. 1982).

GROEBNER and ZOELLNER (1977) have demonstrated that foodstuffs containing predominantly ribonucleic acid raise serum and urinary uric acid levels more markedly than do those mainly containing desoxyribonucleic acid. In addition, we must consider not only the purine content of food per unit weight but also the content per unit energy value. Protein should not exceed 12–15% total calory intake, since an increase in dietary protein will also stimulate purine synthesis.

The observation of DANIELSON et al. (1982) may be important in relation to possible mechanism of nucleation. These workers noted that patients on a high protein diet (142 g/2000 Kcal) all increased their urinary titratable acid, ammonium ion and net acid levels, presumably as a result of the acid group content in protein, with urinary pH consequently falling to low values. Standard bicarbonate was also noted to be low, although within the normal range on all occasions. The acid load was again thought to be the cause of this effect. Increased acidity lowers urinary calcium complexing power. Furthermore, one must not lose sight of the effect on uric acid nucleation of the observed pH of 5.2 combined with the increased uric acid intake implicit in a high protein diet.

A history of *vegetarianism* is extremely important. In a nationwide survey of UK vegetarians ROBERTSON et al. (1979, 1981) found an incidence of urolithiasis only 40–60% of that predicted for an age/sex/social class matched group in the population at large. Similarly, the recurrence rate was reduced to 60–70% of that in a matched non vegetarian group over the same follow-up period.

Any preference for *oxalate* rich foods should be recorded. We asked all our patients about their consumption of such material as chocolate, rhubarb and spinach. It emerged that most people include varying amounts of these foodstuffs in their diets, without there being any clear cut pattern to distinguish the habits of stone formers from those of normal persons (HESSE et al. 1970; STRENGE 1982; VAHLENSIECK et al. 1982; SINGH et al. 1985).

By using standardised diets under steady state conditions we were able to demonstrate that a meal of 200 g *spinach* markedly raised oxalic acid excretion and will thus increase the risk of stone formation. 52% of our patients ate normal quantities of spinach 1 to 4 times weekly throughout the year. Under the same conditions a meal of 200 g *rhubarb* also markedly raised urinary oxalate excretion. 37% of our patients had rhubarb every week during the season, the portions often being over 200 g.

170 g of *chocolate* with a high cocoa content moderately increased oxalate excretion under our test conditions. 42% of our patients gave a history of occasional chocolate consumption in the 25–100 g/day range, whereas 43% rarely consumed even small amounts. 15% said they ate none.

Carbohydrate intake is also important. As long ago as 1965 HODGKINSON and HEATON demonstrated that oral carbohydrate could increase renal calcium excretion. BARILLA et al. (1978) observed increased urinary calcium levels in patients with renal hypercalciuria following a glucose load. BLACKLOCK (1976) suggested that the increased incidence of urolithiasis seen in recent years might be due to a trend towards the consumption of increasingly refined carbohydrate. ROBERTSON et al. (1978) and ROBERTSON (1985) have, however, pointed out that no definite relationship can be established between sugar intake and incidence of stones within various socioeconomic groups. It was THOM et al. (1981) who finally demonstrated a carbohydrate load to raise the urinary calcium concentration, although a concomitant rise in oxalate concentration did not reach statistical significance. The work of JOOST et al. (1982) has shown us that glucose increases proximal tubular reabsorption of sodium in exchange for calcium.

It is worth remembering in this context that the acute administration of large quantities of fructose will lead to temporary uric acid overproduction. Similar effects have been claimed for sorbitol, xylitol and ethanol (ZOELLNER 1976).

Dietary *salt* is a subject of considerable importance. SCHMIDT-GAYK et al. (1977) have pointed out that increase salt intake will tend to swell the extracellular space, which will in turn reduce the tubular reabsorption of a variety of substances, including phosphate. It had already been noted (HENNEMANN et al. 1958) that many patients with absorptive hypercalciuria and calcium lithiasis have low serum phosphate levels. Then, in 1976, DOMINGUEZ et al. showed that a fall in serum and tissue phosphate levels leads to increased synthesis of (OH)2-D from 25-(OH)-D. The consequence is increased intestinal absorption of calcium and absorptive hypercalciuria. RAO et al. (1985) demonstrated that urinary calcium can be reduced by dietary salt restriction, particularly in patients with concomitant hypernatriuria.

Finally, patients should be asked about periods of *fasting*. Although absolute starvation causes hyperuricemia there is also a fall in urinary uric acid excretion. When the fast is broken the hyperuricosuria of refeeding ensues (KRIZEK and SADILEK 1982).

II. Examination

1. Physical Examination

When a patient presents with colic, or if one is called to the bedside during an attack, careful observation of the patient and of his behaviour may provide valuable diagnostic information. Obvious overweight will of itself suggest urolithiasis, and one should consider both pure uric acid lithiasis and the induction of calcium oxalate stones by increased uric acid excretion. The German Society for Nutrition has presented evidence that 35% of persons in the FRG over the age of 14 may be expected to be substantially overweight. Conversely the spectacle of an underweight patient with reduced skin turgor should call the possibility of dehydration and concentrated urine to mind, with their inherent risk of crystal precipitation.

During an episode of colic patients are usually pale and often cold and sweating or clammy, have shallow respirations and exhibit considerable restlessness. Not infrequently the patient will adopt a posture favoring the affected side, or he may prefer to keep his legs drawn up.

Nausea, vomitting and abdominal distension should increase the clinical suspicion of urinary colic, most particularly if the patient or his relatives claim the symptoms to be of sudden onset or if there is a past history of urolithiasis. On the other hand, a long drawn out history of vague intermittent or continuous backache or of dragging pain radiating from the loin to the abdominal wall may be equally suggestive of urolithiasis. Occasionally elevation of the ipsilateral testis or some other change in the scrotal contents may be a feature of low ureteric calculi. Exacerbation of pain on getting up from the supine position and exquisite percussion tenderness of the renal bed virtually confirms the diagnosis, unless marked pyrexia points to pyelonephritis. Palpation and gentle percussion of the renal bed will generally suffice to clarify which side is affected, – patients who have been in severe pain for some time are not always able to provide this information themselves.

In any such situation the next step must be to administer a spasmolytic analgesic intravenously in a dosage adequate on the one hand to control the colic and small enough on the other to leave the patient cooperative and responsive to the examiner. Opiates should only be used in exceptional cases; complications such as respiratory depression, exacerbation of ileus or retention of urine may otherwise occur. The induction of drug dependence is also a hazard to be taken seriously wherever repeated analgesia is called for – not infrequently the case in attacks of ureteric colic. For recurrent colic spasmolytic analgesia should be provided throughout the period of diagnosis and be continued thereafter wherever the stone is thought capable of passing spontaneously.

Proper pain control greatly facilitates abdominal examination. Auscultation may reveal a silent abdomen if the colic has led to ileus, whereas in mechanical intestinal obstruction at least a few tinkling bowel sounds will continue to be heard despite analgesia. The rigid abdomen of urinary colic is relaxed by analgesics; in intestinal obstruction distended loops of intestine will remain palpable.

Acute urinary obstruction by a stone nearly always gives rise, at least early on, to unequivocal percussion tenderness in the loin and tenderness on palpation of the kidney. The same will be true where a renal stone is complicated by pyelonephritis on in perinephric abscess.

If the pain is right sided it will be important to exclude biliary colic. Patients with the latter usually complain of right upper quadrant pain radiating to the scapular region. They will often give a history of several previous similar episodes, perhaps in relation to certain types of food. Careful palpation from the lower abdomen up towards the costal margin during deep in- and expiration is also more likely to give a positive Murphy's sign than it is in pain of renal origin.

Acute appendicitis tends to present with the typical history of epigastric pain shifting to the right iliac fossa and simultaneously increasing in severity, a pattern rarely seen in urinary colic. Percussion tenderness of the right renal bed only occurs with the relatively rare high retrocaecal appendix, and the Psoas irritation sign, elicited by extending the flexed hip or hyperextending it from the neutral, is usually strongly positive. This sign may also be the positive in impacted ureteric calculi with surrounding inflammation. Localized tenderness over McBurney's point, rebound tenderness and a positive Rovsing's sign all point to appendicitis rather than ureteric colic. Acute inflammation of a long appendix hanging down into the pelvis may give rise to pain when the pouch of Douglas is palpated rectally. Although this is rarely so in cases of ureteric calculi, it is just possible where a low-lying ureteric calculus has provoked a marked peritoneal reaction. Such low calculi are more easily assessed per vaginam in women, as rectally in men. Pelvic examination should be carried out with the patient supine, the hips fully flexed. Even so, the length of the examining finger, obesity and strong musculature will limit the scope of examination.

A marked difference between axillary and rectal temperature, combined with leucocytosis, is strongly in favor of appendicitis.

An inflamed Meckel's diverticulum, oophoritis, torsion of an ovarian cyst and ruptured tubal ectopic are also causes of severe abdominal pain. Past history, the exact localization of pain, symptoms of an acute abdomen, rebound tenderness, bimanual findings, presence or absence of pyrexia, leucocytosis and normal urine generally allow early exclusion of urinary colic on clinical grounds.

2. Blood Pressure

The blood pressure must always be taken. 53% of our cases with upper tract calculi had concomitant hypertension. In many cases, no doubt, there is hypertension pre-existing the episode of urolithiasis, a fact of which the patient may have been blissfully unaware. Nevertheless, impaction of a calculus with urinary obstruction may acutely raise the blood pressure. This concept is born out be our observation that in 26 out of 66 (approx 40%) patients with a ureteric calculus and hypertension, the latter resolved as soon as the stone was removed (VAHLENSIECK 1971). Established or previous hypertension will require investigation in its own right and quite apart from the issue of the calculus.

III. Imaging Studies

1. Ultrasound

Although technical details are not to be discussed, it must be said at this point that ultrasound examination has nowadays become the first line of investigation, often avoiding more invasive, expensive and labor-intensive techniques (BARNET and MORLEY 1972; KRATCHOWIL 1977; POLLACK et al. 1978; BACH 1979; BRENNAN et al. 1980; BARTELS 1981; COGGS 1981; GRIMS and HOCURSCAK 1982; HOFFMAN et al. 1982; UTIKALOVA et al. 1982; GOETZ 1983; SCHNEEKLOTH et al. 1983). This is true of a whole variety of aspects of urolithiasis and its investigation. Both radiolucent and radioopaque stones give rise to brilliant echoes with a typical shadow zone (HOLMES 1974; BARTELS 1981; BRAUN et al. 1981). Problems arise chiefly in connection with size and site of the calculus and in terms of instrument sensitivity. GLAZER et al. (1982) have presented some interesting cases of medullary nephrocalcinosis overlooked on the abdominal plain film but clearly seen on sonography.

On the other hand it is frequently difficult to detect calculi less than 8 mm in diameter, so that ureteric stones may not be demonstrated (BARNET and MORLEY 1972; KUNIT and SCHMOLLER 1977; BARTELS 1981).

Ultrasound may be of particular value where a plain KUB film has failed to confirm a calculus and the patients is allergic to contrast media. It is also able to determine whether a pelvicalyceal calculus lies in a dorsal or a ventral calyx. Finally, ultrasound offers rapid and accurate information on the presence of upper tract obstruction and the degree of ectasia.

The development of portable equipment has made examination independent of a fixed facility. The technique is easily tolerated by patients and the absence of radiation makes it especially suitable for use in children and during pregnancy. When investigating pregnant women it is well to bear the physiologic ectasia of the urinary tract in mind, although this situation is normally easy to distinguish from marked obstruction due to a stone, particularly where there are typical symptoms of colic and an abnormal urine to support the diagnosis (BARTELS 1981; BICHLER et al. 1982; KUNTZ and SCHUETZ 1982). If the obstruction is of extreme degree and is unrelieved by spasmolytic analgesics, the lumen of the obstructed system can be catheterised percutaneously under ultrasound control as a temporary diversion (HUTSCHENREITER et al. 1979; VELANAVARRET 1982; STADIE et al. 1982).

Ultrasound offers the additional capability to distinguish an obstructed system from renal cysts and mixed tumors.

The technique is particularly successful at distinguishing between primary uric acid calculi, blood clots and urothelial tumors, a feat virtually impossible on routine radiology (KUNIT and SCHMOLLER 1977; MULHOLLAND et al. 1979; MARBERGER 1983).

Sonography provides a simple, noninvasive technique for following a calculus on its way down the urinary tract and for confirming the resolution of obstruction when stones have passed spontaneously or were removed by endoscopy or open surgery.

Finally ultrasound has greatly contributed to the location of intrarenal calculi at surgery (ROSENBERG et al. 1971). The technique is convenient in the operating room, employing compact equipment to detect and accurately localize calculi of only 2–3 mm diameter. Alone, or in combination with special radiology, sonography thus helps to a far greater degree than would be possible by direct inspection or by radiology alone to reduce the hazard of leaving residual calculi in situ at the end of operation (SCHLEGEL et al. 1961; ANDALORD et al. 1976; COOK and LYTTON 1977; EDELL and ZEGEL 1978; LYTTON and COOK 1979; MARSHALL et al. 1981; SIGEL et al. 1982; THUERHOFF et al. 1982).

2. Radiology

Although ultrasound has to some extent taken over as primary confirmation that a stone is present and may even allow first therapeutic measures to be initiated, further radiologic investigations are usually indispensible for gathering more precise diagnostic information (DE VRIES 1961; FLOCKS et al. 1962; DEUTIKE 1965; EMMET and WITTEN 1971; BRETLAND 1972; OLSSON 1973; LOEHR et al. 1976; ANDERSSON 1977; PYRAH 1979; VAHLENSIECK 1979; WICKHAM 1979; TERHORST 1980; MONTAGUE and STYRAFFON 1981; SMITH 1981; MARBERGER 1983).

a) Abdominal Plain Film

All radiology should start with a plain film showing the entire abdominal cavity and pelvis. If such a control film is omitted a certain number of staghorn calculi will be seen on subsequent studies as area of contrast, whilst small calculi may be completely masked by contrast.

After episodes of colic, large areas of superimposed intestinal gas may render the position, contour and size of the renal shadows difficult to assess and make the detection of small calculi in the kidneys and upper tract virtually impossible. Tomography then comes into its own. Alternatively one may opt to wait until the administration of either a gas absorbing agent or a purgative has cleared the intestine of gas and feces and the abdomen is largely dull to percussion. The intestine of young children virtually always contains gas, but if the stomach is filled with a radiolucent liquid, the bowel may be displaced downward so as to gain radiologic access to the kidney region.

The visualization of a renal or upper tract calculus on the plain film will depend on whether its X ray absorption coefficient is greater than 1, i.e. greater than that of the surrounding soft tissue. This is definitely the case for all calcific calculi but has also been reported for pure cystine stones (GEBHARDT et al. 1977). On the other hand pure uric acid stones are radiolucent and are thus never seen on plain films. The detection of mixed calculi sometimes presents considéral difficulties, depending on the thickness of stone material in the beam path and on the porosity of the stone. One occasionally comes across stones made up of concentric layers of varying density or with a radiolucent core and a calcific mantle. Either appearance is characteristic of mixed calculi, the radiolucent nucleus of which may be either a blood clot or uric acid. It should be apparent from these remarks that a plain film can provide a variety of clues but no exact information on the phase composition of calculi.

Gallstones are usually projected to an area outside the renal parenchymal shadow and a lateral view will place them in a markedly more ventral plane. Calcified mesenteric lymph nodes are easy to recognize by their irregular contour and dense contrast as well as by their marked movement with changes of posture. The same is true of foreign bodies in the intestine (tablets, tablet residues, lead shot, etc.). Calcified costal cartilage and atheroma of the pelvic vasculature are easy to recognize by their linear appearance and offer no renal source of confusion for calculi. Small bone islands in the region of the sacroiliac joint may present rather greater problems, as may phleboliths, despite the round smooth contour of the latter and their usual proximity to the symphysis pubis.

Careful attention should be paid to the area of the prostatic urethra in men; one not infrequently sees collections of prostatic calculi in this vicinity. Although these calculi consist of the same groups of compounds and have similar aggregation patterns to those typical of renal stones (GACA and DOSCH 1981; SPECTOR et al. 1981) they appear to have no direct relationship to urolithiasis as a whole. On the other hand prostatic calculi may provide an important clue to the existence of a subvesical outflow obstruction (sclerosing hyperplasia of the prostate).

b) Intravenous Urography

Unless rapidly recurring colic, general condition and serum creatinine present strong contraindications, it is always of value to perform an intravenous urogram (synonyms: excretion urogram = EU; intravenous pyelogram = IVP), in order to gain further information on urinary tract morphology and function. This is particularly important in cases of suspected urolithiasis where the plain film is negative and ultrasound has proved inconclusive.

Before any contrast medium is given, all possible complications must be carefully explained to the patient. Any tendency to allergic drug reactions should be most carefully enquired after. If there is a corresponding history, or if there has been a previous specific reaction to contrast medium, other techniques of investigation will have to be considered. If the IVU is truly indispensible all the usual precautions (test dose, steroid cover) should be employed and preparations made for the immediate and effective treatment of complications.

In the interest of the patient the relevant radiological protection rules should be strictly adhered to. Prior to injection the renal bed should be carefully examined for percussion tenderness; some other technique is to be preferred, if the latter is marked. The forced diuresis due to the contrast may so severely raise upper tract pressure as to lead to forniceal rupture and pyelointerstitial reflux. Alternatively, urine and contrast may be extravasated into the perinephric and retroperitoneal spaces, where they might excite secondary fibrosis and upper tract compression or, if the urine is infected, result in a perinephric abscess or at least in a phlegmon (GINSBERG 1965; BONK et al. 1966; HARROW 1966; MITCHINSON et al. 1966; RABINOWITZ et al. 1966; SCHWARTZ et al. 1966; GUENTHER and MARX 1968; JUNGMAN 1968; FISCHER 1969; BURGHELE and PROCA 1970; MARQUARDT et al. 1971; HUG and SCHMITT 1972; MELCHIOR and TERHORST 1973; BERNARDINO and MCCLENNAN 1976; KHAN and MALEK 1976; BRAUN et al. 1979; DE RIDDER 1982). The same risk attaches to the technique of ureteric compression, which should therefore not be employed in the investigation of urolithiasis.

During asymptomatic period improved definition can be achieved by increasing the dose of contrast medium or by infusion urography, giving contrast medium by drip over a 2–4 hour period (VAN WAES 1972; NABER et al. 1975).

In the nonobstructed patient standard 5 and 10 minute films will suffice to delineate the upper tracts, and the bladder may be partly filled. Radioopaque calculi can be demonstrated to lie within the lumen of the tract by areas of denser contrast and irregular contour at the level of holdup. Occasionally additional lateral views are helpful in this respect. Calculi either not or only poorly seen on the control film are usually visualized as filling defects in the contrast image. Ureteric calculi generally appear as a holdup in the flow of contrast at the level of impaction and the proximal contour of the calculus is usually demonstrated. These appearances are important evidence for the existence of a stone wherever calcific calculi are masked by bony structures of where the stone is itself radiolucent. The same picture may also denote the presence of a ureteric tumor, although the symptoms are usually different.

The appearance of a prevesical or intramural ureteric calculus is also quite characteristic: the proximal ureter is blown up and the ipsilateral bladder contour more or less markedly flattened.

On the other hand, small ureteric calculi may be so completely bathed in contrast as to become invisible. The recurrence of symptoms after a negative IVU should lead one to suspect this state of affairs, although bouts of crystalluria will produce similar effects.

It is always advisable to take an after-micturition film once the urinary tract has been completely delineated. Low stones and short segments of proximal ureteric distension may have been missed behind a bladder full of contrast, but are likely to be revealed once the bladder is empty. The same film also yields data on any coexisting degree of retention that might require treatment to restore normal urodynamic conditions.

If the bladder or any other part of the urinary tract are incompletely seen at 5 and 10 minutes, a further film should be taken at 30 minutes. If there is then still only a faint image of the pelvicalyceal system but a marked accumulation of contrast in the renal parenchyma (nephrogram) it will be sufficient to take further films every 4–6 hours. These delayed films often give the optimum image at 12–24 hours. If no acceptable view is obtained even after such a substantial delay and if there is no nephrogram (nonfunctioning kidney), some other form of investigation is indicated.

c) Retrograde Pyelography

The retrograde pyelogram is the investigation of choice to determine whether nonfunction of a kidney is due to ureteric obstruction or whether there is a congenital absence of kidney and ureter. The preferred technique is to fill the ureter by a Chevassu catheter inserted into its orifice, since damage to the ureteric wall is thus minimised and calculi cannot pass unnoticed. If on the other hand contrast medium delineates holdup above a level accessible to loop catheters, it may be justified to insert an olivary-tipped catheter further into the ureter in the hope of sliding past the calculus and thus temporarily decompressing the upper tract. Once the latter has been achieved, it becomes possible to demonstrate the pelvicalyceal system on the affected side. The very strictest attention must be paid to aseptic procedure, if fulminating suppurative anuric pyelonephritis is not to be triggered by this maneuver should decompression be unsuccesful or if the catheter should become blocked and obstruction thus recur

(KARCHER 1959; RENYI-VAMOS 1960; KARCHER and VAHLENSIECK 1964; VAHLENSIECK 1973; STOEBER 1983).

d) Antegrade Pyelography

This technique is suitable for cases where the clinical findings suggest an obstructing calculus, where the kidney is nonfunctioning on IVU and where retrograde pyelography has confirmed a block. As an alternative to retrograde ureteric catheterisation, and if ultrasound or CT confirms an obstructed system, percutaneous needle nephrostomy may be performed under local anesthetic. Once again, decompression can then be followed by antegrade pyelography. The same approach is valid for cases in which a stone and marked obstruction have been demonstrated but some other serious problem prohibits immediate loop catheterisation of the ureter or open ureterolithotomy (HUTSCHENREITER et al. 1979; STADIE et al. 1982; STABLES 1982).

e) Computerized Tomography

The extreme sensitivity of computer tomography for variations in absorbance (0.5% as against 5% in conventional radiography) has secured it a special place in the investigation of urolithiasis. Furthermore it is markedly less susceptible to artifacts generated by intestinal gas or by bone. On the other hand any critical assessment of the indication for CT must take account of the failure rate, X-ray dose and cost, compared to ultrasound (AMMON et al. 1979; FREITAG et al. 1982; MOHEBBI et al. 1982; RATHERT and BRAND 1982).

Thin slice collimators permit the demonstration of calculi in the 2–3 mm diameter range. Evaluation of characteristic attenuation levels may even allow qualitative statements to be made about the composition of a calculus, although mixed calculi are problematic. Uric acid calculi produce attenuation in the 346–400 Hounsfield unit (HU) range, whereas xanthine gives 391 HU, cystine 586 HU and calcium oxalate 510 HU. Because of its resolving power for mass density, CT is better at detecting calcific structures than is conventional radiography, but only as long as the calculus occupies the entire tomographic slice. Magnesium ammonium phosphate, uric acid, cystine and xanthine calculi may be demonstrated in addition to calcium oxalate and phosphate (SEGAL et al. 1978; WEGENER 1981; JELINEK et al. 1982). A useful feature of the technique is its ability to distinguish radioopaque and radiolucent calculi from urothelial tumors and blood clots (FEDERLE et al. 1981; STIRIS 1981; BOSNIAK et al. 1982; GREENBERG et al. 1982; LAZICA et al. 1982).

Calcific shadows in the region of the renal sinus must be distinguished from renal artery calcification, although the latter tends to be linear along the course of the artery. Calcified renal artery aneurysms mostly give rise to coarser concentric calcific shadows outwith the renal pelvis (HATTERY et al. 1977; WEGENER 1981).

No doubt future developments will see the entry of nuclear magnetic resonance imaging into clinical usage, possibly to replace classical CT. The former not only provides excellent anatomical and functional data but also obviates any exposure to ionising radiation.

f) Renal Angiography

Where less invasive procedures have failed to clarify the cause of a non-functioning kidney, it may be useful to demonstrate the renal circulation, if only the pyelogram phase is recorded at the same time. Tomograms and perhaps CT may be employed to clarify details. Where surgery is contemplated for staghorn calculi, or in cases of massive hydronephrosis, the distribution and calibre of vessels seen on angiography may be of prime importance in deciding what strategy to adopt (HRADEK et al. 1982). Equally invaluable assessments may be made in the same way of parenchymal thickness.

Renal angiography assumes additional importance from the points of view of pathogenesis and treatment: One third of patients with renal artery stenosis and hypertension can also be shown to have nephrolithiasis (VAHLENSIECK and MAURER 1965).

g) Micturating Cystogram

All cases of staghorn calculus without obvious predisposing factors should be investigated for vesicoureteric reflux. It is by no means rare for reflux to be a significant factor in affected individuals, either simply as a urodynamic abnormality or by facilitating the infection involved in stone formation.

3. Nuclear Medical Studies

The techniques of nuclear medicine may also be a valuable aid to the investigation of urolithiasis. The procedures are generally noninvasive and involve a low level of exposure to ionizing radiation. If the correct investigation is carried out after scrupulous consideration of the relative indications, the results are usually accurate and specific (ZUM WINKEL 1964; BLAUFOX 1972; PABST 1976; PFANNENSTIEL 1977; BACH and DOPPELFELD 1979; HOER and HEIDENREICH 1980; POWEL and BARNETT 1981; VAHLENSIECK et al. 1982; VOIGT 1982).

Where intravenous urography has failed to give an image or where there is known contrast allergy the simple existence of a kidney is conveniently demonstrated by *static renal scintigraphy.*

Urolithiasis is occasionally due in part to the abnormal urodynamics of a rotated or low lying ectopic kidney. If an erect film was omitted from the IVU series in patients with staghorn calculi, this could theoretically be made good by a subsequent plain KUB film. Lying and standing scintigraphy, on the other hand, allows not only ectopia to be confirmed but also a more accurate assessment to be made of the parenchyma than is possible on IVU.

Where nephrolithotomy is envisaged for a staghorn calculus, scintigraphy gives valuable information on the least destructive approach. By the same token, large filling defects on the scintiscan may represent areas of nonfunction worthy of partial nephrectomy. Although the final decision can often not be taken until the time of surgery, operative strategy may nevertheless be considerably influenced by such preoperative knowledge.

Static scintigraphy is of special values in verifying horseshoe or L kidneys containing abnormally placed calculi, a diagnosis often suspected but occasionally unconfirmed on IVU alone.

Where pelvicalyceal distortion suggests some other space occupying lesion (solitary renal cyst, polycystic kidneys, tumor) in addition to a stone, scintigraphy may clarify the situation.

Finally, static scintigraphy allows parenchymal loss and preservation of functioning tissue to be assessed following nephrotomy. *Dynamic scanning* is, however, considerably more suitable for any such investigation, permitting as it does the simultaneous demonstration of anatomy, function and outflow.

Dynamic scanning is quite invaluable in monitoring the passage of calculi under conservative treatment and in checking postoperative recovery. Alternatively such monitoring may be carried out by unilateral radioiodinated hippuran clearance studies. These techniques offer the advantages of a markedly reduced radiation dose compared to repeated intravenous urography and of repeatability in the face of contrast sensitivity. Furthermore, they provide information on both renal function and upper tract flow conditions, as well as – in the case of dynamic scanning – of renal anatomy.

Percussion tenderness of the renal bed is generally quite a fair guide to the degree of obstruction above a calculus. Where stones are slow to pass and conservative treatment with prolonged use of spasmolytic analgesics is punctuated by cycles of obstruction and decompression, it is wise to reassess renal function at regular intervals, since percussion tenderness will decrease during the decompression phase. Prolonged analgesia may also mask persistent obstruction and deteriorating renal function. The correct moment for intervention is thus easily missed.

Even in the absence of obstruction, staghorn calculi are not infrequently associated with marked parenchymal loss. In this situation dynamic scanning aids the decision between organ preservation and partial or total nephrectomy.

The question whether to preserve an obstructed kidney remains difficult to answer by dynamic scanning. On the one hand function may be underestimated, i.e. the scan gives little information on the potential for recovery after decompression. The risk is thus ever present of sacrificing a kidney potentially worthy of preservation, perhaps because a reduction in renal blood flow by the raised intrarenal urine pressure leads to reduced glomerular filtration. This effect would be potentially reversible by surgery to decompress the kidney and restore intrarenal bloodflow. Function could then recover to a greater degree than the renal scan alone suggests, especially in cases of acute obstruction. There are, on the other hand, situations where the dynamic scan may overestimate function. In chronic obstruction some degree of renal decompression appears to occur by a lymphatic pathway, possibly allowing some isotope to accumulate in the parenchyma. The delayed clearance of stored isotope would then convey a false impression of glomerular and tubular function. The best functional assessment of obstructed kidneys may be by the 99^{m}-Tc-DMSA technique of MARISS et al. (1977).

It should be emphasized that renal scanning also provides a far more accurate impression of contralateral renal anatomy and function than is available from intravenous urography. In particular, marked functional compensation by the opposite kidney will render nephrectomy less daunting than would evidence of bilaterally deteriorating function.

Where only function is to be considered, *unilateral catheterless 131-I-hippuran clearance* will be the investigation of choice.

This technique is supremely suitable for monitoring renal function while a stone is being passed. In this connection it should be born in mind that unrelieved complete obstruction leads to irreversible loss of function within three weeks, whereas uninfected partially obstructed kidneys will survive over long periods (MAY 1973). Repeated hippuran clearance estimations offer an ideal basis for deciding when to abandon conservative treatment in favor of early intervention.

When surgery is planned to a staghorn calculus in an unobstructed kidney, the exact relative function of the two kidneys may be the deciding factor in terms of organ preservation, partial or total nephrectomy. As already pointed out, dynamic scanning is to be preferred for bilateral function studies, although both techniques may be employed in combination where there is any doubt.

The problems surrounding the preservability of obstructed kidneys have already been discussed in relation to the dynamic scan, and similar difficulties of over- or underestimation are prone to arise with unilateral catheterless 131-I-hippuran clearances (DOPPELFELD et al. 1978; DOPPELFELD and WEISSBACH 1979). Comparative function studies in obstructed kidneys by unilateral catheterless 131-I-hippuran clearance and by the 99^{m}-Tc-DMSA technique mentioned above, suggest that hippuran clearance gives significantly higher values. Nevertheless, the statistically significant difference in mean function between the two study groups is considered of secondary clinical importance (MOSER et al. 1980). In individual cases, however, considerable discrepancies may arise between results obtained by the two methods, the hippuran clearance generally implying more renal function (DOPPELFELD and WEISSBACH 1979). In doubtful cases, therefore, obstructed kidneys should be assessed in the joint light of radiohippuran clearance and DMSA uptake. It remains to be seen whether perfusion studies will in future be able to resolve this conundrum.

Attempts at *labeling stones with radionuclides* represent a particularly interesting field for future development. By these techniques it may become possible to localize calculi with quite small scintillation counters, although any clinical value will depend on finding substances of suitably specific affinity for different types of calculus to achieve adequate labelling levels (NOBLE et al. 1981; BARKER et al. 1982).

IV. Laboratory Investigations

Before embarking on the laboratory investigation of any given patient with urolithiasis, careful consideration should be given to the basal condition appertaining in that individual, to the specific investigations needed to answer relevant questions, to the samples required for those investigations and to the conservation of that material.

1. Basal Condition

Baseline investigations of stone patients should always be carried out with patients on their usual diet and fluid intake and continuing with any medication. In this way basal conditions will be established that truly apply to the patient in question.

It will then become important to document any departure from this pattern at the time of followup investigations or special studies. If there has been a change in medication, diet or fluid intake, comparisons can be made with baseline values and conclusions drawn as to the influence of individual factors.

2. Sample Collection

Samples should always be collected at equivalent times of day, so as to cut out spurious effects of food intake and biorhythms. Except where profiles are to be established, blood tests should always be taken in the morning (8–9 am) under starving conditions. By the same token early morning urine should be used, its physiologically higher concentration yielding the greatest return of cellular components, bacteria and crystals.

It has become standard to perform most *blood chemistry* on serum, although FRIEDL and MATTENHEIMER (1970) have pointed out that coagulation may cause artifacts by liberating intracellular components and they have therefore recommended the use of plasma. On the other hand, the anticiagulants required for plasma conservation may themselves interfere with the studies, quite apart from the extra workload involved in sample preparation (HESSE and BACH 1982).

Venipuncture technique must be standardised. Firstly the position of the patient is important, since the serum calcium of a supine patient is lower than that of an erect one. On standing up from the supine position fluid is filtered out of the vascular compartment into the interstitial extracellular compartment, leading to a shift in plasma volume of up to 10%. The cellular and high molecular weight constituents of blood are unchanged and their concentration therefore rises. This affects total calcium, because protein bound calcium rises against an unchanged ionized fraction (KREUTZ 1973). Thus blood samples should always be drawn with patients in the same standard position, be it sitting or supine.

It is also advisable to take blood samples exactly under the same conditions either always with or always without compression. Any venous obstruction leads to loss of fluid into the interstitial space, thus raising the apparent concentration of non-filtered constituents in proportion to the duration of obstruction. 10 minutes venous occlusion may raise plasma protein concentration by as much as 20%, resulting in a 10% rise in total calcium (PRELLWITZ 1976; BRAUN 1982). Wherever possible blood should therefore be taken from an unoccluded vein. If compression is unavoidable, it should be for a standardized period, and its effect should be taken into account when interpreting values at the limit of normal.

Glass tubes are preferable to plastic, since the latter may cause hemolysis. Furthermore, polyethylene and polypropylene delay normal coagulation and clot retraction (GUDER 1980).

All *urine samples* sould be collected into absolutely clean sterile containers. Residues of cleaning or disinfectant agents may contain oxidising agents and result in diagnostic errors. Suitably prepared and properly stoppered disposable ware is therefore to be preferred.

Adults and older children should always be asked to provide a midstream specimen. Men must be told to retract the foreskin and women to part the labia minora, so that the area around the external meatus can be cleaned with soap and water prior to micturition. In women the additional use of vaginal tampons is particularly helpful in eliminating vaginal contaminants. Sterile plastic bags are used to collect samples from infants (BRUEHL 1970).

Because it is so important to confirm or exclude infection in stone sufferers, it may be necessary to crosscheck a finding of bacteruria in the midstream specimen against a catheter specimen (in women) or against a suprapubic aspiration specimen (in men, women or children) (EGERT et al. 1971; FIGEL et al. 1972; THIELER et al. 1972; WIEBEL et al. 1972; FUCHS et al. 1982).

24 hour urine collections are required wherever the daily excretion of urinary lithogens is to be established. The early morning (7–8 am) urine should be discarded on the first day of collection and included as the last contribution on the second. Great importance attaches to scrupulous collection by the patient and to accurate determination of volume, since the output of important lithogenic factors such as calcium, uric acid and oxalate has been shown to increase with rising urine output. Oxalic acid excretion exhibits the most marked volume dependent variation (HESSE and BACH 1982). The completeness of a 24 hour collection can (and indeed must) be confirmed by estimating the total urinary creatinine (TISELIUS 1980; HESSE and BACH 1982; ROSE 1982). It should also be born in mind that 24 hour collections contain only the total quantity excreted over the period of collection, without giving any information on rhythmic variations within that time.

The diurnal rhythms of stone formation parameters are only accessible to profile studies, i.e. to repeated estimation of urinary lithogen concentrations at 3–4 hours intervals (ALKEN et al. 1981; HARTUNG et al. 1981; MATOUSCHEK and HUBER 1982). If studies of this type are carried out under steady state conditions, they will not only detect inherent diurnal rhythms but also reveal the effect of various dietary loads or of medication (BACH et al. 1978, 1979, 1981; VAHLENSIECK et al. 1981, 1982).

3. Sample Preservation

The transport of *venipuncture* samples should be as free from vibration and extremes of high or low temperature as possible, so as minimize hemolysis. Serum should be drawn off at the earliest opportunity, certainly within 2 hours. Centrifugation aids (e.g. kaolin coated plastic beads) do not seem to interfere with routine chemistry (HESSE and BACH 1982) and fluorinated hydrocarbons may safely be used to clear lipemic sera (VOIGT 1977).

Where serum is to be stored for prolonged periods (followup or supplementary studies), it should be kept in carefully sealed containers (prevention of secondary contamination) at refrigerator temperatures. Serum is stable under these conditions for up to 4 days, but will become unsuitable for ammonia, bilirubin, glucose, phosphate or acid phosphate estimation. Deep frozen serum may be kept for longer periods with less deterioration, but once again it should be carefully sealed against the ingress of ice (which would dilute the thawed material). Thawed serum must be carefully mixed.

Specimens of urine must kept in carefully cleaned and sterilised containers, thus avoiding contamination and secondary infection. Wherever possible, urine should be examined immediately. If this is not practicable, if the specimen is to be transported or if the specimen is to be kept for comparison with later samples, some form of preservative is indispensible. 0.5 ml of 10% thymol in isopropyl alcohol should be added for every 100 ml of urine, but it is important to remember the bactericidal and pH stabilising action of this manoeuver. A more permanent conservation may be achieved by adding 25% hydrochloric acid to lower the pH below 2.0 (unsuitable for chloride estimation) or by freezing to below -18 °C (HESSE and BACH 1982).

4. Nature and Extent of Investigations

When planning the scope of laboratory investigations for a given case one must distinguish between first attack and recurrences. PAK (1982) demonstrated absorptive hypercalciuria in 55.9% of his patients presenting with solitary episodes of stone disease. Another 11.8% had renal hypercalciuria, 2.9% had primary hyperparathyroidism and 8.8% suffered from hyperuricosuric calcium oxalate lithiasis. Finally 20.8% could not be showm to have any metabolic abnormality at all. He concluded: "The results suggest that the same physiological and environmental disturbances characterize stone formation in patients with a single stone episode as in those with recurrent stone formation and indicate the need for diagnostic evaluation."

A prospective trial by LJUNGHALL et al. (1981) has ably shown the futility of launching into detailed investigations after a first attack, since no additional information on the likelihood of recurrence can be gained by this approach over and above what is available on routine investigation. In the same context SMITH (1982) has commented: "When we see a patient with the first stone, usually with colic, we have no idea when the stone was made and whether he will have more. After hyperparathyroidism, gout and urinary infection have been ruled out perhaps the single most important question is whether additional stone formation will occur in the patient whom you follow in a continuing fashion on increased fluid intake and elimination of dietary excess. If specific treatment is started before the metabolic activity of stone formation is known, you will never know if the treatment is necessary unless it is ineffective. This conservative approach in recurrent stone formers involving fluid and diet has prevented new stone formation in 64 to 70% of the patients with longterm followup, the "stone clinic effect". The single stone former might be expected to show an even better response."

At his point, cost effectiveness must also be drawn into the equation (GUNZER et al. 1982; VAHLENSIECK 1982).

Apart from analysis of the stone itself, investigation of a first episode may be kept within the general confines of what is possible in any general practice (basic screen). Wherever possible, however, this should be supplemented by a more advanced panel of investigations, and where the tests involved cannot be carried out in a general practice setting the help of larger laboratories (multi-user labs and district general hospital) must be sought. By contrast, research projects and patients with recurrent stones will require more intensive and more sensitive investigation (maximum panel).

a) The Basic Screen

The investigations any basic screening panel should comprise are given in *Table 1*.

α) Serum studies

Table 2 lists the *methods* by which the serum levels of important urolith constituents are usually estimated. Technical details are to be found in the more influential reviews (HESSE and BACH 1982; ROSE 1982) and are only discussed in the following considerations to the extent that they are of special significance for the result. Note that the techniques are not infrequently either modifications of or a complete departure from traditional methods. Unusual findings or serious discrepancies with the work of other authors should therefore always prompt one to look carefully at the analytical techniques, conditions and normal ranges given.

In connection with *Table 3* note that the establishment of a *normal range* must take account not only of age, sex, genetic, geographical and occupational variations, but also of quirks of diet and fluid intake. The best control group is a cohort of healthy subjects, investigated first on their habitual individual diet and fluid regimes and subsequently under steady state conditions, i.e. after 5–10 days consistent intake of a standardized and physiologically optimized

Table 1. Basic screening investigations for stone patients

Serum	Urine
Calcium	pH
Chloride	Specific gravity
Creatinine	Red cells
Magnesium	Pus cells
Inorganic phosphate	Protein
Potassium	Sugar
Sodium	Bacteria
Uric acid	Crystals

Table 2. Methods of assaying serum parameters involved in the investigation of urolithiasis

Calcium	
total	Fluorimetry, flame photometry, atomic absorption spectroscopy
ionized	Ion selective electrode, nomogram
Chloride	Coulometry
Creatinine	Jaffe's reaction
Magnesium	Atomic absorption spectroscopy, photometry
Inorganic phosphate	Phosphomolybdate reaction
Potassium	Flame photometry
Sodium	Flame photometry
Uric acid	Uricase reaction and ultraviolet absorption spectrophotometry, uricase catalase color reaction ("Urica-quant"), periodochrome color reaction strips

Table 3. Normal ranges from healthy subjects of serum parameters (group A) not changed with (group B) controlled diet. Deviation of calcium oxalate stone patients from the normal range (group C) not changed with (group D) dietary control (A = Healthy subjects (n = 24) on their own diet fluid intake. B = Healthy subjects (n = 24) on standard diet and fluid intake (2400 ml/24 hours). C = Calcium oxalate stone sufferers (n = 65) on their own diet and fluid intake. D = Calcium oxalate stone sufferers on standard diet and fluid intake (2400 ml/24 hours))

Pro-bands	n	Ca milli Mol/l	Creat. micro Mol/l	Mg milli Mol/l	P milli Mol/l	Pot. milli Mol/l	Sod. milli Mol/l	Uric acid micro Mol/l
A	24	2.35±0.10	66.3±15.9	0.83±0.27	1.08±0.35	4.28±0.44	140.0±2.3	271 ±57.7
B	24	2.39±0.09	68.9±12.3	0.82±0.23	1.11±0.18	4.17±0.25	140.4±2.33	270.6±59.5
C	65	2.44±0.08	78.7±24.8	0.87±0.15	0.97±0.20	4.2 ±0.4	141.0±3	315.0±77
D	65	2.42±0.10	83.1±24.8	0.88±0.13	1.06±0.19	4.2 ±0.3	141.0±3	316.0±79

quantity of food and drink. The table shows serum values substantially the same on individual regimes as on standardised intake, suggesting that the normal range of these serum parameters is largely unaffected by variations of food and drink.

Total serum calcium is best estimated by fluorimetry, emission flame photometry, atomic absorption spectrophotometry, and sensitive electrodes (TRUDEAU and FREIER 1967).

The normal range for total serum or plasma calcium lies between 2.0 and 2.6 mMol/l. The ultrafilterable fraction is 1.3 – 1.55 mMol/l (mean = 1.41) (ROBERTSON and PEACOCK 1968), with the protein bound calcium being around 0.99 mMol/l (PUTMAN 1972). Tests yielding borderline results should be repeated, several times if necessary, since reproducible borderline high values may denote hyperparathyroidism. Values consistantly above 2.5 mMol/l virtually confirm the diagnosis.

Plasma protein and/or albumen estimation is mandatory in this context, since changes in blood protein content will so distort the calcium concentration as to simulate an abnormality. If the serum calcium is normal in the presence of a low protein, some corrective computation is required (ROSE 1982).

Coulometric evidence of *hyperchloremia* should call the possibility of renal tubular acidosis to mind. Normal serum chloride levels are within the range 97 – 108 mMol/l.

Bicarbonate is also an indicator of acid base balance and should therefore be estimated in conjunction with chloride whenever possible (ROSE 1982).

Serum *creatinine* estimation is essential to any assessment of renal function. Cases of unilateral urolithiasis may exhibit considerable contralateral functional compensation. The alkaline picrate technique has become the method of choice in autoanalysers (CHASSON et al. 1968), the normal range being 25 – 100 mMol/l.

Atomic absorption spectrophotometry has rendered serum *magnesium* estimation a simple matter (HANSEN and FREIER 1967). The normal range for total magnesium is usually 0.61 – 1.10 mMol/l with an ionised fraction of 0.46 – 0.56 mMol/l (HEATON 1967). 0.5 – 0.72 mMol/l are ultrafilterable (SCHWILLE and ERNSTBERGER 1972); 0.20 – 0.30 mMol/l are protein bound and 0.14 mMol/l held in complexes (WALSER 1961; HEATON 1967).

The normal range for serum *inorganic phosphate* is 0.81 – 1.29 mMol/l with 10 – 13% protein binding. These values are subject to considerable age and sex differences as well as to day on day variations. A constant sampling time is therefore of special importance (ROSE 1981).

Serum *potassium* estimation is important because hypokalemia may be evidence of renal tubular acidosis. The normal range is 3.1 – 5.5 mMol/l.

Sodium is the main determinant of osmotic equilibrium in the extracellular fluid, and variations in extracellular sodium concentration are associated with various abnormalities of water homeostasis. Sodium deficiency may lead to dehydration and thus cause a concentrated urine with this inherent general risk of stone formation. Normal serum sodium is between 135 and 154 mMol/l.

If *uric acid* is determined by the uricase method (KAGEYAMA 1971), with a "Urica-quant" kit or by periodochrome color reaction strips, normal serum levels for men will lie in the 0.24–0.5 mMol/l range and for women between 0.15 and 0.44 mMol/ l. In view of the significance of urinary uric acid excretion for the pathogenesis of both uric acid and calcium oxalate stones, any stone former whose serum uric acid is in the high normal or above normal range should have repeated estimations and a 24 hour uric acid profile, perhaps combined with urinary uric acid excretion studies.

β) Urine Studies

Table 4 gives a variety of parameters influencing the lithogenicity of the urine along with the commonest methods of estimating them.

Indicator paper is convenient for monitoring urinary *pH*. The paper can be mounted on a dipstick, is easily used by the patient at home and detects variations of the order of 0.2 units. The technique has the distinct advantage of being applicable to freshly collected urine and is thus proof against pH changes due to delay in testing. This latter point is relevant to the otherwise far more accurate measurement of hydrogen ion potential with a glass electrode (Hesse and Bach 1982).

It is important to repeat urinary pH measurements at regular intervals (Gasser et al. 1979). Urine whose pH remains below 5.5 is said to exhibit "fixed acidity", the origin of this phenomenon being still largely unknown (Scholz et al. 1981). Under these conditions there will be a risk of uric acid precipitation even where urinary uric acid levels are within the normal range. If, however, urine pH is consistently greater than 6.8, phosphate precipitation becomes a real hazard. Tiselius (1983) has demonstrated rapid onset of calcium phosphate precipitation above pH 6.5. If infection has been excluded, secondary renal tubular acidosis should seriously be suspected, and an ammonium chloride tolerance test (see below) must be performed.

Where a urometer is used to determine *specific gravity*, care must be taken to ensure the urine is at the temperature for which the instrument is calibrated (usually 20 °C). Temperature mismatch can be corrected for by adding or subtracting one division of scale (0.001) per 3 °C. Once again, the technique has the advantage that it can be used at home by the patient, who can then make

Table 4. Methods of assaying urine parameters involved in the pathogenesis of urolithiasis

pH	Indicator paper, glass electrode potentiometry
Specific Gravity	Urometer, Dip sticks
Red cells	Dip sticks, microscopy of sediment
Pus cells	Dip sticks, microscopy of sediment
Protein	Dip sticks
Sugar	Dip sticks
Bacteria	Nitrite test strips, Griess' reaction, microbiology
Crystals	Light microscopy of sediment

the necessary adjustments to his fluid intake to maintain a specific gravity below 1015 g/cm³. If unusually high values persist in the face of adequate fluid intake, excess excretion of glucose, protein, urinary contrast media or drugs may be responsible. If early morning testing regularly shows hypersthenuria, renal tubular acidosis must be suspected.

The estimation of urine *red cells, leucocytes, protein and sugar* are of special significance in the investigation of urolithiasis. The exact delay between sample collection and estimation or variations in measuring technique may substantially affect the findings (RUPP 1959; STANSFELD 1962; GADEWOLD 1964; TRIGER and SMITH 1966; BRUEHL et al. 1967; GADEHOLT 1968; ALWALL 1973; KELLER and REUTER 1976; BRUEHL et al. 1979; GAARD et al. 1980).

Once again the use of *dipsticks* offers an elegant solution, both being simple and providing rapid and accurate evidence of pathologic change. Combination dipsticks are particularly useful, since they enable a whole battery of important parameters to be measured and recorded in a single operation. The sensitivity and the accuracy of this technique have been documented, and it is worth noting that hemolysis does not interfere with red cell detection (BRUEHL et al. 1979; FUCHS 1980; KUTTER 1980; BONARD et al. 1982; COLOMBO et al. 1982).

The precision of dipstick testing can be further enhanced by incident light photometry, which largely eliminates the spurious effects of varying illumination, background color and individual powers of discrimination in subjective color grading. The measured signal is fed to a microprocessor and the result printed as a peak on a urine profile form or sent to an electronic data bank (COLOMBO et al. 1980; SOJKA 1980).

Dipsticks are quite adequate to provide preliminary data or monitor progress, but where exact quantification is needed of the rate of cell extrusion, red cells and leucocytes must be counted directly from fresh urine samples, either by hemocytometer or by Coulter counter.

If the presence of red cells or leucocytes is confirmed and evidence of pyelo- or glomerulonephritis is sought in the form of casts, some urine must be centrifuged and its sediment examined by microscopy.

Asymptomatic urinary tract infection is a distinct entity, and chronic pyelonephritis may equally enter into an asymptomatic silent phase. Therefore all stone patients should be investigated for *bacteriuria*. E. coli is by far the commonest pathogen, but Proteus, Klebsiella, Aerobacter, Citrobacter and salmonella ssp along with some enterococci, Pseudomonas and staphylococci all share its ability to reduce urinary nitrate to nitrite (RENNEBERG 1967). Nitrite can be tested for by dipstick, or by a field on a combination stick, based on the Griess reaction. A positive test for nitrite is thus indirect evidence of nitrite forming organisms within the purlieus of the urinary tract. The detection rate is 70% for freshly passed daytime urine, 90% in the early morning urine and better than this for repeated testing (FUCHS and GUTENSOHN 1967; BOEHNE 1969; SALLMANDER 1969: CZERWINSKI 1971; FUCHS and GUTENSOHN 1971; ALWALL et al. 1973).

Note that a negative nitrite test does not prove the absence of infection, since the pathogen may not be a nitrite former. Dipinoculum or classical urine culture is therefore mandatory in every case as the only adequate method of excluding infection. In positive cultures the organism must be identified and its antibiotic sensitivity established where indicated by the number of organisms.

Any basic screening panel should also include light microscopy of urine sediment for *crystals*. Urine should be freshly passed and untreated, preferably an early morning specimen, since its higher concentration will enhance the likelihood of crystal detection. Crystalluria depends on urine volume and on often irregular rhythms in the excretion of lithogens and inhibitors, so a number of separate samples must be examined.

Microscopy of urine passed at the end of a 12–24 hour period of fluid restriction ("cristalluria provoquée") (RUGENDORFF et al. 1981) will frequently provide evidence of crystalluria.

Cleanliness of collecting vessels is once again of paramount importance, since residues of cleaning agents and urine preservatives may otherwise lead to considerable artifacts in the sediment, including even complete dissolution of crystals. Delays in examining the sample are to be avoided whenever possible, since changes in pH and temperature may cause secondary crystallisation.

A 10 ml aliquot from a freshly passed and well mixed specimen is quite sufficient, centrifuged at 3000 rpm. In order to secure standardised counting conditions, the resulting pellet should be resuspended in exactly 0.5 ml supernatant. One drop of this preparation is placed on a slide, mounted with a coverslip and viewed on a standard light microscope, several fields being examined at magnifications of the order of 100–300×.

The aim is first and foremost of confirm or exclude the presence of crystals, since confirmation always denotes urine supersaturation and a risk of stone formation. A typical history of pain will further strengthen a diagnosis of urolithiasis, which must also always be entertained where the urine is at either extreme of the pH range. In addition, LESKOVAR (1977) and LESKOVAR et al. (1978) have been able to show that 41.9% of cases of crystalluria also had microscopic hematuria.

Any crystals found in the urine must be classified by type before their pathogenesis can be understood or any treatment planned. Picture atlases are a valuable aid to this task and a great deal of such material has been published (CIFUENTES DELATTE 1974; ELLIOT and RABINOWITZ 1978, 1980; BERG et al. 1980; MATOUSCHECK and HUBER 1981; BERG and SZABO-FOELDVARI 1982).

A positive finding of uric acid crystals is of considerable significance, since plain radiographs will not detect uric acid lithiasis and small uric acid stones may be enveloped in dye on contrast studies. We have seen, furthermore, how increased urinary uric acid levels, perhaps even the crystals themselves, are able to provoke calcium oxalate precipitation. Suspected cystine crystals may be rendered more obvious by adding acetic acid, in which they are insoluble (SMITH et al. 1981). Whewellite crystals are normally quite rare in urine and their presence denotes marked hyperoxaluria with a risk of calcium oxalate stone formation. If such a stone has already been detected but not yet removed, the estimation and classification of crystals may yield solid data on the composition of the calculus and its growth behavior. Finally, careful followup studies enable the effectiveness of treatment to be assessed.

We must remember, however, that normal individuals also have bouts of crystalluria and that the presence of the latter is in itself by no means proof of a stone forming diathesis or of any significant risk of stone formation (DYER and NORDIN 1967; ROBERTSON et al. 1968, 1973; FLEISCH and MONOD 1973; FLEISCH 1973; ELLIOT and RABINOWITZ 1976; ROSE 1977; WERNESS et al. 1981; ROSE 1982).

Nonetheless, stone sufferers have greater quantities of crystals in their urine, these crystals are of certain specific types and they may be aggregated in clusters, although such subtleties require special investigative techniques (ROBERTSON 1969; ROBERTSON et al. 1968; ROBERTSON and PEACOCK 1972; VALYASẸVI and DHANAMITTA 1974; HALLSON and ROSE 1976; BAUMANN 1978; BRANDES et al. 1981; WERNESS et al. 1981).

Although actual crystal size can only be measured by elaborate techniques (see "maximum panel"), in practical terms some degree of comparison can be made to the size of red blood cells (7 micron diameter) (BAUMANN 1978).

b) Advanced Test Panel

Table 5 gives a list of more advanced studies, desirable to supplement the basic screen.

α) *Serum Studies*

No additional investigations are needed over and above those already discussed for the basic panel.

β) *Urine Studies* (Table 6)

Calcium should always be estimated by atomic absorption spectrophotometry (TRUDEAU and FREIER 1967), since flame photometry is subject to interference by sodium (HESSE and BACH 1982).

Chloride, creatinine, magnesium, phosphorus, potassium, sodium and *uric acid* should be estimated by the same technique as was employed for serum, the urine being diluted as necessary (HESSE and BACH 1982; GRAEF et al. 1985).

The *citric acid* assay of GREENBAUM and PACE (1970) has stood the test of time (NORDENVALL 1982). DOSCH (1978, 1980, 1982), on the other hand, has recommended gas chromatography. Urine should always be assayed without delay, since some citric acid may otherwise be lost to bacterial breakdown (HESSE and BACH 1982; LESKOVAR et al. 1982).

Every urine should at least be screened for *cystine*, since opaque calculi on plain X ray tend to be automatically classified as calcium oxalate or calcium phosphate. In urine of fixed acidity these stones are then reinterpreted as mixed calcium/uric acid calculi.

The classical method is Brand's reaction (sodium cyanide and nitroprusside). Prior decoloration of the urine with activated charcoal improves the

Table 5. Advanced panel of investigations

Serum	Urine	
Parameters of basic screen not measured so far	Calcium	Magnesium
	Chloride	Oxalic acid
	Citric acid	Phosphorus
	Creatinine	Potassium
	Cystine	Sodium
		Sulfate
		Uric acid

Table 6. Methods of quantifying more sophisticated urine parameters wich are important for stone formation

Calcium	Atomic absorption spectrophotometry
Chloride	Coulometry
Citric acid	Enzymatic spectrophotometry
Creatinine	Jaffe's reaction
Cystine	Amino acid chromatography, polarography
Magnesium	Atomic absorption spectrophotometry
Oxalic acid	Chromotropic acid technique, enzymatic oxidase method, gas chromatography, ion chromatography, isotachophoresis
Phosphorus	Molybdic acid color reaction
Potassium	Flame photometry
Sodium	Flame photometry
Uric acid	Uricase reaction and ultraviolet absorption spectrophotometry, uricase catalase color reaction ("Urica-quant"), periodochrome color reaction strips
Ammonia	Photometry, ion selective electrode

sensitivity of this technique (KRIZEK and KUZEL 1982), the principal disadvantage of which lies in the constant requirement for fresh reagents and in the use of poisonous cyanide.

KELLY et al. (1972) have recommended a technique employing nitroprusside and borohydride. Although it is sensitive at the 0.3 mMol/l (7 mg%) level, this method is technically demanding. Indeed ROSE (1982) has pointed out that the use of corrosive acids and alkalis along with considerable heat and hydrogen gas render this approach little less hazardous than would the use of cyanide.

BEHRENDT et al. (1975) have, however, obviated these difficulties by giving us the cystine spot test based on salicylic aldehyd under alkaline conditions. The test is quick and relatively simple.

TAKEMOTO et al. (1974) developed a method in which nickel converts cystine to cysteine, resulting in the formation of colored complexes. This technique is somewhat less sensitive than the classical nitroprusside test (KALLISTRATOS et al. 1977; KINOSHITA et al. 1979; HOFFMAN et al. 1982).

Manual or semiautomatic autoanalyser colorimetry is also available for quantitative studies (MOENCH and JIEMS 1970). If the urine contains substances bearing –SH groups or –S–S– bonds in abnormal quantities, chromatography can be used to separate out the individual amino acids involved.

The advantages of quantitative urine amino acid chromatography have been extolled by RAMOS et al. (1973), DOSCH (1980, 1982), DRAWZ et al. (1982), HOFFMANN et al. (1982), and by LUBS et al. (1982). HESSE and BACH also recommend the technique for rapid and reliable urinary cystine estimation.

Polarography (KUZEL 1973; ASPER et al. 1978) has also been put forward as a simple, reliable way of measuring urinary cystine.

ASPER et al. (1978) have indeed developed an electrochemical line assay in which cystine and cysteine are estimated in separate free flow cells.

The pathogenetic significance of even mild *hyperoxaluria* lends special emphasis to the estimation of urinary oxalic acid. The chromotropic acid method (DEMPSEY et al. 1960; HODGKINSON and WILLIAMS 1972; HESSE et al. 1977; ROBERTSON and RUTHERFORD 1981) or its modification by TISELIUS (1977) is of adequate accuracy for routine work (TISELIUS et al. 1978; NORDENVALL 1982). The same is true of the enzymatic technique (HALLSON and ROSE 1974; CONSTABLE et al. 1978; BICHLER et al. 1978; AKCAY and ROSE 1979; CHALMERS 1979; KOHLBECKER and BUTZ 1979; LAKER et al. 1980; BUTZ and KOHLBECKER 1981; ROSE 1982; BAIS et al. 1985; PUNDIR et al. 1985; BEUTLER et al. 1985). With proper mastery of the apparatus equally accurate results may indeed be achieved by gas chromatography (RHODE and ZILLIKEN 1977; DOSCH 1978, 1979, 1980; OFFNER and URING 1979; GELOT et al. 1980; HESSE et al. 1980; DOSCH 1982; STRENGE and HESSE 1982). Direct measurements of urinary oxalate may be made by the simple and accurate technique of ion chromatography, for which minimal preparation and only about 20 minutes analysis time are required per sample (SMALL et al. 1975; MAHLE and MENON 1982; ORWELL et al. 1982; SCURR et al. 1985). LARSSON et al. (1985) as well as SUGIMOTO et al. (1985) underlined the value of the high-performance liquid chromatography.

Finally, isotachophoresis (SCHMIDT et al. 1979, 1980) has nowadays become a routine technique of adequate reliability (TSCHOEPE and RITZ 1981; BRUCHELT and SCHMIDT 1983; TSCHOEPE et al. 1983; SCHMIDT and BRUCHELT 1983; STRENGE and HESSE 1983).

Table 7 gives normal ranges for a variety of parameters relevant to stone formation. These figures were compiled from test results on normal subjects either taking their usual food and drink or under steady state conditions on standard diet and fluid intake of 1400 ml or 2400 ml respectively.

c) **Maximum Test Panel** (Table 8)

This range of investigations should be regarded as supplementary to those in the advanced panel.

These investigations are intended to be brought into play wherever the basic screen and advanced panel have failed to explain recurrent stone formation, or where recurrence prevention has been unsuccessful. Furthermore the investigations in this group aim at providing new insights into pathogenesis and pathophysiology, as well as at monitoring the efficacy of diet and medication.

Table 7a. 24 hour urine values affecting stone formation, measured in healthy control subjects on their own diet and under steady state conditions on 1400 ml fluid/24 hours (figures are mean ± std. deviation)

Parameter	Individual diet	Standardized diet with 1400 ml fluid	
		day 5	day 7
Volume (ml)	1252±455	1637±219	1716±267
pH	6.09±0.19	6.36±0.19	6.42±0.16
Density (g/cm³)	1017±0.006	1009±0.002	1009±0.003
Na (mMol)	174.5±52.3	121.8±30.9	118.9±40.6
K (mMol)	75.1±38.3	83.2±32.7	90.5±43.9
Ca (mMol)	5.03±2.15	3.80±1.65	3.68±1.92
Mg (mMol)	4.97±1.72	4.29±1.32	4.48±2.16
Cl (mMol)	165.8±52.7	87.0±27.3	98.5±28.3
Inorganic phosphate (mMol)	30.2±4.3	25.2±5.0	24.0±5.4
Inorganic sulphate (mMol)	19.4±5.7	18.9±2.7	16.9±3.0
Uric acid (mMol)	3.03±0.37	2.66±0.51	2.63±0.69
Oxalic acid (mMol)	0.349±0.202	0.362±0.179	0.366±0.175
Citric acid (mMol)	2.55±1.42	3.12±1.01	3.20±1.05
Creatinine (mMol)	19.3±7.1	14.28±4.09	14.72±4.73

Table 7b. 24 hour urine values affecting stone formation, measured in healthy control subjects on their own diet and under steady state conditions on 2400 ml fluid/24 hours (figures are mean ± std. deviation)

Parameter	Individual diet	Standardized diet with 2400 ml fluid	
		day 5	day 7
Volume (ml)	1359±577	2576±253	2629±188
pH	6.16±0.40	6.57±0.28	6.48±0.24
Density (g/cm³)	1015±0.005	1006±0.002	1005±0.002
Na (mMol)	146.7±68.1	113.4±47.7	106.6±41.4
K (mMol)	39.8±15.5	37.4±24.9	35.2±9.89
Ca (mMol)	4.34±2.28	3.33±1.85	3.47±2.14
Mg (mMol)	3.57±1.80	3.79±1.16	3.80±1.10
Cl (mMol)	133.8±53.7	88.9±44.7	79.6±29.5
Inorganic phosphate (mMol)	26.5±7.8	22.1±7.8	24.6±7.2
Inorganic sulphate (mMol)	21.2±7.6	20.9±1.01	23.4±1.37
Uric acid (mMol)	3.44±0.99	2.80±0.69	2.77±0.53
Oxalic acid (mMol)	0.385±0.141	0.385±0.181	0.376±0.141
Citric acid (mMol)	2.54±1.42	3.59±1.81	3.74±1.47
Creatinine (mMol)	11.5±5.5	12.4±5.3	12.8±2.6

α) *Special Serum and Urine Investigations*

If the preceding studies repeatedly show serum calcium at the upper limit of the normal range, serum *parathormone* estimation is indicated. Problems arise from the phenotypic diversity of parathormone, both in its immunogenicity and in its molecular weight. Furthermore, the hormone exhibits different properties, depending on the physiologic conditions. This may be the explanation for

Table 8. Maximum test panel for investigation of stone patients

Serum	Urine	
Ionized calcium	Ionized calcium	Amino acids
Parathormone	cAMP	Uromucoid
Calcitonin	Glycollates	beta-2-micro globulin
Vitamin D metabolites	Saturation state	Proteases
Glycollates	Precipitation	Peptidases
	Quant. crystalluria	
	Crystal growth	
	Aggregation	
	Loading Studies	
	Ammonium chloride	
	Calcium	
	Oxalate	
	Purine	
Steady State Investigations		

the observation by ROSE (1982) that many patients with borderline calcium levels nevertheless have normal parathormone values. CARMIGNANI et al. (1982) also stress the fact that their NH_2 specific antiserum yielded 48% false negative results. Undoubtedly the availability of antisera for both the C-terminal and the N-terminal sequences of the molecule have improved the diagnostic accuracy of parathormone assays (ARNAUD et al. 1971; HEHRMANN et al. 1974; SCHWILLE et al. 1978; BROADUS 1979; CARMIGNANI et al. 1982; HESSE and BACH 1982; v. LILIENFELD-TOAL 1982; KOHRI et al. 1982).

CARMIGNANI et al. (1982) have pointed out that carboxyl specific antisera gave 100% specificity against specially drawn blood samples.

Vitamin D and its metabolites are the focus of ever increasing interest (BRONNER et al. 1976; DE LUCCA 1976; LEHMANN et al. 1976; SUTTON et al. 1976; GRAY et al. 1977; KAPLAN et al. 1977; SHEN et al. 1977; CANTERBURY et al. 1978; ONO et al. 1980; VAN DEN BERG et al. 1980; PEACOCK et al. 1981; RASMUSSEN et al. 1981; COE et al. 1982; JONGEN 1983; v. LILIENFELD-TOAL et al. 1984).

BELSEY et al. (1974) have described a rapid assay for 25-OH-vitamin D_3 without preparative chromatography, and EISMANN et al. (1976) report on a sensitive, precise and convenient method for determining 1,25 hydroxy vitamin D in human plasma.

JONGEN et al. (1981) have given us a rapid and reliable technique for the simultaneous estimation of 25-OH-D, 24,25-$(OH)_2$-D and 1,25-$(OH)_2$-D.

Calcitonin can nowadays also be estimated by radioimmunoassay (BROADUS 1979). According to KOHRI et al. (1983) calcitonin is moderately elevated after a period of fasting only in patients with absorption hypercalciuria, and it is only this group which significantly raise their serum calcitonin in response to a calcium load. Serum *ionized calcium* can be measured by an ion selective calcium electrode. Serum ionized calcium is usually quoted as 1.02 – 1.32 mMol/l (mean = 1.17) (FREANY et al. 1974). HERING and LUTZEYER (1978) and SOLZESZ et al. (1982) both report elevated ionized calcium fractions in recurrent stone formers. According to ROBERTSON et al. (1978) ionized calcium is raised in primary and secondary hyperparathyroidism, even in the presence of normocalciuria.

The investigation of oxalate metabolism has drawn attention to the importance of plasma *glycollate* levels. Glycollate can now conveniently be estimated by an enzymatic colorimetric assay (ROSE and KASIDAS 1979).

Sophisticated *urine chemistry* occupies a special position.

Ionized calcium may once again be measured with a calcium electrode (PASCHEN 1975; FUCHS 1976; ULSHOEFER 1977; ULSHOEFER and PEEMOELLER 1978; PEEMOELLER and ULSHOEFER 1979; ULSHOEFER and PEEMOELLER 1981; SOLTECZ et al. 1982).

Berthelot's reaction provides a simple technique for the direct estimation of urinary *ammonia* (KELLER et al. 1976), although ion selective ammonia electrodes are also available.

The determination of *cyclic adenosine monophosphate* (cAMP) levels will provide indirect data on parathormone activity at the periphery. The method of choice is radioimmunoassay (GILLMANN 1970; BROWN et al. 1971; V. LILIENFELD-TOAL et al. 1974; TOVEY et al. 1974; SCHMIDT-GAYK et al. 1975; SCHWILLE and SAMBERGER 1975; SCHWILLE et al. 1977, 1978; BROADUS 1979; KOHRI et al. 1973; LIEN and KEANE 1983). In the view of SCHWILLE et al. (1977) simultaneous elevation of urinary cAMP and serum ionized calcium is definite evidence of hyperparathyroidism. From the highly significant correlation to 24 hour urinary cAMP excretion KRUSE and KRACHT (1981) were able to demonstrate the usefulness in infants, children and adults of measuring the fasting urinary cAMP/creatinine or cAMP/GFR ratio.

Urinary *glycollates* can also be measured by enzymatic colorimetry, providing useful data for the differential diagnosis of the hyperoxalurias. In the majority of cases of primary metabolic hyperoxaluria glycollate excretion is increased, but not so in dietary excess or steatorrhea (ROSE and KASIDAS 1979).

Uromucoid is a glycoprotein formed in the tubules which can be isolated from urine by salt precipitation (TAMM and HORSFALL 1950) and which is nowadays assayed by quantitative immunochemistry (BICHLER et al. 1973; BICHLER 1974, 1975). Despite earlier reports of raised urinary uromucoid levels in stone formers, neither BICHLER (1975) nor WIKSTROEM and WIESLANDER (1981) were able to confirm raised uromucoid levels in patients with calcium oxalate, calcium phosphate or cystine stones, and in fact they found decreased uromucoid excretion associated with uric acid lithiasis. SAMUELL (1978) introduced a modified electroimmunoassay technique, by means of which both SAMUELL himself (1979) and HALLSON et al. (1981) have been able to demonstrate that stone formers who pass small quantities of urine have higher uromucoid excretion and higher urinary concentrations than do healthy subjects (rapid evaporation technique of HALLSON and ROSE 1978, 1979).

Increasing interest is being generated by urinary *amino acid* levels, although their significance for stone formation is still far from clear.

LIAN et al. (1977) demonstrated the presence of gammacarboxyglutamic acid in calcific renal stones and HAUSCHKA et al. (1975) have characterised this substance as a calcium binding amino acid. Amino acid analyzer studies of 24 hour urine from recurrent stone formers have revealed significantly raised excretion compared to healthy controls (JOOST et al. 1981; RESNICK et al. 1981).

In this context the presence of measurable urinary *protease* activity must be worthy of mention. SCHNEIDER and BOERNER (1981) found stone sufferers to have both raised protease activity and increased enzymatic binding capacity. BOERNER et al. (1982) have studied the effects of proteases on calcium oxalate precipitation from nighttime urine. It seems that proteolytic cleavage of high molecular weight organic material in the urine results in complete disappearance of large crystals, with no change or only a moderate increase in smaller ones.

Beta-2-microglobulin may be detected in the urine by radioimmunoassay. This interesting substance is excreted in increased quantities in tubular lesions (BACKMAN et al. 1976; BICHLER et al. 1981, 1982). LJUNGHALL et al. (1982) detected increased excretion overall in about 10% of their stone patients, the highest levels occurring in patients with renal tubular acidosis.

Tubular damage can also be confirmed by estimating urinary *alanine aminopeptidase* (AAP), but pyelonephritis must first be excluded as an alternative source of raised urinary AAP activity. SPENGLER and MOSCHUETZ (1982) found markedly raised AAP activity in the urine of stone patients who were free of any renal inflammatory process, and it is therefore debatable whether the tubular lesion is cause or effect of urolithiasis.

Saturation. The degree of urine saturation is also of great diagnostic import (NANCOLLAS 1985). Some understanding of lithogen and lithogen complex solubility in urine has been gained by adding test substances to natural and synthetic urines under controlled conditions and recording the parameters leading to precipitation. From concentration curves constructed in this way it has been possible to delineate the supersaturated state, i.e. activity greater than the solubility product. Within this region the breadth of the metastable and unstable zones have also been defined. Metastability is characterised by a range of concentrations lying between the absolute limiting solubility product and the degree of saturation at which spontaneous precipitation (nucleation) occurs. Within this range precipitation only occurs in the presence of some trigger factor (seed, nucleating agent). In the unstable region, on the other hand, the concentration is around the precipitation point or higher, so that precipitation always occurs when these concentrations are attained. If a known quantity of test substance is added and equilibrium between precipitate and supernatant allowed to set in, the ionic concentration in the supernatant can be compared with that of other experiments. Such an arrangement allows the effects of diluting the test solution or of changing the concentrations of its constituents to be evaluated in a controlled fashion (DENT and SUTOR 1971; SUTOR 1973; FINLAYSON et al. 1973; BABIC et al. 1976; ROBERTSON et al. 1976; MATOUSCHEK and HUBER 1977; BURNS and FINLAYSON 1981; TEW and MALIS 1981; TISELIUS and LARSSON 1981; TISELIUS et al. 1981; FINLAYSON 1982; NANCOLLAS et al. 1982; SARIG et al. 1982; ZECHNER et al. 1984; WHITE et al. 1983).

From the pH-dependent concentrations of ionised calcium, magnesium, phosphate and sulfate, and from the total concentrations of calcium, magnesium, sodium, potassium, ammonium, phosphate, oxalate, citrate and sulfate, the stability constants of various soluble urinary complexes have been calculated on a suitable computer program. There is no significant difference in the mean values for stone formers and healthy subjects, but many stone formers had raised urinary activity products, denoting a high risk situation (RAAFLAUB 1963; ROBERTSON et al. 1968; ROBERTSON 1969; DANIELS and MARANGELLA 1981).

A dedicated computer program has also been used to calculate the saturation level from total sodium, potassium, (ammonium), calcium, magnesium, phosphate, sulfate, oxalate, citrate, (urate), chloride and pH. Strikingly, a 1% increase in oxalate concentration did more to raise saturation than did calcium, and furthermore the inhibitory effect of citrate on calcium oxalate precipitation ranked higher than did that of sodium, phosphate, magnesium, sulfate, potassium or chloride (FINLAYSON 1977; FINLAYSON and REID 1978; HERING et al. 1981).

NORDENVALL (1982) has also used a computer program similar to that of ROBERTSON (1969) and of FINLAYSON (1977) to determine ionic activity products.

Similar studies of complex chemistry using urine ionic equilibrium programs have been carried out by ELLIOT (1973), MARSHALL and BARRY (1973), GILL (1974), ACHILLES et al. (1976), ERWIN et al. (1976), HESSE et al. (1977), TISELIUS et al. (1978), BRUNDIG et al. (1980), DANIELS and MARANGELLA (1981), HARTUNG et al. (1981), RAPADO et al. (1981), MATOUSCHEK and HUBER (1982), TISELIUS and LARSSON (1982), VOGEL et al. (1984), BAUMANN et al. (1985) and ACHILLES and ULSHOEFER (1985).

ROBERTSON (1969) attempted to reduce the number of measurements required by estimating the calcium oxalate, octacalcium phosphate and magnesium ammonium phosphate activity products. By comparing their urine values with the saturation product of the corresponding salt in aqueous solution, the degree of saturation could be determined. This method required a computer program but had the advantage of measuring simultaneously the activity products of three salts.

PAK (1973) measured the activity product of brushite only and determined the degree of urine saturation with this salt by comparing the brushite activity products before and after overnight incubation of the urine with synthetic brushite. The ratio was then calculated of the pre- and postincubation brushite activity products. A ratio of less than 1 suggested undersaturation and greater than 1 suppersaturation. This technique involved fewer chemical determinations and no computer.

OREOPOULOS et al. (1976) have used both techniques in a comparative study.

Saturation can also be expressed in terms of ratios between urine concentrations of various substances involved in lithogenesis. Suitable ratios are calcium/creatinine, calcium × oxalate/creatinine × magnesium, calcium/citrate × magnesium × sodium or sodium/calcium (TISELIUS et al. 1978; HARTUNG et al. 1979; TISELIUS 1979; BERG 1981; NORDENVALL 1982; MATOUSCHEK and HUBER 1983; ERWIN et al. 1985). BUTZ and SCHULTE (1982) found 68% of their stone patients to have a mean matutinal urinary calcium/citrate ratio of 1.57, whereas healthy individuals had a mean of only 0.86. Single episode and recurrent stone formers were also separated by differences in the magnesium/calcium × oxalate ratio (Robertson 1976). Robertson et al. (1981) have stressed the importance of the oxalate/calcium ratio, whilst Tiselius (1983) has pointed out that, in the routine investigation and followup of calcium oxalate stone formers the mathematical expression $Ca^{0.71} \times Ox$, is of great value in expressing urinary calcium oxalate supersaturation (with or without a volume factor). However, for more detailed analysis and in therapeutic situations where effects on urinary magnesium and citrate are expected, as well as in research work, the more complex index, including calcium, oxalate, magnesium and citrate will probably be of greater use. The chief disadvantage of this term is that it omits uric acid and glycosaminoglycans, both important factors in stone formation, and indeed apart from calcium and oxalate the only ones found by repeated estimation of a panel of twelve urine parameters to be significantly different in stone formers and non-formers (Robertson et al. 1978). Urinary protease activity is also neglected.

Nomograms offer a far less elaborate means of determining urine saturation and show good agreement with the results of computer calculations (Marshall and Robertson 1976; Nordenvall 1982; Hesse and Bach 1982; Tiselius 1984).

In any consideration of urine saturation studies note that healthy individuals also have periods of urine supersaturation by various lithogens, i.e. that not every proven case of supersaturation is hard evidence of urolithiasis. Such supersaturation of urine from healthy individuals with calcium oxalate has been recorded by Elliot and Ribeiro (1967), Gill et al. (1974), Pak and Holt (1976), Robertson (1976), Robertson et al. (1968, 1971).

Robertson et al. (1968, 1971) have recorded similar bouts of hydroxyapatite and octacalcium phosphate supersaturation.

The brushite supersaturation found in the urines of healthy persons by Pak (1969) and by Pak et al. (1969) was less pronounced.

On the other hand uric acid and sodium or ammonium urate supersaturation is not atall uncommon in the urine of normal people (Pak et al. 1977; Robertson et al. 1976).

Magnesium Ammonium Phosphate supersaturation has only been seen in the urine of healthy persons where prior infection had led to urine alkalinisation (Robertson et al. 1968).

Crystalluria. Certain more elaborate techniques yield pathogenetic data over and above that available from the advanced panel of crystalluria studies.

Polarised light microscopy is an excellent method for the *qualitative identification* of crystals, since most crystals exhibit interference colors of varying brilliance when viewed under polarised light with crossed filters. The great advantage of the technique is its ability to distinguish crystal phases of the same typical habit but of differing chemical composition and to elicit data from amorphous crystallisates (Cifuentes Delatte 1974; Schneider 1974; Elliot and Rabinowitz 1978, 1980; Berg and Szabo-Foeldvary 1982).

Haber (1972, 1981) has identified crystals by a combination of polarising-, interference- and phase contrast microscopy.

Infrared spectroscopy, scanning electron microscopy and x-ray diffractometry offer further means of examining crystals in greater detail (CIFUENTES DELATTE 1970, 1971; ELLIOT et al. 1976; ELLIOT and RABINOWITZ 1978; FUSS et al. 1976; ALKEN and SCHAEFER 1978; GEBHARDT 1978; BLOMEN 1981, 1982; BERG and SZABO-FOELDVARI 1982).

Quantitative estimation of crystalluria and measurement of crystal size is almost as important as crystal type in determining the risk of stone formation and in assessing therapeutic outcome (DYER and NORDIN 1967; ROBERTSON et al. 1969; SUTOR 1969; SUTOR and WOOLEY 1970; TEOTIA and SUTOR 1971; WELSHMAN and MCGEOWN 1972; HABER 1972; FLEISCH and MONOD 1973; HALLSON and ROSE 1976; PAK and HOLT 1976; SZABO-FOELDVARI et al. 1976; MILLER et al. 1977; ROSE 1977; DRACH et al. 1978).

Coulter counter technology offers one means of counting crystals and of estimating their volume: Particles passing through a capillary gate trigger electrical signals which can be processed by online computing equipment. Other similar instruments use light scatter by crystals or the interruption of a light beam shining across a glass capillary tube to generate electrical signals (ROBERTSON et al. 1968, 1969, 1971, 1972, 1973; ROBERTSON and PEACOCK 1972; HALLSON and ROSE 1976; FLEISCH et al. 1977; ROSE 1977; LESKOVAR and HARTUNG 1978; BRANDES et al. 1981; HARTUNG et al. 1981; HERING et al. 1981; BERG and SZABO-FOELDVARI 1982; RYALL et al. 1985).

A simple, inexpensive, accurate and readily available technique involving petrographic analysis of millipore filtrates has been described by VAN DEN BERG et al. (1976). Urine is voided into a metal urinal held at 37° C and two millilitres of this fresh sample are immediately suction filtered through a millipore filter, washed with 4 drops distilled water and dried. The filter is placed under a coverglass and refraction oil added to the edge of the coverslip prior to sealing with mounting medium. The sample is thus preserved indefinitely for further examination and a section of the millipore filter may be kept back for scanning electron microscopy. The crystals are preserved in a good approximation to their original state in freshly voided urine.

WERNESS et al. (1981) have given a further impressive demonstration of this technique, identifying their crystal material by petrographic microscopy and scanning electron microscopy with energy dispersive X-ray spectrometry.

Crystal size can also be determined with a micrometer eyepiece, with a measuring grid in the eyepiece or on a special microscope that projects the image onto a suitable external measuring field, whence data is fed into automatic measuring equipment and processed in an on line computer (SCHULZE et al. 1980; BERG and SZABO-FOELDVARI 1982; BOERNER et al. 1982).

The importance of pathogenetic data gleaned from careful qualitative and quantitative analysis of crystal material for the risk of stones forming from identical material is obvious. In addition, however, it may well be that crystals act as promoters of further crystal precipitation. Such heterogeneous nucleation would have to take place in a metastable domain. It has certainly been shown that calcium oxalate promotes the precipitation of calcium phosphate (PAK et al. 1976; MEYER et al. 1977) and of sodium urate (PAK et al.

1976). Hydroxyapatite induces calcium oxalate (MEYER et al. 1975) and sodium urate precipitation (PAK et al. 1976). Brushite promotes the precipitation of calcium oxalate (PAK et al. 1976; MEYER et al. 1977), whilst monosodium urate has the same effect on both calcium oxalate (COE et al. 1975; PAK and ARNOLD 1975; PAK et al. 1976) and calcium phosphate (PAK et al. 1976).

Inhibitors. Particular importance attaches to the presence in the urine of substances capable of inhibiting precipitation, nucleation, crystal growth or aggregation. The substances are termed inhibitors. Excellect reviews of this entire subject have been given by ISAACSON (1969), RUSSEL and FLEISCH (1969), SMITH and MCCALL (1969), THOMAS (1969), WELSHMAN and MCGEOWN (1972), OHATA and PAK (1973), FINLAYSON (1974), ROSE (1975), ROBERTSON and NORDIN (1976), SMITH (1976), FLEISCH et al. (1977), MILLER et al. (1977), DOREMUS et al. (1978), GARDNER and DOREMUS (1978), PAK (1978), FLEISCH (1978, 1980), BROCKIS et al. (1980), BURNS and FINLAYSON (1980), GARTI et al. (1980), ROBERTSON et al. (1981), TISELIUS and FORNANDER (1981), ROSE (1982), NANCOLLAS (1982), NANCOLLAS et al. (1984) and SALLIS (1985).

The chief distinction to be made is whether a given substance acts as a primary inhibitor or forms complexes with certain lithogens, thus reducing their level of saturation. Inhibitors such as magnesium and citrate appear to act by both mechanisms (ROBERTSON et al. 1981).

Our understanding of the inhibitory action of urine on *precipitation* is due largely to in vitro experiments comparing the effects of various dilutions of urine on formation products. The latter are first determined by the minimum concentration of ions or solutes needed to produce a solid phase in a given length of time (FLEISCH and BISAZ 1962). The extent to which the formation product was depressed was then taken to indicate the inhibitory action of the additive. Results obtained with diluted urine do not, however, necessarily reflect the conditions appertaining in undiluted urine, and indeed inhibitory activity is not related linearly to the concentration of urine used. Many inhibitors exhibit nonlinearity and variability of action, so that their relative importance varies with dilution (FLEISCH 1980).

The measurement of formation products in dilute urine is also not without its problems. Although the concentration of lithogenic substances in such a solution can be measured, their thermodynamic activity cannot, and it is the latter that chiefly governs the product of formation.

PAK et al. (1971) and PAK (1972) have outlined an approach by which measured formation products are related to the solubility products for the solids appearing in the individual urine.

This procedure is only valid so long as the percentage of complexes formed is identical under the two sets of conditions and if the complexing agents are not adsorbed on to the crystal surface when solubility is being measured. However, although this formation ratio is not entirely accurate, it nevertheless gives a valid approximation. A further problem when measuring the formation product in whole urine is that the maximum measurable inhibitor activity will actually be obtained at concentrations lower than those in urine. This loss of sensitivity can be compensated to some extent by adding some form of seed to the system (FLEISCH 1980).

MEYER and NANCOLLAS (1972, 1973) have measured the kinetics of precipitation after a seed is introduced. The effect of inhibitors can be measured by the loss of calcium and inorganic phosphate from a supersaturated solution after seeding. Care must be taken to hold the ionic concentrations of the formation partners constant throughout the test.

BAUMANN et al. (1975) employed a modification of the FLEISCH and BISAZ (1962) technique. Two sets of solutions were made up to have constant pH and ionic concentrations but serially increasing phosphate levels. After incubation for three days at 37° C, either with or without the addition of 3% urine, the supernatant calcium concentration was determined as a measure of the limiting calcium × phosphate product, above which precipitation would occur. Adding urine raises this product, and by subtracting the control values a measure of urinary inhibitor activity can be calculated and expressed in (mg^2).

MEYER et al. (1975) have presented a special technique for use in the calcium oxalate monohydrate–hydroxyapatite system, MEYER and SMITH (1975a, b) a similar one for calcium oxalate.

A technique measuring the quantity of hydroxyapatite needed to precipitate 50% calcium phosphate from supersaturated whole urine has been described by FLEISCH et al. (1977) and by BISAZ et al. (1978). Since inhibitor binds to the seed crystal surface, the seed quantity required to induce precipitation reflects urinary inhibitor activity.

Nucleation inhibition effects can also be detected by Coulter counter/Channelyzer techniques. Passage of crystals through a fine capillary tube of known geometry generates impedance changes, the pulse amplitude being directly proportional to particle number.

Gel crystallization (ACHILLES et al. 1980; ACHILLES 1984; BOTHOR et al. 1984; SCHNEIDER et al. 1984) is also convenient for testing the effects of inhibitors. Calcium and oxalate are dropped onto a gel, where a standard quantitative crystallization pattern can be established. The addition of inhibitors will alter the width and density of the crystallization band, depending on their effectiveness. A photometric extinction profile can be drawn and an inhibition index thus computed.

Pyrosphosphate has definitely been confirmed as an inhibitor of calcium oxalate precipitation (FLEISCH and BISAZ 1964; MEYER and SMITH 1975; DRACH et al. 1978), as have citrate (MEYER and SMITH 1975) and magnesium (MEYER and SMITH 1975).

Macromolecules also play a part as calcium oxalate precipitation inhibitors (GILL and KARESCH 1976; GILL et al. 1977), particularly glycosaminoglycans (ITO and COE 1977) and polypeptides (ITO and COE 1977).

Pyrophosphate inhibits the transformation of amorphous calcium phosphate to the crystalline phase (FLEISCH et al. 1968; FRANCIS 1969).

Crystal growth is an important field of fundamental research, currently focussing on measurements and computations of growth and inhibition kinetics (BLIZNAKOW 1965; FINLAYSON 1972; FINLAYSON and DUBOIS 1973; JUNG et al. 1973; ROBERTSON et al. 1973; NANCOLLAS and GARDNER 1974; MEYER and SMITH 1975; NANCOLLAS 1976; LEAL and FINLAYSON 1977; MILLER et al. 1977; BIJVOET et al. 1978; GARDNER 1978; BLOMEN et al. 1979; TISELIUS 1980;

FUEREDI-MILHOFER 1981; SHEEHAN and NANCOLLAS 1981; BLOMEN 1982; NORDENVALL 1982; JOOST et al. 1985; MEYER 1985, WILSON et al. 1985).

WILL et al. (1976, 1977), BIJVOET et al. (1978), BLOMEN (1982), and BLOMEN et al. (1983) report a technique for studying the effect of urine and various other additives on the growth of calcium oxalate crystals. The basic principle is the measurement of ^{45}Calcium uptake from a supersaturated calcium oxalate solution when calcium oxalate monohydrate crystals are added. The crystal radioactivity retained by a filter after twenty minutes is expressed as a fraction of the total count. Fractional reduction in isotope uptake can be shown to be a measure of fractional growth constant reduction.

WERNESS et al. (1981) used various modified systems to determine the effect of mixed inhibitors.

Inhibitory action on calcium oxalate crystal growth was determined by a modification of the MEYER and SMITH (1975) method: Control runs (no inhibitor) were performed with each test series (inhibitors) by adding 2.0 ml $CaCl_2$ (0.016 M) to 65.0 ml NaCl (0.148 M), equilibrating at 37 °C and slowly stirring in 3.0 ml $K_2C_2O_4$ (0.01 M). The pH was adjusted to 6.0 and a seeding slurry added (approx. 0.2 ml) to give a growth rate of about 600 Mol min^{-1} l^{-1}. Aliquots were removed at 0, 5, 15, 30 and 50 minutes, filtered through an 0.22 micron millipore filter ("Metricel") and assayed for calcium by atomic absorption. Rate constants were then calculated as described by MEYER and SMITH (1975a).

Each inhibitor was tested separately for potency, inhibitors being added to the supersaturated calcium oxalate assay solution before seeding. Al least three concentrations of each inhibitor were used to calculate inhibitory activity by fitting them to the Langmuir adsorption isotherm. When mixtures of inhibitors were tested, data from single inhibitor studies was used to concoct mixtures in which each inhibitor would theoretically contribute an equal inhibitory effect. Solutions were first assayed for calcium and sodium concentration crystal growth assay solutions were adjusted to compensate for sodium and calcium in the added urine. The quantity of oxalate contributed by normal urine was usually negligible and was not compensated for. The inhibitory effect of each urine sample was measured as above and mixtures of urine and inhibitors then tested. All solutions were unbuffered, the pH being monitored continuously and adjusted to stay between 5.9 and 6.1. Calculations were performed by linear regression analysis, as described by MEYER and SMITH (1975a, b).

WERNESS et al. (1981) used a modification of the MEYER and NANCOLLAS (1972) or MEYER et al. (1975) method to determine inhibitory activity toward hydroxyapatite: Control runs (no inhibitor) involved adding 4.86 ml $CaCl_2$ (0.028 M) and 4.88 ml KH_2PO_4 (0.018 M) to 65 ml NaCl (0.15 M) and adjusting the pH to 7.4 with 0.086 M NaOH. The reaction vessel was kept in pH-stat (Metrohm, Combinator-3 D) while 0.1 ml hydroxyapatite seed slurry (approx. 20 mg/ml) were added. The volume of 0.086 M NaOH needed to maintain a constant pH was recorded over the next 60 minutes, and rate constants were then calculated from the amount of base added and from the known stoichiometry of hydroxyapatite precipitation (MEYER and NANCOLLAS 1972). Inhibitors could now be assayed in the same manner as that described for the calcium oxalate monohydrate system. Urines were first assayed for calcium and phosphate concentrations and the crystal growth solutions adjusted if necessary. Complexing of calcium by citrate and of phosphate by magnesium were corrected for in all experiments, thus maintaining a constant initial state of supersaturation, whatever amount of inhibitor was to be added.

In addition, a method was described for measuring uric acid crystal growth. Uric acid seed crystals are added to a supersaturated uric acid solution prepared by equilibrating 0.15 M uric acid solution with solid uric acid at 37 °C and pH 5.8. Excess solid uric acid is filtered out and the pH slowly adjusted to 5.0. Crystal growth rate can then be determined by passing aliquots through an 0.22 micron millipore filter at 0, 10, 25, 50 and 75 minutes, diluting the filtrate 1 : 20 with distilled water and reading absorbance at 294 nm (WERNESS et al. 1982).

In summary it can be said that pyrophosphate exerts pronounced inhibition on calcium oxalate and calcium phosphate crystal growth (FLEISCH and BISAZ 1964; RUSSEL and FLEISCH 1969, 1972; FLEISCH and MONOD 1973; ROBERTSON et al. 1973; BISAZ et al. 1978). Citrate inhibits the growth of calcium oxalate (FINLAYSON 1974) and hydroxyapatite crystals (SMITH et al. 1973).

At concentrations between 10^{-3} and 10^{-6} M magnesium was devoid of inhibitory effect on calcium oxalate (ROBERTSON et al. 1973) but had a weak effect on hydroxyapatite crystal growth (BACHRA and FISCHER 1969).

Crystal aggregation and the inhibition thereof have attracted scrutiny, insofar as aggregates are rarely found in healthy individuals whilst commonly occurring in stone formers (ROBERTSON et al. 1969; ROBERTSON and PEACOCK 1972; ROSE 1977).

Aggregation has been studied in vitro by adding disaggregated crystals to slightly supersaturated solutions and counting the rate of aggregate formation per unit time on a Coulter Channelyser (ROBERTSON 1969; ROBERTSON et al. 1969; ROBERTSON and PEACOCK 1972; FLEISCH and MONOD 1973; FELIX et al. 1976, 1977; HANSEN et al. 1976; HARTUNG and LESKOVAR 1976; CURRERI et al. 1981; RODGERS and GARSIDE 1981; RYALL et al. 1981; RYALL and MARSHALL 1981; BLOMEN 1982; BLOMEN et al. 1983; ROBERTSON et al. 1984).

Channelyzer techniques also permit disaggregating additives to be studied in their effect either on aggregates formed in solution or on added crushed stone material (LESKOVAR and HARTUNG 1977; LESKOVAR et al. 1979).

In 1974 FLEISCH presented his Agglometer, an instrument which counts particles faster, more simply and at less cost than the Coulter counter.

Test fluid is forced through a microfilter of 20 micron pore size under constant pressure. The pore size is chosen to allow individual calcium oxalate crystals to slip through whilst retaining aggregates. The filtration rate over a few seconds is displayed graphically: If there are no aggregates, the graph is a straight line but, flattening of the curve develops as aggregates are arrested in the filter and progressively block it, thereby reducing the filtration rate. The overall volume filtered over a given interval can be expressed as a degree of aggregation.

A number of studies have shown urine to have a more marked inhibitory action on aggregation than on crystallization. ROBERTSON and PEACOCK (1972) made the important observation that the urine of recurrent stone formers was less able to inhibit calcium oxalate aggregation than was that of healthy control subjects.

The calcium oxalate aggregate inhibiting power of urine was found to be dilution dependent, the addition of 10% urine totally abolishing aggregation (FLEISCH 1974; ROBERTSON et al. 1976; FELIX et al. 1977; FLEISCH 1980). 10–20% of this effect was due to citrate and pyrophosphate, magnesium making a lesser contribution (MEYER and SMITH 1975; ROBERTSON et al. 1976; FELIX et al. 1977). The great bulk of inhibitor activity was vested in glycosaminoglycans (ROBERTSON et al. 1976; FELIX et al. 1977; DRACH et al. 1985).

Urine has a similarly powerful inhibitory effect on calcium phosphate aggregation (HANSEN et al. 1976). Once again, citrate, pyrophosphate and glycosaminoglycans proved to be powerful inhibitors, with magnesium and other metals lagging far behind in potency (FLEISCH 1980).

The basic classification of inhibitors is by molecular weight.

Pyrophosphate is a potent low molecular weight inhibitor (FLEISCH and BISAZ 1962; FLEISCH 1973; RUSSELL and FLEISCH 1973; SMITH et al. 1973; OREOPOULOS et al. 1976). Urinary pyrophosphate is conveniently estimated with a sensitive and specific radioenzymic assay originally developed by MCGUIRE et al. (1980) for studying pyrophosphate metabolism in tissue culture (WIKSTROEM et al. 1982).

Stone patients have not so far been shown to be pyrophosphate deficient by comparison with normal people (FINLAYSON 1981; ROBERTSON et al. 1983).

Citrate (see above for assay) also belongs to this group (SMITH et al. 1973; FINLAYSON et al. 1983). Patients with urolithiasis have been shown to excrete lesser quantities than do healthy controls (WELSHMAN and MCGEOWN 1976; BACH et al. 1979; SCHWILLE et al. 1979; ROBERTSON et al. 1983).

Magnesium (see assay above) can at best be regarded as a weak low molecular weight inhibitor (SMITH et al. 1973; SUR and PANDEY 1981). No difference in magnesium content can be demonstrated between the urines of healthy people and stone patients (JOHANNSSON et al. 1980; STRENGE et al. 1980; BACH et al. 1981; ROBERTSON et al. 1984).

High molecular weight constituents of urine are disproportionately important as inhibitors, since their concentration is reduced in the urine of stone patients (ROBERTSON et al. 1978, 1983; RANDOLPH et al. 1981). Three principal groups are recognized:

Glycosaminoglycans (GAGS) comprise the acidic mucopolysaccharides hyaluronic acid, chondroitin sulphate, dermatan sulphate, chondroitin, heparin, heparan sulphate and keratan sulphate. Specific assays have been published by TELLER et al. (1962), VARADI et al. (1976), DI FERRANTE (1969), WESSLER (1971), GOLDBERG and COTLIER (1972), BLUMENKRANZ and ASBOE-HANSEN (1973), WHITEMAN (1973), SCHRIER et al. (1979, 1981), MARTIN et al. (1984), AZOURY et al. (1985), FELLSTROEM et al. (1985), MARTELLI et al. (1985), ROSE and SULAIMAN (1985), SCURR and ROBERTSON (1985), TISELIUS (1985).

GAGS have been identified as potent inhibitors (ROBERTSON and PEACOCK 1972; ROBERTSON et al. 1973; GILL and KARESCH 1976; ROBERTSON et al.

1976; HALLSON and ROSE 1979; SALLIS and LUMLEY 1979; BROCKIS et al. 1980; GARTI et al. 1981; HALLSON et al. 1981; HARTUNG et al. 1981; PINTO et al. 1981; RYALL and MARSHALL 1981; SALLIS et al. 1981; SCURR et al. 1981; DRACH et al. 1982). GAG excretion was found by RYALL and MARSHALL (1981) to be of the same order of magnitude in stone patients as in normals. Using the assay technique of BLUMENKRANZ and ASBOE-HANSEN (1973), BICHLER et al. (1981) were able to demonstrate the GAG excretion of uric acid and calcium oxalate stone patients to lie in the same range as that of healthy subjects. On the other hand, patients with large struvite calcium had substantially lower levels, a finding in accordance with earlier reports by ROBERTSON et al. (1978) that stone patients had lower overall GAG excretions than normal. By contrast, ULSHOEFER and ZENKER (1984) have found elevated mucopolysaccharide concentrations in the urine of stone patients and suggest a stone promoting role for these substances.

Ribonucleic acid (RNA) also has a fundamentally inhibitory effect on calcium oxalate (ITO and COE 1977; ROBERTSON et al. 1984; BROWN et al. 1985). On the other hand WERNESS et al. (1981) were able to demonstrate that RNA mixtures had less inhibitory effect on calcium oxalate monohydrate crystal growth than would be predicted from the activities of the added RNA and urine. It was shown that the inhibition is probably due to hydrolysis of RNA by normal urinary ribonuclease activity. These studies and general considerations of molecular weight led SCHRIER et al. (1981) to propose the existence of RNA-like material, responsible for 10–20% of the urinary inhibitor activity seen in their studies.

Finally, a group of *glycoproteins* has been postulated as inhibiting calcium oxalate (NAKAGAWA et al. 1978, 1979; ROBERTSON et al. 1984). This group would include the TAMM-HORSFALL mucoprotein, detectable by quantitative immunoassay (BICHLER et al. 1973; HAUGEN et al. 1978). SCHRIER et al. (1979) found each of these compounds to be capable of up to 50% inhibition at micromolar concentrations, whereas KITAMURA and PAK speak of a slight inhibition of spontaneous calcium oxalate precipitation and crystal growth. By contrast SOPHASAN et al. (1980) were unable to detect any inhibitory effect of the TAMM-HORSFALL glycoprotein in vitro.

β) Loading Studies

Once hypercalciuria has been demonstrated, proper treatment will require absorptive, resorptive and renal forms to be distinguished one from another.

This can conveniently be achieved by a *calcium tolerance test*, of which various modifications are described in the literature (PAK et al. 1975; HESSE 1979; BROADUS et al. 1978; PAK 1978; SAKHAEE et al. 1979; JOOST and PUSCENDORF 1980; KOHRI 1980; JOOST and PUTZ 1982; KORN and BICHLER 1982; FUTTERLIEB et al. 1984; HESSE et al. 1984; KOHRI et al. 1983; MATOUSCHEK and HUBER 1984; PFAB et al. 1984; VONTOBEL et al. 1984).

The calcium content in the fasting urine of *absorptive hypercalciuria* sufferers has been shown to be normal, whilst it is markedly raised postprandially.

PAK et al. (1974) and PAK (1978) therm this "type I", as distinct from a type II. In the latter a calcium load will cause hypercalciuria, just as in type I, but a reduced calcium intake (low calcium diet) is required to keep calcium excretion within the normal range.

Raised serum calcium, parathormone and phosphate levels together with a raised tubular threshold to phosphate are regarded as evidence of *resorptive hypercalciuria*. The fasting urine has a raised calcium/creatinine ratio and elevated cAMP levels. Oral calcium loads result in increased urinary calcium excretion. Note that in urolithiasis the indices of parathyroid function (parathormone, cAMP) will be unequivocally elevated only in cases of overt primary hyperparathyroidism (SCHWILLE et al. 1981). Furthermore, 10–20% of cases have parathormone and cAMP levels within the normal range or belong to the normocalcemic variant of primary hyperparathyroidism (SCHOLZ and SCHWILLE 1981).

Patients with *renal hypercalciuria* have raised calcium levels in their fasting urine. SCHOLZ and SCHWILLE (1981) have demonstrated a concurrent increase in sodium excretion and postulate an abnormality of tubular membrane transport. Unlike COE et al. (1973) or PAK et al. (1974), SUTTON and WALKER (1981) and SCHOLZ and SCHWILLE (1981) were unable to detect any evidence of increased parathyroid activity.

The differential hypercalciuria test after SCHOLZ et al. (1980) and SCHOLZ and SCHWILLE (1981) is a useful aid to the differential diagnosis of hypercalciuria: Patients are asked to attend in the morning after an overnight fast. They bring with them a 24 hour urine collection and a record of the type and quantities of food and drink consumed the previous day. Blood is taken without venous occlusion (to avoid raising the plasma protein and distorting calcium and phosphate levels) on the morning of the test. The patient is then given 2×300 ml tapwater or distilled water to promote diuresis. Urine is collected for two hours to determine basal creatinine clearance and fasting mineral excretion. Calcium uptake is crudely determined by giving 1000 mg (25 mMol) ionised calcium with a commercially available synthetic feed. Three hours later the urinary calcium/creatinine ratio is determined.

Table 9 lists the parameters of 24 hour urine, fasting blood and fasting and postprandial urine that distinguish the hypercalciurias from one another and from the normal.

HEGEMANN et al. (1982), who conduct the test exactly as described by SCHOLZ et al. (1980), have drawn attention to variability in the normal ranges. They attribute this effect to variations in patient preparation, in hospital routine, size of patient cohort and to a number of other endogenous and exogenous, recommending that every center establish its own normal values. They also suggest that diagnostic discrimination can be improved by calculating the rise in calcium/creatinine ration after an oral calcium load (BROADUS et al. 1978). Note must also be taken of the observation by VONTOBEL et al. (1982) that repeated tests yield inconsistent levels of hypercalciuria. Indeed LIEN and KEANE (1983) have denied the test any value whatever in distinguishing the hypercalciurias.

Table 9. Classification of hypercalciuria by the differential hypercalciuria test of Scholz and Schwille 1981 (–) = no change against the normal range; ↑ = at upper end of normal range; ↓ = at lower end of normal range; ↑↑ = above upper limit of normal; ↓↓ = below lower limit of normal

	Hypercalciuria		
	absorptive	resorptive	renal
Serum			
Total calcium	(–)	↑↑	(–)
Ionised calcium	(–)	↑↑	↑
Parathormone	(–)	↑↑	(–)
Tubular phosphate threshold	↓	↓↓	↓
2 hour fasting urine collection			
calcium/creatinine ratio	↑	↑↑	↑↑
Cyclic AMP	(–)	↑↑	(–)
Postprandial urine (3 hours)			
Calcium/creatinine ratio	↑↑	↑↑	↑
24 hour urine			
Calcium	↑↑	↑↑	↑↑
pH	(–)	↑	(–)

JOOST and PUSCHENDORF (1983) have described a reliable outpatient calcium tolerance test for separating different types of hypercalciuria and yielding results as good as those of the classical procedure.

Calcium absorption studies based on the intestinal uptake kinetics of ^{47}Ca (AVIOLI et al. 1965) have also been put forward as a simple outpatient method for classifying cases of hypercalciuria. The isotope is given by mouth as a loading dose and whole body counts compared with the relative ^{47}Ca levels in blood, urine and feces. No special dietary preparation is required in this technique (ZECHNER et al. 1978; HOFFMANN et al. 1982).

In the proven absence of urease positive bacterial infection a urinary pH consistently above 5.8 strongly suggests renal tubular acidosis, a suspicion to be confirmed or refuted by an *ammonium chloride tolerance test.* If the pH still remains above 5.4 the diagnosis can be further strengthened by blood gas analysis (WRONG and DAVIES 1959; BACKMAN et al. 1976; SOMMERKAMP et al. 1977; ALKEN 1981; DANIELSON et al. 1981; HESSE and BACH 1982; ROSE 1982; THIEL and SASCHOWA 1982).

LJUNGHALL et al. (1982) have developed an abbreviated test using ammonium chloride to generate a metabolic acidosis and relating blood acid base balance to urinary pH. This test procedure is also capable of detecting partial forms of renal tubular acidosis, a finding noted by the authors in approximately 20% of all their patients.

In patients unable to tolerate ammonium chloride by mouth the test dose may be administered by intravenous infusion of an isotonic mixture of 70 mMol/l ammonium chloride and 70 mMol/l sodium chloride over one hour (ROSE 1982).

ALKEN and PRELLWITZ (1981) noted patients with hyperparathyroidism to show a sharp increase in calcium excretion in response to an ammonium chloride challenge, so that the latter offers an additional means of confirming or excluding abnormal parathyroid activity.

There can be no doubt of the pathogenetic significance of latent hyperuricemia or hyperuricosuria for both uric acid and calcium oxalate stone formation. Recurrent formers of this type of calculus who have no other demonstrable metabolic abnormality should be subjected to a *purine tolerance test*. If this procedure results in a persistently raised serum uric acid, latent hyperuricemia is demonstrated (OHLENSCHLAEGER and ULBRICH 1976; BACH et al. 1979; SCHNEEBERGER et al. 1979, 1981; HESSE et al. 1981; LUX et al. 1981, 1982).

PFLUEGER and ZECHNER (1981) have documented a correlation between recurrence rates for calcium oxalate or calcium phosphate stones and elevation of urinary uric acid excretion, whereas uric acid stone patients show the same after-loading pattern as healthy controls.

The value of such loading studies for research into pathogenesis has been demonstrated by PAK et al. (1978), who showed that rising urinary uric acid levels in the wake of an oral purine load increase the spontaneous nucleation rate of calcium oxalate in the urine.

In principle *oxalate tolerance tests* can also be performed where specific aspects of oxalic acid metabolism need clarifying (ROBERTSON et al. 1969; ANDERSSON and GILLBERG 1976; BARILLA et al. 1978; CONSTABLE et al. 1978; HESSE et al. 1979; MATOUSCHEK and HUBER 1979; RAMPTON et al. 1979; HESSE et al. 1981; SINGH et al. 1985). The procedure should, however, be performed with discretion, since the hyperoxaluria occuring during the test may of itself increase the risk of stone formation in oxalate stone patients.

γ) Steady State Investigations

Free diet and fluid intake lead to great variability in the urinary excretion and concentration of lithogens and inhibitors (TISELIUS and ALMGARD 1977; SCHOENBERGER et al. 1978; LOUZENSKY et al. 1982). For this reason steady state conditions of standardized diet and fluid intake may be more appropriate to the clarification of key questions.

Table 10. Investigation flow chart for recurrent stone formers investigated at the Urinary Stone Research Unit, Department of Urology, Bonn University Hospital

I. Out patient on free diet (baseline values)	
Day 0	Serum and 24 hour urine
II. In patient on 12 day standard diet	
Days 1–8	Serum and 24 hour urine
Days 9–10	Circadian rhythms of urinary lithogens
Days 11–12	Loading tests for serum and urine studies

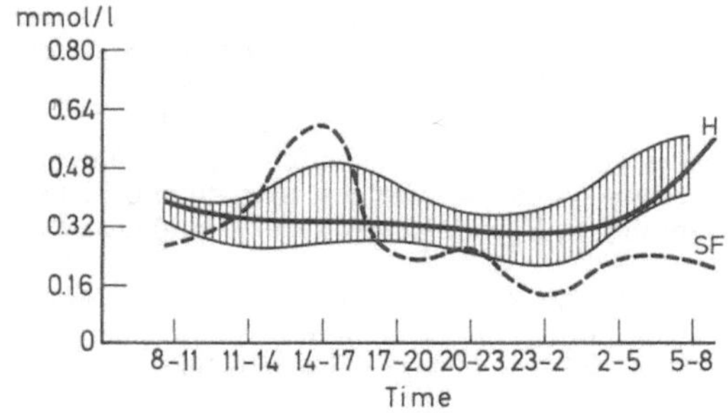

Fig. 1. Circadian rhythm of urinary oxalic acid concentration in a calcium oxalate stone former (*SF*) and in 10 healthy subjects (*H*). The 24 hour urinary oxalic acid concentration of the stone former was 0.250 mMol/l (normal range 0.237 ± 0.067 mMol/l)

Table 10 lists our steady state protocol. It takes 5 days to induce an adequate basal state for studying any parameter of interest (BASTIAN and VAHLENSIECK 1975; BASTIAN et al. 1975; VAHLENSIECK 1979; BACH et al. 1979; HESSE et al. 1979; BACH et al. 1981; VAHLENSIECK et al. 1981, 1982; BACH et al. 1982; STRENGE 1982; VAHLENSIECK et al. 1982; BACH et al. 1984).

First of all, such conditions permit normal values to be determined, by calculating the mean of levels obtained in healthy subjects over a 6–10 day period (see Tables 3 and 7a, b). These normal values form the basis of all further studies on stone patients under identical conditions.

Thus comparison of the levels obtained on free diet and fluids with those under control conditions will reveal the specific effects of the former. Levels persistently higher than normal under basal conditions suggest a non-dietary etiology (PAK 1978; VAHLENSIECK 1979; VAHLENSIECK et al. 1981, 1982; STRENGE 1982).

Considerable interest attends the circadian rhythms exhibited by lithogens and inhibitors on the 9th and 10th days. Typical rhythms occur in healthy individuals and stone formers alike, depending on food intake. Once the normal pattern has been determined for control subjects (shaded zone in Fig. 1), it is possible, following any dietary or fluid load, to demonstrate peaks which will represent risk situations for stone formation. In 24 hour urines such peaks may be masked and be quite undetectable (HESSE et al. 1977; HARGREAVE et al. 1977; TISELIUS 1980; VAHLENSIECK et al. 1981, 1982; HERING et al. 1982; OGAWA et al. 1983; BACH et al. 1984).

From the above it should be clear that the steady state offers optimal conditions for testing the influence of dietary loads (HESSE et al. 1982; STRENGE 1982; STRENGE et al. 1982) and of drugs.

References

Achilles W (1984) Ein neues optisches Mikroverfahren zur Bestimmung relativer Kristallisationsgeschwindigkeiten (Gelkristallisationsverfahren). In: Vahlensieck W, Gasser G (Hrsg) Fortschr Urol Nephrol 22. Steinkopff, Darmstadt, S 377

Achilles W, Ulshöfer B (1985) Calculation of complex chemical equilibria in urine: Estimation of the risk of stone formation and derivation of prophylactic measures. In: Schwille PO, Smith LH, Robertson WG, Vahlensieck W (eds) Urolithiasis and related clinical research. Plenum Press, New York London, p 777

Achilles W, Cumme GA, Scheffel M (1976) Investigation of complex-chemical equilibria in urinary systems with respect to calcium oxalate formation. In: Fleisch H, Robertson WG, Smith LH, Vahlensieck W (eds) Urolithiasis Research. Plenum Press, New York London, p 229

Achilles W, Mergner Ch, Simon M, Berg W, Schneider H-J (1980) Ein neues optisches Mikroverfahren zur Bestimmung von Kristallisationsgeschwindigkeiten. In: Schneider H-J (Hrsg) VI. Jenaer Harnsteinsymposium. Wissenschaftliche Beiträge der Friedrich-Schiller-Universität, Jena, S 61

Ackermann D (1981) Akuter Harnstein: Hausarzt oder Klinik. Notfallmed 7:1248

Ahmed K, Tawashi R (1978) Methylene blue as an inhibitor of stone formation. Urol Res 6:77

Akcay T, Rose GA (1979) The real and apparent oxalate in plasma. In: Rose GA, Robertson WG, Watts RWE (eds) Oxalate in Human Biochemistry and Pathology. Wellcome Found, London, p 82

Alken CE (1969) Gedanken zur Nephrolithiasis. Urologe 8:179

Alken P (1981) Short ammonium chloride loading test for evaluation of hyperparathyroidism. In: Smith LH, Robertson WG, Finlayson B (eds) Urolithiasis. Plenum Press, New York London, p 93

Alken P, Prellwitz W (1981) Calciumausscheidung im Urin nach Ammonium-Chlorid-Belastung. Verh-Ber 32. Tagung Dtsch Ges Urologie, Berlin 1980. Springer, Berlin Heidelberg New York, S 344

Alken P, Schäfer A (1978) Kristallurie beim Cystinsteinpatienten. In: Vahlensieck W, Gasser G (Hrsg) Fortschr Urol Nephrol 11. Steinkopff, Darmstadt, S 183

Alken P, Dosch W, Joost J, Rosenmeiser A (1981) A new approach to oxaluria in nephrolithiasis. In: Brockis JG, Finlayson B (eds) Urinary Calculus. PSG Publ Comp Littleton, p 387

Allwall N (1973) Pyuria: Deposit in high – power microscopic field – WBC/HPF versus WBC/mm³ in counting chamber. Acta Med Scand 194:537

Allwall N, Lohi A, Ekenstam J (1973) Factors affecting the reliability of screening tests for bacteriuria. Acta Med Scand 193:511

Almog R, Shirey TL (1978) A modified orcinol test for the specific determination of RNA. Anal Biochem 91:130

Ammon J, Frick W, Karstens JH, Rübben H, Schoffers J (1982) Ganzkörper-Computertomographie bei Erkrankungen des Urogenitalsystems. Urologe [Ausg A] 18:1

Andaloro VA Jr, Schor M, Marangola JP (1976) Intraoperative localization of a renal calculus using ultrasound. J Urol 116:92

Andersen DA (1973) Enviromental factors in the aetiology of urolithiasis. In: Cifuentes Delatte L, Rapado A, Hodgkinson A (eds) Urinary Calculi. Karger, Basel, p 130

Andersson H (1979) Hyperoxaluria in Malabsorption states. In: Rose GA, Robertson WG, Watts RWE (eds) Oxalate in Human Biochemistry and Clinical Pathology. Proc Int Oxalate Workshop, Wellcome Found, London, p 231

Andersson H, Gillberg R (1976) Urinary oxalate on a high oxalate diet as a clinical test of malabsorption. Lancet II:677

Andersson L (1977) Diagnostic Radiology. Encyclop Urol vol V/1 [Suppl]. Springer, Berlin Heidelberg New York

Arnaud CD, Tsao HS, Littledike T (1971) Radioimmunoassay of human parathyroid hormone in serum. J Clin Invest 50:21

Arnaud CD, Goldsmit RS, Bardier PJ, Sizemore GW (1974) Influence of immunoheterogenity of circulating parathyroid hormone on results of radioimmunoassay of serum in man. Am J Med 56:785

Arora B, Selby PL, Norman RW, Peacock M, Robertson WG (1985) The effect of an increased intake of various constituents of a high animal protein diet on the risk of calcium oxalate stone formation in men. In: Schwille PO, Smith LH, Robertson WG, Vahlensieck W (eds) Urolithiasis and realted clinical research. Plenum Press, New York London, p 85

Asper R, Schmucki O (1979) Measurement of oxalate in urine by high performance liquid chromatography. In: Rose GA, Robertson WG, Watson RWE (eds) Oxalate in Human Biochemistry and Clinical Pathology. Wellcome Found, London, p 76

Asper R, Eggli R, Schmucki O (1978) Simultane elektrochemische Cystein- und Cystinbestimmung im Urin. In: Vahlensieck W, Gasser G (Hrsg) Fortschr Urol Nephrol 11. Steinkopff, Darmstadt, S 178

Avioli LV, McDonald JE, Singer RA, Hennemann PH, Lee SW, Hessman E (1965) A new oral isotopic test of calcium absorption. J Clin Invest 44:128

Azoury R, Goldwasser B, Perlberg S, Wax Y, Garti N, Sarig S (1985) The relative inhibitory potential or urinary macromolecular fractions on Ca Ox precipitation. In: Schwille PO, Smith LH, Robertson WG, Vahlensieck W (eds) Urolithiasis and related clinical research. Plenum Press, New York London, p 839

Babic V, Purgaric B, Despotovic Z, Furedi-Milhöfer H (1976) Precipitation of calcium oxalates from 0,3 M sodium chloride. In: Fleisch H, Robertson WG, Smith LH, Vahlensieck W (eds) Urolithiasis Research. Plenum Press, New York London, p 233

Bach D (1979) Ultraschalldiagnostik. In: Vahlensieck W (Hrsg) Urolithiasis 1. Springer, Berlin Heidelberg New York, S 47

Bach D (1982) Die Stoffwechseluntersuchung beim Harnsteinpatienten. Z Urol Nephrol 75:545

Bach D, Doppelfeld E (1979) Nuclearmedizinische Untersuchungen und ihre Indikation. In: Vahlensieck W (Hrsg) Urolithiasis 1. Springer, Berlin Heidelberg New York, S 40

Bach D, Rohde M, Schneeberger W, Hamm W, Dewes W, Vahlensieck W, Zilliken F (1978) Circadiane Ausscheidung von Calcium, Magnesium und Harnsäure im Urin von Calciumoxalatsteinträgern unter Standardkost. In: Vahlensieck W, Gasser G (Hrsg) Fortschr Urol Nephrol 11. Steinkopff, Darmstadt, S 274

Bach D, Schneeberger W, Hesse A, Vahlensieck W (1979) Erste Erfahrungen mit einem Harnsäure-Belastungstest im Harnstein-Screening. Therapiewoche 29:1482

Bach D, Hesse A, Schneeberger W, Vahlensieck W, Hamm W (1979) Tages- und Nachtrhythmus der Citronensäureausscheidung bei Oxalsteinpatienten und Gesunden. In: Grasser G, Vahlensieck W (Hrsg) Fortschr Urol Nephrol 14. Steinkopff, Darmstadt, S 96

Bach D, Hesse A, Strenge A, Vahlensieck W (1979) Excretion and circadian rhythm of oxalic acid in calcium oxalate stone formers and normal subjects on a standard diet. In: Rose GA, Robertson WG, Watts RWE (eds) Oxalate in human biochemistry and clinical pathology. Wellcome Found, London, p 251

Bach D, Hesse A, Vahlensieck W (1981) Magnesium excretion in urine on condition of individual as well as standard diet in healthy controls and calcium oxalate stone-formers. In: Smith LH, Robertson WG, Finlayson B (eds) Urolithiasis. Plenum Press, New York London, p 45

Bach D, Hesse A, Vahlensieck W (1981) 24-h-excretion and circadian rhythm of citric acid in stone-formers and normal subjects on a standard diet. In: Brockis JG, Finlayson B (eds) Urinary Calculus. PSG Publ Comp, Littleton, p 117

Bach D, Hesse A, Vahlensieck W (1982) Die Vorteile einer Stoffwechseluntersuchung unter Standardkosten in der Harnsteindiagnostik. In: Schneider H-J, Bothor C (Hrsg) VII. Jenaer Harnsteinsymposium. Wissenschaftliche Beiträge der Friedrich-Schiller-Universität, Jena, S 87

Bach A, Hesse A, Strenge A, Vahlensieck W (1982) Normal values of lithogenic and inhibitory substances in urine-evaluation of risk situations for stone formation on the basis of urinary volume. XIX. Congr. Soc. Internat. Urol., San Francisco

Bach D, Hesse A, Dewes W, Vahlensieck W (1984) Die Bedeutung circadianer Rhythmen von Calcium, Oxalsäure und Harnsäure für die Ermittlung von Risikosituationen der Calciumsteinbildung. In: Vahlensieck W, Gasser G (Hrsg) Fortschr Urol Nephrol 22. Steinkopff, Darmstadt, S 336

Bachra BN, Fischer HRA (1969) The effect of some inhibitors on the nucleation and crystal growth of apatite. Calcif Tissue Res 3:348

Backman U, Danielson BG, Sohtell M (1976) A short duration renal acidification test. Scand J Urol Nephrol [Suppl] 35:33

Backman U, Danielson BG, Sohtell M (1976) Beta-2-microglobulin excretion in renal stone-formers. In: Fleisch H, Robertson WG, Smith LH, Vahlensieck W (eds) Urolithiasis Research. Plenum Press, New York London, p 405

Backmann L, Backmann U, Danielson BG, Nordenvall B (1985) Renal tubular function in patients following intestinal By-pass operation. In: Schwille PO, Smith LH, Robertson WG, Vahlensieck W (eds) Urolithiasis and related clinical research. Plenum Press, New York London, p 143

Bais R, Potenzny N, Rofe AM, Conyers RAJ (1985) The measurement of oxalate and glycolate with immobilized enzyme systems. In: Schwille PO, Smith LH, Robertson WG, Vahlensieck W (eds) Urolithiasis and related clinical research. Plenum Press, New York London, p 669

Barilla DE, Townsend J, Pak CYC (1978) An exaggerated augmentation of renal calcium excretion after oral glucose ingestion in patients with renal hypercalciuria. Invest Urol 15:486

Barker MCJ, Noble R, Williams RE (1982) In-vivo labelling of renal calculi with technetium 99m methylene diphosphonate. Br J Radiol 55:39

Barnett E, Morley P (1972) Diagnostic ultrasound in renal disease. Br Med Bull 28:196

Bartels H (1981) Uro-Sonographie. Springer, Berlin Heidelberg New York, S 88

Bastian HP, Vahlensieck W (1975) The value of standard diet in urolithiasis. Europ Urol 1:235

Bastian HP, Vahlensieck W (1976) Nephrolithiasis und Gravidität. Verh. Ber. 27 Tgg. Dtsch. Ges. Urologie, Düsseldorf 1975. Springer, Berlin Heidelberg New York, S 339

Bastian HP, Vahlensieck W, Fillmann B (1975) Die Elektrolytausscheidung im Urin bei Harnsteinpatienten unter Standarddiät. In: Vahlensieck W, Gasser G (Hrsg) Fortschr Urol Nephrol. Steinkopff, Darmstadt, 7:83

Baumann JM (1978) Wert der Sedimentuntersuchung bei Kalziumnephrolithiasis. In: Vahlensieck W, Gasser G (Hrsg) Fortschr Urol Nephrol 11. Steinkopff, Darmstadt, S 192

Baumann JM, Ganz U, Felix R, Fleisch H, Rutishauser G (1975) Die Kristallisationshemmkörper im Urin bei der Calciumlithiasis. In: Vahlensieck W, Gasser G (Hrsg) Fortschr Urol Nephrol 5. Steinkopff, Darmstadt, S 52

Baumann JM, Futterlieb A, Lustenberger FX, Wacker M (1984) Kristallisationsphänomene im Humanurin nach alimentärer Oxalatbelastung. In: Vahlensieck W, Gasser G (Hrsg) Fortschr Urol Nephrol 22. Steinkopff, Darmstadt, S 151

Baumann JM, Futterlieb A, Wacker M, Zingg E (1985) Equations defining urinary crystallization conditions with respect to stone-forming calcium salts. In: Schwille PO, Smith LH, Robertson WG, Vahlensieck W (eds) Urolithiasis and related clinical research. Plenum Press, New York London, p 773

Bavilla DE, Notz C, Kennedy D, Pak CYC (1978) Renal oxalate excretion following oral oxalate loads in patients with ileal disease and with renal and absorption hypercalciurias. Am J Med 64:579

Behrendt WA, Kühn D, Stieh B (1975) Vergleichende Prüfung einiger Farbreaktionen für Cystin auf ihre Brauchbarkeit für die Analyse von Harnkonkrementen. In: Vahlensieck W, Gasser G (Hrsg) Fortschr Urol Nephrol 7. Steinkopff, Darmstadt, S 16

Belsey RE, DeLuca HF, Potts JT Jr (1974) A rapid assay for 25-OH-Vitamin D_3 without preparative chromatography. J Clin Endocrinol Metab 38:1046

Bengtson C, Lennatson J, Lindquist O, Noppa H (1980) Renal stone disease – Experience from a population study of women in Gothenburg, Sweden. In: Danielson BG (ed) Proc. Symp. Urolithiasis. Almqvist Wiksell Period Comp, Stockholm, p 39

Berg W (1981) Bericht über die Jahrestagung der Arbeitsgemeinschaft „Urolithiasis". Z Urol Nephrol 74:149

Berg W, Szabo-Földvari E (1982) Das kristalline Harnsediment. Wissenschaftliche Beiträge der Friedrich-Schiller-Universität, Jena

Berg W, Schneider H-J, Bothor C (1980) Das kristalline Harnsediment als diagnostisches Kriterium einer akuten Harnsteingefährdung. In: Schneider H-J (Hrsg) VII. Jenaer Harnsteinsymposium. Wissenschaftliche Beiträge der Friedrich-Schiller-Universität, Jena, S 105

Berg W, Schneider H-J, Brundig P, Bothor C (1982) Verrechnungsmöglichkeiten von Harnparametern zur Untersuchung von Normalprobanden und Patienten mit Kalziumoxalatlithiasis. In: Gasser G, Vahlensieck W (Hrsg) Fortschr Urol Nephrol 20. Steinkopff, Darmstadt S 21

Berg W, Börner RH, Brundig P, Schulz E, Schneider H-J, Mäurer F, Schorch P, Beck G (1982) Diagnostischer Wert von Gefährdungsformeln für die Erfassung von Bildungsrisiken bei der Kalziumoxalatlithiasis. In: Schneider H-J, Bothor C (Hrsg) VII. Jenaer Harnsteinsymposium. Wissenschaftliche Beiträge der Friedrich-Schiller-Universität, Jena, S 125

Berg W, Bothor C, Erler J, Lange P (1983) Sind Silikate nur Kieselsteine? Z Urol Nephrol 76:319

Bergmann H (1981) The Ureter (sec ed). Springer, New York Heidelberg Berlin, p 255

Bernardino ME, McClennan BL (1976) High dose urography: incidence and relationship to spontaneous peripelvic extravasation. Am J Roentgenol 127:373

Beutler HO, Town MH, Ziegenhorn J, Hammer B (1985) Enzymatic determination of oxalate in urine. In: Schwille PO, Smith LH, Robertson WG, Vahlensieck W (eds) Urolithiasis and related clinical research. Plenum Press, New York London, p 677

Bichler K-H (1974) Uromucoidausscheidung und ihre Bedeutung für die Steinpathogenese. In: Vahlensieck W, Gasser G (Hrsg) Fortschr Urol Nephrol 4. Steinkopff, Darmstadt, S 51

Bichler K-H (1975) Uromucoidausscheidung bei Normalpersonen und Steinbildnern. In: Vahlensieck W, Gasser G (Hrsg) Fortschr Urol Nephrol 5. Steinkopff, Darmstadt, S 32

Bichler K-H, Korn S (1982) GAG – Ausscheidung bei Patienten mit Urolithiasis. In: Vahlensieck W, Gasser G (Hrsg) Fortschr Urol Nephrol 17. Steinkopff, Darmstadt, S 203

Bichler K-H, Haupt H, Uhlemann G, Schwick HG (1973) Human uromucoid. I. Quantitative immunoassay. Urol Res 1:50

Bichler K-H, Ideler V, Bröring S (1978) Erfahrungen mit einer enzymatischen Methode der Oxalatbestimmung im Urin. In: Vahlensieck W, Grasser G (Hrsg) Fortschr Urol Nephrol 11. Steinkopff, Darmstadt, S 214

Bichler K-H, Korn S, Malchow (1979) Oxalic acid excretion and recurrent urolithiasis in patients with small intestinal disease. In: Rose GA, Robertson WG, Watts RWF (eds) Oxalate in Human Biochemistry and Clinical Pathology. Proc Int Oxalate Workshop, Wellcome Found, London, p 243

Bichler K-H, Sallis J, Bröring S (1981) Observations on urinary glycosaminoglycan concentration in relation to the type of calculus and its tissue location, and to tissue tumors. In: Brockis JG, Finlayson B (eds) Urinary Calculus. PSG Publ Comp, Littleton, p 335

Bichler K-H, Korn S, Lämmert J, Haußmann A (1981) β_2 – Microglobulin excretion in patients with uric acid stones. In: Sperling O, Vahlensieck W (eds) Uric acid lithiasis. Steinkopff, Darmstadt, p 110

Bichler K-H, Korn S, Lämmert J (1982) β_2 – Mikroglobulinausscheidung bei Patienten mit Urolithiasis. In: Vahlensieck W, Gasser G (Hrsg) Fortschr Urol Nephrol 17. Steinkopff, Darmstadt, S 80

Bichler K-H, Flüchter StH, Harzmann R, Bachmann F (1982) Erkrankungen der ableitenden Harnwege in der Schwangerschaft. Urologe [Ausg A] 21:218

Bijvoet OL, van der Linden H, Will EJ (1978) Inhibition, diminution and retardation, and the growth of calcium oxalate crystals. In: Vahlensieck W, Gasser G (eds) Fortschr Urol Nephrol 11. Steinkopff, Darmstadt, S 224

Bisaz S, Felix R, Neumann WF, Fleisch H (1978) Quantitative Determination of inhibitors of calcium phosphate precipitation in whole urine. Miner Electrolyte Metab 1:74

Bitter T, Muir MH (1962) A modified uronic acid carbazole reaction. Anal Biochem 4:330

Blacklock NJ (1976) Dietary content of refined carbohydrate: an explanation for the "stonewave" and apparent immunity to renal stone. In: Fleisch H, Robertson WG, Smith LH, Vahlensieck W (eds) Urolithiasis Research. Plenum Press, New York London, p 413

Blackman JE, Gibson GR, Lavan JN, Learoyd HR, Posen S (1967) Urinary calculi and the consumption of analgesics. Br Med J 2:800

Blaufox MD (1972) Evaluation of renal function and disease with radionuclides. In: Potchen EJ, McCready VR (eds) Progress in Nuclear Medicine, vol 2. Karger, Paris London New York Sidney

Bliznakow G (1965) Sur le mécanisme de l'action des additifs adsorbants dans la croissance cristalline. In: Adsorption et Croissance Cristalline. Edition due Centre National de la Recherche Scientifique. Paris, p 291

Blomen LJMJ (1982) Anwendung der Rasterelektronenmikroskopie bei der Urolithiasis. In: Vahlensieck W, Gasser G (Hrsg) Fortschr Urol Nephrol 17. Steinkopff, Darmstadt, S 216

Blomen L (1982) Growth and agglomeration of calcium oxalate monhydrate crystals (Proefschrift). Kanters, Alblasserdam

Blomen LJM, Bijvoet OLM, Will EJ, van der Linden H (1979) Kristallwachstum und Harnsteinerkrankung: Die Wachstumskonstante. In: Gasser G, Vahlensieck W (Hrsg) Fortschr Urol Nephrol 14. Steinkopff, Darmstadt, S 210

Blomen L, Blomen-Kuneken W, Huijsen D, Bijvoet O (1983) Sind Calcium-Komplexe verantwortlich für die Wirkung von HEDP auf Kristallwachstum und Agglomeration? In: Vahlensieck W, Gasser G (Hrsg) Fortschr Urol Nephrol. Steinkopff, Darmstadt (in press)

Blumenkrantz N, Asboe-Hansen G (1973) New method for quantitative determination of uronic acids. Anal Biochem 54:481

Böhne C (1969) Früherkennung von Harnsteininfekten durch Nitritnachweis mit Harn-Teststreifen. Erhöhung der Trefferquote durch orale Nitratsubstitution. Med Klin 64:887

Bonard C, Weber E, Koller U, Willamowski K-D, Bachmann F (1982) Rationalisierung im Urinlaboratorium ohne Verzicht auf diagnostische Sicherheit. Dtsch Med Wochenschr 107:249

Bonk JP, Basch RJ, Cheris DN (1966) Spontaneous rupture of the renal pelvis. Am J Roentgenol 98:54

Börner RH, Berg W, Schneider H-J, Beck G (1982) Experimentelle Untersuchung zum Einfluß der Proteasenaktivität des Harns auf dessen Kristallisationsneigung. In: Schneider H-J, Bothor C (Hrsg) VII. Jenaer Harnsteinsymposium. Wissenschaftliche Beiträge der Friedrich-Schiller-Universität, Jena, S 239

Bosniak MA, Megibow AJ, Ambos MA, Mitnick JS, Lefleur RS, Gordon R (1982) Computed tomography in ureteral obstruction. Am J Roentgenol 138:1107

Bothor C, Berg W, Brien G (1984) Gel-Methode zur Messung von Kristallisations-Inhibitoraktivitäten. In: Vahlensieck W, Gasser G (Hrsg) Fortschr Urol Nephrol 22. Steinkopff, Darmstadt, S 388

Bowyer RC, Brockis JG, McCulloch RK (1981) The role of glycosaminoglycans in the inhibition of calcium oxalate crystal growth and aggregation in urine. In: Brockis JG, Finlayson B (eds) Urinary Calculus. PSG Publ Comp, Littleton, p 329

Boyarski S, Labay P (1972) Ureteral dynamics. Williams and Wilkins, Baltimore, p 430

Brandes L, Oreopoulos DG, Husdan H, Crassweller P (1981) Study of calcium crystals in patients with kidney stones. In: Smith LH, Robertson WG, Finlayson B (eds) Urolithiasis. Plenum Press, New York London, p 23

Braun B, Marberger M, Günther R (1979) Spontanruptur des Nierenbeckens ohne vorherige Kontrastmittelgabe. Fortschr Roentgenstr 131:667

Braun B, Pernice H, Dormeyer HH, Gebauer C, Herzog P, Kujat C (1981) Sonographische Diagnostik bei Nephrolithiasis. DMW 106:1030

Braun J (1982) Laboratoriumsdiagnostik beim Harnsteinleiden. Pharmacotherapy 5:54

Brennan RE, Curtis JA, Kurtz AB, Delton JR (1980) Use of tomography and ultrasound in the diagnosis of nonopaque renal calculi. JAMA 244:594

Bretland PM (1972) Acute ureteric obstruction. Butterworth, London, p 79

Broadus AE (1979) Nephrogenous cyclic AMP as a parathyroid function test. Nephron 23:136

Broadus AE, Dominguez M, Barther FC (1978) Pathophysiological studies in idiopathic hypercalciuria: Use of an oral calcium tolerance test to characterize distinctive hypercalciuric subgroups. J Clin Endocrinol Metab 47:751

Brockis JG, Bowyer RC, McCulloch RK (1980) Macromolecular inhibitors of calcium oxalate crystal growth and aggregation. Scand J Urol Nephrol [Suppl] 53:67

Bronner F, Golub EE, Fischer JA (1976) The effect of vitamin D on renal calcium clearance. In: Fleisch H, Robertson WG, Smith LH, Vahlensieck W (eds) Urolithiasis Research. Plenum Press, New York London, p 383

Brown CM, Senior P, Charest H, Finlayson B (1985) Adsorption of RNA onto aged calcium oxalate monohydrate (COM). In: Schwille PO, Smith LH, Robertson WG, Vahlensieck W (eds) Urolithiasis and related clinical research. Plenum Press, New York London, p 843

Brown LG, Albano JDM, Ekins RP, Sgherzi AM (1971) A simple and sensitive saturation assay for the measurement of adenosine 3-5-cyclic monophosphate. Biochem J 121:561

Bruchelt G, Schmidt K (1983) Analytische Isotachophorese. In: Hesse A (Hrsg) Oxalsäure und Urolithiasis. G-I-T Verlag, Darmstadt, S 29

Brühl P (1970) Methoden der Urinentnahme. Diagnostik 3:119

Brühl P, Müller-Marienburg HWL, Sökeland J (1967) Beurteilung von Harnbefunden in der urologischen Diagnostik. Münch Med Wochenschr 109:1448

Brühl P, Adams E, Straube W (1971) Ergebnisse und Erfahrungen beim Nachweis der Bakteriurie mit Uricult. Urologe [Ausg A] 10:14

Brühl P, Nikolai D, Vahlensieck W (1979) Problemdiagnose Leukozyturie. Urologe [Ausg A] 18:278

Brundig P, Berg W, Neumann J, Hoppe H, Cumme GA, Achilles W, Schneider H-J (1980) Kalzium-Oxalat-Aktivitätsprodukte und diskriminanzanalytische Verrechnungen von Harnparametern als Grundlage eines Kalzium-Oxalat-Screening-Programmes. Urologe [Ausg A] 19:278

Burghele Th, Proca E (1970) Sur l'extravasation périrénale spontanée de l'urine. J Urol (Paris) 76:433

Burns JR, Finlayson B (1980) A proposal for a standard reference artificial urine in in-vitro urolithiasis experiments. Invest Urol 18:167

Burns JR, Finlayson B (1981) The effect of seed crystals on calcium oxalate nucleation. In: Smith LH, Robertson WG, Finlayson B (eds) Urolithiasis. Plenum Press, New York London, p 481

Butz M, Kohlbecker G (1981) Fortschritt in der Oxalatanalytik: Erfahrungen mit der Oxalat-Oxidase-Methode. In: Vahlensieck W, Gasser G (Hrsg) Fortschr Urol Nephrol 17. Steinkopff, Darmstadt, S 181

Butz M, Schulte P, Knispel H (1983) Neue Gesichtspunkte zur Interpretation harnchemischer Befunde beim Harnsteinleiden. Verh. Ber. 34. Tagg Dtsch Ges Urologie, Hamburg 1982. Springer, Berlin Heidelberg New York Tokyo, S 331

Canterbury JM, Lerman S, Clafflin AJ, Henry H (1978) Inhibition of parathyroid hormone secretion by 25-hydroxycholecalciferol and 24,25-dihydrocholecalciferol in the dog. J Clin Invest 61:1375

Carmignani G, Belgrano E, Puppo P, Repetto U, Cichero A, Giusti M, Guiliani L (1982) Erfahrungen mit der selektiven Parathormonbestimmung bei Verwendung verschiedener Antisera und mit Belastungstesten. In: Schneider H-J, Bothor C (Hrsg) VII. Jenaer Harnsteinsymposium. Wissenschaftliche Beiträge der Friedrich-Schiller-Universität, Jena, S 202

Chalmers RA (1979) Quantitative determination of urinary oxalate concentrations by analytical isotachophoresis. In: Rose GA, Robertson WG, Watts RWE (eds) Oxalate in human biochemistry and clinical pathology. Wellcome Found, London, p 61

Chasson AL, Grady HJ, Stanley MA (1961) Determination of creatinine by means of automatic chemical analysis. Am J Pathol 35:83

Churchill DN, Maloney CM, Bear JC, Bryant DG, Fodor G, Gault MH (1981) Urolithiasis – a study of drinking water hardness and genetic factors. In: Smith LH, Robertson WG, Finlayson B (eds) Urolithiasis. Plenum Press, New York London, p 347

Cibert J, Massoumi J, Mohadjer R (1972) Symptomatologie bruyante de certains calculs caliciels. J Urol Nephrol 78:197

Cifuentes-Delatte L (1974) El laboratorio del urologo. Salvat Edition, Barcelona

Cifuentes Delatte, L, Medina JA, Santos M, Rodriguez J (1978) Lithiasis urinaria de silice ($SiO_2 \cdot n\ H_2O$) en los animales y en la especie humana. Rev Clin Espan 151:343

Coe F (1977) Treated and untreated recurrent calcium nephrolithiasis in patients with idiopathic hypercalcuria, hyperuricosuria, or no metabolic disorder. Ann Intern Med 87:404

Coe FL, Canterburry FM, Firpo JJ, Reiss E (1973) Evidence for secondary hyperparathyroidism in idiopathic hypercalcuria. J Clin Invest 52:134

Coe F, Lawton L, Goldstein RL, Tembe RB (1975) Sodium urate accelerates precipitation of calcium oxalate in vitro. Proc Soc Exp Biol Med 149:926

Coe FL, Moran E, Kavalich AG (1976) Animal protein and urolithiasis. J Chronic Dis 29:793

Coe FL, Farus MJ, Crockett S, Strauss AL, Parks JH, Porat A, Gantt CL, Sherwood LM (1982) Effects of low calcium diet on urine calcium excretion, parathyroid function and serum 1,25 $(OH_2)D_3$ levels in patients with idiopathic hypercalciuria and in normal subjects. Am J Med 72:25

Coggs GC (1981) Ultrasonic examination of the urinary tract. In: Smith DR (ed) General Urology, 10th edition. Los Altos, Lange Med Publ, p 82

Cole FE, Snyder S, Bennett DJ, Gladden KM, Frohlich ED, Erwin DT (1981) Evaluation of a new oxalate assay. In: Smith LH, Robertson WG, Finlayson B (eds) Urolithiasis. Plenum Press, New York London, p 767

Colombo J-P, Gorgels JPMC, Kaltwasser F, van Oudheusden APM, Peddler J, Peheim E, Weißhaar D, Poppe WA, Koller PU, Bablock W (1980) Urinanalyse mit urotron. Ergebnissen aus der klinischen Erprobung. Med Lab Sci 33:85

Colombo J-P, Peheim E, Keller H, Kutter D, Bostjanic W, Woschnagg B, Siest G, Henny J, Kaehler H, Oette K, Schindler J, Wisser H, Poppe WA, Koller PU (1982) Zeitverkürzte Erfassung von Urinleukozyten mit einem neuen Leukozyten-Teststreifen. Eine kooperative Studie an 8 Zentren. Dtsch Med Wochenschr 107:853

Constable AR, Jaekes AM, Kasidas GP, O'Reigan P, Rose GA (1978) Plasma level and renal clearance of oxalate in normal subjects and in patients with primary hyperoxaluria and for chronic renal failure. In: Vahlensieck W, Gasser G (eds) Fortschr Urol Nephrol 11. Steinkopff, Darmstadt, S 207

Cook JH, Lytton B (1977) Intraoperative localization of renal calculi during nephrolithotomy by ultrasound scanning. J Urol 117:543

Costello F (1979) The effect of ascorbic acid on oxalate metabolism. In: Rose GA, Robertson WG, Watts RWE (eds) Oxalate in Human Biochemistry and Clinical Pathology. Proc. Oxalate Workshop. Wellcome Found, London, p 270

Crabtree EG (1942) Urological Diseases of Pregnancy. Little Brown, Boston

Curreri PA, Onoda GY jr, Finlayson B (1981) The electric double layer at calcium oxalate-water interfaces. In: Smith LH, Robertson WG, Finlayson B (eds) Urolithiasis. Plenum Press, New York London, p 411

Czerwinski AW, Wilkerson RG, Merrilt JA, Braden B, Colmore JP (1971) Further evaluation of first morning urine to detect significant bacteriuria. Am J Obstet Gynecol 110:42

Dahlberg P-J, van den Bergh CJ, Kurzt SB, Wilson DM, Smith LH (1977) Clinical features and managment of cystinuria. Mayo Clin Proc 52:533

Daniels PG, Marangella M (1981) Equilibrium – based computer model for the estimation of urine saturation. In: Smith LH, Robertson WG, Finlayson B (eds) Urolithiasis. Plenum Press, New York London, p 437

Danielson BG, Backman U, Fellström B, Johansson G, Ljunghall S, Wikström B (1981) Experience with the short ammonium chloride test. In: Smith LH, Robertson WG, Finlayson B (eds) Urolithiasis. Plenum Press, New York London, p 71

Danielson BG, Fellström B, Lithell H, Ljunghall S, Vessby B (1982) The effects of animal protein on the urinary excretion of citrate and on acid base status. Fortschr Urol Nephrol 17:96

Daudon M, Reveillaud RJ (1985) Drug nephrolithiasis: An unrecognized and underestimated pathology. In: Schwille PO, Smith LH, Robertson WG, Vahlensieck W (eds) Urolithiasis and related clinical research. Plenum Press, New York London, p 371

DeLuca HF (1976) Recent advances in our understanding of the vitamin D endocrine system. J Lab Clin Med 87:7

DeLuca HF (1976) Vitamin D metabolism and its relationship to pathologies of calcium metabolism. In: Fleisch H, Robertson WG, Smith LH, Vahlensieck W (eds) Urolithiasis Research. Plenum Press, New York London, p 165

Dempsey EF, Forbes AP, Melick RA, Hennemann PH (1960) Urinary oxalate excretion. Metabolism 9:52

Dent CE, Sutor DJ (1971) Presence or absence of inhibitor of calciumoxalate crystal growth in urine of normals and stone-formers. Lancet II:775

Deuticke P (1965) Die Röntgenuntersuchung der Niere und des Harnleiters. Banaschewski, München, S 379–442

De Ridder PA (1982) Spontaneous urinary extravasation associated with renal colic. Urology 19:97

Deutsche Gesellschaft für Ernährung (1980) Ernährungsbericht 1980. Frankfurt, Druckerei Heinrich

Di Ferrante NJ (1969) Acid and mucopolysaccharides in normal human urine. J Lab Clin Med 61:533

Dobbins JW (1985) Nephrolithiasis associated with intestinal disease. In: Schwille PO, Smith LH, Robertson WG, Vahlensieck W (eds) Urolithiasis and related clinical research. Plenum Press, New York London, p 119

Dominguez JH, Gray RW, Lemann J jr (1976) Dietary phosphate deprivation in women and men: effects on mineral and acid balances, parathyroid hormone and the metabolism of 25-OH-Vitamin D. J Clin Endocrinol Metab 43:1056

Doppelfeld E, Weißbach L (1979) Untersuchungen zum Einfluß von Harnabflußstörungen auf die Ergebnisse der katheterlosen seitengetrennten Bestimmung der renalen Hippuran-Clearance. Akt Urol 10:85

Doppelfeld E, Hanisch K, Weißbach L, Breuel H-P, Wesener K, Winkler C (1978) Einfluß von Harnabflußstörungen auf Ergebnisse der katheterlosen seitengetrennten Bestimmung der 131-J-Hippuran-Clearance. ROFO 129:223

Doremus RH, Teich S, Siluis PX (1978) Crystallization of calcium oxalate from synthetic urine. Invest Urol 15:469

Dorsey TE, McDonald DW, Roels OA (1977) A heated Biuret-Folin protein assay which gives equal absorbance with different proteins. Anal Biochem 78:156

Dosch W (1978) Simultane gaschromatographische Bestimmung urologisch wichtiger Metabolite als Routineverfahren. In: Vahlensieck W, Gasser G (Hrsg) Fortsch Urol Nephrol 11. Steinkopff, Darmstadt, S 199

Dosch W (1979) Gaschromatographie als Standardmethode für Metabolitenbestimmungen. In: Gasser G, Vahlensieck W (Hrsg) Fortschr Urol Nephrol 14. Steinkopff, Darmstadt, S 266

Dosch W (1979) Rapid and direct gaschromatographic determination of oxalic acid in urine. Urol Res 7:227

Dosch W (1980) Gaschromatographie in der Urologie. In: Schneider H-J (Hrsg) VI. Jenaer Harnsteinsymposium. Wissenschaftliche Beiträge der Friedrich-Schiller-Universität, Jena, S 119

Dosch W (1981) New glass capillary gas-chromatographic methods for metabolites in urine and serum. In: Smith LH, Robertson WG, Finlayson B (eds) Urolithiasis. Plenum Press, New York London, p 977

Dosch W (1982) Prächromatographische Methoden und Säulenumschalttechniken in der Gaschromatographie. In: Schneider H-J, Bothor C (Hrsg) VII. Jenaer Harnsteinsymposium. Wissenschaftliche Beiträge der Friedrich-Schiller-Universität, Jena, S 226

Drach GW, Randolph AD, Miller JD (1978) Inhibition of calcium oxalate dihydrate crystallization by chemical modifiers: I. Pyrophosphate and Methylene blue. J Urol 119:99

Drach GW, Kraljevich Z, Randolph AD (1982) Effects of high molecular weight urinary macromolecules on crystallization of calcium oxalate dihydrate. J Urol 127:805

Drach GW, Springman K, Gottung B, Randolph A (1985) Effects of human urine on aggregation of calcium oxalate crystals: Normal persons versus stone-formers. In: Schwille PO, Smith LH, Robertson WG, Vahlensieck W (eds) Urolithiasis and related clinical research. Plenum Press, New York London, p 875

Drawz G, Wiechert P, Hoffmann L, Drawz B, Tittelbach-Helmrich W, Erdmann Th (1982) Die quantitative Aminosäurebestimmung im Harn bei Zystinsteinpatienten. In: Schneider H-J, Bothor C (Hrsg) VII. Jenaer Harnsteinsymposium. Wissenschaftliche Beiträge der Friedrich-Schiller-Universität, Jena, S 163

Dyer R, Nordin BEC (1967) Urinary crystals and their relation to stone formation. Nature 215:751

Edell S, Zegel H (1978) Ultrasonic evaluation of renal calculi. Am J Roentgenol 130:261

Egert H, Breitfellner G, Holzhey P (1971) Ergebnisse der diagnostischen Blasenpunktion. Wien Klin Wochenschr 83:180

Eisman JA, Hamstra AJ, Kream BE, DeLuca HF (1976) A sensitive, precise, and convenient method for determination of 1,25 hydroxy vitamin D in human plasma. Arch Biochem Biophys 176:235

Elliot JR jr, Gordon JO, Evans JW, Platt L (1975) A stone season. A 10-year retrospective study of 768 surgical stone cases with respect to seasonal variations. J Urol 114:574

Elliot JS (1973) A comparison of the chemical composition of urine in normal subjects and in patients with calcium oxalate urinary calculi. In: Cifuentes Delatte L, Rapado A, Hodgkinson A (eds) Urinary Calculi. Karger, Basel München Paris London New York Sidney, p 24

Elliot JS, Rabinowitz JN (1976) Crystal habit, structure and incidence in the urine of a hospital population. In: Fleisch H, Robertson WG, Smith LH, Vahlensieck W (eds) Urolithiasis Research, p 257

Elliot JS, Rabinowitz JN (1978) Diagnostik der Harnkristalle. Extracta Urol 1:11

Elliot JS, Rabinowitz JN (1980) Calcium oxalate crystalluria: Crystal size in urine. J Urol 123:324

Elliot JS, Ribeiro M (1967) Calcium oxalate solubility in urine. The state of relative saturation. Invest Urol 5:361

Elliot JS, Rabinowitz JN, Silvert M (1976) Calcium oxalate crystalluria. J Urol 116:773

Elomaa J, Karonen S, Kairento A, Pelkonen R (1981) Seasonal Variation of Urinary Calcium and Oxalate Excretion. Serum 25(OH)D_3 and Albumine Level in Relation to Renal Stone Formation. Fortschr Urol Nephrol 17:121

Emmett JL, Witten DM (1971) Clinical Urography I–III. Saunders, Philadelphia London Toronto

Erwin DT, Roberts JA, Sledges G, Benett DJ, Finlayson B (1976) Estimating urine supersaturation, a comparison of the results of two methods evaluating changes induced by drinking milk. In: Fleisch H, Robertson WG, Vahlensieck W (eds) Urolithiasis Research. Plenum Press, New York London, p 261

Erwin DT, Bennett DJ, Gladden MKM, Cole FE (1985) A comparison of the Tiselius risk index (Ri) and relative saturation (RS) of calcium oxalate (CaOx) in stone formers. In: Schwille PO, Smith LH, Robertson WG, Vahlensieck W (eds) Urolithiasis and related clinical research. Plenum Press, New York London, p 769

Ettinger B (1979) Recurrence of Nephrolithiasis. Am J Med 67:245

Ettinger B, Oldroyd NO, Sörgel F (1981) Renal Calculi in Triamterene users. In: Smith LH, Robertson WG, Finlayson B (eds) Urolithiasis. Plenum Press, New York London, p 131

Federle MP, McAnich JW, Kaiser JA, Goodman PC, Roberts J, Mall JC (1981) Computed tomography of urinary calculi. Am J Radiol 136:255

Felix R, Bisaz S, Hansen MM, Fleisch H (1976) Aggregation and disaggregation of hydroxyapatite crystals. In: Fleisch H, Robertson WG, Smith LH, Vahlensieck W (eds) Urolithiasis Research. Plenum Press, New York London, p 265

Fellström B, Danielson BG, Lithell H, Ljunghall S, Vessby B (1982) The effect of dietary animal protein on calcium metabolism. Fortschr Urol Nephrol 17:112

Fellström B, Danielson BG, Karlström B, Lithell H, Ljunghall S, Vessby B (1982) The effect of dietary protein on urate metabolism. Fortschr Urol Nephrol 20:369

Fellström B, Danielson BG, Ljunghall S, Wikström B (1985) The inhibition of calcium oxalate crystal growth by chondroitin sulphates, heparin, pentosan polysulphate and Tamm-Horsfall glycoprotein. In: Schwille PO, Smith LH, Robertson WG, Vahlensieck W (eds) Urolithiasis and related clinical research. Plenum Press, New York London, p 887

Fellström B, Danielson BG, Karlström B, Lithell H, Ljunghall S, Vessby B (1985) Dietary history and dietary records in renal stone patients and controls. In: Schwille PO, Smith LH, Robertson WG, Vahlensieck W (eds) Urolithiasis and related clinical research. Plenum Press, New York London, p 73

Fiegel P, Höffler D, Ringelmann R (1972) Die Bedeutung der Blasenpunktion in der nephrologischen Diagnostik. Med Welt 23:1705

Finlayson B (1974) Renal lithiasis in review. Urol Clin North Am 1:181

Finlayson B (1977) Calcium stones: some physical aspects. In: David DS (ed) Metabolism in renal failure and nephrolithiasis. John Wiley and Sons. New York London Sidney Toronto, p 337

Finlayson B (1981) Die derzeitige Vorstellung über die Urolithiasis. Extr Urol 4:13

Finlayson B (1982) Evaluation of additivity in the context of a Langmuir inhibitor adsorption process. J Urol 127:816

Finlayson B, Reid F (1978) The expectation of free and fixed particles in urinary stone disease. Invest Urol 15:442

Finlayson B, Roth R, DuBois L (1973) Calcium oxalate solubility studies. In: Cifuentes Delatte L, Rapado A, Hodgkinson A (eds) Urinary Calculi. Karger, Basel München Paris London New York Sidney, p 1

Fischer E (1969) Pyeloxinöse Refluxe bei der Ausscheidungsurographie. Fortschr Roentgenstr 108:40
Fitzpatrick JM, Kasidas GP, Rose GA (1979) A complication of transurethral resection of the prostate: Hyperoxaluria due to intra-operative glycine absorption. In: Rose GA, Robertson WG, Watts RWE (eds) Oxalate in Human Biochemistry and Clinical Pathology. Proc Int Oxalate Workshop, Wellcome Found, London, p 277
Fleisch H (1973) Pyrophosphat und Diphosphonate. In: Schneider H-J (Hrsg) III. Jenaer Harnsteinsymposium. Wissenschaftliche Beiträge der Friedrich-Schiller-Universität, Jena, S 84
Fleisch H (1974) Die Aggregation von Calciumoxalatkristallen. In: Vahlensieck W, Gasser G (Hrsg) Fortschr Urol Nephrol 4. Steinkopff, Darmstadt, S 47
Fleisch H (1980) Mechanisms of stone formation: role of promotors and inhibitors. Scand J Urol Nephrol [Suppl] 53:53
Fleisch H (1980) Different estimates of the risk of calcium oxalate crystallization in urine. Eur Urol 9:231
Fleisch H, Bisaz S (1962) Isolation from urine of pyrophosphate, a calcification inhibitor. Am J Physiol 203:671
Fleisch H, Bisaz S (1964) The inhibitory effect of pyrophosphate on calcium oxalate precipitation and its relation to urolithiasis. Experientia 20:276
Fleisch H, Monod A (1973) A new technique for measuring aggregation of calcium oxalate crystals in vitro: effect of urine, magnesium, pyrophosphate and diphosphonates. In: Cifuentes Delatte L, Rapado A, Hodgkinson A (eds) Urinary Calculi. Karger, Basel München Paris London New York Sidney, p 53
Fleisch H, Russell RGG (1973) Inhibition on urinary stone disease: Role of diphosphonates. In: Cifuentes Delatte L, Rapado A, Hodgkinson A (eds) Urinary Calculi. Karger, Basel, p 296
Fleisch H, Russell RGG, Bisaz S, Termine JD, Posner AS (1968) Influence of pyrophosphate on the transformation of amorphous to crystalline calcium phosphate. Calcif Tissue Res 2:49
Fleisch H, Bisaz S, Felix R (1977) Neue Technik zur quantitativen Bestimmung der Hemmkörper der Calciumphosphat-Ausfällung im Vollurin. In: Gasser G, Vahlensieck W (Hrsg) Fortschr Urol Nephrol 9. Steinkopff, Darmstadt, S 41
Flocks RH, Jönsson, G, Lindblom K, Olsson O, Romanus R, Winter CC (1962) Diagnostic Radiology. Encyclop Urol, vol V/1. Springer, Berlin Göttingen Heidelberg
Francis MD (1969) The inhibition of calcium hydroxyapatite crystal growth by polyphosphonates and polyphosphates. Calcif Tissue Res 3:151
Fraser D, Russell RGG, Pohler O, Robertson WG, Fleisch H (1972) The influence of disodium ethane-1-hydroxy-1,1-diphosphonate (EHDP) on the development of experimentally induced urinary stones in rats. Clin Sci 42:197
Freany R, O'Donohoe P, Bergin R, Bernard J, Maughan G, Muldowney FP (1974) Serum ionised calcium determination by ion specific electrode, and its value in clinical metabolic disorders. Irish J med Sci 143:286
Freitag J, Freitag G, Müller GW (1982) Ergebnisse computertomographischer Nierendiagnostik. Z Urol Nephrol 75:821
Friedel R, Mattenheimer H (1970) Release of metabolic enzymes from platelets during blood clotting in man, dog, rabbit and rat. Clin Chim Acta 30:37
Froeling PGAM, Bijvoet OLM (1976) Acute acid loads with different anions in patients with renal stones. In: Fleisch H, Robertson WG, Smith LH, Vahlensieck W (eds) Urolithiasis Research. Plenum Press, New York London, p 439
Fuchs C (1976) Ionenselektive Elektroden in der Medizin. Thieme, Stuttgart
Fuchs T (1980) Moderne Harndiagnostik und ihre klinische Bedeutung bei Nierenkrankheiten. Medica 1:987
Fuchs T, Gutensohn G (1967) Wert und Grenzen des Nitrit-Testes bei der Diagnostik einer Pyelonephritis. Dtsch Med Wochenschr 18:343
Fuchs T, Gutensohn G (1971) Die Bedeutung des Zeitfaktors bei der Harndiagnostik mit dem Nitrit-Teststreifen. Med Welt 22:1093
Fuchs T, Nübling H, Granold R, Willamowski K-D, Koller PU, Banauch D (1982) Klinische Bedeutung der Probengewinnung bei Leukozyturie. Dtsch Med Wochenschr 107:424

Füredi-Milhofer H, Skrtić HD, Marković M, Komunjer LJ (1981) Crystal growth and aggregation of calcium oxalate in high ionic strength solutions. In: Smith LH, Robertson WG, Finlayson B (eds) Urolithiasis. Plenum Press, New York London, p 401

Fuss M, Vanlanduyt P, Jedwab J (1976) A routine method for the integrated study of microcrystals in urine by light and scanning electron microscopy, electron microprobe and micro-X-ray diffraction. In: Fleisch H, Robertson WG, Smith LH, Vahlensieck W (eds) Urolithiasis Research. Plenum Press, New York London, p 269

Fuss M, Simon J, Fontinoy N, Coussaert E (1979) High Fluid-Low Calcium Intake: Not all renal stone formers adhere to this simple treatment. Eur Urol 5:97

Futterlieb A, Baumann JM, Lustenberger FX, Wacker M (1984) Hyperkalzurieabklärung unter physiologischen Bedingungen oder im Pak-Test? In: Vahlensieck W, Gasser G (Hrsg) Fortschr Urol Nephrol 22. Steinkopff, Darmstadt, S 326

Gaca A, Dosch W (1981) Konkremente der Prostata. In: Vahlensieck W, Gasser G (Hrsg) Fortschr Urol Nephrol 17, Steinkopff, Darmstadt, S 50

Gadeholt H (1964) Quantitative estimation of urinary sediment, with special regard to sources of error. Br Med J 1:1547

Gadeholt H (1968) Counting of cells in urine. Acta Med Scand 183:9

Gadeholt H (1968) Quantitative estimation of cells in urine. Acta Med Scand 183:369

Gardner GL, Doremus RH (1978) Crystal growth inhibitors in human urine: effect on calcium oxalate kinetics. Invest Urol 15:478

Garti N, Sarig S, Tibika F (1980) Retardation of calcium oxalate formation by polyacidic peptides. Invest Urol 13:36

Garti N, Tibika F, Sarig S, Perlberg S (1981) The inihibitory effect of polymeric carboxylic amino-acids and urine on calcium oxalate crystallization. In: Smith LH, Robertson WG, Finlayson B (eds) Urolithiasis. Plenum Press, New York London, p 657

Gasser G, Preisinger A, Eidler R, Kläring W (1979) Kontinuierliche pH-Messung. In: Gasser G, Vahlensieck W (Hrsg) Fortschr Urol Nephrol 14. Steinkopff, Darmstadt, S 84

Gebhardt M (1978) Kristallographische Untersuchungen zur Harnsteinbildung unter besonderer Berücksichtigung von Epitaxie und Fixation. In: Schneider H-J (Hrsg) V. Jenaer Harnsteinsymposium. Wissenschaftliche Beiträge der Friedrich-Schiller-Universität, Jena, S 54

Gebhardt M, Bastian HP, Vahlensieck W (1977) Was kann das Röntgenschattenbild über die Zusammensetzung eines Harnsteins aussagen? In: Gasser G, Vahlensieck W (Hrsg) Fortschr Urol Nephrol 9. Steinkopff, Darmstadt, S 243

Gelot MA, Lavoue G, Belleville F, Nabet P (1980) Determination of oxalates in plasma and urine using gas chromatography. Clin Chim Acta 106:279

Gill WB, Karesh JW (1976) Demonstration of protective (inhibitory) effects of urinary macromolecules on the crystallization of calcium oxalate. In: Fleisch H, Robertson WG, Smith LH, Vahlensieck W (eds) Urinary Research. Plenum Press, New York London, p 277

Gill WB, Silvert MA, Roma MJ (1974) Supersaturation levels and crystallization rates from urines of normal humans and stone-formers determined by a ^{14}C-oxalate technique. Invest Urol 12:203

Gill WB, Karesh JW, Garsin L, Roma MJ (1977) Inhibitory effects of urinary macromolecules on the crystallization of calcium oxalate. Invest Urol 15:95

Gill WB, Jonas KW, Ruggiero KJ, Fromes MC (1981) Calcium oxalate crystallization in urothelial-lined systems. In: Smith LH, Robertson WG, Finlayson B (eds) Urolithiasis. Plenum Press, New York London, p 497

Gilman AG (1970) A protein binding assay for adenosine 3',5'-monophosphate. Proc Natl Acad Sci 67:305

Ginsberg SA (1965) Spontaneous urinary extravasation in association with renal colic. J Urol 94:192

Glaser GM, Callen PW, Filly RA (1982) Medullary nephrocalcinosis: sonographic evaluation. Am J Roentgenol 138:55

Goebel F-D (1980) Beteiligung der Nieren. In: Zöllner N (Hrsg) Hyperurikämie und Gicht 2. Springer, Berlin Heidelberg New York, S 68

Gödde St, Vahlensieck W (1965) Klinik und Therapie von Harnsteinen während der Gravidität. Urologe 4:216

Gödde St, Vahlensieck W (1965) Komplikationen in der Gravidität durch Nieren- und Harnleitersteine. Zentralbl Gynäkol 87:1681

Goldberg JM, Cotlier (1972) Specific isolation and analysis of mucopolysaccharides (glycosaminoglycans) from human urine. Clin Chim Acta 41:19

Götz A-J (1983) Kompendium der medizinisch-diagnostischen Ultrasonographie. Enke, Stuttgart

Graef V, Schmidtmann H, Jarrar K (1985) On the preservation of urines for the determination of citrate. In: Schwille PO, Smith LH, Robertson WG, Vahlensieck W (eds) Urolithiasis and related clinical research. Plenum Press, New York London, p 689

Gray RW, Wilz DR, Caldas AE, Lemann J jr (1977) The importance of phosphate in regulating plasma 1,25 $(OH)_2$-Vitamin D levels in humans: studies in healthy subjects, in calcium stone formers and in patients with primary hyperparathyroidism. J Clin Endocrinol Metab 45:299

Greenbaum BW, Pace N (1970) Determination of citric acid in microliter quantities of urine. Micro Chem J 15:673

Greenberg M, Falkowski WS, Sakowicz BA, Neuman HL, Schaeffer AJ (1982) Use of computerized tomography in the evaluation of filling defects of the renal pelvis. J Urol 127:1172

Grims P, Hocurscak J (1982) Ultraschalldiagnostik bei Harnsteinleiden. In: Schneider H-J, Bothor C (Hrsg) VII. Jenaer Harnsteinsymposium. Wissenschaftliche Beiträge der Friedrich-Schiller-Universität, Jena, S 329

Gröbner W, Zöllner N (1977) Harnsäuresteine und Ernährung. Akt Ernährungsmed 3:82

Guder WG (1980) Einflußgrößen und Störfaktoren bei klinisch-chemischen Untersuchungen. Internist (Berlin) 21:533

Günther HF, Marx F (1968) Pyelorenaler Reflux im Ausscheidungsurogramm. Radiol Diagn (Berl) 9:565

Gunzer K, Bothor C, Berg W (1982) Stoffwechseluntersuchungsprogramm bei rezidivierenden Calcium-Oxalat-Steinpatienten. In: Gasser G, Vahlensieck W (Hrsg) Fortschr Urol Nephrol 20. Steinkopff, Darmstadt, S 271

Gutman AB, Yü TF (1968) Uric acid nephrolithiasis. Amer J Med 45:756

Haber MH (1972) Interference contrast microscopy for identification of urinary sediments. Am J Clin Pathol 57:316

Haber MH (1981) Urinary sediment: A textbook atlas. Am Soc Clin Pathol 57:316

Hahn E, Sökeland J, Wolters A (1979) Kolikbehandlung und pharmazeutische Harnsteinaustreibung. In: Vahlensieck W (Hrsg) Urolithiasis 2. Springer, Berlin Heidelberg New York, S 1

Hallson PC, Rose GA (1974) Plasma oxalate measurement by enzymatic method. Clin Chim Acta 55:29

Hallson PC, Rose GA (1976) Crystalluria in normal subjects and in stone formers with and without thiazides and cellulose phosphate treatment. Br J Urol 48:515

Hallson PC, Rose GA (1978) A new urinary test for stone "activity". Br J Urol 50:442

Hallson PC, Rose GA (1979) Uromucoids and urinary stone formation. Lancet I:1000

Hallson PC, Rose GA, Samuell CT (1981) Inhibitors of calcium oxalate and calcium phosphate crystal formation in urine – a critique and reappraisal. In: Smith LH, Robertson WG, Finlayson B (eds) Urolithiasis. Plenum Press, New York London, p 589

Hallson PC, Rose GA, Samuell CT (1981) The role of uromucoids in urinary stone formation. In: Brockis JG, Finlayson B (eds) Urinary Calculus. PSG Publ Comp, Littleton, p 285

Hansen JL, Freier EF (1967) The measurement of serum magnesium by atomic absorption spectrophotometry. Am J Med Technol 33:158

Hansen NM, Felix R, Bisaz S, Fleisch H (1976) Aggregation of hydroxyapatite crystals. Biochim Biophys Acta 451:549

Hargreave TB, Sali A, Mackay C, Sullivan M (1977) Diurnal variation in urinary oxalate. Br J Urol 49:597

Harris RE, Dunnihoo DR (1967) The incidence and significance of urinary calculi in pregnancy. Am J Obstet Gynecol 99:237

Harrow BR (1966) Spontaneous urinary extravasation associated with renal colic causing a perinephric abscess. Am J Roentgenol 98:47

Hartung R (1981) Die Klinik der Nephrolithiasis bei der Gicht. In: Zöllner N (Hrsg) Hyperurikämie und Gicht 3. Springer, Berlin Heidelberg New York, S 45

Hartung R, Leskovar P (1976) Studies about crystalluria of stone-formers and controls – experiments on crystal growth. In: Fleisch H, Robertson WG, Smith LH, Vahlensieck W (eds) Urolithiasis Research. Plenum Press, New York London, p 289

Hartung R, Leskovar P, Siebert A (1979) Langzeitstudie: Ausscheidung von Natrium, Gesamtcalcium und ionisierten Calcium bei Patienten mit rezidivierender Harnsteinbildung und bei gesunden Kontrollpersonen. In: Gasser G, Vahlensieck W (Hrsg) Fortschr Urol Nephrol 14. Steinkopff, Darmstadt, S 160

Hartung R, Leskovar P, Allgayr R, Schneider H, Bender O, Wellnhofer E, Simmel M (1981) Inhibited precipitation and growth of ca-oxalate crystals in the presence of the alkaline salts of sone polyhydroxycarboxylic acids. In: Smith LH, Robertson WG, Finlayson B (eds) Urolithiasis. Plenum Press, New York London, p 663

Hartung R, Leskovar P, Riedel J, Schneider H, Siebert A, Kratzer M (1981) Classification of stone-patients and healthy persons. In: Smith LH, Robertson WG, Finlayson B (eds) Urolithiasis. Plenum Press, New York London, p 35

Haschek H, Schmidt W (1975) Nierenschäden durch Phenacetinabusus. Med Klin 70:313

Haschek H, Schumann F (1971) Frühzeitige lebensrettende Nephrektomie bei Sepsis durch gramnegative Erreger. Wien Med Wochenschr 121:868

Hattery RR, Williamson B, Stephens DH (1977) Computed tomography of renal abnormalities. Radiol Clin North Am 15:401

Haugen H, Akessin H, Enger E, Meberg A (1978) Uromucoid in normal urine. Scand J Clin Lab Invest 38:49

Hauschka PV, Lian JB, Gallop PM (1975) Direct identification of the calcium binding amino acid, γ-carboxyglutamic acid, in mineralized tissue. Proc Natl Acad Sci USA 72:3925

Heaton FW (1967) The determination of ionized magnesium in serum and urine. Clin Chim Acta 15:139

Hegemann M, Pfab R, Böttger J, Pullmann F, Schütz W (1982) Normalwerte beim oralen Calciumbelastungstest nach Pak und ihre Bedeutung für die Differentialdiagnose der Calcium-Urolithiasis. In: Gasser G, Vahlensieck W (Hrsg) Fortschr Urol Nephrol 20. Steinkopff, Darmstadt, S 286

Hehrmann R, Wilke R, Nordmeyer JP, Hesch RD (1974) Hochsensitiver, C-terminal-spezifischer Radioimmunassay für menschliches Parathormon als Routinemethode. Dtsch Med Wochenschr 101:1726

Hehrmann R, Tidow G, Hesch RD (1980) Primärer Hyperparathyreoidismus. Pharmacotherapy 3:164

Hennemann PH, Benedict PH, Forbes AP, Dudy HR (1958) Idiopathic hypercalciuria: importance of dietary calcium in the definition of hypercalciuria. N Engl J Med 259:802

Hering F, Lutzeyer W (1978) Bestimmung des ionisierten Serum-Calciums bei verschiedenen Formen der Hypercalciurie und unter der Therapie mit Kationenaustauschen und Thiaziden. In: Vahlensieck W, Gasser G (Hrsg) Fortschr Urol Nephrol 11. Steinkopff, Darmstadt, S 246

Hering F, Burschardt WG, Pyhel N, Lutzeyer W (1981) The relation between relative supersaturation and crystal aggregation in urine – a SEM study and a computerized calculation of the ion equilibrium. In: Smith LH, Robertson WG, Finlayson B (eds) Urolithiasis. Plenum Press, New York London, p 441

Hering F, Friedrich R, Ratyczak H, Lutzeyer W (1982) Risikofaktoren beim Calciumoxalatstein – Ergebnisse des Aachener Harnsteinregisters. In: Gasser G, Vahlensieck W (Hrsg) Fortschr Urol Nephrol 20. Steinkopff, Darmstadt, S 15

Herman JR, Goldberg AS (1960) New type of urinary calculus caused by antacid therapy. J Am Med Ass 174:1206

Hesse A (1979) Laboruntersuchungen – Harn und Serumuntersuchungen. In: Vahlensieck W (Hrsg) Urolithiasis 1. Springer, Berlin Heidelberg New York, S 49

Hesse A, Bach D (1982) Harnsteine – Pathobiochemie und klinisch-chemische Diagnostik. In: Breuer H, Büttner H, Stamm D (Hrsg) Klinische Chemie in Einzeldarstellungen. Thieme, Stuttgart New York, Band 5

Hesse A, Schneider H-J, Schweder P, Flach W, Rebentisch W, Suntheim L, Weber C, Taubert F, Köhler H, Klemm D (1977) Das Harnsteinleiden in der DDR. Untersuchungen zur altersabhängigen und territorialen Verteilung. Dtsch Gesundh Wesen 32:900

Hesse A, Berg W, Schneider H-J, Hienzsch E (1977) Erarbeitung eines Ca-Oxalatstein-Screening-Programms auf der Grundlage biochemischer Meßdaten. In: Gasser G, Vahlensieck W (Hrsg) Fortschr Urol Nephrol 9. Steinkopff, Darmstadt, S 278

Hesse A, Bach D, Schneeberger W, Hamm W, Vahlensieck W (1979) Zitronensäureausscheidung bei Harnsteinkranken und Gesunden unter Normalkost und Standardkost. In: Gasser G, Vahlensieck W (Hrsg) Fortschr Urol Nephrol 14. Steinkopff, Darmstadt, S 100

Hesse A, Bach D, Strenge A, Hicking W, Vahlensieck W (1979) The effect of dietary oxalate loads on urinary oxalate excretion. In: Rose GA, Robertson WG, Watts RWE (eds) Oxalate in Human Biochemistry and Clinical Pathology. Wellcome Found, London, p 100

Hesse A, Strenge A, Bach D, Vahlensieck W (1980) Gaschromatographische Bestimmung von Oxalsäure im Harn unter normaler und oxalatreicher Ernährung. Fresenius Z Anal Chem 301:183

Hesse A, Schneeberger W, Bach D, Dewes W, Vahlensieck W (1981) Latent hyperuricemia and hyperuricosuria – a risk factor for some stone formation – diagnosis with purine loading test. In: Sperling O, Vahlensieck W (eds) Fortschr Urol Nephrol 16. Steinkopff, Darmstadt, S 81

Hesse A, Strenge A, Bach D, Vahlensieck W (1981) Oxalate loading test for the diagnosis of oxalate hyperabsorption. In: Smith LH, Robertson WG, Finlayson B (eds) Urolithiasis. Plenum Press, New York London, p 779

Hesse A, Strenge A, Bach D, Vahlensieck W (1982) Einfluß von Nahrungsbelastungen auf die Ausscheidung von lithogenen Substanzen im Harn. In: Gasser G, Vahlensieck W (Hrsg) Fortschr Urol Nephrol. Steinkopf, Darmstadt 20:67

Hesse A, Bach D, Vahlensieck W (1982) Labordiagnostisches Stufenprogramm beim Harnsteinleiden. In: Schneider H-J, Bothor C (Hrsg) VII. Jenaer Harnsteinsymposium. Wissenschaftliche Beiträge der Friedrich-Schiller-Universität, Jena, S 79

Hesse A, Schneeberger W, Strenge A, Vahlensieck W (1984) Differenzierung von Hyperkalzurietypen bei Kalziumoxalat-Steinpatienten durch Anwendung des Ca-Belastungstestes. In: Vahlensieck W, Gasser G (Hrsg) Fortschr Urol Nephrol 22. Steinkopff, Darmstadt, S 314

Hodgkinson A, Heaton FW (1965) The effect of food ingestion on the urinary excretion of calcium and magnesium. Clin Chim Acta 11:354

Hodgkinson A, Williams A (1972) An improved colorimetric procedure for urine oxalate. Clin Chim Acta 36:127

Hoffmann L, Brügmann E, Erdmann Th (1982) Die Bedeutung der Ultraschalldiagnostik beim Harnsteinleiden. In: Schneider H-J, Bothor C (Hrsg) VII. Jenaer Harnsteinsymposium. Wissenschaftliche Beiträge der Friedrich-Schiller-Universität, Jena, S 322

Hoffmann L, Drawz G, Bast R, Wiechert P, Tittelbach-Helmrich W, Erdmann Th (1982) Wertigkeit der diagnostischen Parameter für die Erkennung des Zystinsteinleidens und für die Verlaufskontrolle unter der Behandlung. In: Schneider H-J, Bothor C (Hrsg) VII. Jenaer Harnsteinsymposium. Wissenschaftliche Beiträge der Friedrich-Schiller-Universität Jena, S 158

Hoffmann L, Esther G, Bast R, Neumann J, Seiter H, Kampehl H-J, Erdmann Th (1982) Erste Ergebnisse der Bestimmung der enteralen Kalziumabsorption und Kalziumkinetik mit 47 – Ca bei Patienten mit chronisch-rezidivierenden Harnsteinleiden. In: Schneider H-J, Bothor C (Hrsg) VII. Jenaer Harnsteinsymposium. Wissenschaftliche Beiträge der Friedrich-Schiller-Universität, Jena, S 121

Holmes JH (1974) Ultrasonic nephrosonography. In: King DL (ed) Diagnostic ultrasound. St. Louis, Mosby

Hör G, Heidenreich P (1980) Nierendiagnostik in der Nuclearmedizin. Konstanz, Schnetztor

Hradec E, Skrivanova V, Kocvara R (1982) Nierenangiographie beim Nierensteinleiden. In: Schneider H-J, Bothor C (Hrsg) VII. Jenaer Harnsteinsymposium. Wissenschaftliche Beiträge der Friedrich-Schiller-Universität, Jena, S 311

Hufnagle KG, Khan SN, Penn D, Cacciarelli A, Williams P (1982) Renal calcifications: A complication of Long-Term Frusemide therapy in preterm infants. Pediatrics 70:360

Hug JP, Schmitt HE (1972) Das peripelvine Urinextravasat bei renalen Koliken. Radiol Clin Biol 41:198

Hütschenreiter G, Alken P, Klippel KF (1979) Ultraschall-gesteuerte perkutane Nephrostomie. Urologe 18:157

Ilievski PM, Ilievska SS (1985) Drinking water quality and urolithiasis. In: Schwille PO, Smith LH, Robertson WG, Vahlensieck W (eds) Urolithiasis and related clinical research. Plenum Press, New York London, p 105

Isaacson LC (1969) Urinary composition in calcific nephrolithiasis. Invest Urol 6:356

Ito H, Coe FL (1977) Acidic peptide and polyribonucleotide crystal growth inhibitors in human urine. Am J Phys 235:455

Jelinek A, Hyrsl L, Girl J (1982) Beitrag der Computer-Tomographie zur Diagnostik der Nephrolithiasis. In: Schneider H-J, Bothor C (Hrsg) VII. Jenaer Harnsteinsymposium. Wissenschaftliche Beiträge der Friedrich-Schiller-Universität, Jena, S 332

Joekes AM, Rose GA, Sutor J (1973) Multiple renal silicate calculi. Br Med J 1:146

Johansson G, Backman U, Danielson BG, Fellström B, Ljunghall S, Wickström B (1980) Magnesium metabolism in renal stone formers. Effect of therapy with magnesium hydroxide. In: Danielsen BG (ed) Proc Symp Urolithiasis. Wellcome, Stockholm, p 125

Jongen MJM (1983) The role of vitamin D in the pathogenesis of urinary calcium-stone disease. Jurriaans bv, Amsterdam

Jongen MJM, van der Viggh WJF, Willems HJJ, Netelenbos JC, Lips P (1981) Simultaneous determination of 25-hydroxyvitamin D, 24,25-dihydroxyvitamin D, and 1,25-dihydroxyvitamin D in plasma or serum. Clin Chem 27:1757

Joost J, Marberger H (1982) Urolithiasis im Kindesalter. Urologe [Ausg A] 21:133

Joost J, Puschendorf B (1980) Hyperkalzurie-Diagnostik bei Kalziumnephrolithiasis. Dtsch Med Wochenschr 105:988

Joost J, Puschendorf B (1983) Ambulante Diagnostik der Hyperkalzurie bei Kalziumnephrolithiasis. Akt Urol 14:30

Joost J, Putz A (1982) Diagnostische und therapeutische Problematik der Hypercalciurie. In: Gasser G, Vahlensieck W (Hrsg) Fortschr Urol Nephrol 20. Steinkopff, Darmstadt, S 348

Joost J, Jarosch E, Egger G, Hohlbrugger G (1981) γ-carboxyglutamic acid in recurrent calcium stone-formers. In: Brockis JB, Finlayson B (eds) Urinary Calculus. PSG Publ Comp, Littleton, p 129

Joost J, Silbernagl S, Jarosch E (1981) Excretion of the Ca-binding amino acid, γ-carboxyglutamate, in stone-formers. In: Smith LH, Robertson WG, Finlayson B (eds) Urolithiasis. Plenum Press, New York London, p 81

Joost J, Lang F, Egger G, Pastner D (1982) Beeinflussung der renalen Calcium-Ausscheidung durch Glukose. Fortschr Urol Nephrol 17:114

Joost J, Lusser M, Kleboth K (1985) Calcium oxalate crystal growth: Investigations on inhibitory activity of model compounds and urine samples. In: Schwille PO, Smith LH, Robertson WG, Vahlensieck W (eds) Urolithiasis and related clinical research. Plenum Press, New York London, p 851

Jung A, Bisaz S, Fleisch H (1973) The binding of pyrophosphate and two diphosphates by hydroxyapatite crystals. Calcif Tissue Res 11:269

Jungmann K (1968) Der pyelo-interstitielle Reflux. Urol Int 23:289

Kageyama N (1971) A direct colorimetric determination of uric acid in serum and urine with the uricase-catalase system. Clin Chim Acta 31:421

Kales AN, Phang JM (1971) Effect of divided calcium intake on calcium metabolism. J Clin Endocrinol Metab 32:83

Kallistratos G, Panteliadis C, Marketos S (1977) Zystinurienachweis mit Hilfe des „Urocystin"-Tests. In: Gasser G, Vahlensieck W (Hrsg) Fortschr Urol Nephrol 9. Steinkopff, Darmstadt, S 210

Kaplan RA, Haussler MR, Deftos LJ, Bone H, Pak CYC (1977) The role of 1α,25 dihydroxyvitamin D in the mediation of intestinal hyperabsorption of calcium in primary hyperparathyroidism and absorptive hypercalciuria. J Clin Invest 59:756

Karcher G (1959) Iatrogene ascendierende anurische Pyelonephritis. Langenbecks Arch Chir 291:35

Karcher G, Vahlensieck W (1964) Zur „iatrogenen, ascendierenden, anurischen Pyelonephritis". Urologe 3:22

Keller H, Müller-Beissenhirtz W, Neumann E (1967) Eine Methode zur Ammoniakbestimmung im Capillarblut. Klin Wochenschr 45:147

Kelly S, Leckhim E, Desjardins L (1972) A qualitative spot test for cystinuria. Clin Chim Acta 39:469

Khan U, Malek RS (1976) Spontaneous urinary extravasation. J Urol 116:161
Kierkegaard H, Feldt-Rasmussen U, Hørder M, Andersen H-J, Jørgensen PJ (1980) Falsely negative leucocyte counts due to delayed examination. Scand J Clin Lab Invest 40:259
Kim Y, Linksweiler HM (1979) Effect of level of protein intake on calcium metabolism and on parathyroid and renal function in the adult human male. J Nutr 109:1399
Kinoshita K, Takemoto M, Itatani H, Yachiku S, Kotake T, Sonoda T (1979) A new method for cystinuria: A simple and safe screening kit. Urol Int 34:369
Kitamura T, Pak CYC (1982) Tamm and Horsfall glycoprotein does not promote spontaneous precipitation and crystal growth of calcium oxalate in vitro. J Urol 127:1024
Klemperer E, Oppenheimer GD (1960) Urological complications in Pregnancy. In: Gutt G (Hrsg) Medical Surgical and Gynaecological Complications of Pregnancy. Baltimore
Kohlbecker G, Butz M (1979) A new method for determination of oxalate in blood serum by gas chromatography. In: Rose GA, Robertson WG, Watts RWE (eds) Oxalate in Human Biochemistry and Clinical Pathology. Wellcome Found, London, p 87
Kohri K (1980) Endocrinological studies on pathogenesis of urolithiasis. IV. Pathophysiological studies in hypercalciuric stone formers: Use of calcium restricted test and an oral calcium tolerance test. Jpn J Urol 71:1349
Kohri K, Kataoka K, Iguchi M, Kurita T (1983) Oral calcium tolerance test and serum calcitonin in calcium stone formers. Urol Res 11:33
Korn S, Bichler K-H (1981) Erfahrungen mit dem Kalziumbelastungstest nach Pak. In: Vahlensieck W, Gasser G (Hrsg) Fortschr Urol Nephrol 17. Steinkopff, Darmstadt, S 192
Kratochwil A (1977) Ultraschalldiagnostik in der Inneren Medizin. Chirurgie und Urologie. Thieme, Stuttgart, S 117
Kremling H (1977) Schwangerschaft und Harnorgane – Krankheiten der Harnorgane – Harnsteine. In: Kremling H, Lutzeyer W, Heintz R (Hrsg) Gynäkolog. Urologie und Nephrologie. Urban und Schwarzenberg, München Wien Baltimore, S 304
Kreutz FH (1973) Auswirkungen der Probennahme auf klinisch-chemische Untersuchungsergebnisse. In: Lang H, Rick W, Roka L (Hrsg) Optimierung der Diagnostik. Springer, Berlin Heidelberg New York, S 149
Krizek V, Kuzel K (1982) Screening der Zystinurie. In: Schneider H-J, Bothor C (Hrsg) VII. Jenaer Harnsteinsymposium. Wissenschaftliche Beiträge der Friedrich-Schiller-Universität, Jena, S 218
Krizek V, Sadilek L (1982) Die Hyperurikurie nach dem Fasten als Risikofaktor der Harnsäuresteinkrankheit. Fortschr Urol Nephrol 17:62
Kruse K, Kracht U (1982) Urinary adenosine 3′,5′-monophosphate excretion in childhood. J Clin Endocrinol Metab 53:1251
Kunit G, Schmoller HJ (1977) Zur Diagnostik des Uratsteinsleidens. In: Gasser G, Vahlensieck W (Hrsg) Fortschr Urol Nephrol 9. Steinkopff, Darmstadt, S 154
Kuntz RM, Schütz W (1982) Untersuchungen mit Ultraschall und ionisierenden Strahlen bei Harnsteinleiden während der Schwangerschaft. Med Klin 77:718
Kutter D (1980) Teststreifen zur Rationalisierung der mikroskopischen Harnuntersuchung. Dtsch Med Wochenschr 105:1246
Kuzel K (1973) Simple polarographic determination of cystine in urine with cystinuria. Clin Chim Acta 48:377
Kuzuku EY (1970) Methoxyflurane, tetracycline, and renal failure. JAMA 211:1162
Laberke H-G (1982a) Analgetika – Nephropathie. DMW 107:448
Laberke H-G (1982b) Persönliche Mitteilung
Laker MF, Hofmann AF, Meense BJD (1980) Spectrophotometric determination of urinary oxalate oxidase prepared from moss. Clin Chim 26:827
Lanzalaco AC, Sheehan ME, White DJ, Nancollas GH (1982) The mineralization inhibitory potentials of urines: a constant composition approach. J Urol 128:845
Larsson L, Libert B, Asperud M (1985) Determination of urinary oxalate by reversed-phase ion-pair "High-Performance" liquid chromatography. In: Schwille PO, Smith LH, Robertson WG, Vahlensieck W (eds) Urolithiasis and related clinical research. Plenum Press, New York London, p 661
Latal D (1975) Steinleiden und Gravidität. Verh Ber 27 Tagg. Dtsch. Ges. Urologie, Düsseldorf 1975. Springer, Berlin Heidelberg New York, S 369

Lazica M, Volkmer H-P, Treutler HJ (1982) Die Computertomographie als Hilfsmittel bei der Differentialdiagnose nichtschattengebener Konkremente und Tumoren der oberen Harnwege. Urologe [Aus A] 21:362

Leal JJ, Finlayson B (1977) Adsorption of naturally occurring polymers onto calcium oxalate crystal surface. Invest Urol 14:278

Lemann J (1985) Urinary calcium excretion and net acid excretion: effects of dietary protein, carbohydrate and calories. In: Schwille PO, Smith LH, Robertson WG, Vahlensieck W (eds) Urolithiasis and related clinical research. Plenum Press, New York London, p 53

Lemann J, Gray RW, Dominguez JH (1976) 25-OH-vitamin D metabolism in calcium stoneformers. In: Fleisch H, Robertson WG, Smith LH, Vahlensieck W (eds) Urolithiasis Research. Plenum Press, New York London, p 467

Leskovar P, Hartung R (1977) Experimentelle Untersuchungen über den Einfluß der Harnsäure auf die Kalziumoxalatsteinbildung. Therapiewoche 27:1152

Leskovar P, Hartung R (1977) Hemmung der Nucleisierung und des Wachstums von Ca-Oxalat-Kristallen durch Al, Fe(II), La-, Nd-, Y-, Yb-, Eu-, Mu- und Zn-Ionen. In Gasser G, Vahlensieck W (Hrsg) Fortschr Urol Nephrol 9. Steinkopff, Darmstadt, S 30

Leskovar P, Hartung R (1978) Beeinflussung des metastabilen Bereiches harnsteinbildender Salze durch Kristalle begleitender, schwerlöslicher Harnkomponenten. Z Urol Nephrol 71:601

Leskovar P, Hartung R, Santoso I (1978) Kristallurie, Mikroerythrurie und Prokinurie: Häufigkeit des Vorkommens und der Koinzidenz. Fortschr Urol Nephrol 11:307

Leskovar P, Santoso I, Hartung R (1979) Inhibition of ca-oxalate crystal growth in the presence of some dye-stuffs. In: Rose GA, Robertson WG, Watts RWE (eds) Oxalate in Human Biochemistry and Clinical Pathology. Wellcome Found, London, p 33

Leskovar P, Vogel E, Wellnhofer E (1982) Vergleich der Citraterhöhung im Harn durch Harnalkalisierende Substanzen und citratstimulierende Verbindungen. In: Vahlensieck W, Gasser G (Hrsg) Fortschr Urol Nephrol 20. Steinkopff, Darmstadt, S 352

Lian JB, Prien EL jr, Glimcher MJ (1977) The presence of protein bound γ-carboxyglutamatic acid in calcium-containing renal calculi. J Clin Invest 59:1151

Lien J, Keane P (1983) Urinary cAMP and calcium excretion in the fasting state and their response to oral calcium loading in patients with calcium urolithiasis. J Urol 129:401

Lilienfeld-Toal vH, Hesch RD, Hüfner M, McIntosh C (1974) Excretion of cyclic 3–5-adenosine monophosphate in renal insuffiency and primary hyperparathyroidism after stimulation with parathyroid hormone. Horm Metab Res 6:314

Lilienfeld-Toal vH, Bach D, Hesse A, Franck H, Issa S (1982) Parathyroid hormone is normal in renal stone patients with idiopathic hypercalciuria and high fasting urinary calcium. Urol Res 10:205

Lilienfeld-Toal vH, Gerlach J, Klehr KU, Issa S, Keck E (1982) Immuno reactive parathyroid hormone in early and advanced renal failure. Nephron 31:116

Lilienfeld-Toal vH, Schwille PO, Issa S (1984) Bedeutung des 1,25 $(OH)_2D_3$ bei der Klassifizierung von Nierensteinträgern. In: Vahlensieck W, Gasser G (Hrsg) Fortschr Urol Nephrol 22. Steinkopff, Darmstadt, S 348

Ljunghall S (1978) Incidence and natural history of renal stone disease and its relationship to calcium metabolism. Eur Urol 4:424

Ljunghall S (1985) Incidence of renal stones in western countries. In: Schwille PO, Smith LH, Robertson WG, Vahlensieck W (eds) Urolithiasis and related clinical research. Plenum Press, New York London, p 31

Ljunghall S, Backman U, Danielson BG, Johansson G, Wikström B (1981) Epidemiology of renal stones in Sweden. In: Brockis G, Finlayson B (eds) Urinary Calculus. PSG Publ Comp, Littleton Mass, p 13

Ljunghall S, Danielson BG, Källsen R, Fritjofsson A (1981) Prediction of stone recurrences. In: Smith LH, Robertson WG, Finlayson B (eds) Urolithiasis. Plenum Press, New York London, p 13

Löhr E, Mellin P, Rodeck G, Rohen JW (1976) Atlas der urologischen Röntgendiagnostik. Schattauer, Stuttgart New York

Louzensky G, Moderova M, Kocvara R, Smuclerova J (1982) Normalwerte von steinbildenden Stoffen im Urin bei Kindern und Jugendlichen. In: Schneider H-J, Bothor C (Hrsg) VII.

Jenaer Harnsteinsymposium. Wissenschaftliche Beiträge der Friedrich-Schiller-Universität, Jena, S 180

Lubs H, Würfel S, Knapp A, Fiedler R (1982) Aminosäurenausscheidungsmuster zur Typisierung der Zystinurie – eine Untersuchung an 5 Familien. In: Schneider H-J, Bothor C (Hrsg) VII. Jenaer Harnsteinsymposium. Wissenschaftliche Beiträge der Friedrich-Schiller-Universität, Jena, S 170

Lux B, May P (1982) Langzeitbeobachtung bei Kindern mit Cystinsteinen unter Vitamin-C-Therapie. Fortschr Urol Nephrol 20:383

Lux B, Braun J, May P (1982) Results of examination in renal stone formers after purine load. In: Gasser G, Vahlensieck W (eds) Fortschr Urol Nephrol 16. Steinkopff, Darmstadt, S 75

Lux B, Braun J, May P (1982) Purinbelastungstest bei Calcium-Oxalat-Steinbildnern. Urologe [Aus A] 21:147

Lytton B, Cook JH, III (1979) In: Resnick MJ, Sanders RC (Hrsg) Ultrasound in Urology. Williams and Wilkins, Baltimore, Chapt 17, p 340

Maguire M, Fituri M, Keogh B, Costello J (1981) The effect of storage on serum oxalate values. In: Smith LH, Robertson WG, Finlayson B (eds) Urolithiasis. Plenum Press, New York London, p 963

Mahle CJ, Menon M (1982) Determination of urinary oxalate by ion chromatography: preliminary observation. J Urol 127:159

Marberger M (1983) Klinik und operative Therapie der Steinerkrankungen. In: Hohenfellner R, Zingg EJ (Hrsg) Urologie in Klinik und Praxis, Bd. II. Thieme, Stuttgart New York, S 749–753

Mariß P, Thiede G (1977) Abschätzung der seitengetrennten Nierenfunktion mittels der 99m-Tc-DMSA-Aufnahme. ROFO 126:442

Marquardt H, Hemmati A, Krüger J (1971) Fornixrupturen bei der Ausscheidungsurographie. Fortschr Roentgenstr 115:233

Marshall FF, Smith NA, Murphy JB, Menon M, Sanders RC (1981) A comparison of ultrasonography and radiography in the localization of renal calculi: Experimental and operative experience. J Urol 126:576

Marshall RE, Robertson WG, Nordin BEC (1972) The role of urine saturation in stone disease of the urogenital tract. WHO Symp on Vesical Calculus, Bangkok

Marshall RW, Barry H (1973) Urine saturation and the formation of calcium-containing renal calculi: the effect of various forms of therapy. In: Cifuentes Delatte L, Rapado A, Hodgkinson A (eds) Urinary Calculi. Karger, Basel München Paris London New York Sidney, p 164

Marshall RW, Robertson WG (1976) Nomogram for the estimation of saturation of urine with calcium oxalate, calcium phosphate, magnesium ammonium phosphate, uric acid, sodium acid urate, ammonium acid urate and cytine. Clin Chim Acta 72:253

Martelli A, Marchesini B, Buli P, Lambertini F, Rusconi R (1985) Urinary excretion pattern of main glycosaminoglycans in stone formers and controls. In: Schwille PO, Smith LH, Robertson WG, Vahlensieck W (eds) Urolithiasis and related clinical research. Plenum Press, New York London, p 355

Martin X, Werness PG, Bergert JH, Smith LH (1984) Pentosan polysulfate as an inhibitor of calcium oxalate crystal growth. J Urol 132:786

Matouschek E, Huber R (1977) Über die Löslichkeit von Calciumoxalatmonohydrat in natürlichen und künstlichen Harnen jeweils gleicher ionischer Zusammensetzung. In: Gasser G, Vahlensieck W (Hrsg) Fortschr Urol Nephrol 9. Steinkopff, Darmstadt, S 25

Matouschek E, Huber R (1979) The influence of the oral administration of oxalate, calcium ion-exchanger on the 24-hour urinary excretion of oxalate and calcium. In: Rose GA, Robertson WG, Watts RWE (eds) Oxalate in Human Biochemistry and Clinical Pathology. Wellcome Found, London, p 111

Matouschek E, Huber R (1981) Urolithiasis – Pathogenese, Diagnostik, Therapie. Schattauer, Stuttgart New York, S 21

Matouschek E, Huber R (1982) Computer-Berechnungen zum Einfluß von Magnesium und Citrat auf die Sättigungsverhältnisse des Calciumoxalats im Harn. In: Gasser G, Vahlensieck W (Hrsg) Fortschr Urol Nephrol 20. Steinkopff, Darmstadt, S 190

Matouschek E, Huber R-D (1984) Calcium-Kreatinin-Quotienten im Harn von Calciumoxalatsteinträgern. In: Vahlensieck W, Gasser G (Hrsg) Fortschr Urol Nephrol 22. Steinkopff, Darmstadt, S 307

May P (1973) Die Harnstauungsniere. In: Vahlensieck W (Hrsg) Fortschr Urol Nephrol. Steinkopff, Darmstadt, Bd 3

McGuire MB, Colman CH, Baghat N, Russel RGG (1980) Radiometric measurement of pyrophosphate in cell cultures. Biochem Soc Trans 8:537

McVann RM (1964) Urinary calculi associated with pregnancy. Am J Obstet Gynecol 89:314

Medina JA, Rodriguez J, Santos M, Cifuentes Delatte L (1978) Cálculo renal de silice en un hombre (undécima observación mundial). Rev Clin Esp 151:411

Medina JA, Sanchidrian JR, Cifuentes Delatte L (1981) Silica in urinary calculi. In: Smith LH, Robertson WG, Finlayson B (eds) Urolithiasis. Plenum Press, New York London, p 923

Melchior H (1981) Urologische Funktionsdiagnostik. Thieme, Stuttgart, S 63

Melchior H, Terhorst B (1973) Urologische Komplikationen der Infusionsurographie. Akt Urol 4:99

Meyer JL (1974) Formation constants for interaction of citrate with calcium and magnesium ions. Anal Biochem 62:295

Meyer JL (1985) The relative importance of calcium phosphate urinary inhibitors. In: Schwille PO, Smith LH, Robertson GW, Vahlensieck W (eds) Urolithiasis and related clinical research. Plenum Press, New York London, p 811

Meyer JL, Nancollas GH (1972) The effect of pH and temperature on the crystal growth of hydroxyapatite. Arch Oral Biol 17:1623

Meyer JL, Nancollas GH (1973) Effect of stannous and fluoride ions on the rate of crystal growth of hydroxyapatite. Calcif Tissue Res 13:295

Meyer JL, Smith LH (1975) Growth of calcium oxalate crystals. I. A model for urinary stone growth. Invest Urol 13:21

Meyer JL, Smith LH (1975) Growth of calcium oxalate crystals. II. Inhibition by natural urinary crystal growth inhibitors. Invest Urol 13:36

Meyer JL, Berger JH, Smith LH (1975) Epitaxial relationship in urolithiasis: the calcium oxalate monohydrate-hydroxyapatite system. Clin Sci Urol Med 49:369

Meyer JL, Bergert JH, Smith LH (1977) Epitaxial relationship in urolithiasis: the brushite-whewellite system. Clin Sci Mol Med 52:143

Michielsen P, De Schepper PJ, De Broe M, Valkenborgh G, Tricot JP (1972) In: Meyler L, Peck HM (eds) Drug induced Diseases. Excerpta Medica, Amsterdam, p 261

Miller JD, Randolph AD, Drach GW (1977) Observations upon calcium oxalate crystallization kinetics in simulated urine. J Urol 117:342

Mitchinson MJ, Bradley-Watson JD (1966) Peripelvic urine granuloma. Br J Urol 38:453

Mohebbi G, Zimmermann A, Truss F (1982) Operativ gesicherte Fehldiagnosen der Computertomographie. Therapiewoche 32:176

Mönch E, Jiems H (1970) Screening auf Cystinurie und Homocystinurie. Z Klin Chem Biochem 8:516

Montague DK, Straffon RA (1981) Ureteral calculi. In: Bergman H (ed) The Ureter (sec ed) Springer, New York Heidelberg Berlin, p 257

Moser E, Jocham D, Büll U, Chaussy C, Leisner B (1980) 99m-Tc-DMSA versus 131-J-Hippuran: Ergebnisse bei Harnstauung. In: Schmidt-Riccabona: Die klinische Relevanz der Nuclearmedizin. Schattauer, Stuttgart

Mulholland SG, Arger PH, Goldberg BB, Pollack HM (1979) Ultrasonic differentiation of renal pelvic filling defects. J Urol 122:14

Murphy KJ (1968) Calcification of the renal papillae as a sign of analgesic nephropathy. Clin Radiol 19:394

Naber KG, Kuni H, Madsen PO (1975) Continous infusion urography in unilateral hydronephrosis. J Urol 114:337

Nakagawa Y, Kaiser ET, Coe FL (1978) Isolation and characterization of calcium crystal growth inhibitors from human urine. Biochem Biophys Res Commun 84:1038

Nakagawa Y, Margolis HC, Kaiser ET, Coe FL (1979) Isolation and characterization of calcium oxalate crystal growth inhibitors from human urine. Fed Proc 38:655

Nancollas GH (1976) The kinetics of crystal growth and renal stone formation. In: Fleisch H, Robertson WG, Smith LH, Vahlensieck W (eds) Urolithiasis Research. Plenum Press, New York London, p 5

Nancollas GH (1982) Biological mineralization and demineralization. Springer, Berlin Heidelberg New York

Nancollas GH (1985) Urine supersaturation: The nucleation, growth and dissulution of stones. In: Schwille PO, Smith LH, Robertson WG, Vahlensieck W (eds) Urolithiasis and related clinical research. Plenum Press, New York London, p 749

Nancollas GH, Salimi MH, de Rooig JF (1984) Aspects of calcium phosphate crystallization under urinary conditions. In: Vahlensieck W, Gasser G (eds) Fortschr Urol Nephrol 22. Steinkopff, Darmstadt, S 198

Nancollas GH, White DJ, Lanzalaco AC (1982) The formation of stone minerals. In: Gasser G, Vahlensieck W (eds) Fortschr Urol Nephrol 20. Steinkopff, Darmstadt S 98

Nanra RS (1980) Clinical and pathological aspects of analgesic nephropathy. Br J Clin Pharmacol 10:359

Nielsen SP, Trap-Jensen J, Hartling O, Christiansen TF (1976) Ionized calcium concentration measured by a new double-membrane calcium sensitive electrode. In: Fleisch H, Robertson WG, Smith LH, Vahlensieck W (eds) Urolithiasis Research. Plenum Press, New York London, p 491

Noble RL, Barker MCJ, Williams RE (1981) The location of urinary calculi using radionuclide imaging. Br J Urol 53:513

Nordenvall B (1982) Hyperoxaluria and Urolithiasis. Diss Kongl Carolinsk Med Chir Inst, Stockholm, p 26

Offner M, Uring B (1979) A new method for determination of oxalate in blood serum by gas chromatography. In: Rose GA, Robertson WG, Watts RWE (eds) Oxalate in Human Biochemistry and Clinical Pathology. Wellcome Found, London, p 90

Ogawa J, Kitagawa R, Umeyama T (1983) Diurnal variation of calcium, phosphorus, and magnesium in normal and calcium oxalate stone-forming urine. Jpn J Nephrol (in press)

Ohata M, Pak CYC (1972) Disphosphonate and kidney stones: inhibition of brushite in vitro. Meet Int Soc Nephrol, Mexico City

Ohlanschläger GH, Ulbrich H (1976) Ambulante und klinische Erfahrungen mit einem neuen Harnsäurebelastungstest. Therapiewoche 26:1254

Olsson O (1973) Roentgen diagnosis of the urogenital system. Encyclop Med Radiology, vol XIII/1. Springer, Berlin Heidelberg New York

Ono J, Kobayashi K, Maeda K (1980) Vitamin D and calcium metabolism in renal diseases. In: Berlyne GM, Giovannetti S, Thomas S (eds) Contributions to Nephrology. Karger, Basel München Paris London New York Sidney, vol 22

Oreopoulos DG, Wilson DR, Husdan H, Pylypchuk G, Rapoport A (1976) Comparison of two methods for measuring activity products of calcium salts in urine. In: Fleisch H, Robertson WG, Smith LH, Vahlensieck W (eds) Urolithiasis Research. Plenum Press, New York London, p 325

Oreopoulos PG, Roncari DAK, Akriotis C, Husdan H, Rapoport A (1976) Urinary inhibitors of calcification. In: Fleisch H, Robertson WG, Smith LH, Vahlensieck W (eds) Urolithiasis Research, p 321

Orwell RL, Scurr DS, Robertson WG (1982) Measurement of oxalate in urine and urinary calculi by a new ion-chromatographic technique – a preliminary report. In: Gasser G, Vahlensieck W (eds) Fortschr Urol Nephrol 20. Steinkopff, Darmstadt S 263

Pabst HW (1976) Einführung in die Nuclearmedizin. Fischer, Stuttgart

Pak CYC (1969) Physicochemical basis for formation of renal stones of calcium phosphate origin: Calculation of the degree of saturation of urine with respect to brushite. J Clin Invest 48:1914

Pak CYC (1972) Effects of cellulose phosphate and of sodium phosphate on the formation product and activity product of brushite in urine. Metabolism 21:447

Pak CYC (1978) Calcium urolithiasis. In: Avioli LV (ed) Topics in bone and mineral disorders. Plenum Publ Corp, New York

Pak CYC (1982) Should patients with single renal stone occurence undergo diagnostic evaluation? J Urol 127:855

Pak CYC, Arnold LH (1975) Heterogeneous nucleation of calcium oxalate by seeds of monosodium urate. Proc Soc Exp Biol Med 149:930

Pak CYC, Holt K (1976) Nucleation and growth of brushite and calcium oxalate in urine of stone formers. Metabolism 25:665

Pak CYC, Diller EC, Smith GW, Howe ES (1969) Renal stone of calcium phosphate: Physicochemical basis for their formation. Proc Soc Exp Biol Med 130:753

Pak CYC, Ohata M, Lawrence EC, Snyder W (1974) The hypercalciurias. Causes, parathyroid function, and diagnostic criteria. J Clin Invest 54:382

Pak CYC, Kaplan RA, Bone H, Townsend J, Waters O (1975) A simple test for the diagnosis of absorption, resorption and renal hypercalciurias. N Engl J Med 292:497

Pak CYC, Arnold LH, Hayashi Y (1976) Heterogenous nucleation with urate, calcium phosphate and calcium oxalate. Proc Soc Exp Biol Med 153:83

Pak CYC, Waters O, Arnold LH, Holt K, Cox C, Barilla D (1977) Mechanism for calcium urolithiasis among patients with hyperuricosuria: Supersaturation of urine with respect to monosodium urate. J Clin Invest 59:426

Pak CYC, Barilla DE, Holt K, Brinkley L, Tolentino R, Zerwekh JE (1978) Effect of oral purine load and allopurinol on the crystallization of calcium salts in urine of patients with hyperuricosuric calcium urolithiasis. Am J Med 65:593

Papaloucas AH, Haliassos DA, Zervor SZ (1970) Lithiasis of the urinary tract during pregnancy. Urologie (Treviso) 37:367

Paschen K (1975) Bestimmung des Calciums und seiner Fraktionen im Serum. Thieme, Stuttgart

Peacock M, Heyburn PJ, Barnet M, Taylor GA, Brown WB, Davies AEJ (1981) Plasma $1{,}25(OH)_2D$ in idiopathic and hyperparathyroid stone-formers. In: Smith LH, Robertson WG, Finlayson B (eds) Urolithiasis. Plenum Press, New York London, p 825

Peemöller A, Ulshöfer BM (1979) Calciumbestimmung in Serum und Urin, Vergleich verschiedener Methoden und klinischer Wertigkeit. In: Gasser G, Vahlensieck W (Hrsg) Fortschr Urol Nephrol 14. Steinkopff, Darmstadt S 285

Pendse AK, Purchit AK, Ghosh R, Goyal A, Singh PP (1985) The effect of ingestion of megadoses of ascorbic acid on urinary oxalate excretion in normal subjects and stone formers. In: Schwille PO, Smith LH, Robertson WG, Vahlensieck W (eds) Urolithiasis and related clinical research. Plenum Press, New York London, p 225

Peterlik M (1979) Vitamin D und intestinale Calcium- und Phosphatresorption. Fortschr Urol Nephrol 14:154

Peters HJ (1978) Pathophysiologie der Nierenkolik und ihre medikamentöse Behandlung. Med Welt 29:46–49

Pfab R, Hegemann M, Böttger I (1984) Diagnostische Kriterien und die metabolische Klassifikation von 100 Patienten mit rezidivierender Ca-Urolithiasis. In: Vahlensieck W, Gasser G (Hrsg) Fortschr Urol Nephrol 22. Steinkopff, Darmstadt, S 320

Pfannenstiel P (1977) Nuclearmedizinische Verfahren bei Erkrankung der Nieren und Harnwege. Konstanz, Schnetztor

Pflüger H, Zechner B (1981) Die orale Purinbelastung in der Routinediagnostik von Harnsteinpatienten. Helv Chir Acta 48:485

Pinto B, Paternain JL (1981) Isolation of the oxalate binding protein. In: Smith LH, Robertson WG, Finlayson B (eds) Urolithiasis. Plenum Press, New York London, p 807

Pinto B, Pujol J (1981) Identification of a small molecular weight inhibitor of oxalate precipitation. In: Smith LH, Robertson WG, Finlayson B (eds) Urolithiasis, Plenum Press, New York London, p 637

Pinto B, Bernshtam J, Paternain JL (1981) Mechanism of the heterogeneous nucleation by a urinary mucoprotein. In: Smith LH, Robertson WG, Finlayson B (eds) Urolithiasis. Plenum Press, New York London, p 697

Pinto B, Paternain JL, Bernshtam J (1981) Isolation of a urinary mucoprotein capable of precipitating oxalate. In: Smith LH, Robertson WG, Finlayson B (eds) Urolithiasis. Plenum Press, New York London, p 651

Pollack HM, Arger PH, Goldberg BB, Mulholland SG (1978) Ultrasonic detection of nonopaque renal calculi. Radiology 127:233

Powell MR, Barnett CA (1981) Radioisotopic kidney studies. In Smith DR (ed) General Urology (10th ed) Lange Med Publ, Los Altos

Prellwitz W (1976) Klinisch-chemische Diagnostik. Thieme, Stuttgart

Pundir CS, Nath R, Thind SK (1985) Enzymatic assay of oxalate using oxalate oxidase from Sorghum leaves. In: Schwille PO, Smith LH, Robertson WG, Vahlensieck W (eds) Urolithiasis and related clinical research. Plenum Press, New York London, p 657

Putman JM (1972) A routine method for determining plasma ionised calcium and its application to the study of congenital heart disease in children. Clin chim Acta 32:33
Pyrah LN (1979) Renal calculus. Springer, Berlin Heidelberg New York, S 190
Raaflaub J (1963) Komplexchemische Gundlagen der Harnsteingenese. Helv Med Acta 49:724
Rabinowitz JG, Keller RJ, Wolf BS (1966) Benign peripelvic extravasation associated with renal colic. Radiology 86:220
Ramos F, Vivanco F, Difuentes Delatte L, Rapado A (1973) Cystine lithiasis: determination of amino acids in blood and urine. In: Cifuentes Delatte L, Rapado A, Hodgkinson A (eds) Urinary Calculi. Karger, Basel München Paris London New York Sidney, p 72
Rampton DS, Kassidas GP, Rose GA, Sarner M (1979) The oxalate loading test – a screening test for steatorrhoea. In: Rose GA, Robertson WG, Watts RWE (eds) Oxalate in Human Biochemistry and Clinical Pathology. Wellcome Found, London, p 264
Randolph AD, Kraljewich ZF, Drach G (1981) Effect of urinary macromolecules on calcium oxalate dihydrate crystal growth and nucleation rates. In: Smith LH, Robertson WG, Finlayson B (eds) Urolithiasis. Plenum Press, New York London, p 427
Rao PN, Faraghar EB, Buxton A, Prendiville V, Blacklock NJ (1985) Is salt restriction necessary to reduce the risk of stone formation? In: Schwille PO, Smith LH, Robertson WG, Vahlensieck W (eds) Urolithiasis and related clinical research. Plenum Press, New York London, p 429
Rapado A, Castrillo JM, Diaz-Curiel M (1981) Saturation of urine in primary hyperparathyroidism: its role in renal stone formation. In: Smith LH, Robertson WG, Finlayson B (eds) Urolithiasis. Plenum Press, New York London, p 99
Rasmussen H, Fontain O, Matsumoto T, Goodman DBP (1981) On the mechanism of action of 1,25 $(OH)_2D_3$ in the intestine. In: Smith LH, Robertson WG, Finlayson B (eds) Urolithiasis. Plenum Press, New York London, p 727
Rathert P, Brandt H (1982) Ultraschall und Computertomographie: Fehlleistungen in der Diagnostik. Therapiewoche 32:723
Remzi D, Calmak F, Erhan I (1979) A study on the urolithiasis incidence in Turkish schoolage children. Proc VIII Congress Society International Urology, Tome 2, p 57
Renneberg W (1967) Nitritnachweis im Harn. Medizin Heute 16:286
Renyi-Vamos F, Gellinek H, Frang D, Rosdy E (1960) Über die Wirkung von Infektionen und Verschluss des Nierenhohlsystems auf die kontralaterale Niere. Acta Chir Hung 3:321
Resnick MJ, Gammon CW, Sorrell MB, Boyce WH (1981) Urinary calcium binding proteins and renal calculi. In: Smith LH, Robertson WG, Finlayson B (eds) Urolithiasis. Plenum Press, New York London, p 675
Robertson WG (1969) A method for measuring calcium crystalluria. Clin Chim Acta 26:105
Robertson WG (1969) Measurement of ionized calcium in biological fluids. Clin Chim Acta 24:149
Robertson WG (1976) Physico-chemical aspects of calcium stone-formation in the urinary tract. In: Fleisch H, Robertson WG, Smith LH, Vahlensieck W (eds) Urolithiasis Research. Plenum Press, New York London, p 25
Robertson WG (1985) Dietary factors important in calcium stone formation. In: Schwille PO, Smith LH, Robertson WG, Vahlensieck W (eds) Urolithiasis and related clinical research. Plenum Press, New York London, p 61
Robertson WG, Peacock M (1972) Calcium oxalate crystalluria and inhibitors of crystallization in recurrent renal stone-formers. Clin Sci 43:499
Robertson WG, Rutherford A (1981) Aspects of the analysis of oxalate in urine – a review. Scand J Urol Nephrol [Suppl] 53:85
Robertson WG, Peacock M, Nordin BEC (1968) Activity products in urine. In: Hodgkinson A, Nordin BEC (eds) Renal stone research Symposium. Churchill, London, p 221
Robertson WG, Peacock M, Nordin BEC (1968) Activity products in stone-forming and non-stone-forming urine. Clin Sci 34:579
Robertson WG, Peacock M, Nordin BEC (1969) Calcium crystalluria in recurrent renal stone formers. Lancet 5:21
Robertson WG, Peacock M, Nordin BEC (1971) Calcium oxalate crystalluria and urine saturation in recurrent renal stone-formers. Clin Sci 40:365

Robertson WG, Peacock M, Knowles CF (1973) Calcium oxalate crystalluria and inhibitors of crystallization in recurrent renal stone-formers. In: Cifuentes. Delatte L, Rapado A, Hodgkinson A (eds) Urinary Calculi. Karger, Basel München Paris London New York Sidney, p 302

Robertson WG, Peacock M, Nordin BEC (1973) Inhibitors of crystal growth and aggregation of calcium oxalate crystal in vitro. Clin Chim Acta 43:31

Robertson WG, Peacock M, Marshall RW, Speed R, Nordin BEC (1975) Seasonal variations in the composition of urine in relation to calcium stone formation. Clin Sci Urol Med 49:597

Robertson WG, Marshall RW, Peacock M, Knowles F (1976) The saturation of urine recurrent idiopathic calcium stone-formers. In: Fleisch H, Robertson WG, Smith LH, Vahlensieck W (eds) Urolithiasis Research. Plenum Press, New York London, p 335

Robertson WG, Knowles F, Peacock M (1976) Urinary acid mucopolysaccharide inhibitors of calcium oxalate crystallization. In: Fleisch H, Robertson WG, Smith LH, Vahlensieck W (eds) Urolithiasis Research. Plenum Press, New York London, p 331

Robertson WG, Peacock M, Heyburn PJ, Speed R, Hanes F (1978) The role of affluence and diet in the genesis of calcium-containing stones. Fortschr Urol Nephrol 11:5

Robertson WG, Peacock M, Heyburn PJ, Marshall DH, Clark PB (1978) Risk factors in calcium stone disease of the urinary tract. Br J Urol 50:449

Robertson WG, Heyburn PJ, Peacock M, Hanes FA, Swaminathan R (1979) The effect of high protein intake on the risk of calcium stone formation in the urinary tract. Clin Sci 57:285

Robertson G, Peacock M, Heyburn PJ, Hanes FA, Rutherford A, Clementson E, Swaminathan R, Clark PB (1979) Should recurrent calcium oxalate stone formers become vegetarians? Br J Urol 51:427

Robertson WG, Peacock M, Heyburn PJ, Hanes FA (1980) Epidemiological risk factors in calcium stone disease. In: Danielson BG (ed) Proc Symp Urolithiasis. Almquist Wiksell Period Comp, Stockholm, p 15

Robertson WG, Peacock M, Heyburn PJ, Hanes FA, Ruimet D, Rutherford A, Sergeant VJ (1981) Should recurrent calcium oxalate stone formers eat less animal protein? In: Smith LH, Robertson WG, Finlayson B (eds) Urolithiasis. Plenum Press, New York London, p 359

Robertson WG, Peacock M, Heyburn PJ, Hanes FA, Swaminathan R (1981) The risk of calcium stone formation in relation to affluence and dietary animal protein. In: Brockis JG, Finlayson B (eds) Urinary calculus. Littleton, Mass, PSG Comp

Robertson WG, Peacock M, Quimet D, Heyburn PJ, Rutherford (1981) The main risk factor for calcium oxalate stone disease in man: Hypercalciuria or mild Hpyeroxaluria. In: Smith LH, Robertson WG, Finlayson B (eds) Urolithiasis. Plenum Press, New York London, p 3

Robertson WG, Peacock M, Heyburn PJ, Rutherford A, Sergant VJ, Bambach CP (1981) A risk factor model of stone formation: application to the study of epidemiological factors in the genesis of calcium stones. In: Smith LH, Robertson WG, Finlayson B (eds) Urolithiasis. Plenum Press, New York London, p 303

Robertson WG, Scurr DS, Bridge CM (1981) Factors influencing the crystallization of calcium oxalate in urine – critique. J Cryst Growth 53:182

Robertson WG, Peacock M, Marshall DH, Speed R (1982) The prevalence of urinary stone disease in practising vegetarians. Fortschr Urol Nephrol 17:6

Robertson WG, Latif AB, Scurr DS, Sergeant V (1984) Inhibitors of calcium oxalate crystallization in urine from stone-formers and normals. In: Vahlensieck W, Gasser G (eds) Fortschr Urol Nephrol 22. Steinkopff, Darmstadt, S 169

Rodgers A, Garside J (1981) The effect of some urinary constituents on the in vitro nucleation and growth kinetics of calcium oxalate. In Smith LH, Robertson WG, Finlayson B (eds) Urolithiasis. Plenum Press, New York London, p 641

Rohde M, Zilliken F (1977) Methodik der Oxalsäurebestimmung im Urin und Tagesprofile der Oxalatausscheidung. In: Gasser G, Vahlensieck W (eds) Fortschr Urol Nephrol 9. Steinkopff, Darmstadt S 142

Rollins R, Finlayson B (1973) Mechanism of prevention of calcium oxalate encrustation by methylene blue and demonstration of the concentration dependence of its action. J Urol 110:459

Rose GA (1977) The value of studying crystalluria in the management of calcium-rich stone-formers. In: Gasser G, Vahlensieck W (eds) Fortschr Urol Nephrol 9. Steinkopff, Darmstadt S 60

Rose GA (1982) Urinary stones: Clinical and laboratory aspects. MTP Press, Lancaster, p 135

Rose GA (1985) Advances in analysis of urinary oxalate: The ascorbate problem solved. In: Schwille PO, Smith LH, Robertson WG, Vahlensieck W (eds) Urolithiasis and related clinical research. Plenum Press, New York London, p 637

Rose GA, Kassidas GP (1979) New enzymatic method for measurement of plasma and urinary glycollate and its diagnostic value. In: Gasser G, Vahlensieck W (eds) Fortschr Urol Nephrol 14. Steinkopff, Darmstadt S 252

Rose GA, Sulaiman (1985) Macromolecules in whole urine that promote calcium oxalate and phosphate crystal formation. In: Schwille PO, Smith LH, Robertson WG, Vahlensieck W (eds) Urolithiasis and related clinical research. Plenum Press, New York London, p 883

Rose MB (1975) Renal stone formation. The inhibitory effect of urine on calcium oxalate precipitation. Invest Urol 12:428

Rosenberg J, Weiss B, Hernberg J (1971) Nephrosonography – a new diagnostic tool. J Urol 106:127

Ross J-A, Edmond P, Kirkland IS (1972) Behaviour of the Human Ureter in Health and Disease. Churchill Livingstone, Edinburgh u. London, p 58

Rugendorf EW, Kornmann S, Kornmann G (1982) Screening-Methode zur Erkennung der Kristallisationsneigung im Harn. In: Vahlensieck W, Gasser G (eds) Fortschr Urol Nephrol 17. Steinkopff, Darmstadt S 211

Rummel HH, Walch E (1963) Harnsteinleiden und Gravidität. 2. Geburtshilfe Frauenheilkd 160:105

Rupp W (1959) Kritik der cytologischen Harndiagnostik. Arztl Wochenschr 14:113

Russell RGG, Fleisch H (1969) Pyrophosphate and stone formation. In: Hodgkinson A, Nordin BEC (eds) Renal stone research Symposium. London, Churchill, p 165

Russell RGG, Fleisch H (1973) Inhibitors in urinary stone disease: role of pyrophosphate. In Cifuentes Delatte L, Rapado A, Hodgkinson A (eds) Urinary Calculi. Karger, Basel München Paris London New York Sidney, p 307

Rutishauser G (1970) Druck und Dynamik in den oberen Harnwegen, Steinkopff, Darmstadt, S 61

Ryall RL, Marshall VR (1981) The effect of normal and stone-forming urine on the growth and aggregation of calcium oxalate crystals in relation to urinary glycosaminoglycans and urate concentrations. In: Smith LH, Robertson WG, Finlayson B (eds) Urolithiasis. Plenum Press, New York London, p 611

Ryall RL, Marshall VR (1981) The effect of urine and other inhibitors on the growth and aggregation of calcium oxalate crystals in vitro. In: Smith LH, Robertson WG, Finlayson B (eds) Urolithiasis. Plenum Press, New York London, p 631

Ryall RL, Marshall VR (1981) Separate estimation of the growth and aggregation of calcium oxalate crystals using the Coulter Counter – effect of pyrophosphate and urine. In: Brockis JG, Finlayson B (eds) Urinary Calculus. PSG Publ Comp, Littleton, p 309

Ryall RL, Marshall VR (1981) The interpretation of particle size distribution curves obtained from the Coulter Counter in relation to the inhibition of crystal growth and aggregation. In: Brockis JG, Finlayson B (eds) Urinary Calculus. PSG Publ Comp, Littleton, p 297

Ryall RL, Harnett RM, Marshall VR (1985) The effect of uric acid on the inhibitory activity of glycosaminoglycans and urine. In: Schwille PO, Smith LH, Robertson WG, Vahlensieck W (eds) Urolithiasis and related clinical research. Plenum Press, New York London, p 855

Ryall RL, Hibberd GM, Mazzachi BC, Marshall VR (1985) A whole urine system for studying nucleation, growth and aggregation of calcium oxalate crystals. In: Schwille PO, Smith LH, Robertson WG, Vahlensieck W (eds) Urolithiasis and related clinical research. Plenum Press, New York London, p 761

Sakhaee K, Peterson R, Northcutt C, Pak CYC (1979) Critical appraisal of oral calcium load test for indirect assessment of intestinal calcium absorption. Urology 14:251

Sallis JD (1985) Inhibitors of the precipitation of stone-forming urinary constituents: Are the established inhibitors effective in preventing stone formation and growth or is a moss-covered stone inevitable? In: Schwille PO, Smith LH, Robertson WG, Vahlensieck W (eds) Urolithiasis and related clinical research. Plenum press, New York London, p 803

Sallis JD, Lumley MF (1979) On the possible role of glycosaminoglycans as natural inhibitors of calcium oxalate stones. Invest Urol 16:296

Sallis JD, Bichler K-H, Korn S, Haußmann A (1981) Urinary glycosaminoglycan excretion in patients with urolithiasis. In: Smith LH, Robertson WG, Finlayson B (eds) Urolithiasis. Plenum Press, New York London, p 619

Sallmander U, Öst C-R, Wallmark G (1969) Asymptomatisk bakteriuri hos hälsoundersökta kvinnor. Lakartidningen 66:1669

Samuell CT (1978) A modified electroimmune assay technique for uromucoid in urine. Clin Chim Acta 85:285

Samuell CT (1979) Uromucoid excretion in normal subjects, calcium stone-formers and in patients with chronic renal failure. Urol Res 7:7

Sarig S, Gartin N, Azoury R, Wax Y, Perlberg S (1982) A method for discrimination between calcium oxalate stone-formers and normals. J Urol 128:645

Schlegel JU, Diggdon P, Cuellar J (1981) The use of ultrasound for localizing renal calculi. J Urol 86:367

Schmidt K, Bruchelt G (1983) Oxalatbestimmung im Harn mittels analytischer Isotachophorese. In: Hesse A (Hrsg) Oxalsäure und Urolithiasis. G-I-T-Verlag, Darmstadt, S 51

Schmidt K, Bruchelt G, Hagmaier V (1979) Quantitative determination of urinary oxalate concentrations by analytical isotachophoresis. In: Rose GA, Robertson WG, Watts RWE (eds) Oxalate in human biochemistry and clinical pathology. Wellcome Found, London, p 67

Schmidt K, Hagmaier V, Hornig D, Vuilleumier JP, Rutishauser G (1981) High dose intake of Ascorbic Acid and oxalate excretion in man measured by analytical isotachophoresis. In: Brockis JG, Finlayson B (eds) Urinary Calculus. PSG Publ. Comp., Littleton, p 395

Schmidt K, Hagmaier V, Hornig D, Rutishauser G (1981) Absorption und Metabolisierung als limitierende Faktoren bei der Oxalatbildung aus Ascorbinsäure. Fortschr Urol Nephrol 17:137

Schmidt K, Hagmaier V, Hornig D, Rutishauser G (1982) Absorption und Metabolisierung als limitierende Faktoren bei der Oxalatbildung aus Ascorbinsäure. Fortschr Urol Nephrol 17:137

Schmidt K-H, Hagmaier V, Bruchelt G, Rutishauser G (1980) Analytical isotachophoresis: A rapid and sensitive method for determination of urinary oxalate. Urol Res 8:177

Schmidt-Gayk H, Haueisen H, Stengel R, Schmückle W (1975) Der Nachweis von cAMP (cyclischem Adenosinmonophosphat) zur Diagnostik des primären Hyperparathyreoidismus bei Nephrolithiasis. In: Vahlensieck W, Gasser G (eds) Fortschr Urol Nephrol 7. Steinkopff, Darmstadt, S 180

Schmidt-Gayk H, Tschöpe W, Ritz E, Eberhard K, Schellenberg B (1977) Calcium-Stoffwechsel, Calciumsteine und Ernährung. Akt Ernährungsmed 3:86

Schneeberger W, Bach D, Hesse A, Dewes W, Vahlensieck W (1981) Circadian excretion of uric acid on condition of standard diet after purine load in calcium oxalate stone-formers and healthy controls. In: Smith LH, Robertson WG, Finlayson B (eds) Urolithiasis. Plenum Press, New York London, p 51

Schneekloth G, Frank Th, Albers G (1983) Ultraschalltomographie abdomineller Organe und der Schilddrüse (2. ed). Enke, Stuttgart

Schneider H-J, Berg Ch (1981) Epidemiologische Aussagen zum Harnsteinleiden auf der Grundlage von 100 000 Harnsteinanalysen unter besonderer Berücksichtigung der Rezidive. Fortschr Urol Nephrol 17:33

Schneider HJ, Börner R-H (1981) Proteolytic activity and organic substances in urine. In: Smith LH, Robertson WG, Finlayson B (eds) Urolithiasis. Plenum Press, New York London, p 691

Schneider HJ, Hienzsch E (1979) Epidemiologie der Urolithiasis. Proc VIII. Congress Society International Urology, Tome 1, p 87

Schneider HJ, Röhrborn Cl, Rugendorff EW (1984) Untersuchungen zur Hemmbarkeit der Kalziumoxalatkristallisation im Gel. In: Vahlensieck W, Gasser G (eds) Fortschr Urol Nephrol 22. Steinkopff, Darmstadt, S 365

Scholz D, Schwille PO (1981) Klinische Laboratioriumsdiagnostik der Urolithiasis. DMW 106:999

Scholz D, Schwille PO, Husemann B, Engelhardt W, Herzog T (1979) Changes of mineral metabolism and oxaluria in patients treated for obesity by jejunoileal bypass. In: Rose GA, Robertson WG, Watts RWE (eds) Oxalate in Human Biochemistry and Clinical Pathology. Proc Ont Oxalate Workshop, Wellcome Found, London, p 235

Scholz D, Schwille PO, Sigel A (1980) Zur metabolischen Klassifikation und Metaphylaxe der häufigsten Lithiasisformen. Urologe [Ausg A] 19:202

Scholz D, Schwille PO, Engelhardt W, Sigel A (1981) Idiopathic uric acid lithiasis – some less known epidemiologic and metabolic findings. In: Gasser G, Vahlensieck W (eds) Fortschr Urol Nephrol 16, Steinkopff, Darmstadt S 66

Scholz D, Schwille PO, Sigel A (1981) Ernährungsgewohnheiten von Patienten mit Urolithiasis. Fortschr Urol Nephrol 17:83

Schönberger B, Willig J, Brien G (1978) Tagesrhythmik der Ausscheidung von Harnsäure, Kalzium, Phosphat, Magnesium, Kalium und Natrium bei steintragenden und gesunden Kindern. In: Schneider H-J (ed) V. Jenaer Harnsteinsymposium. Wissenschaftliche Beiträge der Friedrich Schiller Universität Jena, S 187

Schrier EE, Lee KE, Rubin J-L, Werness PG, Smith LH (1979) Macromolecular inhibitors of calcium oxalate crystal growth and aggregation in urine. In: Rose GA, Robertson WG, Watts RWE (eds) Oxalate in Human Biochemistry and Clinical Pathology. Wellcome Found, London, p 22

Schrier EE, Rubin JL, Lee KE, Wermess PG, Smith LH (1981) Characterization of the calcium oxalate crystal growth inhibitors in human urine. In: Smith LH, Robertson WG, Finlayson B (eds) Urolithiasis. Plenum Press, New York London, p 579

Schulz E, Börner R, Schneider H-J (1980) Methoden zur differenzierten Analyse des Harnsediments. In: Schneider H-J (ed) VI. Jenaer Harnsteinsymposium. Wissenschaftliche Beiträge der Friedrich Schiller Universität Jena, S 133

Schuster J, Finlayson B, Schaefer R, Sierakowski R, Zoltek J, Dzegede S (1982) Water hardness and urinary stone disease. J Urol 128:422

Schwartz A, Cainer M, Hermann G, Bittermann W (1966) Spontaneous renal extravasation during intravenous urography. Am J Roentgenol 98:27

Schwille PO, Ernstberger W (1972) Ultrafiltrables Calcium und Magnesium im Serum von Gesunden und Nierensteinkranken. Clin Chim Acta 38:379

Schwille PO, Samberger NM (1975) Cyclic adenosinemonophosphate (3′,5′-cAMP) in urine and plasma of stone formers. Acta Endocrinol [Suppl] (Copenh) 193, 33

Schwille PO, Bonhof C, Sigel A (1977) Erhöhung des renalen zyklischen AMP (cAMP) – bisher zuverlässigster Indikator der Diagnose Hperparathyreoidismus (HPT). In: Gasser G, Vahlensieck W (eds) Fortschr Urol Nephrol 9. Steinkopff, Darmstadt S 183

Schwille PO, Bonhof C, Thun R, Scholz D, Bötticher R, Schellerer W, Sigel A (1978) Bewertung von renalem zyklischen Adenosinmonophosphat, Serum-Parathormon und Phosphat-Rückresorption bei rezidivierender Calcium-Urolithiasis, Gesunden und Hyperparathyreoidismus. Klin Wochenschr 56:601

Schwille PO, Paulus MO, Scholz D, Sigel A (1979) Urin-Citrat bei Calcium-Urolithiasis. In: Gasser G, Vahlensieck W (eds) Fortschr Urol Nephrol 14. Steinkopff, Darmstadt S 94

Schwille PO, Scholz D, Engelhardt W (1981) Parameters of parathyroid gland activity in subgroups of calcium urolithiasis. Acta Endocrinol [Suppl] (Copenh) 240:32

Schwille PO, Scholz D, Engelhardt W, Schwille K, Schreiber B, Goldberg I, Sigel A (1981) Cyclic nucleotides and related variables in urolithiasis. In: Smith LH, Robertson WG, Finlayson B (eds) Urolithiasis. Plenum Press, New York London, p 835

Scott R, Freeland R, Mowat W, Paterson PJ, Orr PS, Yates AJ, Mills EA (1981) The prevalence of renal stones in a random population and a volunteer population. In: Brockis G, Finlayson B (eds) Urinary Calculus. PSG Publ Comp, Littleton Mass, p 65

Scurr DS, Robertson WG (1985) Studies on the mode of action of polyanionic inhibitors of calcium oxalate crystallization in urine. In: Schwille PO, Smith LH, Robertson WG, Vahlensieck W (eds) Urolithiasis and related clinical research. Plenum Press, New York London, p 835

Scurr DS, Bridge CM, Robertson WG (1981) Studies on inhibitors and promoters of the crystallization of calcium oxalate in urine and in matrix from calcium oxalate stones. In: Smith LH, Robertson WG, Finlayson B (eds) Urolithiasis. Plenum Press, New York London, p 601

Scurr DS, Januzovich N, Smith A, Sergeant VJ, Robertson WG (1985) A comparison of three methods for measuring urinary oxalate – with a note on ascorbic acid interference. In: Schwille PO, Smith LH, Robertson WG, Vahlensieck W (eds) Urolithiasis and related clinical research. Plenum Press, New York London, p 645

Segal AJ, Spatavo RF, Linke CA, Frank I (1978) Diagnosis of nonopaque calculi by computed tomography. Radiology 129:447

Sheehan M, Nancollas GH (1981) A constant composition method for modelling urinary stone formation. In: Smith LH, Robertson WG, Finlayson B (eds) Urolithiasis. Plenum Press, New York London, p 391

Shen FH, Baylink DJ, Nielsen RL, Sherrard DJ, Ivey JL, Haussler MR (1977) Increased serum 1,25-dihydroxyvitamin D in idiopathic hypercalciuria. J Lab Clin Med 90:955

Sierakowski P, Finlayson B, Landes R (1979) Stone incidence as related to water hardness in different geographic regions of the United States. Urol Res 7:157

Sigel B, Coelho JCU, Sharifi R, Waters WB, Spigos DG (1982) Ultrasonic scanning during operation for renal calculi. J Urol 127:421

Silverberg DS, Mc Intyre JWR, Ulan RA, Gain EA (1971) Oxalic acid secretion after methoxyfluorane and halothane anaesthesia. Can Anaesth Soc J 18:496

Simmonds HA, Van Acker KJ, Potter CF, Webster DR, Kasidas GP, Rose GA (1981) Influence of purine content of diet and Allopurinol on uric acid and oxalate excretion levels. In: Smith LH, Robertson WG, Finlayson B (eds) Urolithiasis. Plenum Press, New York London, p 363

Singh PP, Pendse AK, Jain AK (1985) Urolithiasis in Southern Rajasthan: Contribution of dietary oxalate to urinary oxalate. In: Schwille PO, Smith LH, Robertson WG, Vahlensieck W (eds) Urolithiasis and related clinical research. Plenum Press, New York London, p 77

Small H, Stevens LS, Bauman WC (1975) Novel ion exchange chromatographic method using conductimetric detection. Anal Chem 47:1801

Smith A, Yu JS, Brown DA (1981) The significance of cystine crystalluria in childhood. In: Brockis JB, Finlayson B (eds) Urinary Calculus. PSG Publ Comp Littleton, p 161

Smith DR (1981) Urinary stones. In: Smith DR (ed) General Urology. Los Altos, Lange Med Publ, p 227

Smith LH (1982) Editorial comment. J Urol 127:858

Smith LH, McCall JT (1969) Chemical nature of peptide inhibitors isolated from urine. In: Hodgkinson A, Nordin BEC (eds) Renal Stone Research Symposium. Churchill, London, p 153

Smith LH, Meyer JC, McCall JT (1973) Chemical nature of crystal inhibitors isolated from human urine. In: Cifuentes Delatte L, Rapado A, Hodgkinson A (eds) Urinary Calculi. Karger, Basel München Paris London New York Sidney, p 318

Smith LH, Werness PG, Wilson DM (1979) Enteric hyperoxaluria: Associated metabolic abnormalities that promote formation of renal calcuii. In: Rose GA, Robertson WG, Watts RWE (eds) Oxalate in Human Biochemistry and Clinical Pathology. Proc Int Oxalate Workshop, Wellcome Found, London, p 224

Sökeland J, May P (1969) Physiologische und pathophysiologische Gesichtspunkte der Elektromanometrie und Elektromyographie. In: Lutzeyer W, Melchior H (eds) Ureterdynamik. Thieme, Stuttgart, S 114

Sörgel F, Ettinger B, Benet LZ, Schwille PO (1985) Triamterene solubility and metabolism are not causative factors of triamterene nephrolithiasis. In: Schwille PO, Smith LH, Robertson WG, Vahlensieck W (eds) Urolithiasis and related clinical research. Plenum Press, New York London, p 375

Sojka BK (1980) Urotron^R: Ein halbautomatischer Reflexionsphotometer zur Auswertung von Harnteststreifen; Aufbau und Funktionsweise. Med Lab Sci 33:93

Solomon EM (1954) Urinary calculi in pregnancy. Am J Obstet Gynecol 67:1351

Soltész J, Varga A, Szabo E, Pinter J (1982) Diagnostischer Wert der Bestimmung von ionisiertem Kalzium bei Patienten mit kalziumenthaltenden Harnsteinen. In: Schneider H-J, Bothor C (eds) VII. Jenaer Harnsteinsymposium. Wissenschaftliche Beiträge der Friedrich Schiller Universität Jena, S 118

Sommerkamp H (1977) Diagnostik der renalen tubulären Azidose. In: Gasser G, Vahlensieck W (eds) Fortschr Urol Nephrol 9. Steinkopff, Darmstadt, S 165

Sophasan S, Chatasingh S, Thanphaichitr P, Ohanamitta S (1980) Tamm Horsfall mucoprotein in urine potential bladder stone-formers. J Urol 124:522

Spector M, Magura CE, Lilga JC (1981) Prostatic calculi. In: Smith LH, Robertson WG, Finlayson B (eds) Urolithiasis. Plenum Press, New York London, p 943

Spengler B, Moschütz H-R (1982) Die Alaninaminopeptidase (AAP) beim Harnsteinleiden – eine vorläufige Verlaufsstudie. In: Schneider H-J, Bothor C (eds) VII. Jenaer Harnsteinsymposium. Wissenschaftliche Beiträge der Friedrich Schiller Universität Jena, p 243

Stables DP (1982) Percutaneous nephrostomy: techniques, indications and results. Urol Clin North Am 9:15

Stadie G, Möller A, Baumann W (1982) Die transkutane Nephropyelostomie – Indikationen, Komplikationen und Ergebnisse. Z Urol Nephrol 75:799

Stansfeld JM (1962) The measurement and meaning of pyuria. Arch Dis Child 37:257

Stiris MG (1981) CT evaluation of non-opaque renal calculus – a case report. Scand J Urol Nephrol 15:341

Stöber U (1983) Entwicklung von Pyonephrose und Urosepsis. Urol Int 38:44

Strenge A (1982) Einfluß der Ernährung auf lithogene und inhibitorische Substanzen. Inaug Urol Dissertation Bonn

Strenge A (1982) Einfluß der Ernährung auf die Harnsteinbildung. Inaug Urol Dissertation, Bonn

Strenge A, Hesse A (1982) Oxalatbestimmung im Harn, Methodenvergleich Gaschromatographie–Isotachophorese. In: Hesse A (Hrsg) Oxalsäure und Urolithiasis. G-I-T-Verlag, Darmstadt, S 63

Strenge A, Hesse A, Bach D, Vahlensieck W (1980) Mg-Ausscheidung im Harn unter Normal- und Standardkost bei Gesunden und Harnsteinpatienten. Magnesium Bull 2:103

Strenge A, Hesse A, Vahlensieck W (1982) Veränderungen von Ernährungsgewohnheiten und Urinparametern bei Kalziumoxalat-Steinpatienten nach diätischer Beratung. In: Gasser G, Vahlensieck W (Hrsg) Fortschr Urol Nephrol 20. Steinkopff, Darmstadt, S 328

Sugimoto T, Blömer J, Jungling E, Recker F, Funae Y, Hautmann R (1985) The value of oxalate determination by high performance liquid chromatography in clinical practice. In: Schwille PO, Smith LH, Robertson WG, Vahlensieck W (eds) Urolithiasis and related clinical research. Plenum Press, New York London, p 673

Sur BK, Pandey HN (1981) Effect of different urinary constituents on inhibiting or accelerating calcium oxalate crystallization. In: Smith LH, Robertson WG, Finlayson B (eds) Urolithiasis. Plenum Press, New York London, p 607

Sutor DJ (1969) Growth studies of calcium oxalate in the presence of various ions and compounds. Br J Urol 41:171

Sutor DJ (1973) Experiments on the nucleation and growth of calcium oxalate in normal and stone-formers urine. In: Cifuentes Delatte L, Rapado A, Hodgkinson A (eds) Urinary Calculi. Karger, Basel München Paris London New York Sidney, p 313

Sutor DJ, Wooley SE (1970) Growth studies of calcium oxalate in presence of various compounds and ions – Part II. Br J Urol 42:296

Sutton RAL, Walker VR (1980) Responses to hydrochlorothiazide and acetazolamide in patients with calcium stones. N Engl J Med 302:709

Sutton RAL, Quamme GA, Burnatowska M, Wong NLM, Dirks JH (1976) Effects of vitamin D and parathyroid hormone on renal tubular calcium reabsorption. In: Fleisch H, Robertson WG, Smith LH, Vahlensieck W (eds) Urolithiasis Research. Plenum Press, New York London, p 395

Szabo E, Berg W, Hesse A, Schneider H-J (1976) Experimentelle und kristalloptische Betrachtungen zur Kalzium-Oxalatsteingenese. Act Urol 7:325

Tabor H, Hastings AB (1943) The ionization constant of secondary magnesium phosphate. J Biol Chem 148:627

Takameto M, Itatani H, Yashiku S, Kotake T, Kinoshita K, Sonoda T (1974) A simple, safe and qualitative screening method for cystinuria. Hinyo Kiyo 20:837

Tamm I, Horsfall FL jr (1950) Characterization and separation of an inhibitor of viral haemagglutination in urine. Proc Soc Exp Biol Med 74:108

Teller WM, Burke EC, Rosevear JW, McKenzie BF (1962) Urinary excretion of acid mucopolysaccharides in normal children and patients with gargolism. J Lab Clin Med 59:95

Teotia M, Sutor DJ (1971) Crystallization of ammonium acid urate and other uric derivatives from urine. Br J Urol 43:381

Terhorst B (1980) Röntgenuntersuchung. In: Hautmann R, Lutzeyer W (Hrsg) Harnsteinfibel. Deutscher Ärzteverlag, Köln, S 120

Terhorst B (1980) Symptomatologie, Diagnose und Differentialdiagnose des Harnsteinleidens. In: Hautmann R, Lutzeyer W (Hrsg) Harnsteinfibel. Deutscher Ärzteverlag, Köln, S 114

Tew WP, Malis CD (1981) Calcium electrode measurements of calcium oxalate mineralization: the effects of urine and other inhibitors. In: Smith LH, Robertson WG, Finlayson B (eds) Urolithiasis. Plenum Press, New York London, p 421

Thiel U, Sachowa P (1982) Distale renale tubuläre Azidose (RTA) und Nephrolithiasis. In: Schneider H-J, Bothor C (eds) VII. Jenaer Harnsteinsymposium. Wissenschaftliche Beiträge der Friedrich Schiller Universität Jena, S 173

Thieler H, Witzleb W, Färber J, Wachtel D (1972) Die Bedeutung der suprapubischen Blasenpunktion für die bakterielle Diagnostik. Wien Klin Wochenschr 84:313

Thom JA, Morris JE, Bishop A, Blacklock NJ (1981) Increased availability of dietary carbohydrate: a factor in the genesis of idiopathic calcium oxalate urolithiasis? In: Smith LH, Robertson WG, Finlayson B (eds) Urolithiasis. Plenum Press, New York London, p 369

Thomas WC jr (1969) Inhibitors of mineralization and renal stones. In Hodgkinson A, Nordin BEC (Hrsg) Renal Stone Research Symposium. London, Churchill, p 141

Thüroff JW, Alken P, Riedmiller H, Hohenfellner R (1982) Doppler and real-time ultrasound in renal stone surgery. Eur Urol 8:298

Tiselius H-G (1977) Excretion of 4-pyridoxic acid and oxalic acid in patients with urinary calculi. Invest Urol 15:5

Tiselius H-G (1979) Relationship between the severity of renal stone disease and urine composition. Eur Urol 5:323

Tiselius H-G (1980) Inhibition of calcium oxalate crystal growth in urine during treatment with allopurinol. Br J Urol 52:189

Tiselius H-G (1980) Practical aspects of the handling of samples and evaluation of laboratory data. Scand J Urol Nephrol [Suppl] 53:105

Tiselius H-G (1983) Different estimates of the risk of calcium oxalate crystallization in urine. Eur Urol 9:231

Tiselius H-G (1984) Urinary pH and calcium oxalate crystallization. In: Vahlensieck W, Gasser G (eds) Fortschr Urol Nephrol 22. Steinkopff, Darmstadt, S 184

Tiselius HG (1985) The effect of sodium sulfopentosan on the crystallization of calcium oxalate. In: Schwille PO, Smith LH, Robertson WG, Vahlensieck W (eds) Urolithiasis and related clinical research. Plenum Press, New York London, p 895

Tiselius H-G, Almgard L-E (1977) The diurnal urinary excretion of oxalate and the effect of pyridoxine and ascorbate on oxalate excretion. Eur Urol 3:41

Tiselius H-G, Fornander AM (1981) Evaluation of a routine method for determination of calcium oxalate: crystal growth inhibition in diluted urine samples. Clin Chem 27:565

Tiselius H-G, Larsson L (1981) Inhibition of calcium oxalate crystal growth in patients with urolithiasis. In: Smith LH, Robertson WG, Finlayson B (eds) Urolithiasis. Plenum Press, New York London, p 623

Tiselius H-G, Larsson L (1982) Die Zusammensetzung des Harns bei Patienten mit Kalziumsteinbildung. In: Schneider H-J, Bothor C (eds) VII. Jenaer Harnsteinsymposium. Wissenschaftliche Beiträge der Friedrich Schiller Universität Jena, S 134

Tiselius H-G, Almgard LE, Larsson L, Sörbo B (1978) A biochemical basis for the grouping of patients with urolithiasis. Eur Urol 4:241

Tiselius H-G, Ahlstrand C, Larsson L, Nilsson M, Thoren-Johansson (1981) Studies on the inhibition of calcium oxalate crystal growth in patients with urolithiasis. In: Brockis JG, Finlayson B (eds) Urinary Calculus. PSG Publ Comp, Littleton, p 321

Tovey KC, Oldham GN, Whelan JAM (1974) A simple direct assay of cyclic AMP in plasma and other biological samples using an improved competitive protein binding technique. Clin Chim Acta 56:221

Triger DR, Smith JWG (1966) Survival of urinary leucocytes. J Clin Pathol 19:443

Trudeau DL, Freier EF (1967) Determination of calcium in urine and serum by atomic absorption spectrophotometry. Clin Chem 13:101

Tschöpe W, Ritz R (1981) Isotachophoretic determination of oxalate in unprocessed urine. In: Smith LH, Robertson WG, Finlayson B (eds) Urolithiasis. Plenum Press, New York London, p 951

Tschöpe W, Schellenberg B, Schlierf G, Ritz E (1981) Calcium-Phosphat-Stoffwechesel unter oralen Antikonzeptiva. Fortschr Urol 17:118

Tschöpe W, Manz F, Ritz E (1983) Isotachophorese und Urolithiasis In: Hesse A (Hrsg) Oxalsäure und Urolithiasis. G-I-T-Verlag, Darmstadt, S 41

Übelhör R (1976) Reno-renale Reflexe. In: Übelhör R, Figdor PP (eds) Urologische Nephrologie. Urban und Schwarzenberg, München Berlin Wien, p 63

Ulshöfer B (1977) Die direkte Messung des ionisierten Calciums in der Diagnostik des primären Hyperparathyreoidismus. In: Gasser G, Vahlensieck W (Hrsg) Fortschr Urol Nephrol 9. Steinkopff, Darmstadt S 178

Ulshöfer BM, Peemöller A (1981) Direct measurment of ionized calcium (standardization, normales values and clinical results). In: Smith LH, Robertson WG, Finlayson B (eds) Urolithiasis. Plenum Press, New York London, p 969

Ulshöfer B, Zenke J (1984) Saure Mucopolysaccharide im 24-h-Urin bei Gesunden und Steinträgern. In: Vahlensieck W, Gasser G (Hrsg) Fortschr Urol Nephrol 22. Steinkopff, Darmstadt, S 137

Unger G, Thiel C (1977) Die Urolithiasis im Kindesalter. V. Jenaer Harnsteinsymposium 1977. Wissenschaftliche Beiträge der Friedrich Schiller Universität Jena, S 232

Utikalova A, Bana J, Charouzek J, Kucera J (1982) Die Bedeutung des Ultraschalls in der Diagnostik der Urolithiasis. In: Schneider H-J, Bothor C (Hrsg) VII. Jenaer Harnsteinsymposium. Wissenschaftliche Beiträge der Friedrich Schiller Universität Jena, S 326

Vahlensieck W (1969) Behandlung des „akuten Harnsteines". Dtsch Med Wochenschr 94:2381

Vahlensieck W (1970) Symptomatik, Diagnostik und Therapie des „akuten Harnsteines". Dtsch Med Wochenschr 21:499

Vahlensieck W (1970) Methodik der peroralen Chemolitholyse und Dauer der Prophylaxe bei Harnsäuresteinen. Med Welt 21:1559

Vahlensieck W (1971) Häufigkeit und Prognose eines Hypertonus bei urologischen Patienten. Verh Berlin 23. Tagung der Deutschen Gesellschaft für Urologie. Springer, Berlin Heidelberg New York

Vahlensieck W (1973) Das Harnsteinleiden. Wien Med Wochenschr 123:561

Vahlensieck W (1973) Die hochdosierte antibakterielle Chemotherapie in der Urologie. In: Klosterhalfen H (Hrsg) Antibakterielle Chemotherapie in der Urologie. Thieme, Stuttgart, 7

Vahlensieck W (1978) Konservative Therapie der Urolithiasis. Med Welt 29:49

Vahlensieck W (1979) Klinische Untersuchung. In: Vahlensieck W (Hrsg) Urolithiasis 1. Springer, Berlin Heidelberg New York, S 34

Vahlensieck W (1979) Allgemeine Kausal- und Formalgenese. In: Vahlensieck W (Hrsg) Urolithiasis 1. Springer, Berlin Heidelberg New York, S 9

Vahlensieck W (1979) Einfluß der Ernährung auf lithogene Substanzen im Serum und Urin. Report 18. Congr Soc Int Urol, vol II. Grau-Radenez et Joly, Paris, p 72

Vahlensieck W (1979/80) Urolithiasis 1–5. Springer, Berlin Heidelberg New York

Vahlensieck W (1982) Erweiterte Diagnostik bei Harnsteinrezidivbildnern – Methodik, Kostenaufwand und Rechtfertigung. XIX. Congr Soc Internat Urol, San Francisco

Vahlensieck W (1985) Influence of water quality on urolithiasis. In: Schwille PO, Smith LH, Robertson WG, Vahlensieck W (eds) Urolithiasis and related clinical research. Plenum Press, New York London, p 97

Vahlensieck W, Bastian HP (1973) Der „akute" Harnstein. Fortschr Med 91:905–908

Vahlensieck W, Bastian HP (1976) Clinical features and treatment of urinary calculi in childhood. Eur Urol 2:129–134

Vahlensieck W, Maurer H-J (1965) Ist die Nierenarterienstenose ein Kausalfaktor der Harnsteingenese? Fortschr Roentgenstr 102:298

Vahlensieck W, Hesse A, Bach D (1980) Zur Prävalenz des Harnsteinleidens in der Bundesrepublik Deutschland. Urologe [Ausg A] 20:273

Vahlensieck W, Bach D, Hesse A, Schneeberger W (1981) Metabolic investigations in 407 recurrent stone formers and healthy controls on condition of individual as well as standard diet. In: Smith LH, Robertson WG, Finlayson B (eds) Urolithiasis. Plenum Press, New York London, p 29

Vahlensieck W, Bach D, Hesse A (1982) Circadian rhythm of lithogenic substances in the urine. Urol Res 10:195

Vahlensieck W, Bach D, Doppelfeld E, Winkler C (1982) Indikationen und Grenzen nuclearmedizinischer Untersuchungsmethoden für die Urologie. Urologe [Ausg B] 22:12

Vahlensieck EW, Bach D, Hesse A, Strenge A (1982) Epidemiology, pathogenesis and diagnosis of calcium oxalate urolithiasis. Int Urol Nephrol 14:333

Vahlensieck EW, Bach D, Hesse A (1982) Incidence, Prevalence and Mortality of Urolithiasis in the German Federal Republic. Urol Res 10:161

Vainberg ZS, Gimpelson YE (1973) Die Urolithiase bei Schwangeren. Berl Ges Gynäk Geburtsh 10:431

Valyasevi A, Dhanamitta S (1974) Studies of bladder stone disease in Thailand. XVII: effect of exogenous source of oxalate on crystalluria. Am J Clin Nutr 27:877

Van den Berg CJ, Cahill TM, Smith LH (1976) Crystalluria. In: Fleisch H, Robertson WG, Smith LH, Vahlensieck W (eds) Urolithiasis Research. Plenum Press, New York London, p 365

Van den Berg CL, Kumar R, Wilson DM, Heath H III, Smith LH (1980) Orthophosphate therapy decreases urinary calcium excretion and serum 1,25 dihydroxyvitamin D concentrations in idiopathic hypercalciuria. J Clin Endocrinol Metab 51:998

Van Der Vuurst De Vries JHJ (1961) Symptomatologie. In: Boshamer et al. (Hrsg) Die Steinerkrankungen. Handbuch der Urologie Bd. X. Springer, Berlin Göttingen Heidelberg

Van Waes PFGM (1972) High-dose urography in oliguric and anuric patients. Excerpta Medica, Amsterdam

Varadi DP, Cifonelli JA, Dorfman A (1967) The acid mucopolysaccharides in normal urine. Biochim Biophys Acta 141:103

Vela-Navarrete R (1982) Constant pressure flow-controlled antegrade pyelography. Eur Urol 8:265

Vogel W, Leskovar P, Eichhorn R (1984) Isohydrieabhängige Harnmeßgrößen und Ca-bindende Anionen bei Steinpatienten und Kontrollpersonen. In: Vahlensieck W, Gasser G (Hrsg) Fortschr Urol Nephrol 22. Steinkopff, Darmstadt, S 99

Voigt HW (1977) Klärung lipämischer Seren durch ein neues Verfahren. Laboratoriumsblätter 27:168

Voigt R (1982) Zur Diagnostik der Urolithiasis in der Gravidität. In: Schneider H-J, Bothor C (eds) VII. Jenaer Harnsteinsymposium. Wissenschaftliche Beiträge der Friedrich Schiller Universität Jena, S 334

Vontobel HP, Hering F, Haas HG, Rutishauser R (1982) Biologische Reproduzierbarkeit der Hypercalciurieklassifizierung nach Pak. In: Gasser G, Vahlensieck W (Hrsg) Urol Nephrol 20. Steinkopff, Darmstadt, S 292

Vontobel HP, Hering F, Kayser U, Haas HG, Rutishauser G (1984) Biologische Reproduzierbarkeit der Hyperkalziurie – Klassifikation nach Pak. Fortschr Urol Nephrol 22:310

Walser M (1961) Ion association. VI. Interactions between calcium, magnesium, inorganic phosphate, citrate and protein in normal human plasma. J Clin Invest 40:723

Wegener OH (1981) Ganzkörper-Computertomographie. Berlin, Schering

Weinberger A, Schindel B, Liberman UA, Pinkhas J, Sperling O (1982) Calciuric effect of probenecid in gouty patients. Fortschr Urol Nephrol 20:363

Welshman SG, McGeown MG (1972) A quantitative investigation of the effects on the growth of calcium oxalate crystals on potential inhibitors. Br J Urol 44:677

Welshman SG, McGeown MG (1976) Urinary citrate excretion in stone formers and normal controls. Br J Urol 48:7

Werness PG, Bergert JH, Smith LH (1976) Crystalluria. In: Fleisch H, Robertson WG, Smith LH, Vahlensieck W (eds) Urolithiasis Research. Plenum Press, New York London, p 17

Werness PG, Bergert JH, Smith LH (1981) Crystalluria. J Cryst Growth 53:166

Werness PG, Bergert JH, Smith LH (1981) Crystalluria. In: Smith LH, Robertson WG, Finlayson B (eds) Urolithiasis. Plenum Press, New York London, p 17

Werness PG, Bergert JH, Lee LE (1981) Urinary crystal growth: effect of inhibitor mixtures. Clin Sci 61:487

Werness PG, Bergert JH, Smith LH (1982) Triamterene urolithiaisis: solubility, pK, effect on crystal formation, and matrix binding of triamterene and its metabolites. J Lab Clin Med 99:254

Wessler E (1971) The nature of the non-ultrafiltrable glycosaminoglycans of normal human urine. Biochem J 122:373

White DJ jr, Christoffersen J, Hermann TS, Lanzalako AC, Nancollas GH (1983) Effect of urine pretreatment on calcium oxalate crystallization inhibition potentials. J Urol 129:175

Whiteman P (1973) The quantitative determination of glycosaminoglycans in urine with Alcian Blue 8 GX. Biochem J 131:351

Wickham JEA (1979) Urinary calculous disease. Churchill Livingstone, Edinburgh London New York, p 8

Wiebel J, Matz K, Grüttner R, Menking M, Stahnke N, Willig RP (1972) Suprapubische, perkutane Blasenpunktion bei Kindern mit Harnwegsinfekt. Dtsch Med Wochenschr 97:1049

Wikström B, Wieslander J (1981) Excretion of Tamm-Horsfall urinary glycoprotein (uromucoid) in renal calcium stone-formers. In: Smith LH, Robertson WG, Finlayson B (eds) Urolithiasis. Plenum Press, New York London, p 367

Wikström B, Danielson BG, Ljunghall S, McGuire M, Russel RGG (1982) Urinary acidification and pyrophosphat excretion in nephrolithiasis. In: Gasser G, Vahlensieck W (eds) Fortschr Urol Nephrol 20. Steinkopff, Darmstadt S 391

Will EJ, Bijvoet OLM, Te Brake van der Linden H (1976) Inhibition of calcium oxalate crystal growth. A simple method of measurement and preliminary results. In: Fleisch H, Robertson WG, Smith LH, Vahlensieck W (eds) Urolithiasis Research. Plenum Press, New York London, p 367

Will EJ, Bijvoet OLM, Te Brake van der Linden H (1977) Routine measurements of the inhibition of calcium oxalate crystal growth – an evaluation. In: Gasser G, Vahlensieck W (eds) Fortschr Urol Nephrol 9. Steinkopff, Darmstadt S 147

Williams RE (1979) The clinical features and investigation of renal lithiasis. In: Wickham JEA (ed) Urinary Calculous Disease. Churchill Livingstone, Edinburgh London New York, p 96

Wilson JWL, Werness PG, Smith LH (1985) Urinary inhibitors of hydroxyapatite crystal growth: A constant composition approach. In: Schwille PO, Smith LH, Robertson WG, Vahlensieck W (eds) Urolithiasis and related clinical research. Plenum Press, New York London, p 819

Wirths W (1974) Ermittlung des Ernährungszustandes. In: Cremer H-D, Hötzel D (Hrsg) Angewandte Ernährungslehre. Bd. III Ernährungslehre und Diätetik: Cremer et al. (Hrsg) Thieme, Stuttgart, S 50

Wojewski A, Zajaczkowski T (1971) Urolithiasis and pregnancy. Berl Ges Gynäk Geburtsh 102:322

Wrong O, Davies HEF (1959) The excretion of acid in renal disease. R J Med 28:259

Yendt ER (1970) Renal calculi. Canad Med Assoc J 102:479

Yü TF (1978) Uric acid nephrolithiasis. In: Kelley WN, Weiner IM (eds) Uric Acid. Handb Exp Pharm, vol 51. Springer, New York, p 397

Zarembski PM, Hodgkinson A (1962) The oxalic content of English diets. B J Nutr 16:627

Zechner O (1981) Epidemiologische und metabolische Aspekte des Harnsäuresteinleidens. Fortschr Urol Nephrol 17:76

Zechner O, Latal D (1981) Die Problematik der Harnsteinrezidivprophylaxe. Akt Urol 12:103

Zechner O, Scheiber V (1981) Alcohol as an epidemiological risk in urolithiasis. In: Smith LH, Robertson WG, Finlayson B (eds) Urolithiasis. Plenum Press, New York London, p 315

Zechner O, Bergmann H, Kovarik J, Willvonseder R, Heynen G (1978) Die intestinale Kalziumresorption bei Patienten mit hormocalcämischer Hypercalciurie. In: Vahlensieck W, Gasser G (Hrsg) Fortschr Urol Nephrol 11. Steinkopff, Darmstadt S 15

Zechner O, Pflüger H, Latal D, Scheiber V (1981) Der Einfluß epidemiologischer Faktoren auf das Rezidivbildungsverhalten von Harnsteinen. Verh Berl 32. Tagung Dtsch Ges Urologie, Berlin 1980. Springer, Berlin Heidelberg New York, S 342

Zechner O, Loebenstein Th, Pflüger H, Legenstein E, Brandstätter F (1984) Harnsteinwachstum in vitro. In: Vahlensieck W, Gasser G (Hrsg) Fortschr Urol Nephrol 22. Steinkopff, Darmstadt, S 147

Ziegler H (1981) Epidemiologie des Alkoholismus. In: Teschke R, Lieber CS (Hrsg) Alkohol und Organschäden. Baden-Baden, Witzstrock, S 11–18

Zollinger HU (1966) Nieren und ableitende Harnwege. In: Doerr W, Uehlinger E (Hrsg) Spezielle pathologische Anatomie Bd 3. Springer, Berlin Heidelberg New York, S 282

Zöllner N (1976) Influence of diet on urinary uric acid excretion. In: Fleisch H, Robertson WG, Smith LH, Vahlensieck W (eds) Urolithiasis Research. Plenum Press, New York London, p 155

Zöllner N (1980) Das Wesen der Gicht. In: Zöllner N (Hrsg) Hyperurikämie und Gicht 1. Springer, Berlin Heidelberg New York, p 1

Zöllner N (1980) Differentialdiagnose. In: Zöllner N (Hrsg) Hyperurikämie und Gicht 2. Springer, Berlin Heidelberg New York, S 13

Zum Winkel U (1964) Nierendiagnostik mit Radioisotopen. Thieme, Stuttgart

Subject Index

MIX
Papier aus verantwortungsvollen Quellen
Paper from responsible sources
FSC® C105338

If you have any concerns about our products,
you can contact us on
ProductSafety@springernature.com

In case Publisher is established outside the EU,
the EU authorized representative is:
Springer Nature Customer Service Center GmbH
Europaplatz 3, 69115 Heidelberg, Germany

Printed by Libri Plureos GmbH
in Hamburg, Germany